Directory of Unpublished
Experimental Mental Measures

VOLUMES 4-5

BERT A. GOLDMAN

WILLIAM L. OSBORNE

DAVID F. MITCHELL

...

Series Editors: Bert A. Goldman and David F. Mitchell

American Psychological Association, Washington, DC

Copyright © 1996 by the American Psychological Association.
All rights reserved. Except as permitted under the United States Copyright Act of 1976, no part of this publication may be reproduced or distributed in any form or by any means, or stored in a database or retrieval system, without the prior written permission of the publisher.

First printing December 1995
Second printing September 1996
Third printing September 1998

Volume 4 was published in 1985 by Human Sciences Press and Volume 5 in 1990 by Wm. C. Brown Publishers. Reissued in 1996 with a new Introduction.

Copies may be ordered from
APA Order Department
P.O. Box 92984
Washington, D.C. 20090-2984

In the United Kingdom and Europe, copies may be ordered from
American Psychological Association
3 Henrietta Street
Covent Garden
London, WC2E 8LU
England

Composition in Futura Bold and Bodoni Book by Jennifer Ruby, EDTEC Editorial Technologies, Arlington, VA.

Cover and Text Designer: Minker Design, Bethesda, MD
Printer: TechniGraphix, Reston, VA
Technical/Production Editor: Susan Bedford

ISBN: 1-55798-351-8

British Library Cataloguing-in-Publication Data
A CIP record is available from the British Library

Printed in the United States of America

. . .

To our families
B. G.
D. F. M.

To Ed and Gladys Osborne
W. L. O.

Contents

(contents continue on next page)

Introduction

This combined *Directory of Unpublished Experimental Mental Measures* includes Volumes 4 and 5 and marks the second publication of these volumes. Now that the American Psychological Association (APA) has agreed to continue the series of *Directories* by publishing Volume 6, APA acquired the rights to the previously published first five volumes so that all volumes would be made available by one publisher. The authors and publisher believe that there is an ongoing need for directories such as these to enable researchers to determine what types of noncommercial experimental test instruments are currently in use. These reference books provide researchers with ready access to information about experimental measurement scales. The instruments are not evaluated, but the information given about each test should make it possible for researchers to make a preliminary judgment of its usefulness. The *Directories* do not provide all necessary information for researchers contemplating the use of a particular instrument. They do describe basic test properties and in most cases identify additional sources from which technical information concerning an instrument can be obtained.

Bert Arthur Goldman
David F. Mitchell

Directory of Unpublished

Experimental Mental Measures

VOLUME 4

BERT ARTHUR GOLDMAN, EDD
Dean, Academic Advising and Professor of Education
University of North Carolina at Greensboro

WILLIAM LARRY OSBORNE, EDD
Associate Professor of Education
University of North Carolina at Greensboro

Contents

A cumulative subject index to Volumes 1 through 5 appears at the end of this book.

...

Preface

From the Original Printing of Volume 4, 1985

Purpose: This *Directory of Unpublished Experimental Mental Measures* Vol. 4, marks the fourth in a series of publications designed to fill a need for reference tools in behavioral and social science research. The authors recognized the need for the publication of a directory to experimental test instruments, i.e., tests that are not currently marketed commercially. It is intended that this reference provide researchers with ready access to sources of information about recently developed experimental measurement devices. The instruments are not evaluated, however it is anticipated that the directory stimulate further research of these experimental instruments. In essence, this directory provides references to nonstandardized, experimental mental measures currently undergoing development. The directory is not intended to provide evaluation of the instruments, nor is it intended to provide all necessary information for the researcher contemplating the use of a particular instrument; rather it should serve as a reference to enable the reader to identify potentially useful measures and to identify sources from which technical information concerning the instruments can be obtained.

Development: Forty-six relevant professional journals available to the authors were examined. The following list includes those journals which, in the judgment of the authors, contained research involving instruments of value to researchers in education, psychology, and sociology. The list is identical to that of Volume 3. In general, foreign journals were not surveyed for use in this directory, with the exception of the British journal, *Occupational Psychology*. Measures identified in dissertations were excluded as a matter of expediency and because the microfilm abstracts generally contain minimal information.

American Educational Research Journal
American Journal of Economics and Sociology
American Journal of Psychology
American Journal of Sociology
American Sociologist
American Vocational Journal
Behavioral Science
California Journal of Educational Research
Child Development
Colorado Journal of Educational Research
Counseling Psychologist
Counselor Education and Supervision
Developmental Psychology
Education
Educational and Psychological Measurement
Educational Leadership
Elementary School Guidance and Counseling

Gifted Child Quarterly
Human Development
Improving College and University Teaching
International Journal of Comparative Sociology
Journal of Applied Psychology
Journal of College Student Personnel
Journal of Counseling Psychology
Journal of Creative Behavior
Journal of Education
Journal of Educational Measurement
Journal of Educational Psychology
Journal of Educational Research
Journal of Experimental Education
Journal of General Education
Journal of Personality Assessment
Journal of Reading
Journal of School Psychology
Measurement and Evaluation in Guidance
Occupational Psychology
Peabody Journal of Education
Perceptual and Motor Skills
Personnel and Guidance Journal
Personnel Journal
Phi Delta Kappan
Psychological Reports
Reading Research Quarterly
Social Education
Sociology and Social Research
Sociology of Education

This directory lists tests described in the 1974–1980 issues of the previously cited journals. The seven year time span was initiated in this volume in an effort to bring the series into current focus. An attempt was made to omit commercially published standardized tests, task-type activities such as memory word lists used in serial learning reasearch and achievement tests developed for a single, isolated course of study. The reader should not assume that the instruments described herein form a representative sample of the universe of unpublished experimental mental measures.

Organization: Following is a brief description of each of the twenty-three categories under which the authors grouped the measures of Volume 4:

Achievement: Measure learning and/or comprehension in specific areas. Also include tests of memory and tests of drug knowledge.
Adjustment—Educational: Measure academic satisfaction. Also include tests of school anxiety.
Adjustment—Psychological: Evaluate conditions and levels of adjustment along the psychological dimension including, for example, tests of mood, fear of death, anxiety, depression, etc.
Adjustment—Social: Evaluate aspects of interactions with others. Also include tests of alienation, conformity, need for social approval, social desirability, and instruments for assessing interpersonal attraction and sensitivity.

Aptitude: Predict success in given activities.

Attitude: Measure reaction to a variety of experiences and objects.

Behavior: Measure general and specific types of activities such as classroom behavior and drug-use behavior.

Communication: Evaluate information exchange. Also include tests of self-disclosure and counselor/client interaction.

Concept Meaning: Test one's understanding of words and other concepts. Also include tests of conceptual structure, style, and information processing.

Creativity: Measure ability to reorganize data or information into unique configurations. Also include tests of divergent thinking.

Development: Measure emerging characteristics, primarily for preschool ages. Also include tests of cognitive and moral development.

Family: Measure intrafamily relations. Also include tests of marital satisfaction, nurturance, parental interest, and warmth.

Institutional Information: Evaluate institutions and their functioning.

Motivation: Measure goal strength. Also include measures of curiosity.

Perception: Determine how one sees self and other objects. Also include tests dealing with empathy, imagery, locus of control, self-concept, and time.

Personality: Measure general personal attributes. Also include biographical information and defense mechanisms.

Preference: Identify choices. Also include tests of preference for objects, taste preference, and sex role preference.

Problem-Solving and Reasoning: General ability to reason through a number of alternative solutions, to generate such solutions to problems, etc.

Status: Identify a hierarchy of acceptability.

Trait Measurement: Identify and evaluate unitary traits. Also include tests of anger, anxiety, authoritarianism, blame, and cheating.

Values: Measure worth one ascribes to an object or activity. Include tests of moral, philosophical, political, and religious values.

Vocational Evaluation: Evaluate a person for a specific position.

Vocational Interest: Measure interest in specific occupations and vocations as well as interest in general categories of activity.

The choice of the category under which each test was grouped was determined by the purpose of the test and/or its apparent content. The authors attempted to include the following facts regarding each test, however, in many cases not all of these facts were provided in the journal article:

Test Name
Purpose
Description
    Number of items
    Time required
    Format
Statistics
    Reliability (In most cases the particular design used to assess consistency is specified)
    Validity (Includes correlation with other tests, group difference

information, which help to define the characteristic being measured by the test.)

Source

Author

Title

Journal, including date of publication, volume and page number

Related Research

Information identifying publications related to the source.

Volume 4 contains only those tests for which the journal article presented as a minimum: Test Name, Purpose, Source, and at least four facts from either Description, Statistics, or Related Research.

In instances where additional information may be found in Volumes 1, 2, or 3 of the *Directory of Unpublished Experimental Mental Measures,* the reader is referred to *DUEMM* with specific reference following.

Further, the reader is alerted to the fact that the numbers within the Index refer to test numbers rather than to page numbers as was the case with Volume 1. As a convenience to the reader, the authors have incorporated the indices from the three previous volumes in this Index and in so doing they converted all page numbers to test numbers. Thus, numbers 1 through 339 refer to tests of Volume 1, numbers 340 through 1034 refer to tests of Volume 2, numbers 1035 through 1595 refer to tests of Volume 3, numbers 1596 through 2369 refer to tests of Volume 4. Finally, as was the case with Volume 3, a noncumulative author index is included.

The authors express their appreciation to Ms. Debbie Moffitt for typing the manuscript.

Bert Arthur Goldman
William Larry Osborne

CHAPTER 1

Achievement

1596

Test Name: AUDITORY-VISUAL INTEGRATION PERFORMANCE TEST

Purpose: To assess auditory-visual integration performance.

Number of Items: 10

Format: The examiner presents an auditory cue to the subject by tapping on a desk with a pencil in a predetermined sequence and then exposes three separate dot patterns. The subject selects which of the three dot patterns matches the auditory cue.

Validity: With auditory memory, $rs = -.048$ to $.022$; with visual memory, $rs = .003$ to $.188$; with reading vocabulary, $rs = .016$ to $.262$; with reading comprehension, $rs = -.111$ to $.099$.

Author: Jorgenson, G. W., and Hyde, E. M.

Article: Auditory-visual integration and reading performance in lower-social-class children.

Journal: *Journal of Educational Psychology,* October 1974, *66*(5), 718–725.

Related Research: Birch, H., & Belmont, L. (1965). Auditory-visual integration, intelligence, and reading ability in school children. *Perceptual and Motor Skills, 20,* 295–305.

• • •

1597

Test Name: CHECKLIST OF PERCEPTUAL-MOTOR AND LANGUAGE SKILLS

Purpose: To identify specific

perceptual-motor and language skills in developmentally handicapped preschoolers.

Number of Items: 640

Format: Each item is scored *pass* or *fail*.

Reliability: Ranged from .85 to .99.

Validity: Correlation with the Peabody Picture Vocabulary Test was .91.

Author: Burns, W. J., and Burns, K. A.

Article: Checklist of perceptual-motor and language skills for developmentally handicapped preschoolers.

Journal: *Perceptual and Motor Skills,* June 1978, *46*(3, Part 2), 1211–1214.

• • •

1598

Test Name: CLOZE TEST–MODIFIED

Purpose: To measure reading achievement of elementary school English-second-language pupils.

Number of Items: 25

Format: Consists of sets of sentences in which five words from each set are deleted and replaced with blanks. The deleted words are presented in random order in the right margin. The student selects which word to place in each blank.

Reliability: Internal consistency Kuder-Richardson formula 21 for grades 2–5 ranged from .84 to .97.

Validity: Pearson correlations

obtained with the Gates-MacGinitie Reading Test (Primary A, Form 2) for grades 2–5 ranged from .53 to .86, and with the G–M Vocabulary Test ranged from .51 to .90. Correlations with the Marianas English Achievement Test–Reading ranged from .53 to .73 and with the MEAT–Vocabulary ranged from .45 to .88.

Author: Baldauf, R. B., Jr., and Propst, I. K., Jr.

Article: Preliminary evidence regarding the validity of a modified Cloze procedure for lower elementary ESL students.

Journal: *Educational and Psychological Measurement,* Summer 1978, *38*(2), 451–455.

Related Research: Propst, I. K., Jr. (1972). The inappropriateness of the use of U.S. standardized tests for non-native English speakers (Department of Education Bulletin, *1*, 1–6). Pago Pago, American Samoa: Department of Education.

• • •

1599

Test Name: COMPREHENSION OF SOCIAL-MORALS CONCEPTS TEST

Purpose: To test comprehension of social-moral concepts, such as legitimized authority, social contract, and due process.

Number of Items: 40

Format: Ten paragraphs with four interpretative statements for each paragraph. Subject reads the paragraph and then selects the statement that best interprets the paragraph.

Reliability: Test–retest correlation (2 weeks) was .51.

Author: Rest, J. R.

Article: Longitudinal study of the Defining Issues Test of Moral Judgment: A strategy for analyzing developmental change.

Journal: *Developmental Psychology,* November 1975, *11*(6), 738–748.

Related Research: Rest, J. R., et al. (1974). Judging the important issues in moral dilemmas—An objective measure of development. *Developmental Psychology, 10,* 491–501.

■ ■ ■

1600

Test Name: DRUG KNOWLEDGE TEST

Purpose: To measure general knowledge of drugs and their effects.

Number of Items: 31

Format: Five-option multiple-choice.

Reliability: Kuder-Richardson formula 20 reliability coefficient was .76.

Validity: For students in grades 10, 11, and 12, scores on the Drug Knowledge Test correlated .80 with responses to the Drug Knowledge Inventory.

Author: Halpin, G., and Whiddon, T.

Article: Drug education: Solution or problem?

Journal: *Psychological Reports,* April 1977, *40*(2), 372–374.

■ ■ ■

1601

Test Name: EPISODIC LONG-TERM MEMORY QUESTIONNAIRE

Purpose: To measure remote memory.

Number of Items: 74

Format: Written answers to recall questions.

Reliability: Internal consistency reliability (Kuder-Richardson formula 20 variant of coefficient alpha) was .94.

Validity: Correlations with a well-known experimental test of memory, with the verbal subscale of the Shipley-Hartford rated interest in current events, and the Current Events Test are at the .05 level.

Author: Johnson, J. H., and Klingler, D. E.

Article: A questionnaire technique for measurement of episodic long-term memory.

Journal: *Psychological Reports,* August 1976, *39*(1), 291–298.

■ ■ ■

1602

Test Name: FUNDAMENTAL READING COMPETENCIES TEST

Purpose: To assess high school students' functional reading skills.

Number of Items: 65

Format: Includes the following competencies: comprehends main ideas in news articles, comprehends safety warnings, comprehends graphic illustrations, comprehends technical documents, comprehends information and instructions presented on forms and applications, comprehends consumer appeals in advertisements, and uses common reference tools.

Reliability: Test–retest reliabilities ranged from .46 to .71 for individual subtests. Total test score test–retest reliabilities were .83 and .85. Equivalent form

reliabilities ranged from .38 to .79 for individual subtests. Equivalent form reliabilities for total scores were .91 and .94.

Author: Ganopole, S. V.

Article: The Fundamental Reading Competencies Test.

Journal: *Journal of Educational Measurement,* Spring 1980, *17*(1), 71–74.

Related Research: The test is available from the Center for Instructional Design and Evaluation, P.O. Box 3182, Westlake Village, California.

■ ■ ■

1603

Test Name: HYGIENE AND GROOMING TEST

Purpose: To measure social and personal knowledge.

Number of Items: 36

Format: Three alternative multiple-choice items. Two forms.

Reliability: Coefficient alpha .72 (form A) and .73 (form B).

Author: Reynolds, W. M.

Article: The utility of multiple-choice test formats with mildly retarded adolescents.

Journal: *Educational and Psychological Measurement,* Summer 1979, *39*(2), 325–331.

Related Research: Halpern, A., et al. (1975). *Social and prevocational information battery.* Monterey, CA: CTB/McGraw-Hill.

■ ■ ■

1604

Test Name: IDENTICAL FORMS TEST

Purpose: To assess perceptual speed.

Number of Items: 60

Time Required: 4.5 minutes.

Format: Subjects find one of five figures that is exactly like the key figure.

Reliability: .48 (Kuder-Richardson coefficient).

Author: Undheim, J.

Article: Broad ability factors in 12 to 13 year old children, the theory of fluid and crystallized intelligence, and the differentiation hypothesis.

Journal: *Journal of Educational Psychology,* June 1978, *70*(3), 433–443.

Related Research: Guilford, J., & Hoepfner, R. (1971). *The analysis of intelligence.* New York: McGraw-Hill.

• • •

1605

Test Name: INFERENTIAL READING COMPREHENSION TEST

Purpose: To test inferential reading comprehension.

Number of Items: 73

Format: Multiple-choice tests with 14 passages, including the following subtests: detail, main idea, word meaning, character traits, and outcomes.

Reliability: .92

Author: Weintraub, S., et al.

Article: Summary of investigations relating to reading July 1, 1973, to June 30, 1974.

Journal: *Reading Research Quarterly,* 1974–75, *10*(3), 387.

Related Research: Pettit, N. T., & Cockriel, I. W. (1974). A factor study of the Literal Reading Comprehension Test and the Inferential Reading Comprehension Test. *Journal of Reading Behavior, 6,* 63–75.

1606

Test Name: INFORMATION HUNT

Purpose: To test the student's ability to use the library.

Number of Items: 30

Format: Areas included: using the card catalog; using a dictionary; using encyclopedias; using the atlas, globes, and maps; finding fiction and non-fiction books; and using parts of a book. Two forms.

Reliability: Split-half reliabilities were .944 (Form A) and .874 (Form B) with $N = 21$.

Validity: Correlations with: It's fun to think (.73), interpreting data (.65), fluency (.24), flexibility (.25), originality (.18), and elaboration (.31).

Author: Jensen, L. R.

Article: Diagnosis and evaluation of creativity, research and thinking skills of academically talented elementary students.

Journal: *The Gifted Child Quarterly,* Spring 1978, *22*(1), 98–110.

• • •

1607

Test Name: INTERPRETING DATA

Purpose: To test the student's skill in reading various forms of data.

Number of Items: 20

Format: Includes the following subtests: reading graphs; reading charts; reading maps; and probability and statistics.

Reliability: Split-half reliabilities were .930 (Form A) and .896 (Form B) with $N = 21$.

Validity: Correlations with: It's fun to think (.72), information hunt (.65), fluency (.19), flexibility (.16), originality (.13), and elaboration (.26).

Author: Jensen, L. R.

Article: Diagnosis and evaluation of creativity, research and thinking skills of academically talented elementary students.

Journal: *The Gifted Child Quarterly,* Spring 1978, *22*(1), 98–110.

• • •

1608

Test Name: LETTER IDENTIFICATION TEST

Purpose: To assess perceptual speed.

Number of Items: 150

Time Required: 3 minutes.

Format: Subjects identify words that contain the letter *a* in a list of words.

Reliability: .54 (Kuder-Richardson coefficient).

Author: Undheim, J.

Article: Broad ability factors in 12 to 13 year old children, the theory of fluid and crystallized intelligence and the differentiation hypothesis.

Journal: *Journal of Educational Psychology,* June 1978, *70*(3), 433–443.

Related Research: Guilford, J., & Hoepfner, R. (1971). *The analysis of intelligence.* New York: McGraw-Hill.

• • •

1609

Test Name: LITERAL READING COMPREHENSION TEST

Purpose: To test literal reading comprehension.

Number of Items: 101

Format: Multiple-choice test with 18 reading passages and includes the following subtests: detail; main idea; sequence; comprehension;

cause and effect; and character traits.

Reliability: .92

Author: Weintraub, S., et al.

Article: Summary of investigations relating to reading July 1, 1973, to June 30, 1974.

Journal: *Reading Research Quarterly*, 1974–75, *10*(3), 387 (269–543).

Related Research: Pettit, N. T., & Cockriel, I. W. (1974). A factor study of the Literal Reading Comprehension Test and the Inferential Reading Comprehension Test. *Journal of Reading Behavior, 6,* 63–75.

• • •

1610

Test Name: MARKING SPEED TEST

Purpose: To assess motor speed.

Number of Items: 600

Time Required: 4 minutes.

Format: Subjects make as many "11" signs as possible in the time period.

Reliability: .83 (Kuder-Richardson coefficient).

Author: Undheim, J.

Article: Broad ability factors in 12 to 13 year old children, the theory of fluid and crystallized intelligence, and the differentiation hypothesis.

Journal: *Journal of Educational Psychology,* June 1978, *70*(3), 433–443.

Related Research: Guilford, J., & Hoepfner, R. (1971). *The analysis of intelligence.* New York: McGraw-Hill.

• • •

1611

Test Name: MINIMAL READING PROFICIENCY ASSESSMENT

Purpose: To measure functional literacy at the high school level.

Number of Items: 48

Format: Includes 12 skill areas. Multiple choice, criterion referenced test with five possible answers (McDonald & Moorman, 1974).

Reliability: $r = .89$.

Author: Weintraub, S., et al.

Article: Summary of investigations relating to reading July 1, 1973, to June 30, 1974.

Journal: *Reading Research Quarterly*, 1974–75, *10*(3), 461 (269–543).

Related Research: McDonald, T. F., & Moorman, G. B. (1974). Criterion referenced testing for functional literacy. *Journal of Reading, 17,* 363–366.

• • •

1612

Test Name: MUTILATED WORDS TEST

Purpose: To assess speed of closure.

Number of Items: 20

Time Required: 5 minutes.

Format: Subjects identify words in which parts of letters are missing.

Reliability: .70 (Kuder-Richardson coefficient).

Author: Undheim, J.

Article: Broad ability factors in 12 to 13 year old children, the theory of fluid and crystallized intelligence, and the differentiation hypothesis.

Journal: *Journal of Educational Psychology,* June 1978, *70*(3), 433–443.

Related Research: Guilford, J., & Hoepfner, R. (1971). *The analysis of intelligence.* New York: McGraw-Hill.

1613

Test Name: OLGUIN DIAGNOSTIC TEST OF AUDITORY PERCEPTION

Purpose: To provide a diagnostic test of auditory perception for Spanish language-oriented children.

Number of Items: 120

Format: Includes 12 subtests.

Reliability: Kuder-Richardson formula 21 estimates of reliability ranged from .410 to .899.

Validity: Concurrent validity coefficients ranged from −.22 to .55.

Author: Olguin, L., and Michael, W. B.

Article: The development and preliminary validation of the Olguin Diagnostic Test of Auditory Perception for Spanish language-oriented children.

Journal: *Educational and Psychological Measurement,* Winter 1979, *39*(4), 985–999.

Related Research: Olguin, L., & Michael, W. B. (1979). The factorial validity of the Olguin Diagnostic Test of Auditory Perception for Spanish language-oriented students. *Educational and Psychological Measurement, 39,* 1005–1010.

• • •

1614

Test Name: PROPORTION TEST

Purpose: To measure the level of acquisition of the concept of proportion.

Number of Items: 18

Format: For each item the subject must determine which one of two mixtures would produce the stronger tasting mixture.

Reliability: Coefficient of reproducibility ($N = 578$ ages 8–

13) was .93. Minimal marginal reproducibility (N = 578 ages 8–13) was .79.

Author: Cloutier, R., and Goldschmid, M. L.

Article: Individual differences in the development of formal reasoning.

Journal: *Child Development,* March 1976, *47*(1), 1097–1102.

Related Research: Cloutier, R. (1970). *Standardisation de l'epreure des concentrations* (forme collective "C"). Unpublished master's thesis, Université Laval, Quebec.

. . .

1615

Test Name: READING COMPREHENSION TEST

Purpose: To assess reading comprehension of college students.

Number of Items: 32

Format: Four-alternative multiple-choice test.

Reliability: Kuder-Richardson 20 was .75 from 213 college students.

Validity: Item discrimination was .39, average point biserial coefficient was .33.

Author: Bassin, C. B., and Martin, C. J.

Article: Effect of three types of redundancy reduction on comprehension, reading rate and reading time of English prose.

Journal: *Journal of Educational Psychology,* October 1976, *68*(5), 649–652.

. . .

1616

Test Name: READING RETENTION TEST

Purpose: To measure the reading retention of undergraduate college students.

Number of Items: 60

Format: 30–item constructed response test and a matched 30–item multiple-choice test with four alternatives for each item.

Reliability: Kuder-Richardson formula 20 reliability coefficients were .70 and .71.

Author: Ross, S. M., and DiVesta, F. S.

Article: Oral summary as a review strategy for enchancing recall of textual material.

Journal: *Journal of Educational Psychology,* December 1976, *68*(6), 689–695.

Related Research: Anderson, R. C., & Myrow, D. L. (1971). Retroactive inhibition of meaningful discourse. *Journal of Educational Psychology, 62,* 81–94.

. . .

1617

Test Name: STREET GESTALT COMPLETION TEST

Purpose: To assess speed of closure.

Number of Items: 18

Time Required: 6 minutes.

Format: Subjects identify pictured objects having missing segments.

Reliability: .82 (Kuder–Richardson coefficient).

Author: Undheim, J.

Article: Broad ability factors in 12 to 13 year old children, the theory of fluid and crystallized intelligence, and the differentiation hypothesis.

Journal: *Journal of Educational Psychology,* June 1978, *70,* (3), 433–443.

Related Research: Guilford, J., & Hoepfner, R. (1971). *The analysis of intelligence.* New York: McGraw-Hill.

1618

Test Name: SYMBOL IDENTITIES TEST

Purpose: To assess perceptual speed.

Number of Items: 80

Time Required: 3 minutes.

Format: Subjects judge whether pairs of proper names, letters, or numbers are different.

Reliability: .66 (Kuder–Richardson coefficient).

Author: Undheim, J.

Article: Broad ability factors in 12 to 13 year old children, the theory of fluid and crystallized intelligence, and the differentiation hypothesis.

Journal: *Journal of Educational Psychology,* June 1978, *70*(3), 433–443.

Related Research: Guilford, J., & Hoepfner, R. (1971). The analysis of intelligence. New York: McGraw-Hill.

. . .

1619

Test Name: TEST OF SOCIAL INFERENCE

Purpose: An achievement test for the decoding of visual-social cues.

Number of Items: 30 pictures.

Format: Pictures of diverse social situations which are accompanied by standard questions verbally presented by the examiner.

Reliability: Interscorer reliability for trained scorers is in the high .90s. Test–retest reliability for special education groups has ranged from .84 to above .90. For 13-, 14-, and 15-year-old junior-high educable mentally retarded students used in this study, test–retest reliability coefficients exceeded .90. The retest correlations of the short forms of the test were .74 and .75.

Author: Karpf, R. J.

Article: Effects of emotions on altruism and social inference in retarded adolescents.

Journal: *Psychological Reports,* August 1977, *41*(1) 135–138.

Related Research: Edmonson, B., et al. (1971). *Social inference training of retarded adolescents and the Test of Social Inference.* Eugene: University of Oregon Press.

•••

1620

Test Name: TEST WISENESS MEASURE

Purpose: To assess test taking skills.

Number of Items: 16

Format: Measures for test-wise behaviors.

Validity: Correlation with Math Achievement (.35) and with Vocabulary (.32).

Author: Rowley, G.

Article: Which examinees are most favored by the use of multiple choice tests?

Journal: *Journal of Educational Measurement,* Spring 1974, *11*(1), 15–23.

Related Research: Slakter, M., et al. (1970). Grade level, sex, and selected aspects of test-wiseness. *Journal of Educational Measurement, 7,* 119–122.

•••

1621

Test Name: TEST-WISENESS SCALE

Purpose: To measure test-wiseness.

Number of Items: 60

Format: Includes test-wiseness skills of similar-option, absurd-option, and stern-option.

Reliability: Alpha reliability was .73.

Author: Bajtelsmit, J. W.

Article: Test-wiseness and systematic desensitization programs for increasing adult test-taking skills.

Journal: *Journal of Educational Measurement,* Winter 1977, *14*(4), 335–341.

Related Research: Woodley, K. (1973, February). *Test-wiseness program development and evaluation.* Paper presented at the annual meeting of the American Educational Research Association, New Orleans.

•••

1622

Test Name: TRAFFIC SAFETY QUESTIONNAIRE

Purpose: To measure knowledge of accident avoidance and knowledge of the rules of the road.

Number of Items: 40

Time Required: 30 minutes.

Format: A multiple-choice test answered on either a standard answer sheet or punchboard. Two alternate forms are available. A sample item is presented.

Reliability: Alternate-form reliabilities 1 week apart for each of the two parts of the test were .28 and .31.

Author: Schuster, D. H.

Article: Cognitive accident-avoidance training for beginning drivers.

Journal: *Journal of Applied Psychology,* June 1978, *63*(3), 377–379.

Related Research: Schuster, D. H.,

et al. (1971). *Traffic safety questionnaire* (Forms A and B). Unpublished research test, Iowa State University, Department of Psychology.

•••

1623

Test Name: U-TUBE TEST

Purpose: To assess knowledge of a simple hydrostatic principle.

Number of Items: 18

Format: The subject draws the water line in the right portion of a u-shaped tube. Examples are given.

Reliability: Split-half, Spearman-Brown corrected reliabilities ranged from .89 to .99.

Validity: Correlations with Water Level Test ranged from .01 to –.19 (44 men); .08 to –.24 (44 women). Correlations with the Adjective Checklist ranged from .25 to –.03 (44 men); 28 to –.08 (44 women), and with the Concealed Figures Test ranged from .00 to –.05.

Author: Walker, J. T., and Krasnoff, A. G.

Article: The horizontality principle in young men and women.

Journal: *Perceptual and Motor Skills,* June 1978, *46*(3, Part 2), 1055–1061.

•••

1624

Test Name: WATER LEVEL TEST

Purpose: To assess one's understanding of the horizontality principle.

Number of Items: 15

Format: A cognitive-perceptual measure requiring the subject to draw the water level in each drawing of partially filled vertical and tilted containers. Examples are given.

Reliability: .97 (split-half corrected by the Spearman-Brown formula).

Validity: Correlations with the U-Tube Test ranged from .01 to −.19 (44 men); .08 to −.24 (44 women); with the Adjective Checklist ranged from −.04 to −.15 (44 men); .16 to .24 (44 women), and with the Concealed Figures Test were −.28 (44 men); −.42 (44 women).

Author: Walker, J. T., and Krasnoff, A. G.

Article: The horizontality principle in young men and women.

Journal: *Perceptual and Motor Skills,* June 1978, *46*(3, Part 2), 1055–1061.

CHAPTER 2
Adjustment—Educational

1625

Test Name: ACHIEVEMENT ANXIETY TEST

Purpose: To measure test anxiety.

Number of Items: 19

Format: Two subscales: Debilitating Anxiety (9 items) and Facilitating Anxiety (10 items).

Reliability: Reliabilities (Hoyt) under three forms are given and range from .65 to .76 (Facilitative) and from .76 to .86 (Debilitative).

Validity: Multiple correlations of Debilitating and Facilitating scales predicting grade point were .46 (males) and .28 (females); both had a nonsignificant correlation with math achievement of –.30 and with vocabulary of –.42 (see Rowley 1974, below). Significant differences in scores were obtained for the three forms of the test, suggesting that there was an effect in varying the response format. Correlation with score on test in introductory psychology, .31 ($p <$ .01); facilitating test anxiety, –.48 ($p < .01$); debilitating test anxiety, no difference between cheaters/ noncheaters (see Bronzaft et al., 1973, below).

Author: Harper, F.

Article: The comparative validity of the Mandler-Sarason Test Anxiety Questionnaire and the Achievement Test.

Journal: *Educational and Psychological Measurement*, Winter 1974, *34*(4), 961–966.

Related Research: Alpert, R., & Haber, R. (1960). Anxiety in academic achievement situations.

Journal of Abnormal and Social Psychology, 61, 207–215.

Bronzaft, A., et al. (1973). Test anxiety and cheating on college examinations. *Psychological Reports, 32*(1), 149–150.

Huck, S., & Jacko, E. (1974). Effect of varying the response format of the Alpert-Haber Achievement Anxiety Test. *Journal of Counseling Psychology, 21*, 159–163.

Naylor, F. D., & Gaudry, E. (1973). The relationship of adjustment, anxiety, and intelligence to mathematics performance. *Journal of Educational Research, 66*(9), 413–417.

Rowley, G. (1974). Which examinees are most favored by the use of multiple choice tests? *Journal of Educational Measurement, 11*(1), 15–23.

See *DUEMM, 2*, 387.

• • •

1626

Test Name: DEBILITATING ANXIETY SCALE OF THE ALPERT-HABER ACHIEVEMENT ANXIETY TEST

Purpose: To measure anxiety that interferes with students' performance on academic tasks.

Number of Items: 10

Reliability: Test–retest reliabilities were .87 (10-week interval) and .76 (8-month interval).

Validity: With the Mandler–

Sarason Test Anxiety Scale, $r =$ .64; with the Fear of Success Scale, $r = .43$; with the Fear of Success Questionnaire, $r = .54$.

Author: Griffore, R. J.

Article: Validation of three measures of fear of success.

Journal: *Journal of Personality Assessment*, August 1977, *41*(4), 417–421.

Related Research: Alpert, R., & Haber, R. N. (1960). Anxiety in academic achievement situations. *Journal of Personality and Social Psychology, 61*(2), 207–215.

• • •

1627

Test Name: INVENTORY OF TEST ANXIETY

Purpose: To measure the immediate, momentary affective experiences under evaluative stress.

Number of Items: 16

Format: Likert scale with three state anxiety scores: "worry," "emotionality," and a combined "state test anxiety" score.

Reliability: Split-half reliability was .92 (Osterhouse, 1972) and test–retest reliabilities over a 7-week period were .68 for emotionality and .72 for worry (Osipow & Kreinbring, 1971).

Author: Deffenbacher, J. L., et al.

Article: Two self-control procedures in the reduction of targeted and nontargeted anxieties.

Journal: *Journal of Counseling Psychology*, March 1979, *26*(2), 120–127.

Related Research: Osipow, S. H., & Kreinbring, I. (1971). Temporal stability of an inventory to measure test anxiety. *Journal of Counseling Psychology, 18*, 152–154.

Osterhouse, R. A. (1975). Classroom anxiety and the examination performance of test-anxious students. *Journal of Educational Research, 68*(7), 247–249.

Osterhouse, R. A. (1972). Desensitization and study-skills training as treatment for two types of test-anxious students. *Journal of Counseling Psychology, 19*, 301–307.

■ ■ ■

1628

Test Name: LOCUS OF CONFLICT RATING SCALE

Purpose: To provide an index of behavior adjustment in school.

Number of Items: 30

Format: Half the items relate to internalizing behaviors and half relate to externalizing behaviors.

Validity: Correlations with parental locus of control ranged from –.123 to .233.

Author: Ollendick, D. G.

Article: Parental locus of control and the assessment of children's personality characteristics.

Journal: *Journal of Personality Assessment*, August 1979, *43*(4), 401–405.

Related Research: Armentrout, J. A. (1971). Parental child-rearing attitudes and preadolescents' problem behaviors. *Journal of Consulting and Clinical Psychology, 37*, 278–285.

1629

Test Name: MANDLER-SARASON TEST ANXIETY QUESTIONNAIRE

Purpose: To measure test anxiety.

Number of Items: 35

Time Required: 10–30 minutes.

Format: Three subsections: anxiety regarding group IQ tests, individual IQ tests, and course exams.

Validity: Correlation with college grade point was –.26 ($p < .05$) for males but not significant for females. Following treatment, significant ($p < .05$) differences in test anxiety were found between control and an implosive therapy group (see Dawley & Wenrich, 1973). Significant differences ($p < .01$) in test anxiety were found between various treatments (including desensitization) designed to reduce anxiety.

Author: Harper, F.

Article: The comparative validity of the Mandler-Sarason test anxiety questionnaire and the Achievement Anxiety Test.

Journal: *Educational and Psychological Measurement*, Winter 1974, *34*(4), 961–966.

Related Research: Dawley, H., & Wenrich, W. (1973). Massed groups desensitization in reduction of test anxiety. *Psychological Reports, 33*(1), 359–363.

Dawley, H., & Wenrich, W. (1973). Treatment of test anxiety by group implosive therapy. *Psychological Reports, 33*(2), 383–388.

Farley, F. H. (1974). Individual differences in examination persistence and performance. *Journal of Educational Research, 67*(8), 344–346.

Herbert, S., & Sassenrath, J. (1973). Achieve (sic) motivation, test anxiety, achievement conditions, and performance in programmed learning. *California Journal of Educational Research, 24*, 12–22.

Mandler, G., & Sarason, D. (1952). A study of anxiety and learning. *Journal of Abnormal and Social Psychology, 47*, 166–173.

■ ■ ■

1630

Test Name: MATHEMATICS ANXIETY SCALE

Purpose: To assess subjects' anxiety toward mathematics.

Number of Items: 20

Format: Subjects respond either *yes* or *no* to statements such as "do mathematical symbols worry you?"

Reliability: Split-half reliability was .90.

Author: Sepie, A., and Keeling, B.

Article: The relationship between types of anxiety and underachievement in mathematics.

Journal: *Journal of Educational Research*, September/October 1978, *72*(1), 15–19.

Related Research: Levitt, E. (1967). *The psychology of anxiety.* Indianapolis: Bobbs-Merrill.

■ ■ ■

1631

Test Name: SELF-REPORT QUESTIONNAIRE

Purpose: To assess the dynamics of achievement.

Number of Items: 58

Format: 46 of the items require Likert responses, the remaining 12 are forced-choice. There are 8 subscales assessing such factors as fear of failure, locus of control, and incentives to achieve.

Reliability: Average alpha was .70.

Validity: Authors report a predictive test-rate of 77.1%, suggesting that the instrument has "moderately good nomological validity."

Author: Thisanchuk, E.

Article: A model-based prediction of scholastic achievement.

Journal: *Journal of Educational Research*, September/October 1977, *71*(1), 30–35.

• • •

1632

Test Name: SYMPTOM CHECK LIST

Purpose: To measure the extent to which a variety of anxiety symptoms are experienced in preparing for and taking examinations.

Number of Items: 32

Format: Self-report.

Reliability: Reliability coefficient reported was .70.

Validity: Coefficients reported of .70.

Author: Geer, C. A., and Hurst, J. C.

Article: Counselor-subject sex variables in systematic desensitization.

Journal: *Journal of Counseling Psychology*, July 1976, *23*(4), 296–301.

Related Research: Spinelli, P. (1972). *The effect of therapist presence in systematic desensitization.* Unpublished doctoral dissertation, Colorado State University.

• • •

1633

Test Name: TEST ANXIETY INVENTORY

Purpose: To provide a measure of test anxiety.

Format: Includes items from Harleston's measure of test anxiety and items from the Alpert-Haber debilitating anxiety scale.

Reliability: Average interitem correlation corrected for length was .87.

Validity: With vocabulary, $r = -.16$; with ideational fluency, $r = .06$; with formulating hypotheses, $rs = .00, -.03$, and $-.04$; with consequences—obvious, $r = .05$; with consequences—remote, $r = -.07$.

Author: Fredericksen, N., and Evans, F. R.

Article: Effects of models of creative performance on ability to formulate hypotheses.

Journal: *Journal of Educational Psychology*, February 1974, *66*(1), 67–82.

Related Research: Alpert, R., & Haber, R. M. (1960). Anxiety in academic achievement situations. *Journal of Abnormal and Social Psychology, 61,* 207–215.

Harleston, B. W. (1962). Test anxiety and performance in problem-solving situations. *Journal of Personality, 30,* 557–573.

• • •

1634

Test Name: TEST ANXIETY QUESTIONNAIRE

Purpose: To measure the test anxiety of college students.

Number of Items: 11

Format: Five worry and five emotionality items.

Reliability: Coefficient alpha .79 to .88.

Author: Morris, L. W., and Fulmer, R. S.

Article: Test anxiety (worry and emotionality) changes during academic testing as a function of feedback and test importance.

Journal: *Journal of Educational Psychology*, December 1976, *68*(6), 817–824.

Related Research: Liebert, R. M., & Morris, L. W. (1967). Cognitive and emotional components of test anxiety: A distinction and some initial data. *Psychological Reports, 20,* 975–978.

• • •

1635

Test Name: TEST ANXIETY SCALE FOR CHILDREN

Purpose: To measure anxiety in children.

Number of Items: 30

Format: Asks children about their feelings regarding various school tasks and situations.

Reliability: Test–retest correlations obtained for changes over the fourth to the sixth grade were .58 for boys and .49 for girls.

Author: Bauer, D. H.

Article: The effect of instructions, anxiety, and locus of control on intelligence test scores.

Journal: *Measurement and Evaluation in Guidance*, April 1975, *8*(1), 13–19.

Related Research: Bush, E. S., & Dweck, C. S. (1975). Reflections on conceptual tempo: Relationship between cognitive style and performance as a function of task characteristics. *Developmental Psychology, 11,* 562–574.

Related Research: Sarason, S. B., et al. (1960). *Anxiety in elementary school children.* New York: Wiley.

CHAPTER 3
Adjustment—Psychological

1636

Test Name: ACCEPTANCE OF DISABILITY SCALE

Purpose: To measure acceptance of loss.

Number of Items: 50

Format: Six-point Likert scale of agreement–disagreement.

Reliability: Internal consistency coefficient was .93.

Author: Morgan, B., and Leung, P.

Article: Effects of assertion training on acceptance of disability by physically disabled university students.

Journal: *Journal of Counseling Psychology*, March 1980, *27*(2), 209–212.

Related Research: Linkowski, D. C. (1971). A scale to measure acceptance of disability. *Rehabilitation Counseling Bulletin, 14,* 236–244.

■ ■ ■

1637

Test Name: ADULT IRRATIONAL IDEAS INVENTORY

Purpose: To measure the extent to which individuals exhibit the 11 irrational beliefs described by Ellis (1962).

Number of Items: 60

Format: Single statements scored on a 5-point Likert scale, ranging from *strongly agree* to *strongly disagree*.

Reliability: Kuder-Richardson

coefficients were .74 and .78. Test–retest reliability for 110 senior education students over a 3-week period yielded a Pearson correlation of .77.

Author: Morris, G. B.

Article: Beliefs of native teacher trainees.

Journal: *Psychological Reports,* June 1976, *38*(3), 859–862.

Related Research: Davis, R. L. (1970). *Relationship of irrational ideas to emotional disturbance.* Unpublished master's thesis, University of Alberta.

■ ■ ■

1638

Test Name: AFFECTIVE STATES INVENTORY

Purpose: To assess one's emotional dependence, impulse to aggression, overt aggression, depression, anomie, general anxiety, resentment, anxiety and tension, irritability, guilt, and lack of social support.

Number of Items: 63

Format: Five-point Likert scale ranging from 1 *almost always true* to 5 *never true* was used.

Reliability: Internal consistency reliability (coefficient alpha) ranged from .57 to .84.

Author: Burke, R. J., and Weir, T.

Article: Maternal employment status, social support and adolescents' well-being.

Journal: *Psychological Reports,* June 1978, *42*(3), 1159–1170.

Related Research: Bachmann, J. G., et al. (1970). *Youth in transition, 1.* Ann Arbor, MI: Institute for Social Research.

■ ■ ■

1639

Test Name: ALCADD TEST

Purpose: To diagnose the alcoholic addict.

Number of Items: 65

Format: Statements that are answered either *yes* or *no*.

Reliability: Reliability and validity review provided by Jacobson (1976).

Author: Ornstein, P.

Article: The Alcadd test as a predictor of post-hospital drinking behavior.

Journal: *Psychological Reports,* October 1978, *43*(2), 611–617.

Related Research: Jacobson, G. R. (1976). *The alcoholisms: Detection, diagnosis and assessment.* New York: Behavioral Publications.

Manson, M. P. (1949). A psychometric determination of alcoholic addiction. *American Journal of Psychiatry, 106,* 199–205.

■ ■ ■

1640

Test Name: ANOMIE INDEX

Purpose: To measure perceived normlessness.

Number of Items: 6

Format: Items are rated on Likert

scales. All items are presented.

Reliability: Cronbach's alpha was .52.

Author: Kapsis, R. E.

Article: Black ghetto diversity and anomie: A sociopolitical view.

Journal: *American Journal of Sociology,* March 1978, *83*(5), 1132–1153.

Related Research: Lauder, B. (1954). *Toward an understanding of juvenile delinquency.* New York: Columbia University Press.

■ ■ ■

1641

Test Name: ANXIETY QUESTIONNAIRE

Purpose: To measure symptoms commonly associated with tenseness, emotionality, or anxiety in school age children.

Number of Items: 15

Format: Items were rated on a 6-point scale from 1 (*the least anxious*) to 6 (*the most anxious*).

Reliability: Item to total correlations averaged .81 with the lowest being .69. Item–item correlations averaged .50.

Author: Grimm, V. E., and Nachmias, C.

Article: The effect of cognitive style and manifest anxiety on intellectual and vocational interest in adolescents.

Journal: *Journal of Vocational Behavior,* April 1977, *10*(2), 146–155.

■ ■ ■

1642

Test Name: ANXIETY SCALE FOR PRESCHOOL CHILDREN

Purpose: To measure anxiety in young children.

Number of Items: 79

Format: Individually administered test that requires the child to make binary nonverbal responses to a series of 35 ambiguous items and 44 unambiguous items.

Reliability: Test–retest reliability was .77 for a sample of 23 preschool children. Internal consistency coefficient was .75 for 45 children.

Validity: There were no significant correlations between scores on the scale and maternal anxiety or teachers ratings of the children's anxiety.

Author: Hollembeak, N., et al.

Article: Validity of a non-projective anxiety scale for preschool children.

Journal: *Psychological Reports,* August 1977, *41*(1), 212–214.

Related Research: Alpern, J. D. (1959). *The relationship of an objective measure of anxiety for preschool-aged children to two criterion measures.* Unpublished master's thesis, State University of Iowa.

■ ■ ■

1643

Test Name: ANXIETY-STRESS MEASURE

Purpose: To measure anxiety-stress.

Number of Items: 9

Format: Subjects were asked how frequently they "felt bothered" about a number of job-related matters.

Reliability: Coefficient alphas ranged from .67 to .88.

Author: Ivancevich, J. M., and Lyon, H. L.

Article: The shortened workweek: A field experiment.

Journal: *Journal of Applied*

Psychology, February 1977, *62*(1), 34–37.

Related Research: Kahn, R. L., et al. (1964). *Organizational Stress.* New York: Wiley.

■ ■ ■

1644

Test Name: BECK DEPRESSION INVENTORY

Purpose: To measure the severity of depressive symptomatology.

Number of Items: 26

Format: Each item is rated on a separate 3-point scale.

Validity: Correlations with dimensions of the SCL-90 ranged from .46 to .70.

Author: Dinning, W. D., and Evans, R. G.

Article: Discriminant and convergent validity of the SCL-90 in psychiatric inpatients.

Journal: *Journal of Personality Assessment,* June 1977, *41*(3), 304–310.

Related Research: Beck, A. T. (1967). *Depression: Clinical experimental and theoretical aspects.* New York: Hoeber.

■ ■ ■

1645

Test Name: BECK DEPRESSION INVENTORY

Purpose: To measure depression.

Number of Items: 21

Format: Each item is composed of four alternative statements rated in severity from 0 to 3.

Reliability: Split-half reliabilities in the 90s. Coefficient alpha for the present sample was .93.

Author: Steer, R. A., et al.

Article: Structure of depression in Black alcoholic men.

Journal: *Psychological Reports,* December 1977, *41*(3), 1235–1241.

Related Research: Beck, A. T., et al. (1961). An inventory for measuring depression. *Archives of General Psychiatry, 4,* 561–571.

■ ■ ■

1646

Test Name: CHARACTERISTICS OF CLIENT GROWTH SCALE

Purpose: To rate the extent to which clients could experience constructive change.

Number of Items: 3 scales.

Format: Each scale consists of a 5-point rating system with 1.0 being the lowest, 5.0 the highest possible rating, and 3.0 defined as the minimal level at which constructive change can occur. The scales include Owning of Feelings, Client Commitment to Change, and Client Differentiation of Stimuli.

Reliability: Interrater reliability coefficients were .83 (Owning of Feeling), .90 (Commitment to Change), and .94 (Differentiation of Stimuli).

Author: VanNoord, R. W., and Ragan, N.

Article: Stimulated recall and affect simulation in counseling: Client growth reexamined.

Journal: *Journal of Counseling Psychology,* January 1976, *23*(1), 28–33.

Related Research: Ragan, N., et al. (1967). *Studies in human interaction.* East Lansing: Michigan State University Educational Publication Services.

■ ■ ■

1647

Test Name: CHILDREN'S FORM OF THE MANIFEST ANXIETY SCALE

Purpose: To measure the manifest anxiety of fourth, fifth, and sixth-grade children.

Number of Items: 53

Format: Subjects answered *yes* or *no* to declarative statements.

Reliability: Test–retest reliability after a 1-week interval ranged from .70 to .94 for a sample of 361 children.

Author: Cowan, R., et al.

Article: A validity study of selected self-concept instruments.

Journal: *Measurement and Evaluation in Guidance,* January 1978, *10*(4), 211–221.

Related Research: Castenda, A., et al. (1956). A Children's Form of the Manifest Anxiety Scale. *Child Development, 27,* 317–326.

■ ■ ■

1648

Test Name: CONCEPT-SPECIFIC ANXIETY SCALE

Purpose: To measure general anxiety, major choice anxiety, and vocational choice anxiety.

Number of Items: 15

Format: Items are rated on a 7-point scale. Scores range from 15 (low anxiety) to 105 (high anxiety) for each concept rated.

Reliability: Reliability coefficient of .86 is reported.

Author: Hawkins, J. G., et al.

Article: Anxiety and the process of deciding about a major and a vocation.

Journal: *Journal of Counseling Psychology,* September 1977, *24*(5), 398–403.

Related Research: Cole, C. W., et al. (1969). Measurement of stimulus specific anxiety. *Psychological Reports, 25,* 49–50.

1649

Test Name: DEATH ANXIETY SCALE

Purpose: To assess attitude of individual toward own death.

Number of Items: 15

Format: True–false.

Reliability: Correlation with Rescue Scale was .28 (*p* < .05). Correlation with Risk Scale was −.19 (*ns*). Murray (1974) found decreases of anxiety in nurses over the period of a death education workshop.

Author: Tarter, R., et al.

Article: Death Anxiety in suicide attempters.

Journal: *Psychological Reports,* June 1974, *34*(3), 895–897.

Related Research: Murray, P. (1974). Death education and its effect on the death anxiety level of nurses. *Psychological Reports, 35*(3), 1250.

Templer, D. (1970). The construction and validation of a death anxiety scale. *Journal of General Psychology, 82,* 165–177.

Weisman, A., & Worden, J. (1972). Risk rescue rating in suicide assessment. *Archives of General Psychiatry, 26,* 553–560.

See also *DUEMM, 2,* 410.

■ ■ ■

1650

Test Name: DEATH ANXIETY SCALE

Purpose: To measure one's fear of dying.

Number of Items: 20

Format: High scores reflect high levels of death anxiety and low scores indicate low levels of death anxiety.

Reliability: Test–retest reliability is

.85 for a 3-month interval.

Author: Tolor, A.

Article: Some antecedents and personality correlates of health locus of control.

Journal: *Psychological Reports,* December 1978, *43*(3), 1159–1165.

Related Research: Tolor, A., & Reznikoff, M. (1967). Relation between insight, repression-sensitization, internal–external control, and death anxiety. *Journal of Abnormal Psychology, 72*, 426–430.

■ ■ ■

1651

Test Name: DEATH ANXIETY SCALE

Purpose: To measure one's fear of dying.

Number of Items: 35

Format: Thirty-four true–false statements and one Likert item.

Validity: Correlations with the Edwards Personal Preference Schedule were as follows: Succorance, $r = .23$ ($p < .001$); Exhibition, $r = -.14$ ($p < .05$); Endurance, $r = -.16$ ($p < .01$); and Aggression, $r = -.18$ ($p < .01$).

Author: Thorson, J. A.

Article: Variations in death anxiety related to college students' sex, major field of study, and certain personality traits.

Journal: *Psychological Reports,* June 1977, *40*(3), 857–858.

Related Research: Boyer, J. (1964). The construction and partial validation of a scale for the measurement of the fear of death. *Dissertation Abstracts, 25*, 2041.

Templer, D. (1970). The construction and validation of a death anxiety scale. *Journal of General Psychology, 82*, 165–177.

1652

Test Name: DEATH CONCERN SCALE

Purpose: To measure the extent to which an individual consciously contemplates death and evaluates it negatively.

Number of Items: 30

Reliability: Test–retest reliability coefficient of sample of 151 female college students over 8 weeks was .87. Split-half reliabilities were .85 and higher in four separate administrations of the scale to 600 college students.

Author: Klug, L., and Boss, M.

Article: Factorial structure of the Death Concern Scale.

Journal: *Psychological Reports,* February 1976, *38*(1), 107–112.

Related Research: Dickstein, L. S. (1972). Death concern: Measurement and correlates. *Psychological Reports, 30*, 503–571.

Dickstein, L. S. (1975). Self-report and fantasy correlates of death concern. *Psychological Reports, 37*, 147–158.

See *DUEMM, 2,* 1978, 411.

■ ■ ■

1653

Test Name: DEFENSE MECHANISM INVENTORY

Purpose: To assess the relative use of defense mechanisms including turning against object, projection, principalization, turning against self, and reversal (repression, denial, and reaction formation).

Number of Items: 40

Format: Four five-point questions concerning each of 10 stories related to conflict areas of independence, competition, authority, situational factors,

femininity, and masculinity.

Reliability: Test–retest reliabilities range from .61 (Projection) to .93 (Turning against object).

Author: Ross, J. M., and Johnson, R. W.

Article: Social-evaluation anxiety and defensive style.

Journal: *Psychological Reports,* June 1976, *38*(3), 1075–1078.

Related Research: Gleser, G., & Ihilevich, D. (1969). An objective instrument for measuring defense mechanisms. *Journal of Consulting and Clinical Psychology, 33*, 51–60.

■ ■ ■

1654

Test Name: DEPRESSION INVENTORY (Short Form)

Purpose: To diagnose and assess the extent of depression in psychiatric patients.

Number of Items: 13

Format: Self-report format by the patient; each item consists of four statements (graded in severity) from which the patient chooses.

Validity: Beck, A., & Bech, R. (1972) found that with clinician global rating, $r = .61$. In present study a number of different samples were used: correlations between the short and long form were .89, .96 (both $p < .01$); relationships with physician rating were .67, .55, .49, .56 (all $p < .01$).

Author: Beck, A., et al.

Article: Short form of depression inventory: Cross validation.

Journal: *Psychological Reports,* June 1974, *34*(3), 1184–1186.

Related Research: Beck, A. (1972). *Depression: Causes and treatment.* Philadelphia: University of Pennsylvania Press.

Beck, A. (1961). An inventory for measuring depression. *Archives of General Psychiatry, 4,* 561–571.

Beck, A., et al. (1973). Attempted suicide by males and females. *Psychological Reports, 33*(3), 965–966.

Lubin, B. (1967). *Manual for the Depression Adjective Checklist.* San Diego: Educational and Industrial Testing Services.

Martin, W. (1971). *Manual for the Martin S-D Inventory.* Jacksonville, IL: Psychologists and Educators Press.

■ ■ ■

1655

Test Name: DREAM INCIDENT TECHNIQUE

Purpose: To provide a systematic procedure for analyzing dreams.

Number of Items: 77

Format: Includes the following tasks: "reporting the dream, thinking of incidents that happened in one's past that are suggested by the dream, rating each incident on a checklist of items." Includes 12 scales: affection, achievement, dominance, autonomy, adventure, sex, aggression, exhibition, nurturance, play, infavoidance, guilt avoidance.

Reliability: Split-half reliability estimates ranged from .75 to .94 (n = 66).

Author: Robbins, P. R., and Tanck, R. H.

Article: The dream incident technique as a measure of unresolved problems.

Journal: *Journal of Personality Assessment,* December 1978, *42*(6), 583–591.

Related Research: Robbins, P. R. (1966). An approach to measuring psychological tensions by means of

dream associations. *Psychological Reports, 18,* 959–971.

■ ■ ■

1656

Test Name: EMOTIONAL ADJUSTMENT SCALE

Purpose: To assess degree to which terminally ill patients were coping [well] with their illness.

Number of Items: 6

Format: Completed by an observer (Chaplain); rated patient on six questions on a 1–3 scale.

Reliability: Interjudge reliability was .95.

Validity: Emotional adjustment was related to degree of physical comfort.

Author: Carey, R.

Article: Emotional adjustment in terminal patients: A quantitative approach.

Journal: *Journal of Counseling Psychology,* September 1974, *21*(5), 433–435.

■ ■ ■

1657

Test Name: EXISTENTIAL ANXIETY SCALE

Purpose: To assess feeling of lack of meaning in one's life.

Number of Items: 32

Format: True–false measuring of items are given in article.

Reliability: Kuder-Richardson formula 20 was .89 (subjects were undergraduates).

Validity: Nonsignificant difference between males and females. The correlation between this scale and need for achievement scores was −.45, which was in the predicted direction ($p < .001$).

Author: Good, L., and Good, K.

Article: A preliminary measure of existential anxiety.

Journal: *Psychological Reports,* 1974, *34*(1), 72–74.

■ ■ ■

1658

Test Name: FEAR OF SUCCESS QUESTIONNAIRE

Purpose: To measure the motive to avoid success.

Number of Items: 29

Format: True or false items.

Validity: Correlation of .23 ($p < .05$) between Fear of Success Questionnaire and a projective cue (Horner, 1968).

Author: Gibbons, P. A., and Kapelman, R. E.

Article: Maternal employment as a determinant of fear of success in females.

Journal: *Psychological Reports,* June 1977, *40*(3), 1200–1202.

Related Research: Good, L. R., & Good, K. C. (1973). An objective measure of the motive to avoid success. *Psychological Reports, 33,* 1009–1010.

Horner, M. S. (1968). *Sex differences in achievement motive and performance in competitive and non-competitive situations.* Unpublished doctoral dissertation, University of Michigan.

■ ■ ■

1659

Test Name: FEAR OF SUCCESS QUESTIONNAIRE

Purpose: To determine an individual's degree of fear of success.

Number of Items: 83

Format: Yes–no.

Reliability: Kuder-Richardson formula 20 reliability was .89.

Validity: Correlation between the Fear of Success Questionnaire and Debilitating Anxiety Scale was .57; Rotter Internal–External Scale was .24; Rosenberg Self-Esteem Scale was .47; and the Sarnoff Need to Fail Scale was .77.

Author: Konstam, V., and Gilbert, H. B.

Article: Fear of success, sex-role orientation, and performance in differing experimental conditions.

Journal: *Psychological Reports,* April 1978, *42*(2), 519–528.

Related Research: Griffore, R. J. (1977). Validation of three measures of fear of success. *Journal of Personality Assessment, 41*(4), 417–421.

■ ■ ■

1660

Test Name: FEAR OF SUCCESS SCALE

Purpose: To measure fear of success.

Number of Items: 27

Format: Subjects respond to each item by either agreeing or disagreeing. The items are considered indicative of fear of success.

Validity: Correlation with the Fear of Success Questionnaire was .299. Correlation with the Debilitating Anxiety Scale of the Alpert-Haber Achievement Anxiety Test was .43.

Author: Griffore, R. J.

Article: Validation of three measures of fear of success.

Journal: *Journal of Personality Assessment,* August 1977, *41*(4), 417–421.

Related Research: Zuckerman, M., and Allison, S. N. (1976). An objective measure of fear of success: Construction and validation. *Journal of Personality Assessment, 40*, 422–430.

1661

Test Name: HAPPINESS SCALE

Purpose: To measure one's perceived quality of general happiness, along with an estimate of the percentage of time generally spent in happy, unhappy, and neutral moods.

Number of Items: 1

Format: An 11-point happiness scale. Combination score comes from combining the scale score and the happy percentage estimate in equal weights.

Reliability: Test–retest reliability for the combination score was .86 over a 2-week interval and .67 over a 4-month interval.

Author: Fordyce, M. W.

Article: Development of a program to increase personal happiness.

Journal: *Journal of Counseling Psychology,* November 1977, *24*(6), 511–521.

Related Research: Wessman, A. E., & Ricks, D. F. (1966). *Moods and personality.* New York: Holt, Rinehart & Winston.

■ ■ ■

1662

Test Name: HOPELESSNESS SCALE

Purpose: To measure pessimism.

Number of Items: 20

Format: A true–false inventory which includes three factors: affective, motivational, and cognitive.

Validity: Pearson product-moment correlations with Edwards Social Desirability Scale were –.64 for men ($N = 32$) and –.62 for women ($N = 34$).

Author: Fogg, M. E., and Gayton, W. F.

Article: Social desirability and the hopelessness scale.

Journal: *Perceptual and Motor Skills,* October 1976, *43*(2), 482.

Related Research: Beck, A. T., et al. (1974). The measurement of pessimism: The Hopelessness Scale. *Journal of Consulting and Clinical Psychology, 42*, 861–865.

■ ■ ■

1663

Test Name: HOPKINS SYMPTOM CHECKLIST

Purpose: To describe and summarize patients' symptoms.

Number of Items: 58

Format: Self-report; five symptom dimensions: somatization, obsessive compulsive, interpersonal sensitivity, depression, and anxiety; items assigned to each dimension are given in the report.

Reliability: Descriptive item statistics are given in the report; alpha ranged .84 to .87; Test–retest ranged .75 to .84 (1 week); Interrater relability ranged .64 to .80.

Validity: Various construct and criterion related validity studies are reported.

Author: Derogatis, L., et al.

Article: The Hopkins Symptom Checklist (HSCL): A self-report symptom inventory.

Journal: *Behavioral Science,* January 1974, *19*(1), 1–15.

■ ■ ■

1664

Test Name: INDEX OF DEPRESSION

Purpose: To detect depression severe enough to warrant treatment.

Number of Items: 15

Format: Scales include Overt

Depression, Covert Depression, and Healthy.

Validity: Correlations with various scales (Harris & Lingoes, 1955; Wiggins, 1966) range from −.69 to .88.

Author: Rhodes, R. J.

Article: A further look at the Popoff Index of Depression.

Journal: *Psychological Reports,* February 1978, *42*(1), 309–310.

Related Research: Popoff, L. M. (1969). A simple method for diagnosis of depression by the family physician. *Clinical Medicine, 76,* 24–49.

Harris, R. E., & Lingoes, J. C. (1955). *Subscales for the MMPI: An aid to profile interpretation.* San Francisco: University of Southern California.

Wiggins, J. S. (1966). Substantive dimensions of self-report in the MMPI item pool. *Psychological Monographs, 80*(1, Whole No. 630).

■ ■ ■

1665

Test Name: IRRATIONAL BELIEFS TEST

Purpose: To measure irrational beliefs.

Number of Items: 100

Format: Includes 10 belief scales of 10 items each. Subjects respond to each item on a 5-point scale.

Reliability: Test–retest reliability coefficients ranged from .67 to .87 for scales and .92 for full-scale (24 hours). Test–retest reliability coefficients ranged from .48 to .95 for scales and .88 for full-scales (2 weeks).

Validity: Correlations with a 25-item self-report of maladjustment symptoms produced a multiple correlation of .72, and with 16PF

clinical scales, multiple correlations ranged from .43 to .63.

Author: Forman, B. D., and Forman, S. G.

Article: Irrational beliefs and psychological needs.

Journal: *Journal of Personality Assessment,* December 1979, *43*(6), 633–637.

Related Research: Jones, R. G. (1968). *A factored measure of Ellis irrational belief systems with personality and maladjustment correlates.* Unpublished doctoral dissertation, Texas Technological College.

Forman, B. D., & Forman, S. G. (1978). Irrational beliefs and personality. *Journal of Personality Assessment, 42*(6), 613–620.

■ ■ ■

1666

Test Name: JOB-INDUCED ANXIETY MEASURE

Purpose: To assess the existence of tensions and pressures stemming from job requirements.

Number of Items: 7

Format: Subjects respond on a 5-point Likert scale from *strongly agree* to *strongly disagree.* All items are presented.

Reliability: Coefficient alpha was .84.

Author: Fry, L. W., and Greenfeld, S.

Article: An examination of attitudinal differences between policewomen and policemen.

Related Research: House, R. J., & Rizzo, J. R. (1972). Role conflict and ambiguity as critical variables in a model of organizational behavior. *Organizational Behavior and Human Performance, 7,* 467–505.

1667

Test Name: JOB RELATED TENSION INDEX

Purpose: To identify sources of role strain encountered by employees on the job.

Number of Items: 15

Format: Includes four facets of role strain: direct conflicts, job overload, ambiguity, exerting influences without authority. A 5-point Likert scale is used.

Reliability: Coefficient alpha reliabilities ranged from .75 to .83.

Validity: Correlations with a variety of variables ranged from −.39 to .20.

Author: Ivancevich, J. M.

Article: A longitudinal study of behavioral expectation scales: Attitudes and performance.

Journal: *Journal of Applied Psychology,* April 1980, *65*(2), 139–146.

Related Research: MacKinnon, N. J. (1978). Role strain: An assessment of a measure and its invariance of factor structure across studies. *Journal of Applied Psychology, 63,* 321–328.

■ ■ ■

1668

Test Name: LOYOLA SENTENCE COMPLETION BLANK FOR CLERGYMEN

Purpose: To measure adjustment among American Catholic priests.

Number of Items: 72

Format: Includes six areas of adjustment: self, interpersonal relations, psychosexual maturity, church-faith-religion, priesthood, and job satisfaction.

Reliability: Interscorer reliability was .96 for total score.

Validity: Correlations with the

Personal Orientation Inventory ranged from −.18 to −.36 for the subscales with the total score of the LSCBC.

Author: Murphy, T. J.

Article: The relationship between self-actualization and adjustment among American Catholic priests.

Journal: *Educational and Psychological Measurement,* Summer 1980, *40*(2), 457–461.

Related Research: Sheehan, M. A. (1971). *The Loyola Sentence Completion Blank for Clergymen: Construction and validation.* Unpublished master's thesis, Loyola University of Chicago.

■ ■ ■

1669

Test Name: MOOD QUESTIONNAIRE (Shortened version)

Purpose: To assess psychological moods such as anger, happiness, and so forth.

Number of Items: 40

Format: Three choices for response: *not at all* to *mostly or generally.*

Reliability: Test–retest for 3 days to 7-week intervals: Happiness, .55 to .31; Activity, .55 to .37; Depression, .56 to .37; Anger, .56 to .40; Fatigue, .60 to .36.

Validity: With Fear with State Anxiety, $r = .80$ ($p < .05$); with Trait Anxiety, $r = .55$ ($p < .01$). Happiness and Activity Scales correlated with success in a physical training course .40 and .36, both significant.

Author: Ryman, D., et al.

Article: Reliabilities and validities of the Mood Questionnaire.

Journal: *Psychological Reports,* August 1974, *35*(1), 479–484.

Related Research: Nowlis, V. (1965). Research with Mood

Adjective Checklist. In S. S. Tomkins & C. Izard (Eds.), *Affect, cognition and personality* (pp. 352–389). New York: Springer.

■ ■ ■

1670

Test Name: MULTISCORE DEPRESSION INVENTORY

Purpose: To provide a measure of depression.

Number of Items: 118

Format: Includes 10 subscales: sad mood, fatigue, learned helplessness, social introversion, irritability, institutional helplessness, pessimism, low self-esteem, cognitive difficulty, and guilt.

Reliability: Kuder-Richardson reliability was .96 ($N = 200$). Scale reliabilities ranged from .79 to .91.

Validity: Correlation with Beck's Depression Inventory was .69, and with Depression Adjective Checklist was .77.

Author: Berndt, D. J., et al.

Article: Development and initial evaluation of a multiscore depression inventory.

Journal: *Journal of Personality Assessment,* August 1980, *44*(4), 396–403.

Related Research: Berndt, D. J. (1979). *Construction of a multiscore measure of depressive moods and symptoms.* Unpublished master's thesis, Loyola University.

■ ■ ■

1671

Test Name: NEUROPSYCHIATRIC HOSPITAL SUICIDE POTENTIAL SCALE

Purpose: To provide a schedule for prediction of potentiality for

committed suicide among hospitalized neuropsychiatric patients at the time of release from the hospital.

Number of Items: 11

Format: Includes cut-off points high, moderately high, moderately low, and low levels of suicide risk.

Validity: Accuracy of prediction of the high risk group was 95.2%, accuracy of predictions of low risk (controls or nonsuicides) was 80.0%, predictions of the moderately high and moderately low suicide risk groups were 78.6 and 77.1%, respectively. Overall accuracy of the scale was 81.7% (based on weighted percentages scores).

Author: Farberow, N. L., and MacKinnon, D.

Article: Prediction of suicide: A replication study.

Journal: *Journal of Personality Assessment,* October 1975, *39*(5), 497–506.

Related Research: Farberow, N. L., & MacKinnon, D. (1974). A suicide prediction schedule for neuropsychiatric hospital patients. *Journal of Nervous and Mental Disease, 6,* 408–419.

■ ■ ■

1672

Test Name: OCS STRESS REACTION SCALE

Purpose: To identify reaction to stress by officer candidates.

Number of Items: 7

Format: A semiprojective test whereby the candidate is asked to put himself in a situation, numerically rate his emotional reaction, describe what he would do about the situation, and predict the outcome of the situation. Answers are scored for coping failure, solution inadequacy, and unfavorability of the predicted outcomes. Scores from 1 to 5 are assigned, with higher scores indicating greater stress.

Reliability: Interjudge correlations ranged from .75 to .77.

Author: Jennings, J. R., et al.

Article: Stress and performance during and after officer candidate school.

Journal: *Journal of Applied Psychology,* August 1974, *59*(4), 500–503.

Related Research: Goldfried, M. R., & D'Zurilla, T. J. (1969). A behavioranalytic model for assessing competence. In C. D. Spielberger (Ed.), *Current topics in clinical and community psychology.* New York: Academic Press.

■ ■ ■

1673

Test Name: OCS STRESS REACTION SCALE

Purpose: To identify reaction to stress by officer candidates.

Number of Items: 7

Format: A semiprojective test whereby the candidate is asked to put him or herself in a situation, numerically rate his or her emotional reaction, describe what he or she would do about the situation, and predict the outcome of the situation. Answers are scored for coping failure, solution inadequacy, and unfavorability of the predicted outcomes. Scores from 1 to 5 are assigned, with higher scores indicating greater stress.

Reliability: Interjudge correlations ranged from .75 to .77.

Author: Jennings, J. R., et al.

Article: Stress and performance during and after officer candidate school.

Journal: *Journal of Applied Psychology,* August 1974, *59*(4), 500–503.

Related Research: Goldfried, M. R., & D'Zurilla, T. J. (1964). A behavior analytic model for assessing competence. In C. D. Spielberger (Ed.), *Current topics in clinical and community psychology.* New York: Academic Press.

■ ■ ■

1674

Test Name: ONTARIO PROBLEM ASSESSMENT BATTERY

Purpose: To provide an identification of specific problems within several relevant life areas of alcoholics.

Format: Response categories are *not true, slightly true, moderately true, mostly true,* and *completely true.*

Reliability: Split-half reliability indices are typically above .75.

Author: Freedberg, E. J., and Scherer, S. E.

Article: The Ontario Problem Assessment Battery for Alcoholics.

Journal: *Psychological Reports,* June 1977, *40*(3), 743–746.

Related Research: Scherer, S. E., & Freedberg, E. J. (1976). Effects of group videotape feedback on development of assertiveness skills in alcoholics: A follow-up study. *Psychological Reports, 39,* 983–992.

■ ■ ■

1675

Test Name: PICTURE-FRUSTRATION STUDY

Purpose: To assess reactions to frustration by means of a limited projective procedure.

Number of Items: 24

Format: Each item is a cartoon-like picture depicting two persons involved in a mildly frustrating situation of common occurrence.

Reliability: Adult Form, test–retest correlations ($N = 105$) ranged from .45 to .73 for 4-month interval: test–retest correlations ($N = 59$) ranged from .34 to .68 for 4-month interval. Adolescent Form, test–retest correlations ($N = 16$) ranged from .30 to .86 for 1-month interval. Children's Form, test–retest correlations ($N = 45$) ranged from .18 to .55 for 10-month interval: test–retest correlations ($N = 50$) ranged from .56 to .78 for 2.5-month interval.

Author: Rosenzweig, S., et al.

Article: Retest reliability of the Rosenzweig Picture-Frustration Study and similar semiprojective techniques.

Journal: *Journal of Personality Assessment,* February 1975, *39*(1), 3–12.

Related Research: Rosenzweig, S. (1945). The picture-association method and its application in a study of reactions frustration. *Journal of Personality, 14,* 3–23.

■ ■ ■

1676

Test Name: PRELIMINARY FEAR OF SUCCESS SCALE

Purpose: To measure one's fear of success.

Number of Items: 29

Format: True or False.

Validity: Correlates with self-concept ($r = .43, p < .05$) and anxiety ($r = .72, p < .01$).

Author: Reviere, R., and Posey, T. B.

Article: Correlates of two measures of fear of success in women.

Journal: *Psychological Reports,* April 1978, *42*(2), 609–610.

Related Research: Good, L. R., & Good, K. C. (1973). An objective measure of the motive to avoid success. *Psychological Reports, 33,* 1009–1010.

■ ■ ■

1677

Test Name: PSYCHIATRIC SYMPTOM INDEX

Purpose: To assess one's level of stress and ability to cope.

Number of Items: 29

Format: Subjects indicate how often they experienced psychiatric symptoms during the past week from *never* to *once in a while* to *fairly often* to *very often.*

Reliability: Interval consistency alpha coefficients: Psychiatric Symptom Index, .91; Depression, .84; Anxiety, .85; Cognitive Disturbance, .77; Anger, .79.

Validity: Respondents with high scores tended to visit professionals more recently than those with low scores (chi-square test, $p < .01$).

Author: Ilfied, F. W., Jr.

Article: Further validation of a psychiatric symptom index in a normal population.

Journal: *Psychological Reports,* December 1976, *39*(3), 1215–1228.

Related Research: Parloff, M., et al. (1954). Comfort, effectiveness and self-awareness as criteria of improvement of psychotherapy. *American Journal of Psychiatry, 111,* 343–351.

■ ■ ■

1678

Test Name: Q SORT ADJUSTMENT SCALE

Purpose: To measure degree of adjustment.

Number of Items: 95

Format: Q Sort procedure.

Validity: Prisoners classified as high and low self-actualized were significantly different in adjustment.

Author: Mattocks, A., and Jew, C.

Article: Comparison of self-actualization levels and adjustment scores of incarcerated male felons.

Journal: *Educational and Psychological Measurement,* Spring 1974, *34*(1), 69–74.

Related Research: Dymond, R. (1954). Adjustment changes over therapy from self sorts. In C. Rogers, & R. Dymond (Eds.), *Psychotherapy and personality change.* University of Chicago Press.

■ ■ ■

1679

Test Name: RATIONAL BEHAVIOR INVENTORY

Purpose: To provide an overall index of rationality.

Number of Items: 37

Format: Guttman-type scale with subtest scores for 11 factors.

Validity: Pearson coefficient between scores on this test and the Irrational Belief Test (Jones, 1968) was $-.72$ ($p < .001$).

Author: Ray, J. B., and Bak, J. S.

Article: Comparison and cross-validation of the Irrational Belief Test and the Rational Behavior Inventory.

Journal: *Psychological Reports,* April 1980, *46*(2), 541–542.

Related Research: Jones, R. G. (1968). *A factored measure of Ellis' irrational belief system with personality and maladjustment correlates.* Unpublished doctoral dissertation, Texas Tech University.

Shorkey, C. T., & Whiteman, V. L. (1977). Development of the

Rational Behavior Inventory: Initial validity and reliability. *Educational and Psychological Measurement, 37,* 527–534.

■ ■ ■

1680

Test Name: SCHOOL ADMINISTRATOR MORALE MEASURE: III

Purpose: To measure the morale of elementary school principals.

Number of Items: 48

Format: Includes six dimensions of morale: School board operations, superordinate relations, remuneration, community position, security, and peer relations.

Reliability: Kuder-Richardson formula 20 test–retest reliability coefficient was .90.

Author: Nasstrom, R. R., et al.

Article: School board dogmatism and the morale of principals.

Journal: *California Journal of Educational Research,* March 1975, *26*(2), 107–113.

Related Research: Kline, C. E., & Thomas W. (1973). Middle administrator/school board relationships in collective negotiations. *Journal of Collective Negotiations in the Public Sector, 3*(1), 49–55.

■ ■ ■

1681

Test Name: SCL-90

Purpose: To measure psychopathology in medical and psychiatric outpatients.

Number of Items: 90

Format: A self-report symptom inventory containing the following dimensions: somatization, obsessive-compulsive, interpersonal sensitivity, depression, anxiety, hostility, phobic anxiety, paranoid ideation, and psychoticism.

Reliability: Internal reliability coefficients ranged from .77 to .90 (N = 565 psychiatric outpatients).

Validity: Dimensions of the SCL-90 with subscales of the MMPI ranged from −.44 to .60; the Beck Depression Inventory ranged from .46 to .70; the State-Trait Anxiety Inventory ranged from .36 to .69; the Whitaker Index of Schizophrenic Thinking ranged from −.16 to .03.

Author: Dinning, W. D., and Evans, R. G.

Article: Discriminant and convergent validity of the SCL-90 in psychiatric inpatients.

Journal: *Journal of Personality Assessment*, June 1977, *41*(3),304–310.

Related Research: Derogatis, L. R., et al. (1973). The SCL-90, An outpatient psychiatric rating scale. *Psychopharmacology Bulletin, 9,* 13–28.

■ ■ ■

1682

Test Name: SELF-RATING ANXIETY SCALE

Purpose: To measure state anxiety.

Number of Items: 20

Format: Subjects rate each of the items as it applies to them within the past week using a 4-point scale: *none or a little of the time; some of the time; good part of the time; most or all of the time.*

Reliability: Item correlations ranged from −.07 to .51 for normal subjects and −.20 to .57 for psychiatric patients.

Author: Jegede, R. O.

Article: Psychometric attributes of the Self-Rating Anxiety Scale.

Journal: *Psychological Reports,*

February 1977, *40*(1), 303–306.

Related Research: Zung, W. W. K. (1971). A rating instrument for anxiety disorders. *Psychosomatics, 12,* 371–379.

■ ■ ■

1683

Test Name: SITUATIONS INVENTORY

Purpose: To "determine the degree of nervousness felt in a variety of situations."

Number of Items: 73

Format: Subject indicates on a 1–5 scale how he or she feels in each situation.

Validity: Three factors: social, physical, and disorder: correlations of factors with 7 personality measures are given.

Author: Strahan, R.

Article: Situational dimensions of self-reported nervousness.

Journal: *Journal of Personality Assessment*, August 1974, *38*(4), 341–352.

Related Research: Endler, N., et al. (1962). An S-R inventory of anxiousness. *Psychological Monographs, 76*(17).

■ ■ ■

1684

Test Name: SROLE ANOMIE SCALE

Purpose: To measure one's sense of despair and hopelessness.

Number of Items: 5

Format: Likert-type items. All are presented.

Reliability: Cronbach's alpha was .44.

Author: Kapsis, R. E.

Article: Black ghetto diversity and anomie: A sociopolitical view.

Journal: *American Journal of*

Sociology, March 1978, *83*(5), 1132–1153.

Related Research: Srole, L. (1956). Social integration and certain corollaries: An exploration study. *American Sociological Review, 21,* 706–716.

■ ■ ■

1685

Test Name: SROLE ANOMIA SCALE

Purpose: To measure anomia.

Number of Items: 5

Format: A Guttman scale.

Reliability: Coefficient of reproducibility was .90.

Validity: Correlations with the Rational Behavior Inventory ranged from .04 to = −.33 (N = 180).

Author: Whiteman, V. L., and Shorkey, C. T.

Article: Validation testing of the Rational Behavior Inventory.

Journal: *Educational and Psychological Measurement,* Winter 1978, *38*(4), 1143–1149.

Related Research: Robinson, J. P., & Shaver, P. R. (1969). *Measures of social psychological attitudes.* Ann Arbor, MI: The University of Michigan, Institute for Social Research.

■ ■ ■

1686

Test Name: STRAIN MEASURE

Purpose: To measure occupational strain, including anxiety-depression-irritation, psychosomatic symptoms and work satisfaction (amount, interest, and boredom of work).

Number of Items: 35

Format:
Anxiety-depression-irritation scale: 19 items with four anchored

responses; 10 psychosomatic symptoms; work satisfaction: six-item scale using five anchored responses.

Reliability: Reliabilities (coefficient alpha) ranged from .61 to .77.

Author: Gavin, J. F., and Axelrod, W. L.

Article: Managerial stress and strain in a mining organization.

Journal: *Journal of Vocational Behavior,* August 1977, *11*(1), 66–74.

Related Research: Caplan, R. D., et al. (1975). *Job demands and worker health: Main effects and occupational differences.* (Report to the National Institute for Occupational Safety and Health, HEW Publication No. NIOSH 75–160). Washington, DC: Government Printing Office.

■ ■ ■

1687

Test Name: STRESS MEASURE

Purpose: To measure one's stress in the workplace, including such factors as role conflict, role ambiguity, responsibility for others, job security, quantitative workload, participation, job pressure, variation in work load, and utilization of skills.

Number of Items: 36

Format: For all measures except role conflict and variation in workload, items were five-point anchored scales. Role conflict and variation in workload had four-point anchored scales.

Reliability: Reliabilities coefficient alpha) ranged from .20 to .86.

Author: Gavin, J. F., and Axelrod, W. L.

Article: Managerial stress and strain in a mining organization.

Journal: *Journal of Vocational*

Behavior, August 1977, *11*(1), 66–74.

Related Research: Kahn, R. L., et al. (1964). *Organizational stress: Studies in role conflict and ambiguity.* New York: Wiley.

■ ■ ■

1688

Test Name: SUICIDAL INTENT SCALE

Purpose: To assess seriousness of suicide attempt.

Number of Items: 15

Format: Items 1–8 deal with circumstances of an attempt (suicide note, etc.); 9–15 deal with subject's intentions and expectations; observer scores items on 0–2 scale: maximum total score was 30.

Reliability: Interrater reliability was .91.

Validity: Completed suicides had significantly ($p < .001$) higher scores than attempters.

Author: Beck, R., et al.

Article: Cross validation of the suicidal intent scale.

Journal: *Psychological Reports,* April 1974, *34*(2), 445–446.

Related Research: Beck, A., et al. (1973). Development of suicidal intent scales. In A. T. Beck et al. (Eds.), *Measurement of suicidal behaviors.* New York: Charles Press.

■ ■ ■

1689

Test Name: SYMPTOM CHECKLIST

Purpose: To determine one's need for counseling.

Number of Items: 52

Format: Psychiatric symptoms translated into layman's language which the respondent checks if the

symptom applies to her or him.

Reliability: Immediate and delayed reliabilities in the .70s (Van Atta, 1975).

Author: Van Atta, R. E., et al.

Article: Psychological discomfort and its causal attribution in relation to student services program development.

Journal: *Journal of College Student Personnel,* September 1977, *18*(5), 371–375.

Related Research: Van Atta, R. (1975, August). *Epidemiological data as a factor for system change.* Paper presented at the annual convention of the American Psychological Association, Chicago.

■ ■ ■

1690

Test Name: TENSION INDEX

Purpose: To identify sources of tension.

Number of Items: 10

Format: All items are presented.

Reliability: Alpha coefficient was .73.

Author: O'Connell, M. J., et al.

Article: The effects of environmental information and decision unit structure on felt tension.

Journal: *Journal of Applied Psychology,* August 1976, *61*(4), 493–500.

Related Research: Kahn, R. L., et al. *Organizational stress: Studies in role conflict and ambiguity.* New York: Wiley, 1964.

■ ■ ■

1691

Test Name: THREAT INDEX

Purpose: A measure of death threat.

Number of Items: 40 bipolar constructs

Format: Subject records which pole of each bipolar construct applies to self, ideal self and "your own death."

Reliability: Hays (1974) reported a test–retest reliability of .84.

Author: Eckstein, D., and Tobacyk, J.

Article: Ordinal position and death concerns.

Journal: *Psychological Reports*, June 1979, *44*(3), 967–971.

Related Research: Hays, C. (1974). *A methodological investigation of the threat index and an introduction of a short form.* Unpublished senior thesis, University of Florida.

■ ■ ■

1692

Test Name: WAKEFIELD SELF-ASSESSMENT DEPRESSION INVENTORY

Purpose: To measure one's sense of depression.

Number of Items: 12

Format: Items are given and are scored on a 4-point scale and summed to produce a total depression score.

Validity: Correlates .87 with the Hamilton Psychiatric Rating Scale for Depression.

Author: Raymond, E. F., et al.

Article: Prevalence of correlates of depression in elderly persons.

Journal: *Psychological Reports*, December 1980, *47*(3), 1055–1061.

Related Research: Snaith, R. P., et al. (1971). Assessment of the severity of primary depressive illness. *Psychological Medicine, 1,* 143–149.

■ ■ ■

1693

Test Name: WIDOWED ADJUSTMENT SCALE

Purpose: To measure the adjustment-depression of widows and widowers.

Number of Items: 8

Format: Yes–no responses.

Reliability: Internal consistency was .86 using the Kuder-Richardson formula 20 test.

Author: Carey, R. G.

Article: The widowed: A year later.

Journal: *Journal of Counseling Psychology*, March 1977, *24*(2), 125–131.

Related Research: Bornstein, P. E., and Clayton, P. J. (1972). The anniversary reaction. *Diseases of the Nervous System, 33,* 470–471.

■ ■ ■

1694

Test Name: WORRY-EMOTIONALITY SCALE

Purpose: To measure affect under evaluative stress.

Number of Items: 10

Format: Items are rated on a Likert scale to yield (a) a worry score measuring cognitive concern and distraction, (b) an emotionality score assessing self-perceived physiological arousal, and (c) a state test anxiety score composed of the sum of the worry and emotionality scores.

Reliability: Alpha coefficients range from .79 to .88 for worry and emotionality scores (Morris & Fullmer, 1976).

Author: Deffenbacher, J. L., et al.

Article: Comparison of anxiety management training and self-control desensitization.

Journal: *Journal of Counseling Psychology*, March 1980, *27*(2), 232–239.

Related Research: Liebert, R. M., & Morris, L. W. (1967). Cognitive and emotional components of test anxiety: A distinction and some initial data. *Psychological Reports, 20,* 975–978.

Morris, L. W., & Fullmer, R. S. (1976). Test anxiety (worry and emotionality) changes during academic testing as a function of feedback and test importance. *Journal of Educational Psychology, 68,* 817–824.

CHAPTER 4
Adjustment—Social

1695

Test Name: A CLASS PLAY

Purpose: To make a sociometric analysis of students.

Number of Items: 12

Format: Child indicates which student in the class best fits a given positive or negative role as described by the teacher.

Reliability: Test–retest reliability for 108 children was reported to be .92.

Author: Vace, N. A., and Rajpal, P. L.

Article: Comparison of social positions of school children in India and the United States.

Journal: *Psychological Reports,* August 1975, *37*(1), 208–210.

Related Research: Bower, E. M. (1960). *Early identification of emotionally handicapped children in school.* Springfield: Thomas.

. . .

1696

Test Name: ACCULTURATION MEASURE

Purpose: To provide a quantitative measure of acculturation for Chicano adolescents.

Number of Items: 78

Format: Four concepts (mother, father, male, and female) are rated on 18 items covering background information and on 15 pairs of bipolar adjectives that are highly loaded on a potency dimension.

Reliability: Test–retest reliability

coefficients were .84 for a total sample of 129 Chicano and Anglo junior college students in three Southern California communities over 3 weeks, .89 for Chicanos and .66 for Anglos.

Author: Olmedo, E. L., et al.

Article: Measure of acculturation for Chicano adolescents.

Journal: *Psychological Reports,* February 1978, *42*(1), 159–170.

Related Research: Martinez, J. L. Jr., et al. (1976). A comparison of Chicano and Anglo high school students using the semantic differential technique. *Journal of Cross-Cultural Psychology, 7,* 325–334.

. . .

1697

Test Name: AFFILIATIVE TENDENCY

Purpose: To measure social skills conducive to positive and comfortable social exchanges.

Number of Items: 26

Format: Half of the items are negatively worded and half are positively worded. Subjects respond using a 9-point scale ranging from –4 (*very strong disagreement*) to +14 (*very strong agreement*).

Reliability: Kuder-Richardson internal reliability correlation coefficient was .80; 4-week test–retest of one sample of 108 subjects yielded a product–moment correlation coefficient of .89.

Author: Mehrabian, A.

Article: Questionnaire measures of affiliative tendency and sensitivity to rejection.

Source: *Psychological Reports,* February 1976, *38*(1), 199–209.

Related Research: Mehrabian, A., & Epstein, N. (1972). A measure of emotional empathy. *Journal of Personality, 40,* 525–543.

. . .

1698

Test Name: ALIENATION AND DRUG USE QUESTIONNAIRE

Purpose: To measure feelings of frustration with society's goals and norm expectations, as well as its dominance over the future of the individual, and the drug use habits of students and their peers.

Number of Items: 48

Format: Subjects rate each of 24 items (Dean Alienation Scale) on a 5-point scale, yielding three subscales: powerlessness, normlessness, and social isolation. Subjects indicate which drugs they use (Drug Use Scale) and the frequency of use.

Reliability: Reliability coefficient was .78 for the Dean Alienation Scale based on the split-half method corrected by the Spearman-Brown Prophecy formula.

Author: Holtman, A. M., et al.

Article: Alienation and drug use among college students.

Journal: *Journal of College Student Personnel,* July 1975, *16*(4), 277–281.

Related Research: Dean, D. G.

(1961). Alienation: Its meaning and measurement. *American Sociological Review, 26,* 753–758.

Swisher, J. D., & Crawford, J. L. (1971). An evaluation of a short-term drug education program. *School Counselor, 18,* 265–272.

■ ■ ■

1699

Test Name: ALIENATION SCALE

Purpose: To assess feelings of isolation.

Number of Items: 16

Format: Items are rated on 5-point Likert scales.

Reliability: .80 (design not specified).

Author: Abramowitz, S., and Jackson, C.

Article: Comparative effectiveness of there-and-then versus here-and-now therapist interpretations in group psychotherapy.

Journal: *Journal of Counseling Psychology,* July 1974, *21*(4), 288–293.

Related Research: Jessor, R., et al. (1968). *Society, personality, and deviant behavior: A study of a tri-ethnic community.* New York: Holt, Rinehart & Winston.

■ ■ ■

1700

Test Name: ALIENATION SCALES

Purpose: To measure several facets of consumer alienation.

Number of Items: 18

Format: Includes powerlessness, meaninglessness, normlessness, and cultural estrangement.

Reliability: Internal consistency for each of the four scales ranged from .42 to .76.

Validity: Correlations with cognitive differentiation ranged from –.27 to –.34.

Author: Durand, R. M., and Lambert, Z. V.

Article: Cognitive differentiation and alienation of consumers.

Journal: *Perceptual and Motor Skills,* August 1979, *49*(1), 99–108.

■ ■ ■

1701

Test Name: ALIENATION SCALES

Purpose: To measure different types of alienation.

Number of Items: 16

Format: Includes four types of alienation: Powerlessness, self-estrangement, normlessness, and cultural estrangement.

Reliability: Reproducibilities are in the .90s.

Author: Kohn, M. L.

Article: Occupational structure and alienation.

Journal: *American Journal of Sociology,* July 1976, *82*(1), 111–130.

Related Research: Bonjean, C. M., et al. (1967). *Sociological measurement: An inventory of scales and indices.* San Francisco: Chandler.

■ ■ ■

1702

Test Name: ASSERTION SCALE

Purpose: To measure difficulty in expressing personal rights and feelings in a socially acceptable way.

Format: Consists of an under-assertion scale and an over-assertion scale.

Reliability: Split-half reliabilities are above .75.

Validity: Correlations with the Rathus Assertiveness Schedule were generally significant beyond the .02 level.

Author: Scherer, S. E., and Freedberg, E. J.

Article: Effects of group videotape feedback on development of assertiveness skills in alcoholics: A follow-up study.

Journal: *Psychological Reports,* December 1976, *39*(3), 983–992.

Related Research: Freedberg, E. J., & Scherer, S. E. (1976). *Brief schedules for assessing underassertiveness and overassertiveness* (Substudy 760). Toronto, Ontario, Canada: Addiction Research Foundation.

■ ■ ■

1703

Test Name: AVOIDANCE OF THE ONTOLOGICAL CONFRONTATION OF LONELINESS SCALE

Purpose: To identify one's choice of avoidance versus confrontation strategy relative to loneliness.

Number of Items: 20

Format: Subjects respond to each item as either *true for me* or *false for me.*

Reliability: Kuder-Richardson formula 20 correlational coefficient was .81 ($N = 333$). Split-half coefficient corrected for test length was .78.

Validity: Several items on personal cognitions and behaviors relevant to loneliness produced coefficients ranging from .17 to .47.

Author: Thauberger, P. C., and Cleland, J. F.

Article: Avoidance of ontological confrontation of loneliness and some epidemiological indices of social behavior and health.

Journal: *Perceptual and Motor*

Skills, June 1979, *48*(3, Part 2), 1219–1224.

• • •

1704

Test Name: BLECHER EXTENDED LONELINESS SCALE

Purpose: To measure loneliness.

Number of Items: 60

Format: Subjects indicate how often the statements are true of them along a 6-point continuum from 1 (*rarely or almost never true*) to 6 (*true all of the time*).

Reliability: Coefficient alpha was .90 for the 35-item general loneliness scale, .84 for the 19-item alienation scale, and .57 for the 5-item anomie scale. The internal consistency for the total scale is .93.

Author: Solano, C. H.

Article: Two measures of loneliness: A comparison.

Journal: *Psychological Reports,* February 1980, *46*(1), 23–28.

Related Research: Belcher, M. (1973). *The measurement of loneliness: A validation study of the Belcher Extended Loneliness Scale* (BELS). Doctoral dissertation, Illinois Institute of Technology. (University Microfilms No. 74–16, 990)

• • •

1705

Test Name: BRADLEY LONELINESS SCALE

Purpose: To measure the feeling of loneliness.

Number of Items: 38

Reliability: Split-half reliability correlation coefficient was .90. Test–retest reliability coefficient was .82 (1 week interval, *N*= 20).

Validity: Correlation with

MMPI-depression scale was .37. Correlation with Profile of Mood States ranged from –.34 to .71 (*N* = 250).

Author: Loucks, S.

Article: Loneliness, affect, and self-concept: Construct validity of the Bradley Loneliness Scale.

Journal: *Journal of Personality Assessment,* April 1980, *44*(2), 142–147.

Related Research: Bradley, R. (1969). *Measuring loneliness.* Ann Arbor, MI: Washington State University. University Microfilms.

• • •

1706

Test Name: C-SCALE

Purpose: To measure a generally trusting attitude and sense of positive affiliation toward others.

Number of Items: 8

Format: Each item consists of paired alternatives. The subject chooses one of five responses to each pair indicating degree of agreement between A or B as *entirely preferred, somewhat preferred,* or *cannot choose.* All items of the "connectedness" scale are presented.

Reliability: Pretest Hoyt reliability coefficient of .51; posttest Hoyt reliability coefficient of .59.

Author: Shapiro, S. B., and Shiflett, J. M.

Article: Loss of connectedness during an elementary teacher training program.

Journal: *Journal of Educational Research,* December 1974, *68*(4), 144–148.

Related Research: Robinson, J. P., & Shaver, P. R. (1969). *Measures of social psychological attitudes.* Ann Arbor, MI: Institute for Social Research.

1707

Test Name: CHICAGO ACTIVITY INVENTORY

Purpose: To measure the extent to which an individual reports that he or she can and does interact with the environment.

Number of Items: 35

Format: Includes topics such as physical mobility and intimate social contact.

Reliability: Test–retest reliability of .91.

Validity: Correlations with other activity inventories, external checklists, behavior ratings, and the like average around .65.

Author: Harris, J. E., and Bodden, J. L.

Article: An activity group experience for disengaged elderly persons.

Journal: *Journal of Counseling Psychology,* July 1978, *25*(4), 325–330.

Related Research: Cavin, R. S., et al. (1949). *Personal adjustment in old age.* Chicago: Science Research Associates.

• • •

1708

Test Name: CHILDREN'S SOCIAL DESIRABILITY QUESTIONNAIRE

Purpose: To measure the tendency of children in grades three, four, and five to respond in a socially desirable manner.

Number of Items: 47

Format: Direct questions to which participants must respond either *yes* or *no.*

Reliability: Split-half reliabilities for samples at the third, fourth, and fifth grade levels ranged from .69 to .90. Test–retest reliability of 63 children over 1 month was .90.

Author: Cowan, R., et al.

Article: A validity study of selected self-concept instruments.

Journal: *Measurement and Evaluation in Guidance,* January 1978, *10*(4), 211–221.

Related Research: Brannigan, G. (1974). Comparison of yes–no and true–false forms of the children's social desirability scale. *Psychological Reports, 34*(3), 898.

Crandall, V., et al. (1965). A children's social desirability questionnaire. *Journal of Consulting Psychology, 29,* 27–36.

■ ■ ■

1709

Test Name: DEAN'S ALIENATION SCALE

Purpose: To measure one's sense of powerlessness, normlessness, and social isolation.

Number of Items: 24

Format: Items rated on Likert scales.

Reliability: Test–retest over a 7-week period: item reliabilities range from .26 to above .50, subscales vary from .64 to .74, and the total scale is .80.

Validity: Relation of factors indicate lack of correspondence with powerlessness, normlessness, and social isolation using a cut-off point of .60.

Author: Hensley, D. R., et al.

Article: Factor structure of Dean's Alienation Scale among college students.

Journal: *Psychological Reports,* October 1975, *37*(2), 555–561.

Related Research: Dodder, R. A. (1969). A factor analysis of Dean's Alienation scale. *Social Forces, 48,* 252–255.

See *DUEMM, 2,* 1978, 437.

1710

Test Name: GROSS COHESION SCALE

Purpose: To measure group cohesion.

Number of Items: 7

Format: A unidimensional cumulative index of cohesion.

Validity: Schutz (1970) reported a rank order correlation of .31 ($p <$ .05) between the Gross scale and a related measure of cohesion.

Author: Evensen, E. D., and Bednar, R. L.

Article: Effects of specific cognitive and behavioral structure on early group behavior and atmosphere.

Journal: *Journal of Counseling Psychology,* January 1978, *25*(1), 66–75.

Related Research: Schutz, W. C. (1970). *The interpersonal underworld.* Cupertino, CA: Science & Behavior Books.

■ ■ ■

1711

Test Name: GROUP COHESION MEASURE

Purpose: To measure within-group harmony and interpersonal attraction.

Number of Items: 9

Format: A semantic differential containing bipolar adjective pairs. Examples are presented.

Reliability: .87.

Validity: Correlations with a variety of variables ranged from −.22 to .64.

Author: Greene, C. N., and Schriesheim, C. A.

Article: Leader-group interactions: A longitudinal field investigation.

Journal: *Journal of Applied*

Psychology, February 1980, *65*(1), 50–59.

Related Research: Scott, W. E. (1967). The development of semantic differential scales as measures of "morale." *Personnel Psychology, 20,* 179–188.

■ ■ ■

1712

Test Name: GROUP COHESIVENESS SCALE

Purpose: To measure group cohesiveness, or group attractiveness.

Number of Items: 19

Format: Items rated on 5-point Likert scales.

Reliability: Kuder-Richardson formula 20 reliability coefficient was .99.

Validity: There was a correlation of cohesiveness scores with scores on an instrument developed by Aram, Morgan, and Esbeck (1971).

Author: Dailey, R. C.

Article: Relationship between locus of control, perceived group cohesiveness and satisfaction with workers.

Journal: *Psychological Reports,* February 1978, *42*(1), 311–316.

Related Research: Aram, J., et al. (1971). Relationship of collaborative interpersonal relationships to individual satisfaction and organizational performance. *Administrative Science Quarterly, 16,* 289–296.

■ ■ ■

1713

Test Name: GUESS WHO

Purpose: To provide an instrument for sociometric nominations.

Number of Items: 29

Format: The child responds to each item by writing the name of a classmate. All items are presented.

Reliability: Alpha coefficients of internal consistency ranged from .83 to .93.

Validity: Correlations with a self-report instrument and with a teacher rating scale produced correlations ranging from –.50 to .59.

Author: Veldman, D. J., and Sheffield, J. R.

Article: The scaling of sociometric nominations.

Journal: *Educational and Psychological Measurement,* Spring 1979, *39*(1), 99–106.

■ ■ ■

1714

Test Name: INDEX OF RESPONDING

Purpose: To measure one's ability to facilitate human relations.

Number of Items: 8 situations.

Format: Situations included five statements from students (boys), two from houseparents to houseparent, and one from a parent to a houseparent to which one responds as a houseparent.

Reliability: Stability-reliability of the Index of Responding was .90 from test–retest of 147 teacher-trainees of Augusta College.

Author: Bledsoe, J. C., and Layser, G. R.

Article: Effects of human relations training with houseparents on attainment of group facilitation skills.

Journal: *Psychological Reports,* June 1977, *40*(3), 787–791.

Related Research: Carkhuff, R. R. (1969). *Helping and human relations: 1. Selection and*

Training. New York: Holt, Rinehart & Winston.

■ ■ ■

1715

Test Name: INTERPERSONAL DEPENDENCY INVENTORY

Purpose: To assess interpersonal dependency in adults.

Number of Items: 48

Format: Includes three-scales: emotional reliance on another person, lack of social self-confidence, assertion of autonomy. All items are presented.

Reliability: Corrected split-half reliabilities were .87, .78, and .72.

Validity: Correlations with age ranged from .04 to .12 ($N = 400$); with education ranged from –.21 to .10 ($N = 400$); general neuroticism ranged from .01 to .49 ($N = 180$); social desirability ranged from –.09 to –.56 ($N = 180$); anxiety ranged from .06 to .34 ($N = 180$); depression ranged from .08 to .44 ($N = 180$); interpersonal sensitivity ranged from .17 to .53 ($N = 180$).

Author: Hirschfeld, R. M. A., et al.

Article: A measure of interpersonal dependency.

Journal: *Journal of Personality Assessment,* December 1977, *41*(6), 610–618.

■ ■ ■

1716

Test Name: INTERPERSONAL FACILITATIVE FUNCTIONING QUESTIONNAIRE

Purpose: To assess facilitative functioning of people in interpersonal relationships.

Number of Items: 12

Format: Items rated on a 6-point Likert scale completed by observer-raters.

Reliability: Reliability coefficients obtained by an analysis of variance estimate of reliability were self, $r = .79$, other, $r = .88$.

Author: Cabush, D. W., and Edwards, K. J.

Article: Training clients to help themselves: Outcome effects of training college student clients in facilitative self-responding.

Journal: *Journal of Counseling Psychology,* January 1976, *23*(1), 34–39.

Related Research: Truax, C. B., & Carkhuff, R. R. (1967). *Toward effective counseling and psychotherapy.* Chicago: Aldine.

■ ■ ■

1717

Test Name: INTERPERSONAL JUDGMENT SCALE

Purpose: To measure one's judgment of others according to intelligence, knowledge of current events, adjustment, one's desire to have the stranger as a roommate or close neighbor and one's probable liking of the stranger, and the person's desirability as a work partner.

Number of Items: 6

Format: Items were rated on a 7-point scale.

Reliability: Split-half reliability was .85 (Byrne & Nelson, 1965).

Author: Korte, J. R., et al.

Article: Does locus of control similarity increase attraction?

Journal: *Journal of Psychological Reports,* December 1978, *43*(3), 1183–1188.

Related Research: Byrne, D., & Nelson, D. (1965). Attraction as a linear function of proportion of positive reinforcement. *Journal of Personality and Social Psychology, 1,* 659–663.

1718

Test Name: INTERPERSONAL TRUST SCALE

Purpose: To measure one's expectancy that the word, promise, or verbal or written statement of another individual or group can be relied upon.

Number of Items: 40

Format: Likert items with 25 trust items and items designed to disguise the nature of the test.

Reliability: The test–retest reliabilities range from .56 to .68 and the internal consistency reliability coefficient is. 77.

Author: Pereira, M. J., and Austrin, H. R.

Article: Interpersonal trust as a predictor of suggestibility.

Journal: *Psychological Reports,* December 1980, *47*(3), 1031–1034.

Related Research: Rotter, J. B. (1967). A new scale for the measurement of interpersonal trust. *Journal of Personality, 35,* 653–665.

Tedeschi, R. G., & Wright, T. L. (1980). Cross-validation of the Wright-Tedeschi factor of the Interpersonal Trust Scale. *Psychological Reports, 47,* 111–114.

■ ■ ■

1719

Test Name: LIFE EXPERIENCE SCALE

Purpose: To assess social competence in adult males.

Number of Items: 21

Format: Multiple choice; includes such topics as job history, marriage history, and so forth.

Reliability: Test–retest (1 month) reliability was .87.

Validity: Correlation with Ullmann and Giovannoni (1964) Scale was

.84; correlation with ratings for psychiatric disability was –.57.

Author: Wagener, J.

Article: An experimental scale of social competence for adult males.

Journal: *Journal of Personality Assessment,* October 1974, *38*(5), 462–463.

Related Research: Ullmann, L., & Giovannoni, J. (1964). The development of a self-report measure of the process reactive continuum. *Journal of Nervous and Mental Disease, 138,* 38–42.

■ ■ ■

1720

Test Name: LORR INTERPERSONAL BEHAVIOR INVENTORY

Purpose: To assess mode of interpersonal behavior.

Number of Items: 140

Format: Subject rates 140 statements (*not at all* to *quite often*). The inventory has 15 categories: Dominance, Competitiveness, Hostility, Dependence, Detachment, Inhibition, Abasement, Submissiveness, Dependence, Deference, Agreeableness, Nurturance, Affiliation, Sociability, and Exhibition.

Validity: Three factors accounted for 57 to 62% of the variance: Hostility-Affection, Dominance, Submissiveness.

Author: Bochner, A., and Kaminski, E.

Article: Modes of interpersonal behavior: A replication.

Journal: *Psychological Reports,* December 1974, *35*(3), 1079–1083.

Related Research: Lorr, M., & Suziedelis, A. (1959). Modes of interpersonal behavior. *Journal of Abnormal and Social Psychology, 59,* 226–235.

1721

Test Name: MACHIAVELLIANISM SCALE

Purpose: To measure one's generalized tendency to manipulate and exploit others in interpersonal situations.

Number of Items: 20

Format: Items are rated on a Likert scale.

Reliability: Split-half reliability was .79.

Author: Keenan, A., and Clarkson, V.

Article: Machiavellianism and attitudes towards the police.

Journal: *Journal of Occupational Psychology,* 1977, *50*(1), 15–22.

Related Research: Christie, R., & Geis, F. L. (1970). *Studies in Machiavellianism.* New York: Academic Press.

■ ■ ■

1722

Test Name: PERCEIVED DEPTH OF INTERACTION SCALE

Purpose: To evaluate the quality of group interaction.

Number of Items: 10

Format: Items are rated on a Likert scale.

Reliability: Internal consistency alpha was .80 and average item-total scale Pearson product–moment correlation was .56.

Validity: Correlated significantly with the Quad I ($r = -.54, p < .001$) and the Quad IV ($r = .55, p < .001$) measures of the Hill Interaction Matrix-B (Hill, 1965) and the Cohesiveness Subscale of the Group Environments Scale (Moos, 1974; $r = .45, p < .001$).

Author: Rose, G. S., and Bednar, R. L.

Article: Effects of positive and

negative self-disclosure and feedback on early group development.

Journal: *Journal of Counseling Psychology*, January 1980, *27*(1), 63–70.

Related Research: Evensen, P., & Bednar, R. L. (1978). The effects of specific cognitive and behavioral structure on early group development. *Journal of Counseling Psychology, 25*, 18–30.

Hill, W. F. (1965). *HIM: Hill Interaction Matrix.* Los Angeles: University of Southern California, Youth Study Center.

Moos, R. H. (1974). *Preliminary manual for the family, work and group environment scales.* Palo Alto, CA: Consulting Psychologists Press.

■ ■ ■

1723

Test Name: PERCEPTION OF SOCIAL CLOSENESS SCALE

Purpose: To measure degree of acceptance among elementary school students.

Number of Items: 5

Format: The items are social-distance items.

Reliability: Test–retest reliability was .78.

Validity: Correlations with sociogram rankings ranged from .78 to .97 (rho).

Author: Horne, M. D., et al.

Article: Peer status in research and locus of control.

Journal: *Perceptual and Motor Skills,* October 1978, *47*(2), 487–490.

Related Research: Horne, M. D. (1975). *An investigation of teacher and peer attitudes and the effect of achievement on self-concepts and status of learning disabled and non-learning disabled pupils in regular elementary classrooms.* Unpublished doctoral dissertation, Boston University.

■ ■ ■

1724

Test Name: POTENTIAL INTERPERSONAL COMPETENCE SCALE

Purpose: To measure the interpersonal competencies needed by a counselor.

Number of Items: 35

Time Required: 70 minutes.

Format: The items were problem presentations divided equally among the competencies.

Validity: With years of counseling experience, $r = .28$ ($N = 82$); with hours of counseling course work, $r = .56$ ($N = 82$); with GRE-Quantitative score, $r = -.41$ ($N = 82$); with sex, $r = .36$ ($N = 82$).

Author: Remer, R., and Sease, W.

Article: The development of a criterion instrument for counselor selection.

Journal: *Measurement and Evaluation in Guidance,* October 1974, *7*(3), 181–187.

■ ■ ■

1725

Test Name: PSYCHOLOGICAL SCREENING INVENTORY

Purpose: To measure alienation, social nonconformity, discomfort, expression, and defensiveness.

Number of Items: 130

Format: True–false.

Validity: Negative correlations $p <$ .01 with the Marlowe-Crowne Social Desirability Scale.

Author: Pulliam, G. P.

Article: Social desirability and the Psychological Screening Inventory.

Journal: *Psychological Reports,* April 1975, *36*(2), 522.

Related Research: Lanyon, R. I. (1970). The development and validation of Psychological Screening Inventory. *Journal of Consulting and Clinical Psychology Monographs, 35*(1, Part 2).

■ ■ ■

1726

Test Name: SENSITIVITY TO REJECTION

Purpose: To assess weaknesses in social skills.

Number of Items: 24

Format: Items are answered on a 9-point scale from –4 (*very strong disagreement*) to +14 (*very strong agreement*) and half are positively worded.

Reliability: Kuder-Richardson internal reliability coefficient was .83; 4-week test–retest of one sample of 108 subjects yielded a product–moment correlation coefficient of .92.

Author: Mehrabian, A.

Article: Questionnaire measures of affiliative tendency and sensitivity to rejection.

Journal: *Psychological Reports,* February 1976, *38*(1), 199–209.

Related Research: Mehrabian, A., & Epstein, N. (1972). A measure of emotional empathy. *Journal of Personality, 40*, 525–543.

■ ■ ■

1727

Test Name: SOCIAL ISOLATION SCALE—MODIFIED

Purpose: To measure social isolation.

Number of Items: 9

Format: Responses to each item are made on a 4-point continuum: *strongly agree, agree, disagree,* *strongly disagree.* All items are presented.

Reliability: Split-half reliability was .91.

Author: Groat, H. T., et al.

Article: Social isolation and premarital pregnancy.

Journal: *Sociology and Social Research,* January 1976, *60*(2), 188–198.

Related Research: Dean, D. (1961). Alienation: Its meaning and measurement. *American Sociological Review, 26,* 753–758.

■ ■ ■

1728

Test Name: SELF-SOCIAL SYMBOLS TASKS

Purpose: To measure self-other relationships.

Number of Items: 50

Format: A nonverbal test that includes 8 components of the self: esteem, social interest, power, egocentricity, complexity, individuation, inclusiveness, identification. Provides 11 scores.

Reliability: Split-half reliability coefficients corrected for length for the 11 scores ranged from .46 to .92.

Author: Long, B. H., et al.

Article: Self–other orientations of Israeli adolescents reared in kibbutzim and moshavim.

Journal: *Developmental Psychology,* March 1974, *8*(2), 300–308.

Related Research: Long, B. H., et al. (1970). *Manual for the Self-Social Symbols Tasks.* Towson, MD: Goucher College.

■ ■ ■

1729

Test Name: UCLA LONELINESS SCALE

Purpose: To provide a general measure of loneliness.

Number of Items: 20

Format: Subjects respond to each item on a 5-point scale ranging from *much less lonely than others* to *much more lonely than others.* All items are presented.

Reliability: Coefficient alpha was .96 ($n = 239$). Test–retest correlation was .73 over 2-month interval ($n = 102$).

Validity: Correlations with self-ratings of depression, $r = .49$ ($n = 131$), self-ratings of anxiety, $r = .35$ ($n = 131$); Beck Depression Scale, $r = .38$ ($n = 47$); Multiple Affect Adjective Checklist, $r = .43$ ($n = 65$).

Author: Russell, D., et al.

Article: Developing a measure of loneliness.

Journal: *Journal of Personality Assessment,* June 1978, *42*(3), 290–294.

Related Research: Sisenwein, R. J. (1964). *Loneliness and the individual as viewed by himself and others.* Doctoral dissertation, Columbia University. (University Microfilms No. 65–4768)

Solano, C. H. (1980). Two measures of loneliness: A comparison. *Psychological Reports, 46*(1), 23–68.

■ ■ ■

1730

Test Name: UNIVERSITY ALIENATION SCALE

Purpose: To assess feelings of alienation within the context of the university.

Number of Items: 24

Format: Items are rated on a 5-choice *agree–disagree* Likert continuum.

Reliability: Split-half corrected

reliability coefficient for the total scale of .88.

Author: Babbit, C. E., et al.

Article: Organizational alienation among Black college students: A comparison of three educational settings.

Journal: *Journal of College Student Personnel,* January 1975, *16*(1), 53–56.

Related Research: Burbach, K. J. (1972). The development of a contextual measure of alienation. *Pacific Sociological Review, 15,* 225–234.

■ ■ ■

1731

Test Name: WOMEN'S SOCIAL SITUATIONS TEST

Purpose: To measure conformity types, including inner-direction, other-direction, and non-conformity.

Number of Items: 30

Format: Three subscales, including Self-Ideal, Self-Average, and Idiosyncratic. Each item is followed by five response alternatives.

Reliability: Reliabilities by Hoyt's formula (Hoyt, 1941) ranged from .74 to .86.

Author: Sprinthall, R. C., and Bennett, B.

Article: Conformity and nonconformity among married women: The Riesman typologies.

Journal: *Psychological Reports,* June 1978, *42*(3), 1195–1201.

Related Research: Sprinthall, R. C. (1967). *Social conformity in a college fraternity.* Ann Arbor, MI: University Microfilms.

Hoyt, C. J. (1941). Note on a simplified method of computing test reliability. *Educational and Psychological Measurement, 1,* 93–95.

CHAPTER 5
Aptitude

1732

Test Name: AMERICAN UNIVERSITY OF BEIRUT TRIAL APTITUDE BATTERY

Purpose: To predict college grades.

Number of Items: 150

Format: Includes three subtests: English Proficiency Test, Quantitative-Aptitude Test, and Science-Aptitude Test. Responses to each item are made on a 5-choice form.

Reliability: Kuder-Richardson formula 21 coefficients of internal consistency for two forms of the Science-Aptitude Test were .81 and .80.

Validity: Multiple correlations between combinations of subtests and first semester freshman grades ($N = 73$) ranged from .28 to .35. Multiple correlations between combinations of subtests and first semester sophomore grades ($N = 202$) ranged from .30 to .38.

Author: Abu-Sayf, F. K., and Za'Rour, G. I.

Article: Predictive validity of the American University of Beirut Trial Aptitude Battery.

Journal: *Educational and Psychological Measurement,* Summer 1975, *35*(2), 451–454.

• • •

1733

Test Name: DEFENSE LANGUAGE APTITUDE BATTERY

Purpose: To provide a foreign language aptitude test.

Format: Includes three factors.

Reliability: Kuder-Richardson formula 21 reliabilities ranged from .78 to .82 for the three factors and .89 for the total.

Validity: Predictive validities with language courses in Arabic, $r = .56$ ($n = 112$); Mandarin Chinese, $r = .53$ ($n = 70$); German, $r = .55$ ($n = 87$); Russian, $r = .50$ ($n = 111$); Spanish, $r = .57$ ($n = 87$).

Author: Peterson, C. R., and Al-Haik, A. R.

Article: The development of the defense language aptitude battery (DLAB).

Journal: *Educational and Psychological Measurement,* Summer 1976, *36*(2), 369–380.

Related Research: Al-Haik, A. R. (1972). *Exploring the auditory aspects of aptitude for intensive modern foreign language learning.* Unpublished doctoral dissertation, University of California, Berkeley.

• • •

1734

Test Name: FIGURE COPYING TEST

Purpose: To measure mental ability.

Number of Items: 10

Time Required: 10–15 minutes.

Format: Ten geometric forms are presented to the child, who must copy figures (scored 1–3).

Validity: Article states that scores correlated substantially with other IQ tests.

Author: Jensen, A.

Article: The effect of race of examiner on the mental test scores of White and Black pupils.

Journal: *Journal of Educational Measurement,* Spring 1974, *11*(1), 1–14.

Related Research: Ilg, F., & Ames, L. (1964). *School readiness: Behavior tests used at the Gesell Institute.* New York: Harper & Row.

Jensen, A. (1973). Level I and Level II abilities in three ethnic groups. *American Educational Research Journal,* Fall, *10*, 4, 263–276.

• • •

1735

Test Name: HAYES EARLY IDENTIFICATION LISTENING RESPONSE TEST

Purpose: To provide a rapidly administered screening test for readiness for first grades.

Number of Items: 10

Format: Contains a series of psychomotor tasks for which the teacher gives verbal instructions and emphasizes the importance of listening, comprehension, visual perception, and five motor skills. Total possible score is 22 points.

Reliability: Kuder-Richardson formula 20 reliability was .86 ($n = 121$) with a standard error of measurement of 1.73. Interrater reliability was estimated to be .99 through an analysis of variance model.

Validity: Correlation with the Metropolitan Readiness Test was .79.

Author: Hayes, M., et al.

Article: Validity and reliability of a simple screening device for readiness screening.

Journal: *Educational and Psychological Measurement,* Summer 1975, *35*(2), 495–498.

Related Research: Buttram, J., et al. (1976). Prediction of school readiness and early grade achievement by classroom teachers. *Educational and Psychological Measurement, 36,* 543–546.

■ ■ ■

1736

Test Name: JOB INTERVIEW PERFORMANCE EXPECTATIONS SCALE

Purpose: To permit subjects to estimate how well they expect to do in a job interview.

Number of Items: 8

Format: Provides a self-report of how well the subjects expect to do in a job interview. Subjects answer each item on a 5-point scale. Sample items are presented.

Reliability: Internal consistency was .86.

Validity: With Body Satisfaction, r = .24 (N = 87); Self-Cathexis Scale, r = .30; Janis-Field-Eagley Scale, r = .52; Interview Self-ratings, r = .34; Judges' ratings, r = .31; Self-rating discrepancy scores, r = .03.

Author: King, M. R., and Manaster, G. J.

Article: Body image, self-esteem, expectations, self-assessments and actual success in a simulated job interview.

Journal: *Journal of Applied*

Psychology, October 1977, *62*(5), 589–594.

■ ■ ■

1737

Test Name: JOB INVOLVEMENT QUESTIONNAIRE

Purpose: To predict academic performance.

Number of Items: 6

Reliability: Split-half Spearman-Brown corrected reliability coefficient was .64.

Validity: Correlation with age was .13 (n = 107); with SAT Aptitude was .12 (n = 48); with grade point average was .37 (n = 81); with Satisfaction was –.01 (n = 34); with Performance was .43 (n = 34).

Author: Batlis, N. C.

Article: Job involvement as a predictor of academic performance.

Journal: *Educational and Psychological Measurement,* Winter 1978, *38*(4), 1177–1180.

Related Research: Lodahl, T. M., & Kejner, M. (1965). The definition and measurement of job involvement. *Journal of Applied Psychology, 49,* 24–33.

■ ■ ■

1738

Test Name: MENTAL DEXTERITY TEST

Purpose: To measure a wide variety of mental abilities and aptitudes including verbal, numerical, reasoning, space relations, memory, and general information.

Number of Items: 100

Time Required: 1 hour.

Format: A power test of the omnibus type consisting of multiple choice items. Designed as an alternative to the Otis and Wonderlic Tests. Includes two

subtests: verbal comprehension and numerical ability. Two examples are presented.

Reliability: Kuder-Richardson formula 20 reliability coefficient for verbal ability was .89; numerical ability was .82; the total test was .93.

Author: Thumin, F. J.

Article: Factor analysis and reliability of the mental dexterity test.

Journal: *Perceptual and Motor Skills,* June 1974, *38*(3, Part 1), 744–746.

Related Research: Thumin, F. J. (1970). The mental dexterity test: A study of reliability and validity. *Perceptual and Motor Skills, 30,* 163–166.

■ ■ ■

1739

Test Name: MMPI WOMEN'S SCHOLASTIC PERSONALITY SCALE

Purpose: To predict scholastic potential in women.

Number of Items: 68

Format: MMPI items from the standardized test which differentiated between a criterion (National Merit) group and a comparison group.

Validity: Significant differences between criterion groups in scale performance were found.

Author: Clopton, J., and Neuringer, C.

Article: An MMPI scale to measure scholastic personality in women.

Journal: *Perceptual and Motor Skills,* December 1973, *37*(3), 963–966.

■ ■ ■

1740

Test Name: MODIFIED HALL'S MATRICES

Purpose: To predict achievement in mathematics among African children.

Number of Items: 30

Format: Each item is a matrix-completion task consisting of 4 cells in a 2 x 2 matrix.

Validity: Kuder-Richardson formula 20 yielded coefficients of .75 and .78. Test–retest yielded a coefficient of .71.

Validity: Correlations with Experimenter's Mathematics Test was .81 and with Class Teacher's Test was .76.

Author: Adejumo, D.

Article: The reliability and validity of Modified Hall's Matrices (MHM) for predicting mathematics achievement among Nigerian children.

Journal: *Educational and Psychological Measurement,* Summer 1977, *37*(2), 501–503.

● ● ●

1741

Test Name: PRESCHOOL SCREENER

Purpose: To tap school-related skills in children 3 to 5.5 years.

Number of Items: 15

Time Required: 5–10 minutes.

Reliability: Kuder-Richardson formula 20 reliability was .726.

Validity: Total score correlated .562 with age, .777 with Peabody Mental Age, and .740 with Psycholinguistic Age.

Author: Winett, R. A., et al.

Article: A preschool screener test for child care and related evaluation research.

Journal: *Developmental*

Psychology, January 1975, *11*(1), 110.

● ● ●

1742

Test Name: SELF-DIRECTED LEARNING READINESS SCALE–ABBREVIATED FORM

Purpose: To assess self-directed learning readiness.

Number of Items: 10

Format: Subjects respond to each item by indicating agreement, uncertainty, or disagreement. All items are presented.

Validity: Pearson product–moment correlation coefficients with Thinking Creatively About the Future ranged from .18 to .64 for grades 5, 8, 11, and 12.

Author: Torrance, E. P., and Mourad, S.

Article: Self-directed learning readiness skills of gifted students and their relationship to thinking creatively about the future.

Journal: *The Gifted Child Quarterly,* Summer 1978, *22*(2), 180–186.

Related Research: Guglielmino, L. M. (1977). *Self-directed Learning Readiness Scale.* Boca Raton, FL: Author.

● ● ●

1743

Test Name: SERIES LEARNING POTENTIAL TEST

Purpose: To assess learning potential in the primary and elementary grades.

Number of Items: 65

Time Required: 30–40 minutes.

Format: A group test involving the completion of series of pictures or geometric forms arranged in a

pattern in which the figures change systematically. Four concepts may vary in a series: semantic content, size, color, or orientation. Two forms of the test.

Reliability: Alternate form reliability is .84.

Validity: Correlations with teacher ratings range from .22 to .54.

Author: Babad, E. Y., and Budoff, M.

Article: Sensitivity and validity of learning-potential measurement in three levels of ability.

Journal: *Journal of Educational Psychology,* June 1974, *66*(3), 439–447.

● ● ●

1744

Test Name: SYMBOLS TEST

Purpose: To provide a predictor of later reading performance of 5-year-olds.

Number of Items: 24

Format: Items 1 to 13, child decodes short statements and errors are corrected by the examiner; Items 14 to 19, no corrections are made and credit is awarded only if the sentence is correctly memorized; Items 20 to 24 are comprehensive items. An example is given.

Reliability: Test–retest, $r = .76$ ($N = 90$ with a 14–day interval).

Validity: Correlation with Burt Rearranged Graded Word Reading List taken 1 year later was .50.

Author: Ferguson, N.

Article: Pictographs and prereading skills.

Journal: *Child Development,* September 1975, *46*(3), 786–789.

CHAPTER 6
Attitude

1745

Test Name:
ATTITUDE-BEHAVIOR SCALE

Purpose: To measure attitudes and behaviors regarding interracial interaction.

Number of Items: 7 scales.

Format: The scales are Stereotype, Norm, Moral evaluation, Hypothetical behavior, Actual feelings, Actual action, and Life experiences.

Reliability: Reliability figures range between .87 and .95 for the seven scales.

Author: Parker, M., and Wittmer, J.

Article: The effects of a communications training program on the racial attitudes of Black and White fraternity members.

Journal: *Journal of College Student Personnel*, November 1976, *17*(6), 500–503.

Related Research: Jordan, J. E. (1972). *Attitude-Behavior Scale: Blacks/Whites or Whites/Blacks* (mimeo). East Lansing: Michigan State University.

■ ■ ■

1746

Test Name: ATTITUDE OF CONCEPT-EDUCATIONAL RESEARCH

Purpose: To assess the feelings of subjects toward educational research.

Number of Items: 30

Format: 30 adjective pairs describing educational research.

Subjects indicate on a 7-point scale which adjective they agree with and how strongly they agree.

Reliability: Spearman-Brown split-half correlation coefficient, .93 on pretest, .95 for posttest.

Validity: Current validity assessed by correlating with the Attitude Toward Educational Research Scale developed by the same authors.

Author: Napier, J.

Article: An experimental study of the relationship between attitude toward and knowledge of educational research.

Journal: *Journal of Experimental Education*, Winter 1978, *47*(2), 131–134.

■ ■ ■

1747

Test Name: ATTITUDE MEASURE OF SEXUAL BEHAVIOR

Purpose: To assess attitudes toward sexual behavior.

Number of Items: 12

Time Required: 20 minutes.

Format: Seven bipolar dimensions for each item.

Reliability: Test–retest reliability over a period of 1 week for college age subjects ranges from .52 (active–passive) to .78 (good–bad) for the bipolar dimensions.

Author: Fretz, B. R.

Article: Assessing attitudes toward sexual behaviors.

Journal: *The Counseling*

Psychologist, 1975, *5*(1), 100–106.

■ ■ ■

1748

Test Name: ATTITUDE QUESTIONNAIRE

Purpose: To measure one's attitudes toward God, the draft, smoking, birth control, drinking, grading practices, welfare, war, discipline, and careers for women.

Number of Items: 24

Format: Ten relevant items and 14 fillers measured on a 7-point scale from 1 (*unimportant*) to 7 (*very important*).

Reliability: Test–retest reliability coefficients range from .69 on the item about welfare to .95 on the item about God.

Author: Dilendik, J. R.

Article: Attitude similarity and the covert curriculum.

Journal: *Journal of Educational Research*, April 1976, *69*(8), 304–308.

Related Research: Byrne, D. (1971). *The attraction paradigm.* New York: Academic Press.

■ ■ ■

1749

Test Name: ATTITUDE SCALE

Purpose: To measure attitudes.

Number of Items: 60

Format: Each item was responded to in a 5-point Likert scale ranging from *very true* through *undecided* to *definitely untrue*. All items are presented.

Author: Bardo, J. W.

Article: Internal consistency and reliability in Likert-type attitude scales—Some questions concerning the use of pre-built scales.

Journal: *Sociology and Social Research*, July 1976, *60*(4), 403–420.

Related Research: Fessler, D. A. (1970). Community solidarity index. In Delbert C. Miller (Ed.), *Handbook of Research Design and Social Measurement*. New York: David McKay.

■ ■ ■

1750

Test Name: ATTITUDE TOWARD CAPITAL PUNISHMENT SCALE

Purpose: To measure one's attitudes toward capital punishment.

Number of Items: 24

Reliability: Test–retest reliability over 12 days was .92.

Validity: Analysis of variance, *p* < .001.

Author: Moore, M.

Article: Attitude toward capital punishment: Scale validation.

Journal: *Psychological Reports,* August 1975, *37*(1), 21–22.

Related Research: Thurstone, L. L. (1932). *Motion pictures and attitudes of children*. Chicago: University of Chicago Press.

■ ■ ■

1751

Test Name: ATTITUDE TOWARD DISABLED PERSONS SCALE

Purpose: To assess attitude of adolescents toward disabled individuals.

Number of Items: 20

Format: Likert instrument (*agree*

very much to *disagree very much*); in study cited in source, scales modified to include measurement of attitude toward mentally retarded, aged, alcoholic, and mentally ill groups.

Reliability: Yuker (1966) provides reliability data.

Validity: Significant differences between delinquent and nondelinquent male adolescents were found on the scale.

Author: Evans, J.

Article: Attitudes of adolescent delinquent boys.

Journal: *Psychological Reports,* June 1974, *34*(3), 1175–1178.

Related Research: Yuker, H., et al. (1966). *The measurement of attitudes toward disabled persons* (Human Resources Study No. 7). Albertson, NY: Human Resources.

■ ■ ■

1752

Test Name: ATTITUDE TOWARD EDUCATIONAL RESEARCH SCALE

Purpose: To determine subjects' feelings toward educational research.

Number of Items: 26

Format: Subjects respond to statements about educational research on a 5-point scale ranging from *strongly agreed* to *strongly disagreed*.

Reliability: Spearman-Brown split-half correlations were .91 (pretest) and .85 (posttest).

Validity: Concurrent validity was calculated by correlating responses with the Attitude of Concept-Educational Research Scale. 67 (pretest) and .66 (posttest).

Author: Napier, J.

Article: An experimental study of the relationship between attitude

toward and knowledge of educational research.

Journal: *Journal of Experimental Education,* Winter 1978, *47*(2), 132–134.

■ ■ ■

1753

Test Name: ATTITUDE TOWARD EXPRESSING FEELINGS SURVEY

Purpose: To assess one's attitude toward expressing feelings.

Number of Items: 30

Format: Likert scale, ranging from 1 (*strongly agree*) to 7 (*strongly disagree*).

Reliability: Hoyt reliability was reported as .84.

Author: Highlen, P. S., and Gillis, S. F.

Article: Effects of situational factors, sex, and attitude on affective self-disclosure and anxiety.

Journal: *Journal of Counseling Psychology,* July 1978, *25*(4), 270–276.

Related Research: Highlen, P. S., & Voight, N. L. (1978). Effects of social modeling, cognitive structuring, and self-management strategies on affective self-disclosure. *Journal of Counseling Psychology, 25*, 21–27.

■ ■ ■

1754

Test Name: ATTITUDES TOWARD FEMALE PROFESSORS SCALE

Purpose: To measure attitudes toward female professors.

Number of Items: 20

Format: Items are rated on a Likert scale.

Reliability: Split-half reliability

coefficient is .88. Test–retest reliability coefficient determined over a 5-week period is .95.

Validity: Correlates –.63 ($p < .05$) with Rokeach's Dogmatism Scale.

Author: Brant, W. D.

Article: Attitudes toward female professors: A scale with some data on its reliability and validity.

Journal: *Psychological Reports,* August 1978, *43*(1), 211–214.

■ ■ ■

1755

Test Name: ATTITUDES TO FEMALES' SOCIAL ROLES QUESTIONNAIRE

Purpose: To assess women's attitudes to females' social roles.

Number of Items: 35

Format: Items are scored on a 4-point scale (0, 1, 3, and 4) which forces an expression of attitude. Subjects are asked Do you strongly disagree, mildly disagree, mildly agree, or strongly agree? (Questionnaire is included.)

Reliability: Test–retest reliability on 17 of the 20 subjects after 10 days gave $r = .94$ (Spearman rank correlation coefficient). Split-half reliability coefficient (Spearman-Brown) estimated on the original sample was .92.

Validity: Secretaries and nurses achieved higher scores than female university lecturers ($p < .001$). Female university students received higher scores than student members of the University Women's Liberation Group ($p < .001$).

Author: Slade, P., and Jenner, F. A.

Article: Questionnaire measuring attitudes to females' social roles.

Journal: *Psychological Reports,* October 1978, *43*(2), 351–354.

1756

Test Name: ATTITUDES TOWARD THE HANDICAPPED SCALE

Purpose: To measure one's attitudes toward the handicapped.

Number of Items: 6

Format: Open-ended statements that the respondents complete.

Reliability: Split-half reliability was .68.

Author: Dahl, H. G., et al.

Article: Simulation of exceptionalities for elementary school students.

Journal: *Psychological Reports,* April 1978, *42*(2), 573–574.

Related Research: Feldhusen, J. F., et al. (1966). Sentence completion responses and classroom social behavior. *Personnel and Guidance Journal, 45,* 165–170.

■ ■ ■

1757

Test Name: ATTITUDES TOWARD MASCULINE TRANSCENDENCE SCALE

Purpose: To measure what men and women regard as appropriate roles for men in general.

Number of Items: 54

Format: Higher the score, the more liberal the attitudes; the lower the score, the more traditional or stereotypic are the attitudes.

Reliability: Cronbach's alpha internal consistency coefficients for four separate samples have been found to range from .89 to .95.

Author: Harren, V. A., et al.

Article: Influence of gender, sex-role attitudes and cognitive complexity on gender-dominant career choices.

Journal: *Journal of Counseling Psychology,* May 1979, *26*(3), 227–234.

■ ■ ■

1758

Test Name: ATTITUDES TOWARD MATHEMATICS—REVISED

Purpose: To measure attitude toward mathematics.

Number of Items: 10

Format: Items are rated on a Likert scale.

Reliability: Two-day delay, test–retest reliability was estimated to be .98.

Author: Block, J. H., and Tierney, M. L.

Article: An exploration of two correction procedures used in mastery learning approaches to instruction.

Journal: *Journal of Educational Psychology,* December 1974, *66*(6), 962–967.

Related Research: Husén, T. (Ed.). (1967). *International study of achievement in mathematics* (Vol. I). New York: Wiley.

■ ■ ■

1759

Test Name: ATTITUDES TOWARD MENTALLY RETARDED CHILDREN SCALE

Purpose: To measure the attitudes of nonretarded children toward mentally retarded children and nonretarded peers.

Number of Items: 10

Format: 5-point rating scale of 10 adjective pairs.

Reliability: Test–retest correlation based on a randomly selected sample of 50 was .72.

Author: Gottlieb, J.

Article: Attitudes toward retarded

children: Effects of labeling and behavioral aggressiveness.

Source: *Journal of Educational Psychology,* August 1975, *67*(4), 581–585.

Related Research: Gottlieb, J., Cohen, L., & Goldstein, L. (1974). Social contact and personal adjustment as variables relating to attitudes toward EMR children. *Training School Bulletin, 71,* 9–16.

• • •

1760

Test Name: ATTITUDE TOWARD OLD PEOPLE SCALE

Purpose: To measure attitudes toward old people.

Number of Items: 19

Format: Likert scale employing four response categories from *strongly agree* to *strongly disagree.* All items are presented.

Reliability: Cronbach's alpha was .80.

Author: Ward, R. A.

Article: Aging group consciousness: Implications in an older sample.

Journal: *Sociology and Social Research,* July 1977, *61*(4), 496–519.

Related Research: Tuckman, J., & Lorge, I. (1953). Attitudes toward old people. *Journal of Social Psychology, 37,* 249–260.

• • •

1761

Test Name: ATTITUDE TOWARD PUBLIC EXPOSURE TO SEXUAL STIMULI SCALE

Purpose: To measure attitudes toward public exposure to sexual stimuli.

Number of Items: 10

Format: Items are in Likert format

with subjects responding to each item on a 5-point scale from *strongly agree* to *strongly disagree.* All items are presented.

Reliability: Kuder-Richardson coefficients were .87 ($n = 59$) and .84 ($n = 38$).

Validity: With Traditional Family Ideology Scale, $r = -.71$; Religiosity, $r = -.56$; Modernity, $r = .48$.

Author: Crawford, J. E., and Crawford, T. J.

Article: Development and construct validation of a measure of attitudes toward public exposure to sexual stimuli.

Journal: *Journal of Personality Assessment,* August 1978, *42*(4), 392–400.

• • •

1762

Test Name: ATTITUDE TOWARD RETAIL BARGAINING SCALE

Purpose: To measure a person's predisposition toward bargaining in a retail setting.

Number of Items: 18

Format: Used a Likert scaling procedure.

Reliability: Kuder-Richardson formula 20 reliability was .966.

Author: Kahler, R. C., et al.

Article: Bargaining process as a determinant of postpurchase satisfaction.

Journal: *Journal of Applied Psychology,* August 1977, *62*(4), 487–492.

Related Research: Allen, B. H. (1974). *Post-transactional evaluation as a consequence of bargaining in an experimental setting.* Unpublished doctoral dissertation, University of Cincinnati.

1763

Test Name: ATTITUDES TOWARD TEACHING READING IN CONTENT CLASSROOMS SCALE

Purpose: To assess attitudes toward teaching reading in content area classrooms.

Number of Items: 15

Format: Subject responds on a 7-point scale from 1 (*strongly disagree*) to 7 (*strongly agree*). All items are presented.

Reliability: Total scale coefficient of internal consistency (Cronbach's alpha) was .87. Stability coefficient r ranged from .66 to .89.

Validity: Correlation with a scale on attitudes toward open education ranged from .13 to .40.

Author: Vaughan, J. L., Jr.

Article: A scale to measure attitudes toward teaching reading in content classrooms.

Journal: *Journal of Reading,* April 1977, *20*(7), 605–609.

• • •

1764

Test Name: ATTITUDES TOWARD SEEKING PROFESSIONAL PSYCHOLOGICAL HELP SCALE

Purpose: To assess persons' help-seeking attitudes, including recognition of need, stigma tolerance, interpersonal openness, and confidence.

Number of Items: 29

Format: Likert items presented in a 4-point, *agree–disagree* response format and scored 0–3 (reverse keyed for negative items).

Reliability: Internal consistency reliability coefficients range from .83 to .86 and stability r's ranged from .73 to .89.

Author: Cash, T. F., et al.

Article: Help-seeking attitudes and perceptions of counselor behavior.

Journal: *Journal of Counseling Psychology,* July 1978, *25*(4), 264–269.

Related Research: Fischer, E. H., & Turner, J. L. (1970). Orientations to seeking professional help: Development and research utility of an attitude scale. *Journal of Consulting and Clinical Psychology, 35,* 79–90.

∎ ∎ ∎

1765

Test Name: ATTITUDES TOWARD SPEAKERS SCALE

Purpose: To assess effectiveness of speakers in various contexts: teachers, debaters, and so forth.

Number of Items: 22

Time Required: 3–10 minutes.

Format: Two Forms (A and B).

Reliability: Odd–even (corrected) reliability was .85 (A), .84 (B); reliability for Parallel Forms was .86.

Author: Blumenfeld, W.

Article: Development of parallel forms of a generalized scale of attitudes toward speakers.

Journal: *Psychological Reports,* October 1974, *35*(2), 884.

∎ ∎ ∎

1766

Test Name: ATTITUDES TOWARD WOMEN SCALE

Purpose: To assess attitudes regarding women's rights and roles in vocational educational, intellectual, social and sexual activities as well as marital relationships and obligations.

Number of Items: 25

Format: Likert scales scored from

0 to 3, with the high score indicating agreement with contemporary, profeminist responses.

Reliability: Correlations of individual items with the total scale score in earlier studies yielded correlations ranging from .31 to .73.

Author: Follingstad, D. R., et al.

Article: Effects of consciousness-raising groups on measures of feminism, self-esteem, and social desirability.

Journal: *Journal of Counseling Psychology,* May 1977, *24*(3), 223–230.

Related Research: Berman, M. R., et al. (1977, July). The efficacy of supportive learning environments for returning women: An empirical evaluation. *Journal of Counseling Psychology, 24*(4), 324–331.

Kilpatrick, D., & Smith, A. (1974). Validation of the Spence-Helmreich Attitudes Toward Women Scale. *Psychological Reports, 35*(1), 461–462.

Spence, J. T., et al. (1973). A short version of the Attitudes Toward Women Scale (AWS). *Bulletin of the Psychonomic Society, 2,* 219–220.

∎ ∎ ∎

1767

Test Name: ATTITUDES TOWARD WOMEN SCALE

Purpose: To assess one's endorsement of feminist or liberal attitudes.

Number of Items: 12

Format: Seven items related to educational, vocational, and intellectual roles factors and five on marital relations and obligations factors were randomly mixed with 12 filler items concerning morals.

Reliability: Coefficient alpha was .76.

Author: Gilbert, L. A., and Waldroop, J.

Article: Evaluation of a procedure for increasing sex-fair counseling.

Journal: *Journal of Counseling Psychology,* September 1978, *25*(5), 410–418.

Related Research: Spence, J. T., & Helmreich, R. (1972). The Attitudes Toward Women Scale: An objective instrument to measure attitudes toward the rights and roles of women in contemporary society. *JSAS Catalog of Selected Documents in Psychology, 2,* 66–67 (Ms. No. 153).

∎ ∎ ∎

1768

Test Name: ATTITUDES TOWARD WOMEN SCALE

Purpose: To measure the degree of feminist orientation.

Number of Items: 55

Format: Four-point Likert scale ranging from *strongly agree* to *strongly disagree.*

Reliability: Split-half reliability of .92 (Stein & Weston, 1976).

Author: Mezydle, L. S., and Betz, N. E.

Article: Perceptions of ideal sex roles as a function of sex and feminist orientation.

Journal: *Journal of Counseling Psychology,* May 1980, *27*(3), 282–285.

Related Research: Doyle, J. A. (1975). Comparison of Kirkpatrick's and Spence and Helmreich's Attitudes Toward Women Scales. *Psychological Reports, 37*(3), 878.

Etaugh, C., & Gerson, A. (1974). Attitudes toward women: Some geographical correlates.

Psychological Reports, 35(2), 701–702.

Rozsnafszky, J., & Hendel, D. D. (1977). Relationship between ego development and attitudes toward women. *Psychological Reports, 41*(1), 161–162.

Spence, J., and Helmreich, R. (1972). The Attitudes Toward Women Scale: An objective instrument to measure attitudes toward the rights and roles of women in contemporary society. *JSAS Catalog of Selected Documents in Psychology, 2,* 66–67 (Ms. No. 153).

Stein, S., & Weston, L. (1976). Attitudes toward women among female college students. *Sex Roles, 2,* 199–202.

■ ■ ■

1769

Test Name: BLASS SUBJECTIVITY–OBJECTIVITY SCALE

Purpose: To measure objectivity–subjectivity.

Number of Items: 30

Format: Scale consists of a series of statements about hypothetical situations (items are given in article); subjects are asked to rate the situation on a 1 to 5 scale in terms of how pleasant it makes them feel.

Reliability: Odd–even reliability was .77.

Validity: For subjective subjects (as rated on this scale) there were positive and significant correlations between course performance and ratings given to the instructor of the course.

Author: Blass, T.

Article: Measurement of objectivity-subjectivity: Effect of tolerance for imbalance and grades on evaluations of teachers.

Journal: *Psychological Reports,*

June 1974, *34*(3), 1199–1213.

Related Research: Blass, T. (1969). *Personality and situational factors in tolerance for imbalance.* Doctoral dissertation, Yeshiva University. (University Microfilms, No. 69–15,207)

■ ■ ■

1770

Test Name: CHILDREN'S PICTORIAL ATTITUDE SCALE

Purpose: To measure elementary school children's attitudes toward school.

Format: Children are shown a picture and asked how they would feel if they were in the situation.

Reliability: Split-half reliability was .69 (grades 1–6).

Validity: Significant difference between grade levels (the higher the grade the more negative the attitude).

Author: Lewis, J.

Article: A pictorial attitude scale for elementary pupils.

Journal: *Educational and Psychological Measurement,* Summer 1974, *34*(2), 461–462.

Related Research: Lewis, J. (1972). *Children's Pictorial Attitude Scale.* Winona, MN: Winona State College, Bureau of Educational Research.

■ ■ ■

1771

Test Name: CHILDREN'S SCHOOL-RELATED ATTITUDES SELF-REPORT QUESTIONNAIRE

Purpose: To provide a self-report measure of school-related attitudes of 8-year-old children.

Number of Items: 78

Format: Includes three scales: attitude toward school, attitude toward teacher, attitude toward

self, and independence. Examples are given.

Reliability: Internal consistency reliabilities ranged from .25 to .84.

Validity: Correlation with achievement scores ranged from .07 to .33 (*N* = 236).

Author: Khan, S. B.

Article: A comparative study of assessing children's school-related attitudes.

Journal: *Journal of Educational Measurement,* Spring 1978, *15*(1), 59–66.

Related Research: Traub, R. E., et al. (1973). *Openness in schools: An evaluation of the Wentworth County Roman Catholic School Board Schools* (Research Report). Ontario, Canada: The Ontario Institute for Studies in Education.

■ ■ ■

1772

Test Name: CLIENT ATTITUDE QUESTIONNAIRE

Purpose: To measure attitudes toward mental illness.

Number of Items: 20 statements.

Format: High scores (maximum 60) generally reflect psychosocial orientation: low scores (minimum 20), a medical model orientation.

Reliability: Reported reliability coefficient of .90.

Author: Morrison, J. K., and Teta, D. C.

Article: Effect of demythologizing seminars on attributions to mental health professionals.

Journal: *Psychological Reports,* October 1978, *43*(2), 493–494.

■ ■ ■

1773

Test Name: COLLECTIVE BARGAINING ATTITUDE SCALE

Purpose: To measure attitudes toward collective bargaining.

Number of Items: 7

Format: Subjects respond to each item on a 5-point scale from *strongly agree* to *strongly disagree*. All items are presented.

Reliability: Reliability estimated by applying the Spearman-Brown prophecy formula to the mean interitem correlation was .88.

Validity: Correlations with Job Description Index ranged from −.09 to −.35, Job Involvement, −.16; Locus of Control, −.17 Salary, −.41; Age, −.15 ($N = 222$).

Author: Bigoness, W. J.

Article: Correlates of faculty attitudes toward collective bargaining.

Journal: *Journal of Applied Psychology,* April 1978, *63*(2), 228–233.

Related Research: Feville, P., & Blandin, J. (1974). Faculty job satisfaction and bargaining sentiments: A case study. *Academy of Management Journal, 17,* 678–692.

• • •

1774

Test Name: COLOR MEANING TEST II

Purpose: To assess the evaluative responses of preliterate children to the colors white and black.

Number of Items: 24

Format: The child selects white or black animals in response to 24 stories containing evaluative adjectives. The adjectives are listed.

Reliability: Internal consistency $r = .63$.

Author: Williams, J. E., et al.

Article: Evaluative responses of

preschool children to the colors white and black.

Journal: *Child Development,* June 1975, *46*(2), 501–508.

Related Research: Boswell, D. A., & Williams, J. E. (1975). Correlates of race and color bias among preschool children. *Psychological Reports, 36,* 147–154.

• • •

1775

Test Name: COMPETITIVE-COOPERATIVE ATTITUDES SCALE

Purpose: To measure one's attitudes toward competition or cooperation.

Number of Items: 28

Format: Likert scales.

Reliability: Spearman-Brown prophecy correlation coefficient of .82.

Validity: Correlation was .39 ($p < .01$) between scores on the competitiveness scale and Mach IV; Correlation was .29 ($p < .01$) between scores on the competitiveness and Martin-Larsen Approval Motivation Scale.

Author: Martin, H. J., and Larsen, K. S.

Article: Measurement of competitive-cooperative attitudes.

Journal: *Psychological Reports,* August 1976, *39*(1), 303–306.

Related Research: Christie, R., & Geis, F. L. (1970). *Studies in Machiavellianism.* New York: Academic Press.

• • •

1776

Test Name: CONSERVATISM SCALE

Purpose: To assess attitudes

toward preserving the natural environment.

Number of Items: 20

Format: Total scores ranged from 20 to 100.

Reliability: Spearman-Brown (corrected) reliability was .75; test–retest (2 weeks) reliability was .83; interscorer reliability was .99.

Validity: Significant differences between psychology students and forestry students ($p < .01$).

Author: Moffett, L.

Article: Conservatism toward the natural environment.

Journal: *Psychological Reports,* June 1974, *34*(3), 778.

Related Research: Document NAPS-02319, Microfiche Publications, 305 E. 46th St., New York, NY, 10017.

• • •

1777

Test Name: CONSERVATISM SCALE

Purpose: To measure one's conservative attitudes.

Number of Items: 50

Format: Concepts for which subjects indicate whether they favor or believe in by circling *yes*, *no*, or *?* response categories.

Reliability: Item-by-total score correlations ranged from .07 for "computer music" and "pajama parties" to .56 for "church authority."

Author: Hogan, H. W.

Article: Cross-cultural reliability and factor structure of the Wilson-Patterson Conservatism Scale.

Journal: *Psychological Reports,* October 1977, *41*(2), 453–454.

Related Research: Wilson, G. D. (Ed.). (1973). *The psychology of* *conservatism.* New York: Academic Press.

■ ■ ■

1778

Test Name: CURIOSITY TEST

Purpose: To measure attitudes toward curiosity-related behavior.

Number of Items: 42

Format: Pairs of contrasting proverbs.

Reliability: Test–retest coefficient of .91 over 1 week with 70 subjects.

Validity: Correlations between proverbs scores and subtests of Ontario Test of Intrinsic Motivation were ambiguity, .39; complexity, .35; novelty, .35; specific curiosity, .39 ($p < .05$).

Author: Maw, W. H., and Maw, E. W.

Article: Contrasting proverbs as a measure of attitudes of college students toward curiosity-related behaviors.

Journal: *Psychological Reports,* December 1975, *37*(3), 1085–1086.

Related Research: Maw, W. H., & Maw, E. W. (1961). Establishing criterion groups for evaluating measures of curiosity. *Journal of Experimental Education, 28,* 299–306.

■ ■ ■

1779

Test Name: DEATH ATTITUDE SCALE

Purpose: To assess attitude toward death.

Number of Items: 32

Format: Items in Likert format, included in article.

Reliability: Split-half (corrected) reliability was .92.

Validity: Correlation with Bardis Religion Scale was −.21 ($p < .05$).

There was no significant difference between the physician and professor groups.

Author: Larsen, K., et al.

Article: Attitudes toward death: A desensitization process.

Journal: *Psychological Reports,* October 1974, *35*(2), 687–690.

Related Research: Bardis, P. (1961). A religion scale. *Social Science, 36,* 120–123.

■ ■ ■

1780

Test Name: DISABILITY FACTOR SCALE G

Purpose: To measure attitudes toward disabled persons.

Format: Seven dimensions: interaction strain, rejection of intimacy, generalized rejection, authoritarian virtuousness, inferred emotional consequences, distressed identification, and imputed functional limitations.

Reliability: Reliabilities range from .80 to .85.

Validity: Correlations with Attitudes Toward Disabled Persons Scale range from .10 to .64.

Author: Elsberry, N. I.

Article: Comparison of two scales measuring attitudes toward persons with physical disabilities.

Journal: *Psychological Reports,* April 1975, *36*(2), 473–474.

Related Research: Siler, J. (1970). Generality of attitudes toward the physically disabled. *Proceedings: Annual convention of APA, 5,* Part II, 697–698.

■ ■ ■

1781

Test Name: DRUG ATTITUDE QUESTIONNAIRE

Purpose: To ascertain the

respondent's attitude toward the personal use of drugs.

Number of Items: 14

Format: Responses to each item involve agreeing or disagreeing on a 5-point scale. Scores range from 14 (conservative, anti-drug attitude) to 70 (liberal, pro-drug attitude).

Reliability: Split-half reliability of .84, .87.

Author: Hoffman, A. M., and Warner, R. W., Jr.

Article: A comparison of college students' and parents' attitudes toward the abuse of drugs.

Journal: *Journal of College Student Personnel,* September 1973, *14*(5), 430–433.

Related Research: Horan, J. J. (1972). *A reliability study of the drug education evaluation scale.* Unpublished manuscript, Pennsylvania State University.

■ ■ ■

1782

Test Name: EAST–WEST QUESTIONNAIRE

Purpose: To measure traditional Eastern and Western perspectives on reality and man-in-the-world.

Number of Items: 34 pairs of statements.

Format: Items are given and are rated on a 5-point Likert scale from 1 (*agree strongly*) to 5 (*disagree strongly*).

Reliability: Pearson correlation coefficient for test–retest after two weeks was .76.

Validity: The difference between the mean scores on the test of art and philosophy/religion students (54.77) and business majors (47.10) was statistically significant ($p < .0001$).

Author: Gilgen, A. R., and Cho, J. H.

Article: Questionnaire to measure eastern and western thought.

Journal: *Psychological Reports,* June 1979, *44*(3), 835–841.

Related Research: Cho, J. H., & Gilgen, A. R. (1980). Performance of Korean medical and nursing students on the East–West Questionnaire. *Psychological Reports, 47,* 1093–1094.

Gilgen, A. R., & Cho, J. H. (1980). Comparison of performance on the East–West Questionnaire, Zen Scale and Consciousness I, II and III Scales. *Psychological Reports, 47,* 583–588.

Gilgen, A. R., & Cho, J. H. (1979). Performance of Eastern and Western-oriented college students on the Value Survey and Ways of Life Scale. *Psychological Reports, 45,* 263–268.

■ ■ ■

1783

Test Name: EDUCATION ATTITUDE SURVEY

Purpose: To measure teachers' attitudes toward the mainstreaming of handicapped children into regular classrooms.

Number of Items: 16

Format: Response to each item is made on a 5-point Likert scale from *strongly agree* to *strongly disagree.*

Reliability: Test–retest reliability (2–3 week interval) was .70 (subscale I), .80 (subscale II), .85 (total); coefficient alpha was .83 (subscale I), .86 (subscale II), .90 (total).

Validity: Correlations with the Crowne-Marlowe Social Desirability Scale were –.02 (full scale), .01 (subscale I), and –.07 (subscale II).

Author: Reynolds, W. M., and Greco, V. T.

Article: The reliability and factorial validity of a scale for measuring teachers' attitudes towards mainstreaming.

Journal: *Educational and Psychological Measurement,* Summer 1980, *40*(2), 463–468.

■ ■ ■

1784

Test Name: EDUCATIONAL INNOVATION ATTITUDE SCALE

Purpose: To measure one's receptivity toward educational innovation.

Number of Items: 20

Format: Agree–disagree continuum.

Reliability: Test–retest stability reported is .81.

Author: O'Reilly, R. R., and Fish, J. C.

Article: Dogmatism and tenure status as determinants of resistance toward educational innovation.

Journal: *Journal of Experimental Education,* Fall 1976, *45*(1), 68–70.

Related Research: Ramer, B. (1967). *The relationship of belief systems and personal characteristics of chief school administrators and attitudes toward educational innovation.* Doctoral dissertation, State University of New York at Buffalo.

■ ■ ■

1785

Test Name: DRUG ATTITUDE SCALE

Purpose: To measure "adaptive attitudes toward the use of illegal drugs."

Number of Items: 14

Format: Likert items.

Reliability: Internal consistency was .9.

Author: Horan, J., et al.

Article: Drug Usage: An experimental comparison of three assessment conditions.

Journal: *Psychological Reports,* August 1974, *35*(1), 211–215.

Related Research: Horan, J. (1974). Outcome difficulties in drug education. *Review of Educational Research.* In press.

Swisher, J. D., et al. (1973). Four approaches to drug abuse prevention among college students. *Journal of College Student Personnel,* May, *14*(3), 231–235.

■ ■ ■

1786

Test Name: EDUCATIONAL WORK COMPONENTS STUDY

Purpose: To identify attitudes toward intrinsic-extrinsic job outcomes and risk orientations.

Number of Items: 56

Format: Likert items representing six factors: potential for personal challenge and development, competitiveness, desirability and reward of success, tolerance for work pressure, conservative security, willingness to seek reward in spite of uncertainty versus avoidance of uncertainty, and concern for hygienic aspects of the job. A second version referred to as "Work Components Study" is identified. Examples are presented.

Reliability: Cronbach's alpha coefficients as estimates of reliability ranged from .73 to .83 ($N = 683$).

Author: Miskel, C.

Article: Intrinsic, extrinsic, and risk propensity factors in the work attitudes of teachers, educational administrators, and business managers.

Journal: *Journal of Applied Psychology,* June 1974, *59*(3), 339–343.

Related Research: Miskel, C. G., & Heller, L. E. (1973). The educational work components study: An adapted set of measures for work motivation. *Journal of Experimental Education, 42,* 45–50.

■ ■ ■

1787

Test Name: ESTES ATTITUDE SCALE

Purpose: To measure reading attitude of secondary school students.

Number of Items: 20

Format: Consists of eight positive and twelve negative statements to which students respond on a 5-point scale indicating degree of agreement. High scores indicate positive attitudes toward books and reading. Examples are presented.

Validity: Pearson product–moment correlation coefficients with pupil self-rating scores ranged from .36 to .63 and with teacher-rating scores ranged from .33 to .40.

Author: Dulin, K. L., and Chester, R. D.

Article: A validation study of the Estes Attitude Scale.

Journal: *Journal of Reading,* October 1974, *18*(1), 56–59.

Related Research: Estes, T. H. (1971). A scale to measure attitudes toward reading. *Journal of Reading, 15*(2), 135–138.

■ ■ ■

1788

Test Name: FACULTY ORIENTATIONS STUDY

Purpose: To assess faculty attitudes regarding the nature,

purpose, and "process" of a college education.

Number of Items: 48

Format: Six scales (Achievement, Assignment Learning, Assessment, Inquiry, Independent Study, and Interaction) with 8 items per scale. Faculty respond to each item using a 4-point Likert scheme (1 = *strongly disagree*; 2 = *disagree*; 3 = *agree*; 4 = *strongly agree*).

Reliability: Scale internal consistency (coefficient alpha) estimates ranged from .69 to .89 with a median of .80.

Author: Morstain, B. R., and Smart, J. C.

Article: Educational orientations of faculty: Assessing a personality model of the academic professions.

Journal: *Psychological Reports,* December 1976, *39*(3), 1199–1211.

Related Research: Morstain, B. (1973). *The Faculty Orientations Survey: Technical Notes.* Newark: University of Delaware.

■ ■ ■

1789

Test Name: FEM SCALE

Purpose: To measure attitudes toward feminism.

Number of Items: 20

Format: A Likert format with responses ranging from *strongly agree* to *strongly disagree.* All items are presented.

Reliability: Based upon coefficient alpha, reliability was estimated at .91.

Validity: Correlation with Anti-Black Prejudice was –.462; with Dogmatism was –.506; with Identification with the Women's Movement was .638.

Author: Singleton, R., Jr., and Christiansen, J. B.

Article: The construct validation of

a shortform attitudes toward feminism scale.

Journal: *Sociology and Social Research,* April 1977, *61*(3), 294–303.

Related Research: Singleton, R., Jr., & Christiansen, J. B. (1977). The construct validation of a shortform attitudes toward feminism scale. *Sociology and Social Research, 61,* 3, 294–303.

Smith, E. R., et al. (1975). A short scale of attitudes toward feminism. *Social Psychology, 6,* 51–56.

■ ■ ■

1790

Test Name: FEMINISM SCALE

Purpose: To measure attitudes toward changing roles and status of women in the direction of equality with men.

Number of Items: 28

Format: Subject responds on a 4-point scale (*agree very much, agree a little, disagree a little, disagree very much*).

Reliability: Split-half reliability was .976 and parallel forms reliability of Forms A and B was .96. The stability coefficient over a short period of time was .95.

Author: Orcutt, M. A., and Walsh, W. B.

Article: Traditionality and congruence of career aspirations for college women.

Journal: *Journal of Vocational Behavior,* February 1979, *14*(1), 1–11.

Related Research: Dempewolff, J. (1974). Development and validation of a feminism scale, *Psychological Reports, 3*(2), 651–657.

Dempewolff, J. A. (1972). *Feminism and its correlates.* Unpublished doctoral dissertation, University of Cincinnati.

1791

Test Name: FEMINIST–
ANTIFEMINIST
BELIEF-PATTERN SCALE

Purpose: To measure attitudes toward women with respect to their involvement in economic, political, social, and domestic spheres.

Number of Items: 80

Reliability: Correlations with Attitudes Toward Women Scale are .87, .86, and .87.

Validity: Men scored more traditional than women ($p < .01$).

Author: Doyle, J. A.

Article: Comparison of Kirkpatrick's and Spence and Helmreich's Attitudes Toward Women Scale.

Journal: *Psychological Reports,* December 1975, *37*(3), 878.

Related Research: Kirkpatrick, C. (1936). The construction of a belief pattern scale for measuring attitudes toward feminism. *Journal of Social Psychology, 7,* 421–437.

■ ■ ■

1792

Test Name: GENERAL
INTOLERANCE SCALE

Purpose: To measure one's tolerance of other races.

Number of Items: 10

Format: Agree–disagree statements about racial practices.

Reliability: .65.

Author: Katz, P. A., et al.

Article: Perceptual concomitants of racial attitudes in urban grade-school children.

Journal: *Developmental Psychology,* March 1975, *11*(2), 135–144.

Related Research: Gough, H. G., et al. (1950). Children's ethnic attitudes: I. Relationship to certain personality factors. *Child Development, 21*, 83–90.

■ ■ ■

1793

Test Name: GLOBAL SELF
ATTITUDE SCALE

Purpose: To measure a student's global attitude toward self in positive or negative terms.

Number of Items: 6

Format: All items are presented.

Reliability: Coefficient of reproducibility was .90.

Author: Hunt, J. G., and Hunt, L. L.

Article: Racial inequality and self-image: Identity maintenance as identity diffusion.

Journal: *Sociology and Social Research,* July 1977, *61*(4), 539–559.

Related Research: Kaplan, H. B., & PoKorny, A. D. (1969). Self-derogation and psychosocial adjustment. *Journal of Nervous and Mental Disease, 149*, 421–434.

■ ■ ■

1794

Test Name: IMAGE OF SCIENCE
AND SCIENTISTS SCALE

Purpose: To assess high school students' attitudes toward science as a field of study.

Number of Items: 29

Format: Involves a 6-point Likert format.

Reliability: Coefficient alpha was .86.

Author: Smith, J. K., and Krajkovich, J. G.

Article: Validation of the image of science and scientists scale.

Journal: *Educational and Psychological Measurement,* Summer 1979, *39*(2), 495–498.

Related Research: Krajkovich, J. G. (1977). *The development of a science attitude instrument and an examination of the relationships among science attitude, field dependence-independence and science achievement.* Unpublished doctoral dissertation, Rutgers University.

■ ■ ■

1795

Test Name:
INTERNATIONALISM SCALE

Purpose: To measure one's degree of internationalism.

Number of Items: 18

Format: Nine pro-world-minded and nine anti-world-minded items that require a degree of agreement or disagreement on statements concerning immigration, race, education, patriotism, war, the United Nations, or some form of world government and foreign policy.

Reliability: Hoyt estimate of reliability for the Internationalism Scale (11 items) was .74 for the pretest (95 respondents) and .82 for the posttest (88 respondents).

Author: Marion, P. B.

Article: Relationships of student characteristics and experiences with attitude changes in a program of study abroad.

Journal: *Journal of College Student Personnel,* January 1980, *21*(1), 58–64.

Related Research: Lutzker, D. R. (1960). Internationalism as a predictor of cooperative behavior. *Journal of Conflict Resolution, 4,* 426–430.

Sampson, D. L., & Smith, H. P. (1957). A scale to measure worldminded attitudes. *Journal of Social Psychology, 45,* 99–106.

1796

Test Name: INTOLERANCE OF AMBIGUITY

Purpose: To measure one's attitude toward ambiguity.

Number of Items: 16

Format: Likert scale.

Reliability: The reliability of the scale is .49 using Cronbach's alpha (Budner, 1962).

Author: Keenan, A., and McBain, G. D. M.

Article: Effects of Type A behavior, intolerance of ambiguity and locus of control on the relationship between role stress and work-related outcomes.

Journal: *Journal of Occupational Psychology,* December 1979, *52*(4), 277–285.

Related Research: Budner, S. (1962). Intolerance of ambiguity as a personality variable. *Journal of Personality, 30,* 29–50.

■ ■ ■

1797

Test Name: LAW AND ORDER TEST

Purpose: To identify attitudes toward public policy issues.

Number of Items: 15

Format: Subjects indicate on a 5-point scale the degree to which they agree or disagree with each statement.

Reliability: Split-half reliability with Spearman-Brown correction was .89; test–retest correlation for 24 ninth graders was .74.

Validity: Correlation with Defining Issues Test (a measure of moral judgment) was –.23, Correlation with Comprehension of Social-Moral Tests was .12.

Author: Rest, J.

Article: Judging the important

issues in moral dilemmas—An objective measure of development.

Journal: *Developmental Psychology,* July 1974, *10*(4), 491–501.

■ ■ ■

1798

Test Name: LAW-RELATED ATTITUDES TEST

Purpose: To measure law-related attitudes of junior high school students.

Number of Items: 30

Format: A 5-point Likert format is used. Includes 5 dimensions. All items are presented.

Reliability: Alpha reliabilities ranged from .62 to .81.

Author: Fraser, B. J., and Smith, D. L.

Article: Assessment of law-related attitudes.

Journal: *Social Education,* May 1980, *44*(5), 406–409.

Related Research: Fraser, B. J. (1978). Evaluation of inquiry skills. *The Social Studies, 69,* 131–134.

■ ■ ■

1799

Test Name: LIBERTARIAN DEMOCRACY SCALE

Purpose: To study democratic political orientation attitudes.

Number of Items: 5

Format: The subject indicates endorsement on a 5-point scale from *strongly agree* to *strongly disagree*. Scores range from 5 to 25 with the maximum being the most libertarian.

Validity: Correlation with Defining Issues Test (a measure of moral judgment) was .37.

Author: Rest, J.

Article: Judging the important issues in moral dilemmas—An objective measure of development.

Journal: *Developmental Psychology,* July 1974, *10*(4), 491–501.

Related Research: Patrick, J. (1971). *Political education and democratic political orientations of ninth-grade students across four community types.* Unpublished manuscript, Indiana University.

■ ■ ■

1800

Test Name: LIFE STYLES FOR WOMEN

Purpose: To measure attitude towards women's life styles.

Number of Items: 20

Format: Subjects responded on a 5-point Likert scale from *strongly agree* to *strongly disagree*. Items are given in the article (e.g., "I would have a great deal of difficulty being a mother and housewife 24 hours a day").

Reliability: Cronbach's alpha was .829 (men), none reported for women.

Validity: Correlation with expressed interest in feminist activities was –.53 for women ($p < .01$).

Author: Burns, M.

Article: Life styles for women, an attitude scale.

Journal: *Psychological Reports,* August 1974, *35*(1), 227–230.

■ ■ ■

1801

Test Name: MENTAL HEALTH LOCUS OF ORIGIN SCALE

Purpose: To assess beliefs about the etiology of psychological problems.

Number of Items: 20

Format: Includes 13 endogenous and 7 interactional items. Employs a 6-point Likert format. All items are presented.

Reliability: Coefficient alpha was .76.

Validity: Correlation with Rotter's I-E Scale was .18. Correlation with the Mental Health Locus of Control Scale was .40.

Author: Hill, D. J., and Bale, R. M.

Article: Development of the Mental Health Locus of Control and Mental Health Locus of Origin Scales.

Journal: *Journal of Personality Assessment*, April 1980, *44*(2), 148–156.

■ ■ ■

1802

Test Name: MINNESOTA SCHOOL AFFECT ASSESSMENT

Purpose: To measure student attitudes toward school, including cooperation and competition.

Number of Items: 27

Format: Two parts: a series of five-level semantic differential questions and a series of four-level true–false items that were combined into composite scores on the basis of factor analysis.

Reliability: Pooled internal consistency reliability for cooperativeness is .72; for competitiveness, .82.

Author: Johnson, D. W., and Ahlgren, A.

Article: Relationship between student attitudes about cooperation and competition and attitudes toward schooling.

Journal: *Journal of Educational Psychology*, February 1976, *68*(1), 92–102.

Related Research: Johnson, D. W.

(1974). Evaluating affective outcomes of schools. In H. J. Walberg (Ed.), *Evaluating school performance*. Berkeley, CA: McCutchan.

■ ■ ■

1803

Test Name: MOTHER'S ATTITUDE TOWARD DEVIANCE

Purpose: To assess attitudinal tolerance of transgression with regard to both legal and moral norms.

Number of Items: 13

Format: Items include stealing, lying, aggression, drug use, drinking, and extramarital sex. Each item is rated on a 4-point scale of wrongfulness. Scores range from 0 to 39.

Reliability: Scott's homogeneity ratio was .26; Cronbach's alpha was .80.

Validity: With the Problem Behavior Index, –.42 (women), –.13 (men).

Author: Jessor, S. L., and Jessor, R.

Article: Maternal ideology and adolescent problem behavior.

Journal: *Developmental Psychology*, March 1974, *10*(2), 246–254.

■ ■ ■

1804

Test Name: MULTIFACTOR RACIAL ATTITUDE INVENTORY—REVISED

Purpose: To measure change in verbal racial attitude.

Number of Items: 12

Format: Subject responds to each item by rating the strength of agreement or disagreement. All items are presented.

Validity: Correlations of this shortened version with the 120-item full length inventory ranged from .862 to .934.

Author: Ard, N., and Cook, S. W.

Article: A short scale for the measurement of change in verbal racial attitude.

Journal: *Educational and Psychological Measurement,* Autumn 1977, *37*(3), 741–744.

Related Research: Brigham, J. C., et al. (1976). Dimensions of verbal racial attitudes: Interracial marriage and approaches to racial equality. *Journal of Social Issues, 32*, 9–21.

■ ■ ■

1805

Test Name: OPEN OFFICE OPINION INVENTORY

Purpose: To measure attitudes toward the visual layout, the noise level, the communication facility, perceived solidarity, job satisfaction, clarity of work space definition, and so forth.

Number of Items: 53

Format: Likert format includes six factors: greater job satisfaction, more effective communication, greater productivity, lack of auditory privacy, lack of personal privacy, and lack of confidentiality.

Reliability: Contingency coefficient was .72 ($N = 600$); test–retest contingency coefficient of C was .67 ($N = 28$, 24-day interval).

Validity: Overall measure of sampling adequacy was .90; index of factorial simplicity was .78.

Author: McCarrey, M. W., et al.

Article: Landscape office attitudes: Reflections of perceived degree of control over transactions with the environment.

Journal: *Journal of Applied*

Psychology, June 1974, *59*(3), 401–403.

• • •

1806

Test Name: OPINIONNAIRE ON POLITICAL INSTITUTIONS AND PARTICIPATION

Purpose: To measure six dimensions of the overall construct of political attitude.

Number of Items: 48

Format: Includes six subtests. A 5-point response scale is used at the secondary school level and a 3-point response scale is used at the elementary school level.

Reliability: Test–retest reliability was .78.

Author: Hepburn, M. A., and Napier, J. D.

Article: Development and initial validation of an instrument to measure political attitudes.

Journal: *Educational and Psychological Measurement,* Winter 1980, *40*(4), 1131–1139.

Related Research: Hepburn, M. (1979). Reforming political education in the schools: A systems approach. *Teaching Political Science, 6,* 430–450.

• • •

1807

Test Name: OPINIONS ABOUT MENTAL ILLNESS SCALE

Purpose: To determine attitudes toward mental illness.

Format: Includes five factors: (a) Authoritarianism, (b) Benevolence, (c) Mental Health Ideology, (d) Social Restrictiveness, (e) Interpersonal Etiology.

Reliability: Correlations (product–moment) among the scores on the factor scales ranged from −.26 to .88.

Author: Moore, G., and Castles, M. R.

Article: Intercorrelations among factors in Opinions About Mental Illness Scale in scores of nonpsychiatric nurses: Comparison with other studies.

Journal: *Psychological Reports,* December 1978, *43*(3), 876–878.

Related Research: Fracchia, J., et al. (1972). Comparison of intercorrelations of scale scores from the Opinions About Mental Illness Scale. *Psychological Reports, 30,* 149–150.

Koutrelakas, J., et al. (1978). Opinions about mental illness: A comparison of American and Greek professionals and laymen. *Psychological Reports, 43,* 915–923.

• • •

1808

Test Name: PARENT AS A TEACHER INVENTORY

Purpose: To measure critical aspects of a parent's attitudes and behavior that influence child development.

Number of Items: 50

Format: Five subtests of ten items each: creativity; frustration; control; play; teacher-learning. (A complete description of the subtests is given in reference.)

Reliability: .76 alpha coefficient.

Validity: The inventory was administered to 30 intact families. Afterwards the actual behaviors were observed. The correlation between expressed and observed behaviors was .66.

Author: Strom, R., and Slaughter, H.

Article: Measurement of childrearing expectations using the Parent as a Teacher Inventory.

Journal: *Journal of Experimental Education,* Summer 1978, *46*(4), 44–53.

Related Research: Strom, R., & Johnson, A. (1978). Assessment for parent education. *Journal of Experimental Education, 47*(1), 9–16.

• • •

1809

Test Name: PERSONAL ATTRIBUTE INVENTORY

Purpose: To measure one's attitudes toward various individuals and groups.

Number of Items: 100

Format: Fifty positive adjectives and 50 negative adjectives. Subjects check 30 which are most descriptive of a target individual or group.

Reliability: Test–retest correlation over 4 weeks was .83 for 50 college students.

Validity: Correlated .80 ($p < .001$) with responses on the "unfavorable" subscale of the Adjective Check List (Gough, 1952) and −.73 ($p < .001$) with responses on the "favorable" subscale.

Author: Parish, T. S., et al.

Article: The Personal Attribute Inventory as a self-concept scale: A preliminary report.

Journal: *Psychological Reports,* December 1977, *41*(3), 1141–1142.

Related Research: Gough, H. (1952). *The Adjective Check List.* Palo Alto, CA: Consulting Psychologists Press.

Parrish, T., et al. (1976). The Personal Attribute Inventory. *Perceptual and Motor Skills, 42,* 712–720.

Parish, T. S., & Eads, G. M. (1977). The Personal Attribute Inventory as a self-concept scale. *Educational and Psychological*

Measurement, 37(4), 1063–1067.

■ ■ ■

1810

Test Name: POLICEMEN'S ATTITUDES TOWARD CITIZENRY SCALE

Purpose: To measure policemen's attitudes toward citizenry.

Number of Items: 17

Format: Four subscales including Policemen's Views of Citizens' Support, General Faith in People, Police Defensive Posture, and Police Stereotype of Poor People.

Reliability: Internal subscale reliabilities were View of Citizen's Support, .751; Faith in People, .610; Defensive Posture, .733; Stereotyping of Poor People, .871.

Author: Aldag, R. J., et al.

Article: Some correlates of policemen's attitudes toward citizenry.

Journal: *Psychological Reports,* October 1976, *39*(2), 543–548.

Related Research: Kelly, R., et al. (1972). *The pilot police project in Washington, D.C.* Washington, DC: American Institutes for Research and U.S. Government Printing Office.

■ ■ ■

1811

Test Name: POP

Purpose: To measure attitude toward population control.

Number of Items: 30

Format: Likert scale with seven choices (*agree very strongly* to *disagree very strongly*).

Reliability: Spearman-Brown corrected, split-half reliability was .89. Test–retest reliability was .91 (time interval not determined).

Validity: Relationships of scale with age, sex, political preference,

religious affiliation were nonsignificant: relationship with number of children respondents expected to parent was significant, $r = -.48$; correlation with Social Attitude Scale was .46 ($p < .01$).

Author: McCutcheon, L.

Article: Development and validation of a scale to measure attitude toward population control.

Journal: *Psychological Reports,* June 1974, *34*(3), 1235–1242.

■ ■ ■

1812

Test Name: PRESCHOOL RACIAL ATTITUDE MEASURE II

Purpose: To assess racial attitudes in preliterate children.

Number of Items: 24 stories.

Format: Picture-story format in which the child chooses one of two human figures, one with pinkish-tan skin, and one with medium-brown skin, in response to a story containing either a positive or negative evaluative adjective.

Reliability: Test–retest reliability of .55 over a 1-year period.

Author: Boswell, D. A., and Williams, J. E.

Article: Correlates of race and color bias among preschool children.

Source: *Psychological Reports,* February 1975, *36*(1), 147–154.

Related Research: Williams, J. E., et al. (1975). The measurement of children's racial attitudes in the early school years. *Child Development, 46,* 494–500.

■ ■ ■

1813

Test Name: PRESCHOOL RACIAL ATTITUDE MEASURE II

Purpose: To measure racial attitude of first grade children.

Number of Items: 18

Format: Each item consists of an 8 x 10 color photograph which includes two figures. The 12 racial attitude pictures have identical figures except that one figure has brown skin, the other [has] pinkish-tan skin. The sex-role pictures have figures with identical skin and hair color, but one is a male, the other a female. Each picture is accompanied by a story and the subject points to the figure he or she thinks the story is about.

Reliability: Pre- and post-test reliability coefficients were approximately .70. Total reliability estimated to be .80.

Author: Singh, J. M., and Yancey, A. V.

Article: Racial attitudes in White first grade children.

Journal: *Journal of Educational Research,* April 1974, *67*(8), 370–372.

Related Research: Williams, J. E. (1971). *PRAM II* (Technical Report No. 1). Winston-Salem, NC: Wake Forest University, Department of Psychology.

■ ■ ■

1814

Test Name: PRESCHOOL RACIAL ATTITUDE MEASURE II

Purpose: To assess racial bias in pre-literate children.

Number of Items: 36

Format: Includes 36 pictures, 24 of which are used for racial attitudes and 12 for sex-role items.

Reliability: Internal consistency $r = .80$ (Spearman-Brown estimate). Test–retest reliability $r = .55$ (1-year interval).

Author: Williams, J. E., et al.

Article: Preschool Racial Attitude Measure II.

Source: *Educational and Psychological Measurement,* Spring 1975, *35*(1), 3–18.

Related Research: Williams, J. E. (1971). *Preschool Racial Attitude Measure II (PRAM II): General information and manual of directions.* Winston-Salem, NC: Wake Forest University, Department of Psychology.

• • •

1815

Test Name: PROFESSIONAL ATTITUDES SCALE

Purpose: To measure professional attitudes.

Number of Items: 20

Format: Seven-point Likert pattern ranging from *strongly agree* to *strongly disagree* covering five factors: Autonomy, Collegial Maintenance of Standards, Ethics, Professional Commitment, and Professional Identification.

Reliability: Corrected split-half reliabilities were .82 (Autonomy), .82 (Collegial Maintenance of Standards), .79 (Ethics), .75 (Professional Commitment), and .85 (Professional Identification).

Author: Bartol, K. M.

Article: Individual versus organizational predictors of job satisfaction and turnover among professionals.

Journal: *Journal of Vocational Behavior,* August 1979, *15*(1), 55–67.

Related Research: Hall, R. H. (1968). Professionalization and bureaucratization. *American Sociological Reviews, 33,* 92–104.

• • •

1816

Test Name: PROFESSIONALISM AND RESEARCH

ORIENTATION OF STUDENTS INVENTORY

Purpose: To assess attitudes toward professional preparation programs in college student personnel.

Number of Items: 48

Format: Twenty-six of the items comprise a research orientation (RO) scale. Examples of items are given.

Reliability: The RO scale reliability estimate (Cronbach's alpha) was .87.

Validity: The correlation between institutional RO scores and ratings of knowledge production and utilization activities of schools, colleges, and departments of education ($n = 687$) was .47 ($p < .05$).

Author: Kuh, G. D., et al.

Article: Research orientation of graduate students in college student personnel.

Journal: *Journal of College Student Personnel,* January 1979, *20*(1), 99–104.

• • •

1817

Test Name: PROTEST SITUATIONAL ATTITUDE SCALE

Purpose: To measure reactions to various types of protest behavior.

Number of Items: 33

Format: Nine protest situations and 2 due process items. Subjects respond to 3 bipolar semantic differential scales for each situation.

Reliability: Test–retest reliabilities ranged from .44 to .77. Communalities in principal-components factor analysis ranged from .60 to .89.

Validity: Correlations with subjects' previous protest

behavior resulted in 15 significant correlations ($p < .05$) ranging from .15 to .37.

Author: Hopple, G. W.

Article: A new scale for measuring college student attitudes toward protest.

Journal: *Journal of College Student Personnel,* May 1976, *17*(3), 211–214.

Related Research: Sedlacek, W. E., & Brooks, G. C. (1970). Measuring racial attitudes in a situational context. *Psychological Reports, 27,* 971–980.

• • •

1818

Test Name: PROVERBS TEST

Purpose: To measure attitudes toward curiosity-related behavior.

Number of Items: 42

Format: Pairs of proverbs, the subject checks which proverb is characteristic of his or her attitude.

Reliability: Index of stability over 2 weeks was .91.

Validity: Coefficients between Ontario Test of Intrinsic Motivation and the Proverbs Test: Ambiguity, .39; Complexity, .35; Novelty, .35; and Specific Curiosity, .39.

Author: Maw, W. H., et al.

Article: Contrasting proverbs as a measure of attitudes toward curiosity-related behavior of Black and White college students.

Journal: *Psychological Reports,* December 1976, *39*(3), 1229–1230.

Related Research: Maw, W. H., & Maw, E. W. (1975). Contrasting proverbs as a measure of attitudes of college students toward curiosity-related behaviors. *Psychological Reports, 37,* 1085–1086.

1819

Test Name: PUPIL CONTROL IDEOLOGY FORM

Purpose: To tap educators' views on pupil control on a humanistic-custodia continuum.

Number of Items: 20

Format: Likert device using a 5-point response scale ranging from *strongly agree* to *strongly disagree*.

Reliability: Split-half reliabilities are above .90.

Author: Brenneman, O. N., et al.

Article: Teacher self-acceptance, acceptance of others, and pupil control ideology.

Source: *Journal of Experimental Education*, Fall 1975, *44*(1), 14–17.

Related Research: Willower, D. J., et al. (1973). *The school and pupil control ideology* (2nd ed., Penn State Studies No. 24). University Park: Pennsylvania State University.

■ ■ ■

1820

Test Name: PUPIL OPINION QUESTIONNAIRE

Purpose: To measure attitude toward school.

Number of Items: 30

Format: Taps attitudes toward aspects of the school experience: teachers, school in general, school work, and peers. Employs a modified 4-point Likert scale.

Reliability: $r = .84$.

Validity: With Otis Quick-Scoring Mental Abilities Test and Form A, $r = -.01$; and Form B, $r = .07$; with California Reading Test Form W and Form A, $r = .03$, and Form B, $r = .10$; with Tennessee Self-Concept Scale and Form B, $r = .21$; and Form B, $r = -.34$.

Author: Thornburg, H. D.

Article: An investigation of a dropout program among Arizona's Minority Youth.

Journal: *Education*, February–March 1974, *94*(3), 249–265.

■ ■ ■

1821

Test Name: RADICALISM–CONSERVATISM INVENTORY

Purpose: To measure attitudes of radicalism–conservatism.

Number of Items: 20

Format: Likert scale.

Reliability: Hoyt estimate of reliability was .83 for the pretest (95 respondents) and .84 for the posttest (88 respondents).

Author: Marion, P. B.

Article: Relationships of student characteristics and experiences with attitude changes in a program of study abroad.

Journal: *Journal of College Student Personnel*, January 1980, *21*(1), 58–64.

Related Research: Christie, R., et al. (1969). *The new left and its ideology*. New York: Columbia University Press.

Nettler, G., & Huffman, J. (1957). Political opinion and personal security. *Sociometry, 20,* 51–66.

■ ■ ■

1822

Test Name: READING ATTITUDE INVENTORY

Purpose: To measure attitude toward reading for elementary school pupils.

Number of Items: 20

Format: Student responds to each item by indicating *yes, no, or sometimes*. All items are presented.

Reliability: Split-half reliability

coefficients were .75 ($N = 45$, grade 3), .69 ($N = 93$, grade 4), and .72 ($N = 76$, grade 5).

Validity: Correlation with teachers' ratings of apparent enthusiasm for reading was .33.

Author: Lewis, J.

Article: A reading attitude inventory for elementary school pupils.

Journal: *Educational and Psychological Measurement,* Summer 1979, *39*(2), 511–513.

■ ■ ■

1823

Test Name: READING ATTITUDE SURVEY

Purpose: To measure student attitude toward reading.

Number of Items: 35

Format: The maximum score possible was 140.

Validity: Correlations with the Nelson-Denny Reading Test, Form C were $r = .32$ and .63.

Author: Shannon, A. J.

Article: Effects of methods of standardized reading achievement test administration on attitude toward reading.

Journal: *Journal of Reading,* May 1980, *23*(8), 684–686.

Related Research: Kennedy, L. D., and Halinski, R. S. Measuring attitudes: An extra dimension. *Journal of Reading,* 1975, *18* (7), 518–522.

■ ■ ■

1824

Test Name: RHODY SECONDARY READING ATTITUDE ASSESSMENT

Purpose: To assess attitudes toward reading in the secondary schools.

Number of Items: 25

Format: Each item is answered on a 5-point scale from *stongly disagree* to *strongly agree*. All items are presented.

Reliability: Test–retest reliability was .84.

Author: Tullock-Rhody, R., and Alexander, J. E.

Article: A scale for assessing attitudes toward reading in secondary schools.

Journal: *Journal of Reading,* April 1980, *23*(7), 609–614.

Related Research: Rhody, R. (1978). *The development of a reading attitude instrument for grades seven through twelve.* Unpublished doctoral dissertation, University of Tennessee, Knoxville.

■ ■ ■

1825

Test Name: SCHOOL ATTITUDE SCALE

Purpose: To measure students' attitudes or feelings toward school.

Number of Items: 11

Format: Students make a *yes* or *no* response to each question. Examples are presented.

Reliability: Alpha reliability was .81.

Author: Sheenan, D. S.

Article: A study of attitude change in desegregated intermediate schools.

Journal: *Sociology of Education,* January 1980, *53*(1), 51–59.

Related Research: Vitale, M. (1974). *Evaluation of the Title III Dallas Junior High School Career Education Project: 1973–1974* (Research Report No. 74–291). Dallas, TX: Department of Research, Evaluation and Information Systems, Dallas Independent School District.

1826

Test Name: SCHOOL COUNSELOR ATTITUDE INVENTORY

Purpose: To measure attitudes on a continuum ranging from *status quo* to *change agent.*

Number of Items: 20

Format: Test consists of stems that present the respondent with the description of a client problem and six choices of counselor strategies for responding to that problem.

Reliability: Alpha generalization of the Kuder-Richardson formula 20 reliability coefficient of .75.

Author: Baker, S. B., and Slakter, M. J.

Article: Validity and reliability of the *School Counselor Attitude Inventory.*

Source: *Measurement and Evaluation in Guidance,* January 1975, *7*(4), 239–242.

Related Research: Baker, S. B., & Hansen, J. C. (1972). School counselor attitudes on a status quo-change agent measurement scale. *School Counselor, 19*(3), 243–248.

■ ■ ■

1827

Test Name: SCHOOL SURVEY

Purpose: To measure teachers' job-related attitudes.

Number of Items: 105

Format: Includes the following scales: administrative practices, professional work load, non-professional work load, materials and equipment, buildings and facilities, educational effectiveness, evaluation of students, special services, school-community relations, supervisory relations, colleague relations, voice in

educational program, performance and development, and financial incentives.

Validity: Correlations with the External Observation Instrument ranged from .07 to .29.

Author: Payne, D. A., et al.

Article: The development and validation of an observation instrument to assess competencies of school principals.

Journal: *Educational and Psychological Measurement,* Winter 1976, *36*(4), 945–952.

Related Research: Coughlan, R. J., & Cooke, R. A. (1974). Work attitudes. In H. J. Walberg (Ed.), *Evaluating educational performance.* Berkeley, CA: McCutchan.

■ ■ ■

1828

Test Name: SEAT BELT ATTITUDES AND BELIEFS QUESTIONNAIRE

Purpose: To measure attitudes and beliefs concerning seat belt usage.

Number of Items: 59

Format: Seven statements measured attitude to belt usage with respondents indicating on a five-step verbal scale their degree of agreement with each statement. Fifty-two Likert items measured beliefs about seat belts with respondents indicating their degree of agreement on the five-step verbal scale. Item content is presented for several items.

Validity: Correlation between attitude and reported use of seat belts was .56 ($N = 184$).

Author: Fhanér, G., and Hane, M.

Article: Seat belts: Relation between beliefs, attitude, and use.

Journal: *Journal of Applied Psychology,* August 1974, *59*(4), 472–482.

1829

Test Name: SEAT BELT BELIEFS SCALE

Purpose: To measure one's beliefs about the use of automobile seat belts, including the discomfort of seat belts and the effect of wearing them in a car crash.

Number of Items: 7

Format: Items are rated on 5-point Likert scales.

Reliability: Reliabilities in terms of homogeneity using Kuder-Richardson formula 20, .86 for discomfort and .68 for effect.

Author: Fhanér, G., and Hane, M.

Article: Seat belts: Changing usage by changing beliefs.

Source: *Journal of Applied Psychology*, October 1975, *60*(5), 589–598.

Related Research: Fhanér, G., & Hane, M. (1974). Seat belts: Relations between beliefs, attitude, and use. *Journal of Applied Psychology, 59*, 472–482.

■ ■ ■

1830

Test Name: SENTENCE COMPLETION QUESTIONNAIRE

Purpose: To measure attitudes toward authority.

Number of Items: 22

Format: Consists of stems dealing with authority and authority figures. Responses are categorized by judges into six categories: liking, submissive, fearful, disliking, self-assertive, and neutral.

Reliability: Hoyt's correlation of agreement between judges ranged from .83 for liking to .65 for self-assertive.

Author: Matteson, D. R.

Article: Changes in attitudes

toward authority figures with the move to college: three experiments.

Journal: *Developmental Psychology*, May 1974, *10*(3), 340–347.

Related Research: Lindgren, H., & Sallery, R. (1966). Arab attitudes toward authority: A cross-cultural study. *Journal of Social Psychology, 68*, 27–31.

■ ■ ■

1831

Test Name: SEX-ROLE ATTITUDE SCALE

Purpose: To differentiate youth with new and traditional sex-role attitudes.

Format: A Likert scale of 1–5 values.

Reliability: Kuder-Richardson reliability of .85.

Validity: All but one item differentiated male adolescents holding the new and traditional attitudes and all but one item differentiated the female adolescents ($p < .001$).

Author: Tarr, L. H.

Article: Developmental sex-role theory and sex-role attitudes in late adolescents.

Journal: *Psychological Reports*, June 1978, *42*(3), 807–814.

Related Research: Tarr, L. H. (1973). *The relationship of parental variables to sex role attitudes and identity in late adolescents.* Unpublished doctoral dissertation, Ohio State University.

■ ■ ■

1832

Test Name: SOCIAL AND EXISTENTIAL COURAGE SCALE

Purpose: To measure social and existential courage.

Number of Items: 50

Format: Likert response categories with 22 existential courage items and 28 social courage items.

Reliability: Split-half correlation coefficient corrected by the Spearman-Brown prophecy formula was .60 for the social items and .90 for the existential scale.

Validity: Correlation between the social and existential scales was .21 ($p < .05$).

Author: Larsen, K. S., and Giles, H.

Article: Survival or courage as human motivation: Development of an attitude scale.

Journal: *Psychological Reports*, August 1976, *39*(1), 299–302.

■ ■ ■

1833

Test Name: SUCCESS-FAILURE INVENTORY

Purpose: To measure attitudes toward the likelihood of success attainment relative to failure avoidance.

Number of Items: 22

Format: A true–false inventory yielding a difference score between overlapping success- and failure-keyed items.

Reliability: Internal consistency coefficient (odd-even) was .82.

Validity: Correlations with the Pleasant Events Schedule ranged from .29 to .55 ($N = 32$ males) and from .01 to .49 ($N = 42$ females).

Author: Cash, T. F., and Burns, D. S.

Article: The occurrence of reinforcing activities in relation to locus of control, success-failure expectancies, and physical attractiveness.

Journal: *Journal of Personality*

Assessment, August 1977, *41*(4), 387–391.

Related Research: McReynolds, P., & Guevara, C. (1967). Attitudes of schizophrenics and normals toward success and failure. *Journal of Abnormal Psychology, 72,* 303–310.

■ ■ ■

1834

Test Name: THE SEXES: AN ATTITUDE INVENTORY

Purpose: To measure feminist and nonfeminist attitudes.

Number of Items: 40

Format: Seven-point Likert scale to indicate level of agreement or disagreement.

Reliability: Retest reliability coefficient of .84 for 60 students after eight weeks. Internal consistency alpha coefficients (Hoyt, 1941): total, .89; civil rights, .66; marriage, .79; sex roles, .75; and male chauvinism, .76.

Author: McClain, E.

Article: Feminists and nonfeminists: Contrasting profiles in independence and affiliation.

Journal: *Psychological Reports,* October 1978, *43*(2), 435–441.

Related Research: Hoyt, C. J. (1941). Test reliability estimated by analysis of variance. *Psychometrika, 6,* 153–160.

■ ■ ■

1835

Test Name: THUMIN CONSERVATISM–LIBERALISM SCALE

Purpose: To assess liberalism of political viewpoint in college students.

Number of Items: 25

Format: Items scored on scale 1–4.

Validity: When nonstudents were compared with students they were relatively more conservative.

Author: Wildman, R., and Wildman, R.

Article: Liberalism of college students and general public on the Thumin Conservatism-Liberalism Scale.

Journal: *Psychological Reports,* August 1974, *35*(1), 441–442.

Related Research: Thumin, F. (1972). The relation of liberalism to sex, age, academic field and college grades. *Journal of Clinical Psychology, 28,* 160–164.

■ ■ ■

1836

Test Name: UNION ATTITUDE QUESTIONNAIRE

Purpose: To measure attitudes about unions.

Number of Items: 98

Format: Responses were made on a 5-point scale from 1 (*strongly agree*) to 5 (*strongly disagree*).

Reliability: Coefficient alphas ranged from .73 to .92.

Author: Gordon, M. E., et al.

Article: Commitment to the union: Development of a measure and an examination of its correlates.

Journal: *Journal of Applied Psychology Monograph,* August 1980, *65*(4), 479–499.

Related Research: Uphoff, W. H., & Dunnette, M. D. (1956). *Understanding the union member.* Minneapolis: University of Minnesota Press.

■ ■ ■

1837

Test Name: UNION ATTITUDE SCALE

Purpose: To measure affective attitude toward unions in general.

Number of Items: 20

Reliability: Coefficient alpha was .88.

Validity: Correlation with voting for union was .51.

Author: Schriesheim, C. A.

Article: Job satisfaction, attitudes toward unions, and voting in a union representation election.

Journal: *Journal of Applied Psychology,* October 1978, *63*(5), 548–552.

Related Research: Uphoff, W. H., & Dunnette, M. D. (1956). *Understanding the union member.* Minneapolis: University of Minnesota, Industrial Relations Center.

■ ■ ■

1838

Test Name: WOMEN AS MANAGERS SCALE

Purpose: To measure one's attitudes toward women as managers.

Number of Items: 21 statements.

Format: Response alternatives range from *strongly agree* to *strongly disagree.*

Reliability: Split-half reliability was .91.

Author: Herbert, T. T., and Yost, E. B.

Article: Faking study of scores on the Women as Managers Scale.

Journal: *Psychological Reports,* April 1978, *42*(2), 677–678.

Related Research: Gackenbach, J. (1978). The effect of race, sex and career goal differences on sex role attitudes at home and at work. *Journal of Vocational Behavior, 12*(1), 93–101.

Garland, H., & Price, K. H. (1977). Attitudes toward women in management and attributions for their success and failure in a managerial position. *Journal of Applied Psychology, 62*(1), 29–33.

Peters, L. H., et al. (1974). Women as Managers Scale (WAMS): A measure of attitudes toward women in management positions. *JSAS Catalog of Selected Documents in Psychology, 4,* 27(Ms. No. 585).

CHAPTER 7
Behavior

1839

Test Name: ACTIVATION–DEACTIVATION ADJECTIVE CHECKLIST

Purpose: To rate one's momentary states of activation or arousal.

Number of Items: 50 adjectives.

Format: Subject checks those adjectives that apply to himself or herself.

Reliability: Test–retest reliability coefficients for an immediate retest with a short form ranged from .66 to .96. Factor analysis transformations yielded an average coefficient of .71.

Author: Thayer, R. E.

Article: Factor analytic and reliability studies on the Activation–Deactivation Adjective Check List.

Journal: *Psychological Reports,* June 1978, *42*(3), 747–756.

Related Research: Thayer, R. E. (1978). Toward a psychological theory of multidimensional activation (arousal). *Motivation and Emotion, 2,* 1–34.

• • •

1840

Test Name: AGGRESSION ASSESSMENT SCALE

Purpose: To determine a child's level of aggression on the basis of peer reports.

Number of Items: 15

Format: Each child in the class indicated which child best fit each question. All items are presented.

Reliability: Temporal stability, *r* = .82.

Validity: Correlations with preference for aggression–conducive activities ranged from .17 to .36.

Author: Bullock, D., and Merrill, L.

Article: The impact of personal preference on consistency through time: The case of childhood aggression.

Journal: *Child Development,* September 1980, *51*(3), 808–814.

Related Research: Lefkowitz, M. M., et al. (1977). *Growing up to be violent. A longitudinal study of the development of aggression.* New York: Pergamon.

• • •

1841

Test Name: ART AND MUSIC ACTIVITIES SCALE

Purpose: To identify student participation in artistic endeavors and their attitudes toward art and music.

Number of Items: 17

Format: Includes items of how often students participate in various kinds of artistic activities, self-ratings of capability in the arts and enjoyment of artistic activities, the value of artistic experiences, and so forth.

Validity: Correlation with art achievement for 5th graders was .27; for 11th graders it was .38; music achievement for 5th graders was .36, for 11th graders it was .43; mathematics (Comprehensive Test of Basic Skills) for 5th graders was .15, for 11th graders it was .06; socio-economic status

for 5th graders was .27, and for 11th graders it was .23.

Author: Ellison, R. L., et al.

Article: Using biographical information in identifying artistic talent.

Journal: *The Gifted Child Quarterly,* Winter 1976, *20*(4), 402–413.

Related Research: Ellison, R. L., et al. (1975). *Utah statewide educational assessment: General report.* Salt Lake City: Utah State Board of Education.

• • •

1842

Test Name: BAKKER ASSERTIVENESS–AGGRESSIVENESS INVENTORY

Purpose: To measure the probability of both assertive responding and aggressive behavior.

Number of Items: 36

Format: Includes two subscales: one of assertiveness items, the other of aggressiveness items. All items are presented.

Reliability: Test–retest reliability: Pearson product–moment correlation coefficients were .75 (assertiveness) and .88 (aggressiveness). Split-half reliability coefficients were .58 (assertiveness) and .67 (aggressiveness).

Validity: Assertiveness correlated with age, .146; with income, .067; with occupation, −.039; with education, −.110. Aggressiveness correlated with age, −.037; with income, −.032; with occupation, −.249; and with education, −.277.

Author: Bakker, C. B., et al.

Article: The measurement of assertiveness and aggressiveness.

Journal: *Journal of Personality Assessment,* June 1978, *42*(3), 277–284.

■ ■ ■

1843

Test Name: BEHAVIOR CHECKLIST

Purpose: To measure aggressive behavior.

Number of Items: 10

Format: Includes ten examples of aggressive behavior. Counselors check those items the student engaged in during the past 7 days.

Validity: Correlation with a behavior rating scale was .75 and with the Thematic Apperception Test was −.085 (*n* = 76).

Author: Matranga, J. T.

Article: The relationship between behavioral indices of aggression and hostile content on the TAT.

Journal: *Journal of Personality Assessment,* April 1976, *40*(2), 130–134.

Related Research: Mussen, P. H., & Naylor, H. K. (1954). The relationship between overt and fantasy aggression. *Journal of Abnormal and Social Psychology, 49*, 235–240.

■ ■ ■

1844

Test Name: BEHAVIOR-PROBLEM CHECKLIST

Purpose: To identify frequently occurring problem behavior traits in children and adolescents.

Number of Items: 55

Format: Employs a three-point

rating for each trait.

Reliability: Interjudge correlations ranged from .50 to .77.

Validity: Correlation with minor physical anomalies were: for males (*N* = 50) .42; for females (*N* = 50) .24.

Author: Halverson, C. F., Jr., and Victor, J. B.

Article: Minor physical anomalies and problem behavior in elementary school children.

Journal: *Child Development,* March 1976, *47*(1), 281–285.

Related Research: Grieger, R. M., & Richards, H. C. (1976). Prevalence and structure of behavior symptoms among children in special education and regular classroom settings. *Journal of School Psychology, 14*, 27–38.

Quay, H. C., et al. (1966). Some correlates of personality disorder and conduct disorder in a child guidance clinic sample. *Psychology in the Schools, 3,* 44–47.

■ ■ ■

1845

Test Name: BEHAVIOR RATING FORM

Purpose: To measure behaviors "assumed to be an external manifestation of the person's prevailing self-appraisal" (Coopersmith, 1967, p. 11).

Number of Items: 13

Format: Five-point *always* to *never* response format.

Reliability: Test–retest reliability over an 8-week period was reported by Coopersmith to be .96 (p. 11).

Author: Cox, W. D., and Matthews, C. O.

Article: Parent group education: What does it do for the children?

Journal: *Journal of School Psychology,* 1977, *15*(4), 358–361.

Related Research: Coopersmith, S. (1967). *The antecedents of self-esteem.* San Francisco, CA: Freeman.

■ ■ ■

1846

Test Name: BEHAVIORAL STYLE QUESTIONNAIRE

Purpose: To measure temperament dimensions in 3–7 year olds.

Number of Items: 100

Format: Each item is a behavior description rated for frequency on a 6-point scale ranging from *almost never* to *almost always.*

Reliability: Test–retest reliability was .89. Internal consistency ranged from .48 to .80 for temperament categories and .84 for the total instrument.

Validity: Correlations with the Teacher Temperament Questionnaire ranged from .18 to .46. Correlations with behavior observations ranged from .33 to −.33.

Author: Billman, J., and McDevitt, S. C.

Article: Convergence of parent and observer ratings of temperament with observations of peer interaction in nursery school.

Journal: *Child Development,* June 1980, *51*(2), 395–400.

Related Research: McDevitt, S. C., & Carey, W. B. (1978). The measurement of temperament in 3–7 year old children. *Journal of Child Psychology and Psychiatry, 19*, 245–253.

■ ■ ■

1847

Test Name: BELIEFS-ABOUT-BEHAVIOR INVENTORY

Purpose: To assess *extent* of three conceptual approaches to understanding behavior in mental health professionals.

Number of Items: 40

Format: Three conceptual bases for understanding behavior are theology, illness, and psychology; forced-choice inventory.

Validity: When various population groups were compared on the theological scale, the scale failed to differentiate between them unless degrees of conservatism and liberalism were taken into consideration.

Author: Strunk, O., and Larsen, J.

Article: Variability within the theological concept of behavior of the Beliefs about Behavior Inventory.

Journal: *Psychological Reports,* August 1974, *35*(1), 432–434.

Related Research: Shaw, W. (1971). The development of a measure of three conceptual models of behavior. *Canadian Journal of Behavioral Science, 3,* 37–46.

● ● ●

1848

Test Name: BLAKE-MOUTON CONFLICT INSTRUMENT

Purpose: To determine one's mode of handling conflict.

Number of Items: 5 statements.

Format: Each statement describes one mode of handling conflict. Subjects select the single statement which best describes them.

Reliability: Test–retest reliabilities ranged from .14 to .57 for 5 modes with a mean of .39.

Validity: Correlates from –.07 to .37 with Lawrence-Lorsch, .13 to .49 with Hall, and .09 to .59 with Thomas-Kilmann.

Author: Thomas, K. W., and Kilmann, R. H.

Article: Comparison of four instruments measuring conflict behavior.

Journal: *Psychological Reports,* June 1978, *42*(3), 1139–1145.

Related Research: Blake, R. R., & Mouton, J. S. (1964). *The managerial grid.* Houston, TX: Gulf Publications.

Hall, J. (1969). *Conflict management survey: A survey of one's characteristic reaction to and handling of conflicts between himself and others.* Conroe, TX: Teleometrics International.

Thomas, K. W., & Kilmann, R. H. (1974). *Thomas-Kilmann conflict mode instrument.* Tuxedo, NY: Xicom.

● ● ●

1849

Test Name: BRAZELTON NEONATAL BEHAVIORAL ASSESSMENT SCALE

Purpose: To provide neonatal behavioral assessment.

Format: Includes 19 variables.

Reliability: Interrater reliability ranged from .89 to .99.

Validity: Correlations between Brazelton assessments and infant behavior ranged from –.59 to .70.

Author: Osofsky, J. D., and Danzger, B.

Article: Relationships between neonatal characteristics and mother–infant interaction.

Journal: *Developmental Psychology,* January 1974, *10*(1), 124–130.

Related Research: Brazelton, T. B. (1972). *Neonatal behavioral assessment scale.* Unpublished manuscript, Harvard University.

● ● ●

1850

Test Name: BROOKOVER'S SELF-CONCEPT OF ABILITY SCALE

Purpose: To assess behavior in which one indicates to himself (publicly or privately) his ability to achieve in academic tasks as compared with others engaged in the same task (Brookover et al., 1967, p. 8).

Number of Items: 8

Reliability: Coefficient alpha internal consistency reliability was .83.

Validity: Pearson product–moment correlations behavior scores on the scale and grade point average was .58 ($p < .001$) and between the scale and final examination scores was .26 ($p < .005$).

Author: Griffore, R. J., and Samuels. D. D.

Article: Self-concept of ability and college students' academic achievement.

Journal: *Psychological Reports,* August 1978, *43*(1), 37–38.

Related Research: Brookover, W., et al. (1967). *Self-concept of ability and school achievement: III* (Final Report of Cooperative Research Project No. 2831, U.S. Office of Education). East Lansing: Michigan State University, Human Learning Research Institute.

● ● ●

1851

Test Name: CALIFORNIA CHILD Q-SET

Purpose: To describe the child's behavior and psychological characteristics.

Number of Items: 100

Format: Q-sort format.

Reliability: Correlations between teachers ranged from .53 to .74.

Author: Arend, R., et al.

Article: Continuity of individual adaptation from infancy to kindergarten: A predictive study of ego-resiliency and curiosity in preschoolers.

Journal: *Child Development,* December 1979, *50*(4), 950–959.

Related Research: Block, J. (1971). *Lives through time.* Berkeley, CA: Bancroft.

■ ■ ■

1852

Test Name: CHILD STIMULUS SCREENING SCALE

Purpose: To measure the degree to which an individual automatically and selectively responds to stimulation.

Number of Items: 46

Format: Half the items are positively worded and half are negatively worded. Mothers respond to each item on a 9-point scale ranging from +14 (*very strong agreement*) to –4 (*very strong disagreement*).

Reliability: Kuder-Richardson formula 20 reliability coefficient was .92.

Author: Mehrabian, A., and Falender, C. A.

Article: A questionnaire measure of individual differences in child stimulus screening.

Journal: *Educational and Psychological Measurement,* Winter 1978, *38*(4), 1119–1127.

Related Research: Mehrabian, A. (1976). *Manual for the questionnaire measure of stimulus screening and arousability.* Los Angeles: University of California.

■ ■ ■

1853

Test Name: CHILDREN'S REINFORCEMENT SURVEY SCHEDULE

Purpose: To identify positive stimuli which maintain children's behavior.

Number of Items: 55 and 80

Time Required: 20 minutes for Forms A and B; 35 minutes for Form C.

Format: Forms A and B (55 items) are for the early elementary grades and use a Likert scale from *dislike* to *like* to *like very much.* Form C (80 items) is for the upper elementary grades and uses multiple-choice and open-ended questions.

Reliability: Test–retest correlations following 3 weeks ranged from .48 to .72 for all scales (*p* < .02).

Author: Cautela, J. R., and Brion-Meisels, L.

Article: A Children's Reinforcement Schedule.

Journal: *Psychological Reports,* February 1979, *44*(1), 327–338.

Related Research: Cautela, J. R., & Kastenbaum, R. A. (1967). Reinforcement survey schedule for use in therapy, training and research. *Psychological Reports, 20,* 1115–1130.

■ ■ ■

1854

Test Name: CLASSROOM BEHAVIOR INVENTORY

Purpose: To assess task-oriented behavior versus distractibility, hostility versus considerateness, and extroversion versus introversion child behavior.

Number of Items: 18

Time Required: 2 or 3 minutes.

Format: Teachers rate students.

Reliability: Inter-rater reliabilities ranged from .52 to .69 for factor scores and .58 to .79 for algebraically summed raw scores. Stability coefficients based on algebraically summed raw scores for individual factors ranged from .65 to .88. Internal consistency (Cronbach's coefficient alpha) for

individual factors ranged from .71 to .95.

Author: Ryckman, D. B., and Mirante, T. J.

Article: Reliabilities of Schaefer's Classroom Behavior Inventory.

Journal: *Psychological Reports,* December 1977, *41*(3), 1054.

Related Research: Mirante, T. J., & Ryckman, D. B. (1974). Classroom Behavior Inventory: Factor verification. *Journal of Research in Personality, 8,* 291–293.

■ ■ ■

1855

Test Name: CLASSROOM BEHAVIOR RATING SCALE

Purpose: To measure learning-related classroom behaviors.

Number of Items: 40

Format: A Likert scale format is used. Sample items are presented.

Reliability: Cronbach's coefficient alpha was .98.

Validity: Correlations with the Metropolitan Achievement Test ranged from .65 to .87.

Author: Reynolds, W. M.

Article: Development and validation of a scale to measure learning-related classroom behaviors.

Journal: *Educational and Psychologial Measurement,* Winter 1979, *39*(4), 1011–1018.

■ ■ ■

1856

Test Name: COLLEGE CRITERIA QUESTIONNAIRE

Purpose: To describe dimensions of college student performance.

Number of Items: 67

Format: Includes five academic

and eight nonacademic common factors. Responses to each item are made on a 7-point scale. Examples are presented.

Reliability: Median commonality was .50 for the most successful students and .60 for the least successful students.

Validity: Correlations with: SAT-V ranged from −.23 to .29; with SAT-M ranged from −.10 to .29; with Academic rating ranged from −.22 to .29; and with GPA ranged from −.14 to .39.

Author: Taber, T. D., and Hackman, J. D.

Article: Dimensions of undergraduate college performance.

Journal: *Journal of Applied Psychology,* October 1976, *61*(5), 546–558.

■ ■ ■

1857

Test Name: CONFLICT RESOLUTION INVENTORY

Purpose: To measure refusal behavior, a single response class of assertion.

Format: The inventory has a face sheet containing eight global items of which two (Items 7 and 8) are used for screening and a separate section containing 35 specific refusal items that can be used both for screening and the measurement of change.

Reliability: Test–retest reliabilities for three of the four variables used for screening, the assertion score, nonassertion score, and global difficulty in saying "no" (face sheet item 7) were .83, .70, and .56 (*p* < .001), respectively.

Author: Galassi, J. P., et al.

Article: The Conflict Resolution Inventory: Psychometric data.

Journal: *Psychological Reports,* April 1978, *42*(2), 492–494.

Related Research: McFall, R. M., & Lillesand, D. B. (1971). Behavior rehearsal with modeling and coaching in assertion training. *Journal of Abnormal Psychology,* 77, 313–323.

■ ■ ■

1858

Test Name: DRUG KNOWLEDGE, USE, AND ATTITUDE QUESTIONNAIRE

Purpose: To measure drug information, drug use, and attitudes relating to drug use.

Format: Includes three parts: Part 1 asks for self-report of the present and past use of seven classes of drugs; Part 2 measures worry about drugs, the span of drug-related deviance, and drug-related alienation; Part 3 measures the subject's knowledge of the pharmacology, psychological effects, and legal implications of drug use.

Reliability: Part 1 test–retest reliability was .86. Part 2 test–retest reliability was .61, .81, .88; Kuder-Richardson formula was .79, .80, .92. Part 3 test–retest reliability was .85; Kuder-Richardson formula was .96.

Validity: Part 2 with reported use correlation ranged from −.48 to + 20.

Author: Stuart, R. B.

Article: Teaching facts about drugs: Pushing or preventing.

Journal: *Journal of Educational Psychology,* April 1974, *66*(2), 189–201.

Related Research: Stuart, R. B., & Schuman, M. C. (1972). *Tripping and toking in mid-America: A survey of teenage drug abuse in four Michigan communities.* Lansing, MI: Office of Drug Abuse and Alcoholism.

1859

Test Name: FOCUSING TEST

Purpose: To measure the degree to which people can use their emotional experience facilitatively.

Number of Items: 9

Format: Rate the items on a scale from 1 (*definitely did not focus*) to 4 (*definitely did focus*).

Reliability: Interrater reliability of ratings, *r* = .90 (*p* < .01).

Author: Bohart, A. C.

Article: Role playing and interpersonal-conflict reduction.

Journal: *Journal of Counseling Psychology,* January 1977, *24*(1), 15–24.

Related Research: Gendlin, E. T. (1969). Focusing. *Psychotherapy: Theory Research and Practice, 6,* 4–14.

■ ■ ■

1860

Test Name: GROUP INCIDENTS QUESTIONNAIRE

Purpose: To measure skills relevant to leading process groups.

Number of Items: 15

Format: Respondents read each incident, imagine they are leading the group, and rank order the proposed interventions by indicating the response they prefer with a plus (+) and the response they like least with a minus (−).

Reliability: Item-total score correlations ranged from .23 to .54; internal consistency alpha coefficient was .80; test–retest reliability for 35 undergraduate psychology students over 2 weeks was .76.

Validity: Median rankings of trainees correlated .70 with total scores at the end of training.

Author: Stokes, J. P., and Tait, R. C.

Article: The Group Incidents Questionnaire: A measure of skill in group facilitation.

Journal: *Journal of Counseling Psychology*, May 1979, *26*(3), 250–254.

∎∎∎

1861

Test Name: HOSPITAL BEHAVIOR RATING SCALE

Purpose: To measure a patient's reaction to his or her physical illness and hospitalization as judged by others from observations of his or her behavior.

Number of Items: 29

Format: Patient's behavior is described on a 5-point scale, together with 3 adverb check lists that describe the way the patient talks about the illness, about the medical and nursing care he or she is receiving, and about his or her possible death.

Reliability: Split-half reliabilities range from .87 to .92.

Validity: Validity by the known-groups method resulted in significant differences ($p < .001$).

Author: Smith, W. J., and Apfeldorf, M.

Article: Scales which measure behavioral reactions to illness during hospitalization and attitudes toward hospitals.

Source: *Psychological Reports*, June 1975, *36*(3), 719–724.

∎∎∎

1862

Test Name: INPATIENT BEHAVIORAL RATING SCALE

Purpose: To record daily nursing observations of mood and behavior of patients in a clinical setting.

Number of Items: 26

Format: Optical scan sheet on which observer records behavior along an 8-point continuum (0 = *not present*; 1, 2 = *mild*; 3, 4, 5 = *moderate*; 6, 7 = *severe*).

Reliability: Reliability estimate based on an average of four raters is .50 and on most items above .80.

Author: Green, R. A., et al.

Article: The Inpatient Behavioral Rating Scale: A 26-item scale for recording nursing observations of patients' mood and behavior.

Journal: *Psychological Reports*, April 1977, *40*(2), 543–549.

Related Research: Wyatt, R. J., & Kupfer, D. J. (1968). A fourteen-symptom behavior and mood rating scale for longitudinal patient evaluation by nurses. *Psychological Reports, 23*, 1331–1334.

∎∎∎

1863

Test Name: INTERPERSONAL AND ADMINISTRATIVE BEHAVIOR SCALE

Purpose: To measure the interpersonal and administrative behavior of college head residents.

Number of Items: 58

Format: Subjects check the frequency of head resident behavior on a 4-point Likert scale.

Reliability: Test–retest reliability was .82 for the person-oriented items and .88 for the management-oriented items.

Author: Hutchins, D. E., et al.

Article: A comparison of undergraduate and professionally trained head residents.

Journal: *Journal of College Student Personnel*, November 1976, *17*(6), 510–513.

Related Research: Riker, H. C., & DeCoster, D. A. (1971). The educational role in college student housing. *Journal of College Student Housing, 1*, 3–6.

∎∎∎

1864

Test Name: INTERVIEW RATING SCALE

Purpose: To measure critical interview behaviors.

Number of Items: 23 specific critical interview behaviors.

Format: Five-point classification range.

Reliability: Coefficients of concordance of .95 for the pretest total rating score and .83 for the posttest total rating score.

Author: Speas, C. M.

Article: Job-seeking interview skills training: A comparison of four instructional techniques.

Journal: *Journal of Counseling Psychology*, September 1979, *26*(5), 405–412.

Related Research: Venardos, M. G., & Harris, M. B. (1973). Job interview training with rehabilitation clients: A comparison of videotape and role-playing procedures. *Journal of Applied Psychology, 58*, 365–367.

∎∎∎

1865

Test Name: LAWRENCE-LORSCH CONFLICT INSTRUMENT

Purpose: To determine one's mode of handling conflict.

Number of Items: 25 proverbs.

Format: Subjects rate each proverb on the extent to which it describes their own approach to disagreements. Response categories ranged from 1 (*not at all—this behavior never occurs*) to 5 (*to a very great extent—this*

behavior usually occurs).

Reliability: Test–retest reliabilities ranged from .33 to .63 for five modes of handling conflicts. Internal consistency reliabilities ranged from .39 to .73.

Validity: Correlates from –.07 to .37 with Blake-Mouton, from .02 to .47 with Hall, and from .02 to .35 with Thomas-Kilmann.

Author: Thomas, K. W., and Kilmann, R. H.

Article: Comparison of four instruments measuring conflict behavior.

Journal: *Psychological Reports,* June 1978, *42*(3), 1139–1145.

Related Research: Hall, J. (1967). *Conflict management survey: A survey on one's characteristic reaction to and handling of conflicts between himself and others.* Conroe, TX: Teleometrics International.

Lawrence, P. R., & Lorsch, J. W. (1967). *Organization and environment.* Boston: Harvard University, Graduate School of Business Administration.

Thomas, K. W., & Kilmann, R. H. (1974). *Thomas-Kilmann conflict mode instrument.* Tuxedo, NY: XICOM.

■ ■ ■

1866

Test Name: LEADER BEHAVIOR RATING SCALE

Purpose: To rate leader behavior.

Number of Items: 25

Format: Includes areas: support, goal emphasis, work facilitation, interaction facilitation, planning and coordination, upward interaction, and confidence and trust.

Reliability: Alphas ranged from .47 to .81.

Author: Butler, M. C., and Jones, A. P.

Article: Perceived leader behavior, individual characteristics, and injury recurrence in hazardous work environments.

Journal: *Journal of Applied Psychology,* June 1979, *64*(3), 299–304.

Related Research: Jones, A. P., et al. (1975). Perceived leadership behavior and employee confidence in the leader as moderated by job involvement. *Journal of Applied Psychology, 60,* 146–149.

■ ■ ■

1867

Test Name: LEARNING FOCUS INVENTORY

Purpose: To assess the relative student-centeredness of junior high and middle school teachers.

Number of Items: 16

Format: A semantic differential with a 7-point scale.

Reliability: Internal consistency reliability coefficient was .83.

Validity: Correlation with principals' judgments was .47.

Author: Clasen, R. E., and Bowman, W. E.

Article: Toward a student-centered learning focus inventory for junior high and middle school teachers.

Journal: *Journal of Educational Research,* September 1974, *68*(1), 9–11.

■ ■ ■

1868

Test Name: LEARNING TASKS SCALE

Purpose: To determine the types of tasks high school students engage in.

Number of Items: 17

Format: Subjects respond, on a 5-point scale, the extent to which their class engages in various types of tasks.

Reliability: Odd–even reliability for simple tasks, .94; for complex abstract tasks, .92; interactional tasks, .96; and self-expression tasks, .92.

Author: Gosenpud, J.

Article: A learning task classification scheme.

Journal: *Journal of Experimental Education,* Fall 1978, *47*(1), 67–75.

■ ■ ■

1869

Test Name: MATTHEWS YOUTH TEST FOR HEALTH (MYTH-FORM O)

Purpose: To enable the classroom teacher to assess Type A behavior in children.

Number of Items: 17

Format: For each item the teacher indicates how characteristic the item is of the child by using a 5-point scale from 1 (*extremely uncharacteristic*) to 5 (*extremely characteristic*). All items are presented.

Reliability: Correlations ranged from .64 to .86. Cronbach's alpha ranged from .88 to .90.

Author: Matthews, K. A., and Angulo, J.

Article: Measurement of the Type A behavior pattern in children: Assessment of children's competitiveness, impatience–anger, and aggression.

Journal: *Child Development,* June 1980, *51*(2), 466–475.

Related Research: Glass, D. C. (1977). *Behavior patterns, stress, and coronary disease.* Hillsdale, NJ: Erlbaum.

1870

Test Name: MISSOURI CHILDREN'S BEHAVIOR CHECKLIST

Purpose: To rate children's behavior.

Number of Items: 70

Format: The ratings can be converted into behavioral scores in aggression, activity level, somatization, sociability, inhibition, and sleep disturbance.

Reliability: Odd–even item correlations ranged from .50 to .76.

Author: Starr, P.

Article: Facial attractiveness and behavior of patients with cleft lip and/or palate.

Journal: *Psychological Reports,* April 1980, *46*(2), 579–582.

Related Research: Sines, J. O., et al. (1969). Identification of clinically relevant dimensions of children's behavior. *Journal of Consulting and Clinical Psychology, 33,* 728–734.

■ ■ ■

1871

Test Name: PATIENT BEHAVIOR TEST

Purpose: To describe patient behavior in a community setting.

Number of Items: 127

Time Required: 25 to 45 minutes.

Format: Items are rated in terms of rate of occurrence, including almost never, sometimes, frequently, almost always.

Reliability: Equivalent forms comparison between the Katz Adjustment Scale and the family rater form of the Interpersonal Checklist was $p < .001$.

Author: Zimmerman, R. L., et al.

Article: Validity of family informants' ratings of psychiatric patients: General validity.

Journal: *Psychological Reports,* October 1975, *37*(2), 619–630.

Related Research: Katz, M. M., & Lyerly, S. B. (1963). Methods of measuring adjustment and social behavior in the community: 1. Rationale, description, discriminative validity and scale development. *Psychological Reports, 13,* 503–535.

■ ■ ■

1872

Test Name: PRESCHOOL BEHAVIOR QUESTIONNAIRE

Purpose: To serve as a short screening instrument for the identification of preschool children with behavior problems.

Number of Items: 36

Format: Includes three factors: Hostile-Aggressive, Anxious-Fearful, and Hyperactive-Distractable. Employs a 3-point scaling system of *does not apply, applies sometimes,* or *frequently applies.* All items are presented.

Reliability: Overall scale mean interrater reliability was .79; for Factors 1, 2, and 3, mean interrater reliability was .76, .70, and .61, respectively.

Author: Behar, L., and Stringfield, S.

Article: A behavior rating scale for the preschool child.

Journal: *Developmental Psychology,* September 1974, *10*(5), 601–610.

Related Research: Ruter, M. (1967). A children's behaviour questionnaire for completion by teachers: Preliminary findings. *Journal of Child Psychology and Psychiatry, 8,* 1–11.

1873

Test Name: RATHUS ASSERTIVENESS SCALE

Purpose: To assess assertive behavior.

Number of Items: 30 statements.

Format: Subjects respond on a 6-point scale from 3 (*strongly characteristic of me*) to –3 (*strongly uncharacteristic of me*).

Reliability: Test–retest reliability for an undergraduate population was .78 after 8 weeks and split-half reliability was .77.

Validity: Positive correlations with ratings of boldness (.61), outspokenness (.62), assertiveness (.33), aggressiveness (.54), and confidence (.32; Rathus, 1973).

Author: Morgan, B., and Leung, P.

Article: Effects of assertion training on acceptance of disability by physically disabled university students.

Journal: *Journal of Counseling Psychology,* March 1980, *27*(2), 209–212.

Related Research: Harris, T. L., & Brown, N. W. (1979). Congruent validity of the Rathus Assertiveness Schedule. *Educational and Psychological Measurement, 39*(1), 181–186.

Rathus, S. A. (1973). A 30–item schedule for assessing behavior. *Behavior Therapy, 4,* 398–406.

■ ■ ■

1874

Test Name: RATIONAL BEHAVIOR INVENTORY

Purpose: To provide an index of rationality.

Number of Items: 37

Format: Includes 11 factors. The subject responds to each item on a

5-point Likert scale from *strongly agree* to *strongly disagree*.

Reliability: Split-half reliability corrected by the Spearman-Brown formula was .73.

Validity: Correlations with anomia, authoritarianism, dogmatism, and self-esteem ranged from −.36 to .45 (N = 180).

Author: Whiteman, V. L., and Shorkey, C. T.

Article: Validation testing of the Rational Behavior Inventory.

Journal: *Educational and Psychological Measurement,* Winter 1978, *38*(4), 1143–1149.

Related Research: Shorkey, C. T., & Whiteman, V. L. (1977). Development of the Rational Behavior Inventory: Initial validity and reliability. *Educational and Psychological Measurement, 37,* 527–534.

■ ■ ■

1875

Test Name: REPRESSION– SENSITIZATION SCALE

Purpose: To measure subjects' characteristic ways of responding to threatening stimuli.

Number of Items: 156

Format: High scores on the scale are indicative of sensitizing defenses.

Validity: With (N = 158) self-derogation scale, r = .64; MMPI K Scale, r = −.70; Ego-control Scale, r = .24; A-Trait Scale, r = .81.

Author: Rios-Garcia, L. R., and Cook, P. E.

Article: Self-derogation and defense style in college students.

Journal: *Journal of Personality Assessment,* June 1975, *39*(3), 273–281.

Related Research: Byrne, D., et al. (1963). Relation of the revised repression-sensitization scale to measures of self-description. *Psychological Reports, 13,* 323–334.

Chelune, G. J. (1975). Sex differences and relationship between repression-sensitization and self-disclosure. *Psychological Reports, 37,* 920.

Shapiro, D. L., & Rosenwald, G. C. (1975). Free association and repression–sensitization. *Journal of Personality Assessment, 39,* 25–27.

■ ■ ■

1876

Test Name: RESTRAINT SCALE

Purpose: To discriminate between weight-conscious individuals who manifest considerable restraint in their eating habits (restrainers) and individuals who manifest minimal restraint in their eating habits and show little concern about their weight.

Number of Items: 11

Reliability: Test–retest reliability over a 4-week interval for 30 subjects was .93.

Validity: Pearson product– moment correlation between scores on the Restraint Scale and the Edwards Social Desirability Scale was .11.

Author: Kirkham, K., and Gayton, W. F.

Article: Social desirability and the Restraint Scale.

Journal: *Psychological Reports,* April 1977, *40*(2), 550.

Related Research: Herman, C. P., & Mack, D. (1975). Restrained and unrestrained eating. *Journal of Personality, 43,* 647–660.

1877

Test Name: SAMPLE PROFILE

Purpose: To assess styles of loving, including Storgic (friendship), Agapic (giving), Manic (possessive), Pragmatic, Ludic (game-playing), and Erotic.

Number of Items: 53

Format: True–false.

Validity: Correlations with Rubin's (1973) Loving and Liking Scales range from −.09 to .52 for men and women combined on the Loving Scale, and from −.09 to .23 for men and women combined on the Liking Scale.

Author: Rosenman, M. F.

Article: Liking, loving and styles of loving.

Journal: *Psychological Reports,* June 1978, *42*(3), 1243–1246.

Related Research: Rubin, Z. (1973). *Liking and loving: An invitation to social psychology.* New York: Holt, Rinehart & Winston.

■ ■ ■

1878

Test Name: SCHEDULE FOR CLASSROOM ACTIVITY NORMS

Purpose: To record the classroom behavior of students.

Number of Items: 120 observations for each subject.

Format: Classroom behavior is coded into one of 27 discrete categories every 10 seconds.

Reliability: .89 based on 12 5- minute observations across two observers.

Author: McKinney, J. D., et al.

Article: Relationship between classroom behavior and academic achievement.

Source: *Journal of Educational Psychology,* April 1975, *67*(2), 198–203.

Related Research: Spaulding, R. I. (1970). *Classroom behavior analysis and treatment using the Coping Analysis Schedule for Educational Settings* (Cases). Durham, NC: Duke University, Education Improvement Program.

■ ■ ■

1879

Test Name: SEAT BELT USE QUESTIONNAIRE

Purpose: To measure seat belt use.

Number of Items: 18

Format: Subjects responded to each item on a 5-point scale from 1 (*totally agree*) to 5 (*totally disagree*). Items dealt with discomfort, worry, risk, effect, and inconvenience.

Reliability: Kuder-Richardson formula 20 reliabilities ranged from .55 to .86.

Author: Fhanér, G., and Hane, M.

Article: Seat belts: Opinion effects of law-induced use.

Journal: *Journal of Applied Psychology,* April 1979, *64*(2), 205–212.

Related Research: Fhanér, G., & Hane, M. (1975). Seat belts: Changing usage by changing beliefs. *Journal of Applied Psychology, 60,* 589–598.

■ ■ ■

1880

Test Name: SELF-ACCEPTANCE AND ACCEPTANCE OF OTHERS FORM

Purpose: To measure behavior patterns guided by internalized values, life-coping capabilities, sense of self-worth, and an

absence of shyness or self-consciousness.

Number of Items: 64

Format: Likert items with 5 response categories ranging from *true of myself* to *not at all true of myself.*

Reliability: Matched-half reliabilities were .89 or greater, except in one case where a corrected coefficient of .75 was indicated.

Validity: Correlations between judges' ratings of subjects' attitudes about self and attitudes about others with scale scores were .90 for self-acceptance and .73 for acceptance of others.

Author: Brenneman, O. N., et al.

Article: Teacher self-acceptance, acceptance of others, and pupil control ideology.

Source: *Journal of Experimental Education,* Fall 1975, *44*(1), 14–17.

Related Research: Berger, E. M. (1952). The relationship between expressed acceptance of self and expressed acceptance of others. *Journal of Abnormal and Social Psychology, 47,* 778–782.

■ ■ ■

1881

Test Name: SHERMAN-KULHAVY LATERALITY ASSESSMENT INVENTORY

Purpose: To provide an index of cerebral laterality.

Number of Items: 45

Format: A verbal report instrument which assesses both fine and gross motor activities of the hands, arms, legs, and feet.

Reliability: Cronbach's alpha was .97.

Author: Sherman, J. L., et al.

Article: The Sherman-Kulhavy Laterality Assessment Inventory: Some validation data.

Journal: *Perceptual and Motor Skills,* June 1976, *42*(3, Part 2), 1314.

Related Research: Sherman, J. L., & Kulhavy, R. W. (1976). *The assessment of cerebral laterality: The Sherman-Kulhavy Laterality Assessment Inventory* (Laboratory for the Study of Human Intellectual Processes, Technical Report No. 4). Arizona State University.

■ ■ ■

1882

Test Name: TACTICS SCALE

Purpose: To determine the tactics used to influence the boss, co-workers, and subordinates.

Number of Items: 58

Format: Includes eight dimensions of influence. All items are presented.

Reliability: Alpha coefficients ranged from .42 to .81.

Author: Kipnis, D., et al.

Article: Intraorganizational influence tactics: Explorations in getting one's way.

Journal: *Journal of Applied Psychology,* August 1980, *65*(4), 440–452.

Related Research: Michener, A., & Schwertfeger, M. (1972). Liking as a determinant of power tactic preference. *Sociometry, 35,* 190–202.

■ ■ ■

1883

Test Name: TEACHER LOYALTY QUESTIONNAIRE

Purpose: To measure the basic

dimensions of teachers' subordinate loyalty.

Number of Items: 8

Format: Includes cognitive, behavioral, and affective aspects of subordinate loyalty. Likert items scored from 5 to 1, where the higher the score, the more loyal the teacher.

Reliability: Interitem correlation ranged from .357 to .843; coefficient alpha was .92.

Validity: With hierarchical influence, $r = .74$.

Author: Hoy, W. K., and Rees, R.

Article: Subordinate loyalty to immediate superior: A neglected concept in the study of educational administration.

Journal: *Sociology of Education,* Spring 1974, *47*(2), 268–286.

Related Research: Blau, P. M., & Scott, W. R. (1962). *Formal organizations.* San Francisco: Chandler.

Murray, V. V., & Corenblum, A. F. (1966). Loyalty to immediate superior at alternative hierarchical levels in a bureaucracy. *American Journal of Sociology, 2,* 77–85.

● ● ●

1884

Test Name: TEACHER TEMPERAMENT QUESTIONNAIRE

Purpose: To identify classroom behavior of 3- to 7-year-olds.

Number of Items: 64

Format: Children are judged on 8 categories: activity, approach, adaptability, intensity, mood, persistence, distractibility, and threshold.

Validity: Correlations with the Behavioral Style Questionnaire

ranged from .18 to .46. Correlations with behavior observations ranged from .53 to −.43.

Author: Billman, J., and McDevitt, S. C.

Article: Convergence of parent and observer ratings of temperament with observations of peer interaction in nursery school.

Journal: *Child Development,* June 1980, *51*(2), 395–400.

Related Research: Thomas, A., & Chess, S. (1977). *Temperament and development.* New York: Brunner/Mazel.

● ● ●

1885

Test Name: TUCKMAN TEACHER FEEDBACK FORM

Purpose: To provide a quantitative tool for specifying teacher behavior consistent with a psychological model of teaching.

Number of Items: 28

Format: A semantic differential which produces four scores in creativity, dynamism, organized demeanor, and warmth and acceptance. All items are presented.

Reliability: Interrater reliability coefficients ranged from .38 to .77 for the four dimensions. Other interrater reliabilities ranged from ⁻.22 to .75.

Validity: Correlations with the Pedagogic Competency Instrument averaged .60.

Author: Tuckman, B. W.

Article: The Tuckman Teacher Feedback Form.

Journal: *Journal of Educational Measurement,* Fall 1976, *13*(3), 233–237.

Related Research: Tuckman,

B. W. (1974). Teaching: The application of psychological constructs. In R. T. Hyman (Ed.), *Teaching: Vantage points for study* (2nd ed.). Philadelphia, PA: Lippincott.

● ● ●

1886

Test Name: TYPE A BEHAVIOR SCALE

Purpose: To measure a group of attitudes, emotional reactions, and behaviors referred to as the Type A behavior pattern of administrators.

Number of Items: 44

Format: Includes measures of involved striving, persistence, competitive orientation, range of activities, positive attitudes toward pressure, environmental overburdening, sense of time urgency, leadership, and history of past achievements. Subjects responded to each item on a 7-point Likert scale indicating how true a statement was of them.

Validity: Correlations with wives' satisfaction and well-being ranged from −.30 to .38.

Author: Burke, R. J., et al.

Article: Type A behavior of administrators and wives' reports of marital satisfaction and well-being.

Journal: *Journal of Applied Psychology,* February 1979, *64*(1), 57–65.

Related Research: Sales, S. M. (1970). Differences among individuals in affective behavioral, biochemical and physiological responses to variations in work load. (Doctoral dissertation, University of Michigan, 1969). *Dissertation Abstracts International, 31,* 8162A. (University Microfilms No. 69–18098)

CHAPTER 8
Communication

1887

Test Name: APHASIC SPEECH EVALUATION QUESTIONS AND CATEGORIES

Purpose: To evaluate aphasic speech.

Number of Items: 10

Format: Includes open-ended questions and seven response categories. All items and categories are presented.

Reliability: Interjudge agreement ranged from .59 to .94.

Author: Packman, A., and Ingham, R. J.

Article: On-line measurement of aphasic speech.

Journal: *Perceptual and Motor Skills,* December 1978, *47*(3, Part 1), 851–856.

Related Research: Goodkin, R. (1968). Use of concurrent response categories in evaluating talking behavior in aphasic patients. *Perceptual and Motor Skills, 26,* 1035–1040.

Goodkin, R. (1978). Note: Procedure for training judges to score tapes of aphasic speech. *Perceptual and Motor Skills, 47,* 868.

■ ■ ■

1888

Test Name: CREDIBILITY CHECKLIST

Purpose: To permit employees to describe their information milieu.

Number of Items: 18

Format: A bipolar adjective

checklist utilizing a 7-point scale. Assesses safety, expertise, and dynamism.

Validity: Spearman rank-order correlations with 7 communication variables ranged from .17 to .79 (*N* = 20).

Author: O'Reilly, C. A., III, and Roberts, K. H.

Article: Relationships among components of credibility and communication behaviors in work units.

Journal: *Journal of Applied Psychology,* February 1976, *61*(1), 99–102.

Related Research: Berlo, D., et al. (1969). Dimensions for evaluating the acceptability of message sources. *Public Opinion Quarterly, 33,* 563–675.

■ ■ ■

1889

Test Name: GROSS RATING OF FACILITATIVE INTERPERSONAL FUNCTIONING SCALE

Purpose: To measure ability in facilitative communication.

Number of Items: 16

Format: Subjects write responses to an audiotape of client stimulus statements. Scores range from 1.0 (*lowest ability*) to 5.0 (*highest ability*).

Reliability: Interrater reliability coefficients ranged from .84 to .94.

Validity: Correlations with scales of the Personal Orientation Dimensions ranged from .25 to .46.

Author: Omizo, M. M., et al.

Article: Self-actualization measures as predictors of ability in facilitative communication among counselor trainees.

Journal: *Educational and Psychological Measurement,* Summer 1980, *40*(2), 451–456.

Related Research: Carkhuff, R. R. (1969). *Helping and human relations: A primer for lay and professional helpers* (Vol. 1). New York: Holt, Rinehart & Winston.

■ ■ ■

1890

Test Name: GROSS RATINGS OF FACILITATIVE INTERPERSONAL FUNCTIONING SCALE

Purpose: To rate one's communication skills.

Number of Items: 1

Format: Five-level process Likert rating scale, with scores ranging from 1 to 5.

Reliability: Rate–rerate reliabilities are as high as .95.

Author: Parker, M., and Wittmer, J.

Article: The effects of a communications training program on the racial attitudes of Black and White fraternity members.

Journal: *Journal of College Student Personnel,* November 1976, *17*(6), 500–503.

Related Research: Carkhuff, R. R. (1969). *Helping and human relations: A primer for lay and*

professional helpers (2 vols.). New York: Holt, Rinehart & Winston.

■ ■ ■

1891

Test Name: HALO SCALE

Purpose: To measure teacher rapport with students.

Number of Items: 10

Format: 4-point scales ranging from *always, most of the time, sometimes,* to *never.*

Reliability: .89 estimated by analysis of variance procedures.

Author: Good, T. L., and Grouws, D. A.

Article: Teacher rapport: Some stability data.

Source: *Journal of Educational Psychology,* April 1975, *67*(2), 179–182.

Related Research: Rabinowitz, W., & Rosenbaum, I. (1958). A failure in the prediction of pupil-teacher rapport. *Journal of Educational Psychology, 49,* 93–98.

■ ■ ■

1892

Test Name: HIERARCHICAL INFLUENCE INDEX

Purpose: To measure hierarchical influence.

Number of Items: 15

Format: Likert items. Examples are presented.

Reliability: With teacher loyalty, $r = .74$.

Validity: Average correlation between items scores and total index score was .67. Coefficient alpha was .83.

Author: Hoy, W. K., and Rees, R.

Article: Subordinate loyalty to immediate superior: A neglected concept in the study of educational administration.

Journal: *Sociology of Education,* Spring 1974, *47*(2), 268–286.

Related Research: Hills, R. J. (1963). The representative function: A neglected dimension of leadership behavior. *Administrative Science Quarterly, 8,* 83–101.

■ ■ ■

1893

Test Name: INTENSITY OF INTERORGANIZATIONAL SCALE

Purpose: To measure the intensity of interorganizational relations.

Number of Items: 6

Format: Each item is answered *yes* or *no.* All items are presented.

Reliability: Item reproducibility ranged from .85 to .96; coefficient of reproducibility was .91; coefficient of scalability was .66.

Validity: Correlation with the number of joint programs with other organizations was .55.

Author: Rogers, D. L.

Article: Towards a scale of interorganizational relations among public agencies.

Journal: *Sociology and Social Research,* October 1974, *59*(1), 61–70.

■ ■ ■

1894

Test Name: INTERACTION ANALYSIS SYSTEM

Purpose: To permit the analysis of classroom interaction patterns of teacher and students.

Number of Items: 39

Format: Includes four types of subcategories: indirect influence, direct influence, student talk, silence. All items are presented.

Reliability: For major categories .90; for sub-categories .80.

Author: Bailey, G. D.

Article: A study of classroom interaction patterns from student teaching to independent classroom teaching.

Journal: *Educational Leadership,* December 1974, *32*(3), 225–230.

Related Research: Seagren, A. T., et al. (1969). *An evaluation of self-assessment techniques* (Appendix A). Kansas City, MO: Mid-Continent Regional Educational Laboratory.

■ ■ ■

1895

Test Name: INTIMACY OF SELF-DISCLOSURE SCALE

Purpose: To measure depth of self-disclosure.

Number of Items: 21

Format: Statements that subjects rate as *nonintimate, moderately intimate,* or *highly intimate.*

Validity: Correlation of .96 with the Intimacy Rating Scale.

Author: Strassberg, D. S., and Anchor, K. N.

Article: Rating intimacy of self-disclosure.

Journal: *Psychological Reports,* October 1975, *37*(2), 562.

Related Research: Taylor, D. A., & Altman, I. (1966). Intimacy-scaled stimuli for use in studies of interpersonal relations. *Psychological Reports, 18,* 729–730.

■ ■ ■

1896

Test Name: LEADER–MEMBER EXCHANGE MEASURE

Purpose: To assess the quality of leader–member exchange via judgments of the members, not the leaders.

Number of Items: 4

Format: All items are presented.

Reliability: Internal consistency (Kuder-Richardson formula 20) estimates at three successive quarterly intervals were .76, .80, and .84. Test–retest stability coefficients were .90, .89, and .80 between 1st and 2nd quarter, 2nd and 3rd quarter, and 1st and 3rd quarter, respectively.

Author: Graen, G., and Schiemann, W.

Article: Leader–member agreement: A vertical dyad linkage approach.

Journal: *Journal of Applied Psychology*, April 1978, *63*(2), 206–212.

Related Research: Dansereau, F., et al. (1975). A vertical dyad linkage approach to leadership in formal organizations. *Organizational Behavior and Human Performance, 13,* 46–78.

■ ■ ■

1897

Test Name: NEBRASKA SKILL ANALYSIS SYSTEM

Purpose: To permit the analysis of classroom interaction patterns of teacher and students.

Number of Items: 40

Format: Includes 9 types of subcategories: visualization, reinforcement, feedback, questioning, teacher talk, obtaining attending behavior, control of participation, student talk, silence, or confusion. All items are presented.

Reliability: For major categories, $r = .90$; For subcategories, $r = .80$.

Author: Bailey, G. D.

Article: A study of classroom

interaction patterns from student teaching to independent classroom teaching.

Journal: *Educational Leadership,* December 1974, *32*(3), 225–230.

Related Research: Seagren, A. T., et al. (1969). *An evaluation of self-assessment technique* (Appendix B). Kansas City, MO: Mid-Continent Regional Educational Laboratory.

■ ■ ■

1898

Test Name: ORGANIZATIONAL COMMUNICATION SCALE

Purpose: To measure perceived influences of communication.

Format: Includes 4 scales: interpersonal trust, perceived influence of superior, mobility aspirations and promotion within the organization.

Reliability: Reliabilities for the 4 scales ranged from .57 to .90.

Validity: Correlations with self-determination, personal sensitivity, negotiating latitude, initiating structure, consideration with supervision, co-workers, work, and promotion ranged from –.17 to .40.

Author: Adams, E. F.

Article: A multivariate study of subordinate perceptions of and attitudes toward minority and majority managers.

Journal: *Journal of Applied Psychology,* June 1978, *63*(3), 277–288.

Related Research: Roberts, K. H., & O'Reilly, C. A. (1974). Measuring organizational communication. *Journal of Applied Psychology, 59,* 321–326.

■ ■ ■

1899

Test Name: PERCEIVED DEPTH OF INTERACTION SCALE

Purpose: To evaluate perceived depth of self-disclosure and interpersonal feedback.

Number of Items: 10

Format: Verbal-report measure with five possible responses to each item, with 5 reflecting the greatest depth of feedback or self-disclosure.

Reliability: Internal consistency reliability coefficient was .55 ($p < .003$).

Validity: Relationship between the scale and actual rated group behavior was .59 ($p < .01$).

Author: Evensen, E. P., and Bednar, R. L.

Article: Effects of specific cognitive and behavioral structure on early group behavior and atmosphere.

Journal: *Journal of Counseling Psychology,* January 1978, *25*(1), 66–75.

Related Research: Evensen, P. (1976). *The effects of structure and risk taking disposition on early group development.* Unpublished doctoral dissertation, University of Kentucky.

Melnick, J., & Wicher, D. (1977). Social risk taking propensity and anxiety as predictors of group performance. *Journal of Counseling Psychology, 24,* 415–419.

■ ■ ■

1900

Test Name: POTENTIAL INTERPERSONAL COMPETENCE SCALE

Purpose: To measure the potential for interpersonal communication of applicants to counselor training programs.

Number of Items: 35

Format: Each item consists of a counselor situation with four counselor-response options.

Reliability: Hoyt reliability was .87.

Validity: Correlation with amount of counselor training was .67. Attenuated validity coefficient for different stages of training over 4 years was .44 ($N = 570$).

Author: Remer, R.

Article: Three modes of stimulus presentation in a simulation test of interpersonal communication competence.

Journal: *Journal of Educational Measurement,* Summer 1978, *15*(2), 125–130.

■ ■ ■

1901

Test Name: ROBERTS AND O'REILLY ORGANIZATIONAL COMMUNICATION QUESTIONNAIRE

Purpose: To measure organizational communication.

Number of Items: 36

Format: Includes 16 dimensions of organizational communication. Eleven of the dimensions consist of multi-item scales.

Reliability: Coefficient alpha reliability for the 11 multi-item scales ranged from .40 to .93 ($n = 270$).

Author: Muchinsky, P. M.

Article: An intraorganizational analysis of the Roberts and O'Reilly Organizational Communication Questionnaire.

Journal: *Journal of Applied Psychology,* April 1977, *62*(2), 184–188.

Related Research: Roberts, K. H., & O'Reilly, C. A., III. (1974). Measuring organizational communication. *Journal of Applied Psychology, 59,* 321–326.

■ ■ ■

1902

Test Name: SELF-DISCLOSURE INVENTORY

Purpose: To measure self-disclosure.

Number of Items: 16 topic areas.

Format: Respondents are given nine disclosure options ranging in intimacy from *no one* (9), through *closest friend* (7) and *casual friend* (3), to *stranger you have just met and may see again* (1).

Validity: A correlation of .47 ($df = 58$, $p < .001$) was obtained between questionnaire scores and actual self-disclosure.

Author: Domelsmith, D. E., and Dietch, J. T.

Article: Sex differences in the relationship between Machiavellianism and self-disclosure.

Journal: *Psychological Reports,* June 1978, *42*(3), 715–721.

Related Research: Dietch, J. T., & House, J. (1975). Affiliative conflict and individual differences in self-disclosure. *Representative Research in Social Psychology, 6,* 69–75.

CHAPTER 9
Concept Meaning

1903

Test Name: ANAGRAM FLUENCY TEST

Purpose: To assess word fluency.

Number of Items: 2

Time Required: 5 minutes.

Format: Subjects select letters from sets of six letters to make familiar words.

Reliability: .78

Author: Undheim, J.

Article: Broad ability factors in 12 to 13 year old children, the theory of fluid and crystallized intelligence, and the differentiation hypothesis.

Journal: *Journal of Educational Psychology,* June 1978, *70*(3), 433–443.

Related Research: Guilford, J., & Hoepfner, R. (1971). *The analysis of intelligence.* New York: McGraw-Hill.

1904

Test Name: ANTONYMS TEST

Purpose: To assess verbal comprehension.

Number of Items: 26

Time Required: 5 minutes.

Format: Multiple-choice test of antonyms to given words.

Reliability: .86 (Kuder-Richardson coefficient).

Author: Undheim, J.

Article: Broad ability factors in 12 to 13 year old children, the theory of fluid and crystallized intelligence, and the differentiation hypothesis.

Journal: *Journal of Educational Psychology,* June 1978, *70*(3), 433–443.

Related Research: Guilford, J., & Hoepfner, R. (1971). *The analysis of intelligence.* New York: McGraw-Hill.

1905

Test Name: CONCEPTUAL STYLE TEST

Purpose: To evaluate the method of perceptual categorization that children initially use in cognitive processing.

Number of Items: 19

Format: Individually administered with responses recorded on tape and transcribed.

Reliability: Interrater reliability was .96.

Author: Keller, B. B.

Article: Developmental and sex differences in performance on the brief conceptual style test.

Source: *Perceptual and Motor Skills,* October 1975, *41*(2), 419–422.

Related Research: Kagan, J., et al. (1963). Psychological significance of styles of conceptualization. In J. Wright & J. Kagan (Eds.), Basic cognitive processes in children. *Monographs of the society for research in child development, 28* (2 Serial No. 86), 73–112.

1906

Test Name: CONCEPTUAL STYLE TEST—REVISED

Purpose: To identify analytic and nonanalytic responses.

Number of Items: 30

Format: Each item is a card containing line drawings of three pictures. The subject selects two of the pictures that are alike or that go together in some way.

Reliability: The cards randomly divided into two sets produced a correlation of .93.

Author: Zelniker, T., et al.

Article: The relationship between speed of performance and conceptual style: The effect of imposed modification of response latency.

Journal: *Child Development,* September 1974, *45*(3), 779–784.

Related Research: Kagan, J., et al. (1964). Information processing in the child: Significance of analytic and reflective attitudes. *Psychological Monographs,* 78 (1, Whole No. 578).

1907

Test Name: CONSEQUENCES TEST

Purpose: To assess ideational fluency.

Number of Items: 3

Time Required: 9 minutes.

Format: Subjects list the effects of a new and unusual event. All relevant responses are counted.

Reliability: .72 (Kuder-Richardson coefficient).

Author: Undheim, J.

Article: Broad ability factors in 12 to 13 year old children, the theory of fluid and crystallized intelligence, and the differentiation hypothesis.

Journal: *Journal of Educational Psychology*, June 1978, *70*(3), 433–443.

Related Research: Guilford, J., & Hoepfner, R. (1971). *The analysis of intelligence.* New York: McGraw-Hill.

. . .

1908

Test Name: INTERCONCEPT DISTANCE

Purpose: To measure discrimination complexity.

Number of Items: 20

Format: Person concepts that are evaluated by 14 seven-point semantic differential dimensions.

Validity: A loading of .70 on Vannoy's (1965) Factor II.

Author: Lichtenberg, J. W., and Heck, E. J.

Article: Interactional structure of interviews conducted by counselors of different levels of cognitive complexity.

Journal: *Journal of Counseling Psychology*, January 1979, *26*(1), 15–22.

Related Research: Vannoy, J. S. (1965). Generality of cognitive complexity-simplicity as a personality construct. *Journal of Personality and Social Psychology, 2*, 385–396.

. . .

1909

Test Name: OCCUPATIONAL CONCEPT TEST

Purpose: To find which concepts people use when clarifying different occupations.

Number of Items: 20

Format: Subject decides which two of three occupations have something in common that is different from the third and give a name to that factor and its opposite.

Reliability: Test–retest correlations after 6 months for ninth ($N = 56$) and tenth grade ($N = 50$) classes gave significant correlations for all the categories ranging from .35 ($p < .01$) to .80 ($p < .001$) for the ninth grade and up to .88 ($p < .001$) for the tenth grade.

Author: Bloch, T., and Rim, Y.

Article: The latent structure of occupations.

Journal: *Journal of Vocational Behavior,* April 1979, *14*(2), 145–168.

Related Research: Kelly, G. A. (1955). *The psychology of personal constructs* (Vols. I and II). New York: Norton.

. . .

1910

Test Name: PARAGRAPH COMPLETION TEST

Purpose: To measure the degree of "integrative complexity" relative to interpersonal stimuli.

Number of Items: 5

Format: Incomplete sentence stems that subjects complete by adding at least two additional sentences within a 2-minute time limit.

Reliability: Interrater reliability for 33 tests was .77.

Author: Blaas, C. D., and Heck, E. J.

Article: Selected process variables as a function of client type and cognitive complexity in beginning counselors.

Journal: *Journal of Counseling Psychology,* July 1978, *25*(4), 257–263.

Related Research: Harvey, O. J., et al. (1961). *Conceptual systems and personality organization.* New York: Wiley.

. . .

1911

Test Name: SUBJECTS USES TEST

Purpose: To assess ideational fluency.

Number of Items: 4

Time Required: 10 minutes.

Format: Subjects list different uses for which common subjects can be employed (e.g., book, brick, car, tire, and pen).

Reliability: .65 (Kuder-Richardson coefficient).

Author: Undheim, J.

Article: Broad ability factors in 12 to 13 year old children, the theory of fluid and crystallized intelligence, and the differentiation hypothesis.

Journal: *Journal of Educational Psychology*, June 1978, *70*(3), 433–443.

Related Research: Guilford, J., & Hoepfner, R. (1971). *The analysis of intelligence.* New York: McGraw-Hill.

. . .

1912

Test Name: SYNONYMS TEST

Purpose: To assess verbal comprehension.

Number of Items: 23

Time Required: 6 minutes.

Format: Multiple-choice vocabulary test.

Reliability: .84 (Kuder-Richardson coefficient).

Author: Undheim, J.

Article: Broad ability factors in 12 to 13 year old children, the theory of fluid and crystallized intelligence, and the differentiation hypothesis.

Journal: *Journal of Educational Psychology*, June 1978, *70*(3), 433–443.

Related Research: Guilford, J., & Hoepfner, R. (1971). *The analysis of intelligence.* New York: McGraw-Hill.

■ ■ ■

1913

Test Name: TUCKMAN TOPICAL INVENTORY

Purpose: To measure cognitive complexity.

Number of Items: 72

Format: Subject chooses statements closest to own worldview.

Author: Corenblum, B.

Article: Locus of control, latitude of acceptance and attitudes toward abortion.

Journal: *Psychological Reports,* June 1973, *32*(3), 753–754.

Related Research: Tuckman, B. (1966). Interpersonal probing and revealing systems of integrative complexity. *Journal of Personality and Social Psychology, 3,* 655–664.

■ ■ ■

1914

Test Name: UNUSUAL MEANINGS VOCABULARY TEST

Purpose: To measure internal scanning.

Number of Items: 42

Format: Multiple-choice items; two examples are provided.

Reliability: Kuder-Richardson

formula 20 was .90 (*N* = 135); test–retest reliability was .81 (6 to 8 week interval with *N* = 54).

Validity: With Novelty-Experiencing Scale and four subscales (*N* = 135), *r* ranged from –.01 to .22; with Sensation-Seeking Scale (*N* = 135), *r* was .10; with Stroop Color-Word Test (*N* = 54), *r* was –.04.

Author: Gaines, L. S., and Coursey, R. D.

Article: Novelty-experiencing, internal scanning, and cognitive control.

Journal: *Perceptual and Motor Skills,* June 1974, *38*(3, Part I), 891–898.

Related Research: Willner, A. (1965). Impairment of knowledge of unusual meanings of familiar words in brain damage and schizophrenia. *Journal of Abnormal Psychology, 70,* 405–411.

■ ■ ■

1915

Test Name: VERBAL CLASSIFICATION TEST

Purpose: To assess verbal comprehension.

Number of Items: 14

Time Required: 8 minutes.

Format: Subjects assign words to one of two classes (each class is represented by four words).

Reliability: .70 (Kuder-Richardson coefficient).

Author: Undheim, J.

Article: Broad ability factors in 12 to 13 year old children, the theory of fluid and crystallized intelligence, and the differentiation hypothesis.

Journal: *Journal of Educational Psychology,* June 1978, *70*(3), 433–443.

Related Research: Guilford, J., & Hoepfner, R. (1971). *The analysis of intelligence.* New York: McGraw-Hill.

■ ■ ■

1916

Test Name: VERBALIZER–VISUALIZER QUESTIONNAIRE

Purpose: To assess the extent to which one's thinking processes consist of words or self-verbalizations versus pictorial or visual images.

Number of Items: 15

Format: Sample items are presented.

Reliability: Test–retest (3 weeks) coefficients were .49 (male), .29 (female), and .48 (total). Test–retest (7 days) coefficient was .91 (total).

Author: Warren, R., and Good, G.

Article: The verbalizer–visualizer questionnaire: Further normative data.

Journal: *Perceptual and Motor Skills,* April 1979, *48*(2), 372.

Related Research: Paivo, A. (1971). *Imagery and verbal processes.* New York: Holt, Rinehart & Winston.

■ ■ ■

1917

Test Name: WORD FLUENCY TEST

Purpose: To assess word fluency.

Number of Items: 2

Time Required: 3.5 minutes.

Format: Subjects write down words starting with a specified letter (letters *s* and *t* were used).

Reliability: .83 (Kuder-Richardson coefficient).

Author: Undheim, J.

Article: Broad ability factors in 12

to 13 year old children, the theory of fluid and crystallized intelligence, and the differentiation hypothesis.

Journal: *Journal of Educational Psychology*, June 1978, *70*(3), 433–443.

Related Research: Guilford, J., & Hoepfner, R. (1971). *The analysis of intelligence.* New York: McGraw-Hill.

■ ■ ■

1918

Test Name: WORD LISTING TEST

Purpose: To assess word fluency.

Number of Items: 2

Time Required: 3.5 minutes.

Format: Subjects write down three 4-letter words.

Reliability: .73 (Kuder-Richardson coefficient).

Author: Undheim, J.

Article: Broad ability factors in 12 to 13 year old children, the theory of fluid and crystallized intelligence, and the differentiation hypothesis.

Journal: *Journal of Educational Psychology*, June 1978, *70*(3), 433–443.

Related Research: Guilford, J., & Hoepfner, R. (1971). (1971). *The analysis of intelligence.* New York: McGraw-Hill.

■ ■ ■

1919

Test Name: WORD RECOGNITION TEST

Purpose: To measure conceptual tempo.

Number of Items: 20

Format: Includes four types of stimuli. Words in which the initial phonemes are similar (show, shore, shove, shame); words in which the final phonemes are identical (bang, rang, hang, sang, gang); multisyllable words with the same initial phoneme (quagmire, quadrang, quadrate, quartile, quadroon); multisyllable words with the same final phoneme (reflective, additive, sensitive, tentative, creative).

Reliability: Correlations were .710, .730, and .810.

Validity: Correlations with I.Q. ranged from −.376 to .586.

Author: Hall, V. C., and Russell, W. J. C.

Article: Multitrait-multimethod analysis of conceptual tempo.

Journal: *Journal of Educational Psychology*, December 1974, *66*(6), 932–939.

Related Research: Kagan, J. (1965). Reflection-impulsivity and reading ability in primary grade children. *Child Development, 5*(36), 609.

CHAPTER 10
Creativity

1920

Test Name: CONSEQUENCES TEST

Purpose: To measure divergent production.

Format: Each item presents a hypothetical situation (e.g., "What would be the results if people no longer needed or wanted sleep?"). The task is to list possible consequences. Guilford's scoring method produces two scores: Consequences–Obvious and Consequences–Remote.

Reliability: Consequences–Obvious, $r = .85$; Consequences–Remote, $r = .75$. Average item intercorrelation within the total group corrected for the length by the Spearman-Brown formula.

Validity: Correlations with Formulating Hypotheses Scores ranged from $r = -.26$ to $r = .41$.

Author: Fredericksen, N., and Evans, F. R.

Article: Effects of models of creative performance on ability to formulate hypotheses.

Journal: *Journal of Educational Psychology,* February 1974, *66*(1), 67–82.

Related Research: Guilford, J. P. (1967). *The nature of human intelligence.* New York: McGraw-Hill.

. . .

1921

Test Name: CREATIVE ACTIVITY QUESTIONNAIRE

Purpose: To measure one's creative activity in fine arts,

crafts, performing arts, math-science, literature, and music.

Number of Items: 75

Format: Scores on items are 0, 1, 3, or 5. Individual scales range from 8 to 19 items.

Reliability: Scale reliabilities (coefficient alpha) range from .63 to .90.

Author: Hocevar, D.

Article: Dimensions of creativity.

Journal: *Psychological Reports,* December 1976, *39*(3), 869–870.

Related Research: Holland, J., & Nichols, R. (1964). Prediction of academic and extra-curricular achievements in college. *Journal of Educational Psychology, 55,* 55–65.

. . .

1922

Test Name: CREATIVE BEHAVIOR CHECK LIST FOR DISADVANTAGED CHILDREN

Purpose: To allow teachers to assess the creative behavior of disadvantaged children.

Number of Items: 25

Format: All items are presented.

Reliability: Test–retest over a 2-year period was .31 ($N = 32$).

Validity: Correlation with composite reading and arithmetic scores on the Stanford Achievement Test was .39. Correlation with Torrance Test of Creative Thinking was .08.

Author: Swenson, E. V.

Article: Teacher-assessment of creative behavior in disadvantaged children.

Journal: *The Gifted Child Quarterly,* Fall 1978, *22*(3), 338–343.

. . .

1923

Test Name: CREATIVE BEHAVIOR DISPOSITION SCALE

Purpose: To measure behavioral disposition to creativity.

Number of Items: 75

Time Required: 30 minutes.

Format: Paper and pencil adult instrument whereby each item is answered on a scale of 0 to 100. The scale yields 10 subscores from five dispositions and five areas of creativity, an overall summary score, and five profiles.

Reliability: Split-half correlations were .82 to .96.

Validity: Overall score and five subscales with Shostrom's POI scores for self-actualizing values and/or self regard ranged from .42 to .51.

Author: Taylor, I. A., et al.

Article: The measurement of creative transactualization: A scale to measure behavioral dispositions to creativity.

Journal: *Journal of Creative Behavior,* 1974, *8*(2), 114–115.

Related Research: Taylor, I. A. (1972). *A theory of creative transactualization: A systematic approach to creativity with*

implications for creative leadership (Occasional Paper No. 8). Buffalo, NY: Creative Education Foundation.

■ ■ ■

1924

Test Name: CREATIVITY BATTERY

Purpose: To measure creative thinking.

Number of Items: 16

Format: Includes four subtests of four items each.

Reliability: Alpha coefficients ranged from .42 to .84.

Author: Milgram, R. M., et al.

Article: Quantity and quality of creative thinking in children and adolescents.

Journal: *Child Development*, 1978, *49*, 385–388.

Related Research: Wallach, M. A., & Kogan, N. (1965). Modes of thinking in young children: A study of the creativity-in-intelligence distinction. New York: Holt, Rinehart & Winston.

■ ■ ■

1925

Test Name: CREATIVITY/ LEADERSHIP SELF-RATING CHART

Purpose: To provide for self-evaluations of creativity and leadership.

Number of Items: 50

Format: Includes a list of creativity traits and a list of leadership traits.

Reliability: Test–retest reliability coefficient is .91.

Author: Burstiner, I.

Article: Creative management

training for department store middle managers: An evaluation.

Journal: *Journal of Creative Behavior*, Second Quarter 1977, *11*(2), 105–108.

Related Research: Burstiner, I. (1975, November–December). Development and self-evaluation of a workshop in creative management. *College Student Journal, 9*, 315–318.

■ ■ ■

1926

Test Name: DOG AND BONE TEST

Purpose: To measure the child's creative or innovative behavior.

Format: The child is shown two ways of getting the dog to reach its bone and then is invited to demonstrate as many different routes as he or she can create to accomplish the same objective. May earn nine to three points on any one trial.

Reliability: Interrater Correlations of .99.

Validity: With: CATB Matching Familiar Figures, .34; Color Recognition, .38; Weight Gradation, .31; WPPSI–Arithmetic, .49; WPPSI–Comprehension, .41; WPPSI–Sentences, .33; Wide Range Achievement, .15.

Author: Wexley, K., et al.

Article: An evaluation of Montessori and day care programs for disadvantaged children.

Journal: *Journal of Educational Research*, 1974, *68*(3), 95–99.

Related Research: Banta, T. (1970). Data for the evaluation of early childhood education: The Cincinnati Autonomy Test Battery. In J. Hellmuth (Ed.), *Cognitive Studies* (pp. 424–490). New York: Brunner/Mazel.

1927

Test Name: GROUP INVENTORY FOR FINDING CREATIVE TALENT

Purpose: To predict creativity of elementary school children.

Number of Items: 36, also a 25-item version.

Format: Includes three forms to cover primary (grades 1 and 2), elementary (grades 3 and 4), and upper elementary (grades 5 and 6) school. Items are read to grade 1 students. All students respond to each item by circling *yes* or *no*. Items are presented.

Reliability: Hoyt reliability coefficients were .55 (primary), .69 (elementary), and .68 (upper elementary). For the 25–item form the coefficient was .61.

Validity: Correlation with a composite criterion was .30, and for the 25-item version, $r = .34$.

Author: Rimm, S., and Davis, G. A.

Article: GIFT: An instrument for the identification of creativity.

Journal: *Journal of Creative Behavior*, 1976, *10*(3), 178–182.

■ ■ ■

1928

Test Name: HOW DO YOU THINK—FORM B

Purpose: To measure a predisposition to behave creatively.

Number of Items: 102

Time Required: 15–25 minutes.

Format: The test assesses attitudes, motivations, interests, values, and other personality and biographical information. Subjects respond to each item on a 5-point scale indicating the extent to which they agree or disagree with each statement. Some items are presented.

Reliability: Hoyt reliability of the total test was .94; interrater reliability ($N = 37$) was .78.

Validity: For men the correlation with creativity ratings was .64. For women the correlation with creativity ratings was .36. Overall correlation with creativity ratings was .42.

Author: Davis, G. A., and Subkoviak, M. J.

Article: Multidimensional analysis of a personality-based test of creative potential.

Journal: *Journal of Educational Measurement*, Spring 1975, *12*(1), 37–43.

Related Research: Rimm, S., & Davis, G. A. (1976). GIFT: An instrument for the identification of creativity. *Journal of Creative Behavior, 10,* 178–182.

■ ■ ■

1929

Test Name: IDEAL PUPIL CHECKLIST

Purpose: To provide a criterion of the productive, creative person or when modified, to permit persons to describe their own ideal.

Number of Items: 66

Format: Items may be ranked from *most desirable* to *least desirable* or subject may check generally desirable characteristics, double-check most important characteristics, and draw a line through undesirable characteristics. All items are presented.

Reliability: Pre- and posttesting (8 weeks apart) produced a correlation of .91 ($N = 43$).

Validity: Correlations with 199 art educators, .66; 61 nursery

teachers, .39; 1,512 USA teachers, .43; 50 elementary school principals, .42; 125 juvenile court judges, .30; 36 juvenile probation officers, .26; and 50 juvenile police officers, .10.

Author: Torrance, E. P.

Article: Assessing children, teachers, and parents against the ideal child criterion.

Source: *The Gifted Child Quarterly,* Summer 1975, *19*(2), 130–139.

■ ■ ■

1930

Test Name: JUDGING CRITERIA INSTRUMENT

Purpose: To judge student-produced creative ideas in physics.

Number of Items: 18

Format: Creative ideas were scored on a 5-choice continuous scale.

Reliability: Correlation was .62 between peer mean and self score.

Validity: Correlations with the Torrance Tests of Creative Thinking, Figural and Verbal Forms ranged from .24 to .54.

Author: Eichenberger, R. J.

Article: Creativity measurement through the use of judgement criteria in physics.

Journal: *Educational and Psychological Measurement,* Summer 1978, *37*(2), 421–427.

■ ■ ■

1931

Test Name: LINK TOGETHER TEST

Purpose: To measure creativity by remote associations.

Number of Items: 15

Time Required: 7 minutes.

Format: Each item consists of three uses descriptive of things unknown to the respondent. The subjects guess the name of the thing or things that could serve the three uses together.

Author: Ibrahim, A. S.

Article: Sex differences, originality, and personality response styles.

Journal: *Psychological Reports,* December 1976, *39*(3), 859–868.

Related Research: Ibrahim, A. S. (1972). *Originality and its relationship to personality style as measured by response sets techniques.* Unpublished dissertation, Cairo University, Egypt.

■ ■ ■

1932

Test Name: MINISCAT TEST

Purpose: To measure creativity in elementary children.

Number of Items: 20 (Form A), 20 (Form B)

Format: Children are given word doublets and asked to respond with a third word associated with the two stimulus words. Two Forms: A, B; item development information is given.

Reliability: Split-half reliability was .78 (A), .79 (B).

Validity: High and low creative children (as determined by judges) were significantly different in Miniscat performance.

Author: Lynch, M., and Edwards, T.

Article: The Miniscat: Its development and some evidence of its validity.

Journal: *Educational and Psychological Measurement,* Summer 1974, *34*(2), 397–405.

1933

Test Name: NEW SCIENTIFIC USES TEST

Purpose: To measure creative potential of scientists and engineers.

Number of Items: 14

Format: Includes a list of objects, pieces of apparatus, and equipment routinely encountered by research scientists. The subject is to record in the test booklet as many new scientific uses as he or she can think of. All items are presented.

Reliability: Odd–even corrected reliability was .90 (*N* = 45). Median corrected interjudge reliability coefficient was .68 (*N* = 45).

Validity: Correlation with the Kent-Rosanoff Word List was .51 (*N* = 45).

Author: Gough, H. G.

Article: A new scientific uses test and its relationship to creativity in research.

Journal: *Journal of Creative Behavior*, 1975, *9*(4), 245–252.

■ ■ ■

1934

Test Name: STROOP COLOR AND WORD TEST—GROUP FORM

Purpose: To measure creativity.

Number of Items: 300

Time Required: 135 seconds.

Format: Each page consisted of five columns of 20 items each.

Validity: Correlation with the Matchstick Test was .15 (*N* = 75). Correlation with the Improvements Test was .30 (*N* = 133). Correlation with teacher's rating of student's creativity was .42 (*N* = 212).

Author: Golden, C. J.

Article: The measurement of creativity by the Stroop Color and Word Test.

Journal: *Journal of Personality Assessment*, October 1975, *39*(5), 502–506.

Related Research: Golden, J. P. (1975). A group version of the Stroop Color and Word Test. *Journal of Personality Assessment*, *39*, 386–388.

■ ■ ■

1935

Test Name: WHAT KIND OF PERSON ARE YOU? TEST

Purpose: To provide a brief screening device for identifying creatively gifted adolescents and adults.

Number of Items: 50

Format: A forced choice checklist of dichotomous alternatives that are socially desirable or undesirable, and relatively creative or noncreative. Two sample items are provided.

Validity: Correlations with Vividness of Imagery Scale ranged from .01 to .20.

Author: Khatena, J.

Article: Vividness of imagery and creative self perceptions.

Source: *The Gifted Child Quarterly*, Spring 1975, *19*(1), 33–37.

Related Research: Joesting, J. (1975). Relationship of two tests of creativity to freshman English grades, school activities, and number of absences for Black college students. *Psychological Abstracts*, *37*, 69–70.

Joesting, J., & Whitehead, G. I., III. (1976). Equalitarianism curiosity, and creativity: Partial replication. *Psychological Reports*, *38*, 369–376.

Torrance, E. P., & Khatena, J. (1970). *Technical-norms manual for What Kind of Person Are You? test*. Athens: Georgia Studies of Creative Behavior.

...

CHAPTER 11
Development

1936

Test Name: ADULT VOCATIONAL MATURITY INVENTORY

Purpose: To measure vocational maturity.

Number of Items: 40

Format: Likert 5-point scale ranging from 5 (*strongly agree*) to 1 (*strongly disagree*).

Reliability: Sheppard (1971) reports a Spearman-Brown split-half reliability coefficient of .84.

Author: Loesch, L. C., et al.

Article: Vocational maturity among community college students.

Journal: *Journal of College Student Personnel,* March 1979, *20*(2), 140–144.

Related Research: Sheppard, D. I. (1971). The measurement of vocational maturity in adults. *Journal of Vocational Behavior, 1,* 339–406.

...

1937

Test Name: BEHAVIORAL MATURITY SCALE

Purpose: To provide an indication of maturity as perceived by the respondent.

Number of Items: 18

Format: Six items measure academic maturity; six items identify social maturity; and six items measure emotional maturity.

Validity: Total score with Metropolitan Readiness Test, $r =$

.60 ($N = 165$); I Feel-Me Feel Test, $r = .24$ ($N = 165$).

Author: White, W. F., and Simmons, M.

Article: First-grade readiness predicted by teacher's perception of students' maturity and students' perception of self.

Journal: *Perceptual and Motor Skills,* August 1974, *39*(1, Part 2), 395–399.

Related Research: Kim, Y., et al. (1968). The simple structure of social maturity at the second grade level. *Educational and Psychological Measurement, 28,* 145–153.

...

1938

Test Name: COGNITIVE VOCATIONAL MATURITY TEST

Purpose: To assess vocational maturity in youth.

Number of Items: 120

Format: Six areas of maturity: (1) Fields of Work, (2) Job Selection, (3) Work Conditions, (4) Education Required, (5) Attributes Required, (6) Duties.

Reliability: Kuder-Richardson formula coefficients on grades 6–9 for each of six subtests ranged .67 to .91; only 6 of 24 coefficients were below .80 (Westbrook & Mastie, 1973).

Validity: For a delinquent sample, on 5 of 6 areas there were significant differences between

groups whose parents were divorced and who were living together. Westbrook and Mastie (1973) report correlations with California Test of Mental Maturity of .53 to .69.

Author: Woodbury, R., and Pate, D.

Article: The relationship of parental marital status to measures of the cognitive vocational maturity of delinquents.

Journal: *Educational and Psychological Measurement.* Winter 1974, *34*(4), 1013–1015.

Related Research: Westbrook, B., & Mastie, M. (1973). Three issues in vocational maturity: A beginning to know about. *Measurement and Evaluation in Guidance, 6*(1), 8–16.

Westbrook, B., & Parry-Hill, J. (1973). The measurement of cognitive vocational maturity. *Journal of Vocational Behavior, 3,* 239–252.

...

1939

Test Name: DEFINING ISSUES TEST

Purpose: To assess one's ability to determine the issues that influence making a decision about a dilemma.

Number of Items: 72

Format: Six dilemmas, 12 statements for each that the subject ranks in terms of their perceived importance in making a decision about the dilemma.

Reliability: Test–retest correlation (2 weeks) was .81.

Author: Rest, J. R.

Article: Longitudinal study of the Defining Issues Test of moral judgement: A strategy for analyzing developmental change.

Source: *Developmental Psychology*, November 1975, *11*(6), 738–748.

Related Research: Prawat, R. S. (1976). Mapping the affective domain in young adolescents. *Journal of Educational Psychology, 68*, 566–572.

Rest, J. R., et al. (1974). Judging the important issues in moral dilemmas—The objective nature of development. *Developmental Psychology, 10*, 491–501.

■ ■ ■

1940

Test Name: INFANT CHARACTERISTICS QUESTIONNAIRE

Purpose: To provide a screening device for difficultness.

Number of Items: 24

Format: Each item is rated on a 7-point scale from 1 (*optimal temperament*) to 7 (*difficult temperament*). Includes 4 factors: fussy-difficult, unadaptable, dull, and unpredictable.

Reliability: Test–retest (2 to 10 day intervals) ranged from .59 to .68 ($N = 98$–100).

Author: Bates, J. E., et al.

Article: Measurement of infant difficulties.

Journal: *Child Development*, September 1979, *50*(3), 794–803.

Related Research: Robson, K. L., & Moss, H. A. (1970). Patterns and determinants of maternal

attachment. *Journal of Pediatrics, 77*, 976–985.

■ ■ ■

1941

Test Name: INVENTORY OF PSYCHOSOCIAL DEVELOPMENT

Purpose: Measures an individual's level of psychosocial maturity based upon Eriksonian principles.

Number of Items: 60

Format: Five items reflect successful and five reflect unsuccessful resolution of each of Erikson's first six stages of psychosocial development. Short words or phrases rated on a 7-point scale describe how *characteristic* (7) or *uncharacteristic* (1) the phrase is of the subject.

Reliability: Median test–retest correlation coefficient was .70 ($N = 150$) between six subscales of the inventory with 6 weeks between administrations.

Author: Goldman, J. A., and Olczak, P. V.

Article: Effect of an innovative academic program upon self-actualization and psychosocial maturity.

Journal: *Journal of Educational Research*, May/June 1976, *69*(9), 333–337.

Related Research: Constantinople, A. (1969). An Eriksonian measure of personality development in college students. *Developmental Psychology, 1*, 357–372.

Goldman, J. A., & Olczak, P. V. (1975). Relationship between psychosocial maturity and fear of appearing incompetent. *Psychological Reports, 36*, 21–22.

Munley, P. H. (1975). Erik Erikson's theory of psychosocial development and vocational

behavior. *Journal of Counseling Psychology, 22*, 314–319.

See *DUEMM, 2*, 1978, 632.

■ ■ ■

1942

Test Name: LIFE CHANGE INVENTORY

Purpose: To assess the life changes in college students.

Number of Items: 50

Format: Items dealt with changes such as marriage, death of close friend, change in sexual morality, and so forth; each item has scoring weight determined by ratings of college students.

Reliability: Cronbach's alpha was .87, Test–retest reliabilities were .68 and .88 for two samples; time period was 1 week.

Validity: Correlations with subscales of Eysenck Personality Inventory, Profile of Mood States, and Differential Personality Inventory are reported.

Author: Constantini, A., et al.

Article: The Life Change Inventory: A device for quantifying psychological magnitude of changes experienced by college students.

Journal: *Psychological Reports*, June 1974, *34*(3), 991–1000.

■ ■ ■

1943

Test Name: RIGHT–LEFT DISCRIMINATION BATTERY— FORM A

Purpose: To determine the development of right–left concepts in children.

Number of Items: 32

Format: Covers knowledge of right and left on oneself and on others. Twelve are single commands and 20 are double commands.

Validity: Correlations with vocabulary, .82; age, .80; space, .79; and draw-a-man, .76.

Author: Lacoursière-Paige, F.

Article: Development of right–left concept in children.

Journal: *Perceptual and Motor Skills,* February 1974, *38*(1), 111–117.

Related Research: Benton, A. L. (1959). *Right-left discrimination and finger localization: Development and pathology.* New York: Harper.

1944

Test Name: SENTENCE COMPLETION TEST

Purpose: To assess level of ego development.

Format: Total score is an item-sum score determined by scoring each item for ego level, assigning numerical ratings to each ego level, and adding numerical item scores.

Reliability: Interrater, test–retest, and split-half coefficients were in the middle .70s and above.

Validity: With extracurricular activities correlations ranged from −.15 to .45.

Author: Cox, N.

Article: Prior help, ego development, and helping behavior.

Journal: *Child Development,* September 1974, *45*(3), 594–603.

Related Research: Loevinger, J., & Wessler, R. (1970). *Measuring ego development.* San Francisco: Jossey-Bass.

...

CHAPTER 12
Family

1945

Test Name: CHILD STUDY INVENTORY

Purpose: To measure parental motivation.

Number of Items: 18

Format: Each item is a four-choice multiple choice item. Includes five factors: parental fatalism, parental nurturance, children's independence, parental instrumentalism, and children's happiness.

Reliability: Cronbach's alpha ranged from .70 to .92.

Author: Counte, M. A., and Garron, D. C.

Article: Factor structure of Rabin's Child Study Inventory.

Journal: *Journal of Personality Assessment,* February 1979, *43*(1), 59–63.

Related Research: Rabin, A. I., & Greene, R. J. (1968). Assessing motivation for parenthood. *Journal of Psychology, 69,* 39–46.

...

1946

Test Name: HOME EDUCATIONAL ENVIRONMENT INTERVIEW SCHEDULE

Purpose: To measure the dynamic characteristics of the home environment of first-grade children.

Format: Includes 7 environmental themes.

Reliability: Test–retest (after 1 month, $N = 25$) subscale

reliabilities ranged from .91 to 1.00.

Validity: With total achievement scores correlation was .80. With teacher's estimate of achievement, Pearson product–moment correlations for the subscales ranged from .43 to .80.

Author: Skoczylas, R. V.

Article: Bilingual education: An alternative to the traditional all-English curriculum.

Source: *California Journal of Educational Research,* January 1975, *26*(1), 40–51.

Related Research: Dave, R. H. (1963). *The identification and measurement of environmental process variables that are related to educational achievement.* Unpublished doctoral dissertation, The University of Chicago.

...

1947

Test Name: HOME ENVIRONMENTAL MEASURES

Purpose: To measure home environmental variables that relate to I.Q.

Number of Items: 39

Format: Includes three imitation and seven process variables. Some examples are presented.

Validity: For male subjects ($N = 60$) correlations with Binet ranged from $-.19$ to .42. For female subjects ($N = 50$) correlations with Binet ranged from $-.23$ to .63. For total sample ($N = 110$) correlations with Binet ranged from $-.13$ to .45.

Author: Hanson, R. A.

Article: Consistency and stability of home environmental measures related to I.Q.

Source: *Child Development,* June 1975, *46*(2), 470–480.

Related Research: Wolf, R. M. (1965). The measurement of environments. In C. W. Harris (Ed.), *Proceedings of the 1964 invitational conference on testing problems.* Princeton, NJ: Educational Testing Service.

...

1948

Test Name: HOME OBSERVATION FOR MEASUREMENT OF THE ENVIRONMENT

Purpose: To provide an index of the quality and quantity of social, emotional, and cognitive support available to children from birth to age three within the home setting.

Number of Items: 45

Format: Includes the following environmental forces: emotional and verbal responsivity of the mother, avoidance of restriction and punishment, organization of the environment, provision of appropriate play materials, maternal involvement with the child, and opportunities for variety in the daily routine.

Reliability: Internal consistency (Kuder-Richardson formula 20) for the total scale was .89.

Validity: Correlations of total scores with total scores of the Illinois Test of Psycholinguistic

Abilities were .39 for 6 months (N = 74); .61 for 24 months (N = 74).

Author: Elardo, R., et al.

Article: A longitudinal study of the relation of infants' home environment to language development at age three.

Journal: *Child Development,* June 1977, *48*(2), 595–603.

Related Research: Bradley, R. J., & Caldwell, B. M. (1980). The relation of home environment, cognitive competence, and I.Q. among males and females. *Child Development,* December, *51*(4), 1140–1148.

Caldwell, B., et al. (1966, September). *Home observation for measurement of the environment.* Paper presented at the meeting of the American Psychological Association, New York.

■ ■ ■

1949

Test Name: INTENSITY OF PARENTAL PUNISHMENT SCALE

Purpose: To provide a measure of parental punishment intensity.

Number of Items: 33

Format: Each item consists of a description of how a child has misbehaved. Parents are to view the child as their own and on a 7-point scale indicate how they would respond behaviorally and emotionally.

Reliability: Test–retest reliability was .85 (2-month interval).

Author: Gordon, D. A., et al.

Article: A measure of intensity of parental punishment.

Journal: *Journal of Personality Assessment,* October 1979, *43*(5), 485–496.

Related Research: Baumrind, D. (1973). The development of

instrumental competence through socialization. In Anne D. Pick (Ed.), *Minnesota Symposia on Child Psychology* (7). Minneapolis: University of Minnesota Press.

■ ■ ■

1950

Test Name: INTERPERSONAL CONFLICT SCALE

Purpose: To measure the degree of fulfillment of emotional and interaction needs by the marital partners based on the perceptions of those needs.

Number of Items: 90 items (Two forms).

Format: Nine factors.

Reliability: The reliability levels of the factors range between .78 and .98 (Spearman-Brown Prophecy Formula).

Author: Hoskins, C. N., et al.

Article: Social chronobiology: Circadian activation rhythms of married couples.

Journal: *Psychological Reports,* October 1979, *45*(2), 607–614.

Related Research: Hoskins, C. N. (1978). A study of the relationship between level of activation, body temperatures, and interpersonal conflict in family relationships (Doctoral dissertation, New York University, 1978). *Dissertation Abstracts International, 39,* 139. (University Microfilms No. 78–18)

■ ■ ■

1951

Test Name: INVENTORY OF FAMILY FEELINGS

Purpose: To measure interpersonal and family relationships.

Number of Items: 38

Format: Each member of a family

responds to each item by indicating *agree, disagree,* or *neutral.*

Reliability: Test–retest reliability coefficient was .96 (N = 34 over 2-week period).

Author: Lowman, J.

Article: Measurement of family affective structure.

Journal: *Journal of Personality Assessment,* April 1980, *44*(2), 130–141.

Related Research: Lowman, J. (1971). Development and field-testing of a self-administered measure of family functioning (Doctoral dissertation, University of North Carolina at Chapel Hill, 1971). *Dissertation Abstracts International, 32,* 1218B. (University Microfilms No. 71–20, 983)

■ ■ ■

1952

Test Name: INVENTORY OF HOME STIMULATION

Purpose: To measure the child's home learning environment.

Number of Items: 45

Format: Includes six subscales: emotional and verbal responsivity of the mother, avoidance of restriction and punishment, organization of the physical and temporal environment, provision of appropriate play materials, maternal involvement with the child, and opportunities for variety in daily stimulation.

Reliability: Internal consistency coefficients (Kuder-Richardson formula 20; N = 176) for subscales ranged from .44 to .89. Internal consistency for the total scale was .89.

Validity: IHS subscales at 6 months with Bayley Mental Development Index at 6 months ranged from –.008 to .224; at 12 months ranged from –.003 to .263; with Binet at 36 months ranged from .244 to .408. Full scale averaged from .14 to .500. IHS subscales at 12 months with BMDI at 12 months ranged from –.008 to .353, with Binet at 36 months ranged from .241 to .561. Full scale was .252 and .551, respectively. IHS subscales at 24 months with Binet at 36 months ranged from .406 to .635 and IHS full scale with Binet was .695.

Author: Elardo, R., et al.

Article: The relation of infants' home environments to mental test performance from six to thirty-six months: A longitudinal analysis.

Source: *Child Development,* March 1975, *46*(1), 71–76.

■ ■ ■

1953

Test Name: MOTHER–CHILD AFFECTIONATE INTERACTION SCALE

Purpose: To assess the amount and quality of mother–child interaction.

Number of Items: 5

Format: Items referred to amount of time spent together, enjoyment and interest in doing things together, spontaneous expression of affection, and closeness of the relationship. Scores range from 5 to 23.

Reliability: 48; homogeneity was .18.

Validity: With the Problem Behavior Index, $rs = -.28$ (females), –.05 (males).

Author: Jessor, S. L., and Jessor, R.

Article: Maternal ideology and adolescent problem behavior.

Journal: *Developmental Psychology,* March 1974, *10,* 246–254.

1954

Test Name: MOTHER'S CONTROLS AND REGULATIONS SCALE

Purpose: To assess the existence of maternal controls and regulations.

Number of Items: 5

Format: Open-ended, multipart questions regarding maternal regulations concerning doing homework, being in at night, use of leisure time, and drinking. Scores range from 0 to 14.

Reliability: Homogeneity ratio was .18; Cronbach's alpha was .53.

Validity: With the Problem Behavior Index, –.22 (females), –.30 (males).

Author: Jessor, S. L., and Jessor, R.

Article: Maternal ideology and adolescent problem behavior.

Journal: *Developmental Psychology,* March 1974, *10,* 246–254.

■ ■ ■

1955

Test Name: PARENT–CHILD INTERACTION RATING SCALES—MODIFIED

Purpose: To assess perceived parental nurturance.

Number of Items: 20

Format: Includes the following dimensions, each of which is measured by a Likert scale: affection, physical contact, security, and consistency-trust.

Reliability: Split-half reliability reported to be in the .70s.

Author: Nowicke, S., Jr., and Segal, W.

Article: Perceived parental characteristics, locus of control orientation, and behavioral

correlates of locus of control.

Journal: *Developmental Psychology,* January 1974, *10*(1), 33–37.

Related Research: Heilbrun, A. B. (1964). Parent model attributes, nurturant reinforcement and consistency of behavior in adolescents. *Child Development, 35,* 151–167.

■ ■ ■

1956

Test Name: PARENT PERCEPTIONS QUESTIONNAIRE

Purpose: To measure parent perceptions of how they relate to their children, how concerned they are about child behaviors, to what extent they agreed with statements about college, and whether they agreed with their children's religious and political views, morality, money managements, choice of friends, and vocational goals.

Number of Items: 45

Format: Likert items.

Reliability: Internal consistency reliability of .70 for six statements related to the parents' views of their children's religious and political views, morality, money managements, choice of friends, and vocational goals.

Author: Biggs, D. A.

Article: A parental view of the collegiate generation gap.

Source: *Journal of College Student Personnel,* May 1975, *16*(3), 220–225.

Related Research: French, R. J., Jr., & Raven, B. (1959). The bases of social power. In D. Cartwright (Ed.), *Studies in social power* (pp. 159–167). Ann Arbor: University of Michigan Press.

1957

Test Name: STRANGE SITUATION BEHAVIOR INSTRUMENT—REVISED

Purpose: To assess behavior in the home situation.

Number of Items: 6

Format: A controlled observational technique for assessing infants' behavior in their home.

Reliability: Interrater reliability for two independent raters ranged from .84 to .88.

Author: Brookhart, J., and Hock, E.

Article: The effects of experimental context and experiential background on infants' behavior toward their mothers and a stranger.

Journal: *Child Development,* March 1976, *47*(1), 333–340.

Related Research: Ainsworth, M. D., & Bell, S. M. (1970). Attachment, exploration, and separation: Illustrated by the behavior of 1-year-olds in a strange situation. *Child Development, 41,* 49–67.

■ ■ ■

1958

Test Name: WHEN MY CHILD WAS BORN

Purpose: To assess retrospective maternal reactions and the perceived paternal reactions to the birth of the child.

Number of Items: 32

Format: Multiple-choice format.

Validity: Correlations with locus of control ranged from −.114 to −.370 (*n* ranged from 97 to 200).

Author: Brantley, H. T., and Clifford, E.

Article: When my child was born: Maternal reactions to the birth of a child.

Journal: *Journal of Personality Assessment,* December 1980, *44*(6), 620–623.

Related Research: Brantley, H. T., & Clifford, E. (1979). Maternal and child locus of control and field dependence in cleft palate children. *Cleft Palate Journal, 16,* 183.

CHAPTER 13
Institutional Information

1959

Test Name: ADVISING
SATISFACTION
QUESTIONNAIRE

Purpose: To correlate student
perceptions and faculty
perceptions about academic
advising.

Number of Items: 23

Format: Likert items that elicit
information in 10 areas.

Reliability: Coefficient alpha of .99
for the entire 23-item instrument.

Author: Teague, G. V.

Article: Community college student
satisfaction with four types of
academic advisement.

Journal: *Journal of College
Student Personnel*, July 1977,
18(4), 281–285.

Related Research: Grites, T. J.
(1974). *Student perceptions and
self-perceptions of faculty
members in the related roles of
classroom teacher and academic
advisor.* Unpublished doctoral
dissertation, University of
Maryland.

■ ■ ■

1960

Test Name: ATTRIBUTIVE
CAUSATION QUESTIONNAIRE

Purpose: To assess one's
psychosocial environment.

Number of Items: 14

Format: Items are included.

Reliability: Reliability coefficients
for 13 items range from .57 to .91.

Twelve of the 14 items have
reliabilities of .70 or better.

Author: Van Atta, R. E., et al.

Article: Psychological discomfort
and its causal attribution in
relation to student services
program development.

Journal: *Journal of College
Student Personnel*, September
1977, *18*(5), 371–375.

Related Research: Murray, H.
(1938). *Explorations in
personality.* New York: Oxford.

■ ■ ■

1961

Test Name: COLLEGE STUDENT
SATISFACTION
QUESTIONNAIRE

Purpose: To determine one's
satisfaction with college in the
areas of working conditions,
compensation, quality of
education, social life, and
recognition.

Number of Items: 70

Format: Five-choice Likert scale
from 5 (*very satisfied*) to 1 (*very
dissatisfied*).

Reliability: Reliability coefficients
for public universities ranged from
.78 to .84 with a median of .82.

Author: Maxwell, B. A., and
Reilley, R. R.

Article: Creativity, satisfaction,
and orientation of college
freshmen.

Journal: *Psychological Reports*,
June 1978, *42*(3), 859–864.

Related Research: Betz, E. L., et
al. (1971). A dimensional analysis

of college student satisfaction.
*Measurement and Evaluation in
Guidance, 4,* 99–106.

■ ■ ■

1962

Test Name: CONTROL
QUESTIONNAIRE

Purpose: To measure the degree of
influence that each level of the
organization exercised over the
organization's activities.

Format: Five-point scale.

Reliability: Split-half reliabilities
corrected by the Spearman-Brown
formula of .67 and .87.

Author: Hough, R. S., et al.

Article: Senior citizen centers: A
study of control, loyalty and
effectiveness.

Journal: *Psychological Reports*,
October 1977, *41*(2), 354.

Related Research: Price, J. L.
(1972). *Handbook of
organization's measurement.*
Lexington: Heath.

■ ■ ■

1963

Test Name: DIMENSIONS OF
SCHOOLING

Purpose: To quantify program
openness in elementary schools.

Number of Items: 28

Format: Teacher self-report
instrument that assesses
characteristics relating to open
education in 10 program areas.

Reliability: Product–moment

correlation over 8.5 months was .92 and the rank order correlation was .86.

Validity: Concurrent validity rank order coefficient was .75.

Author: Ward, W. D., and Barcher, P. R.

Article: Reading achievement and creativity as related to open classroom experience.

Journal: *Journal of Educational Psychology,* October 1975, *67*(5), 683–691.

■ ■ ■

1964

Test Name: DUSO AFFECTIVITY ASSESSMENT DEVICE

Purpose: To assess whether the objectives of the Developing Understanding of Self and Others programs have been met.

Number of Items: 51

Time Required: 30 minutes.

Format: Each answer space is identified by a picture symbol. The child responds *yes* or *no* to items read aloud. Two forms.

Reliability: Correlation between the total scores on alternate forms of test given one week apart is .77 ($p < .01$).

Validity: Both forms correlate significantly ($p < .05$) with teacher's ranking of children.

Author: Ohnmacht, S., et al.

Article: Practicality, reliability, and validity of the Duso Affectivity Device.

Journal: *Journal of Educational Research,* April 1975, *68*(8), 315–318.

Related Research: Nelson, W. (November 1971/April 1972). The development of a device for assessing the Duso unit objectives. *ARGR Journal, 13,* 23–27.

1965

Test Name: ENVIRONMENTAL SATISFACTION SCALE

Purpose: To measure satisfaction of the living environment in a dormitory situation.

Number of Items: 10

Format: Subjects are asked to evaluate life in their dorm in relation to such factors as support for personal problems, recreation, comfort, and privacy. The items are rated on a 7-point scale.

Validity: A significant correlation ($r = .41$, $p < .01$) was found between scores on the scale and student's decisions to remain in or leave the particular dormitory for the next academic year.

Author: Holahan, C., and Wilcox, B.

Article: Residential satisfaction and friendship formation in high-and-low-rise student housing: An interactional analysis.

Journal: *Journal of Educational Psychology,* April 1978, *70*(2), 237–241.

Related Research: Wilcox, B., & Holahan, C. (1976). Social ecology of the megadorm in university student housing. *Journal of Educational Psychology, 68,* 453–458.

■ ■ ■

1966

Test Name: ISRAELI FEAR SURVEY INVENTORY

Purpose: To assess behavior modification techniques of use in both research and clinical practice.

Number of Items: 97

Format: Subject indicates which situations and objects arouse fear.

Reliability: Test–retest reliability was .80 over 4 weeks.

Author: Goldberg, J., et al.

Article: A factor analysis of the Israeli Fear Survey Inventory.

Journal: *Psychological Reports,* February 1975, *36*(1), 175–179.

Related Research: Wolpe, J., & Lang, P. J. (1964). A fear survey for use in behavior therapy. *Behavioral Research and Therapy, 2,* 27–30.

■ ■ ■

1967

Test Name: JOB CLIMATE QUESTIONNAIRE

Purpose: To measure the achievement features of job climate.

Number of Items: 25

Format: Bipolar items, one pole of which is a description of a job environment likely to satisfy the need of a high achievement manager and the other pole reflects a situation more typically conducive to the need of a low achievement manager.

Reliability: Internal consistency coefficients range from .86 to .88; median item-total correlations from .40 to .42.

Validity: Correlations with Stern's Occupational Climate Index range from .60 to .79; .39 with Hall's Organization Characteristics Questionnaire.

Author: Fineman, S.

Article: The influence of perceived job climate on the relationship between managerial achievement motivation and performance.

Journal: *Journal of Occupational Psychology,* 1975, *48*(2), 113–124.

■ ■ ■

1968

Test Name: JOB PROBLEMS SCALE

Purpose: To identify job problems.

Number of Items: 11

Format: Items are answered on a 4-point scale from *not a problem* (0) to *major problem* (3). A list of the items is presented.

Reliability: Coefficient alpha was .89.

Validity: Correlations with such variables as work sensitivity; self-determination; personal sensitivity; negotiating latitude; initiating structure; consideration; satisfaction with supervision; co-workers, work, promotion; trust; influence; mobility; and promotion in organization ranged from –.56 to .20.

Author: Adams, E. F.

Article: A multivariate study of subordinate perceptions of and attitudes toward minority and majority managers.

Journal: *Journal of Applied Psychology,* June 1978, *63*(3), 277–288.

Related Research: Cashman, J., et al. (1975). Organizational understructure and leadership: A longitudinal investigation of the managerial role-making process. *Organizational Behavior and Human Performance, 13*, 46–78.

■ ■ ■

1969

Test Name: LEARNING STRUCTURE QUESTIONNAIRE

Purpose: To describe classrooms on three scales.

Number of Items: 24

Format: Student rates classroom on 1 to 5 scale; three dimensions and scores; teacher-centered, student-centered, and self-directed.

Validity: None of scales were significantly related to measures of

attitude toward teacher or classroom.

Author: Di Marco, N.

Article: Life style, learning structure, congruence, and student attitudes.

Journal: *American Educational Research Journal,* Spring 1974, *11*(2), 203–209.

Related Research: Vinton, J. (1972). *The relationships among life style, task and structure in university classrooms.* Unpublished doctoral dissertation, Case Western Reserve University.

■ ■ ■

1970

Test Name: LIKERT ORGANIZATIONAL PROFILE

Purpose: To measure organizational characteristics.

Number of Items: 20

Format: Each item is answered on a 20-point scale divided into four sections. An outline of the scale is presented.

Reliability: Test–retest reliability was .52 (6–18 months).

Author: Butterfield, D. A., and Farris, G. F.

Article: The Likert Organizational Profile: Methodological analysis and test of System 4 theory in Brazil.

Journal: *Journal of Applied Psychology,* February 1974, *59*(1), 15–23.

Related Research: Foundation for Research on Human Behavior. (1967). *Sample kit: Profile of organizational characteristics.* Ann Arbor, MI: Institute for Social Research.

■ ■ ■

1971

Test Name: MILITARY MORALE SCALE

Purpose: To measure morale in military units.

Format: Includes eight dimensions of behavior: community relations; teamwork and cooperation; reactions to adversity; superior–subordinate relations; performance and effort on the job; bearing, appearance, and military discipline; pride in unit, army, and country; and use of time during off-duty hours.

Reliability: Interrater reliability for individual morale scales at the platoon level, $r = .55$. Interrater reliability for an overall morale scale, $r = .72$.

Validity: Correlation with measures of motivation: $r = .13$ (platoon morale, $n = 47$); $r = .13$ (company morale, $n = 16$). Overall satisfaction: $r = .24$ (platoon morale $n = 47$); $r = .26$ (company morale, $n - 16$). Satisfaction with job: $rs = .15$ to $.22$ (platoon morale, $n = 47$); $rs = .23$ to $.33$ (company morale, $n = 16$).

Author: Motowidlo, S. J., and Borman, W. C.

Article: Relationships between military morale, motivation, satisfaction, and unit effectiveness.

Journal: *Journal of Applied Psychology,* February 1978, *63*(1), 47–52.

Related Research: Motowidlo, S. J., & Borman, W. C. (1977). Behaviorally anchored scales for measuring morale in military units. *Journal of Applied Psychology, 62*, 177–184.

■ ■ ■

1972

Test Name: ORGANIZATIONAL PRACTICES QUESTIONNAIRE

Purpose: To measure organizational practices relevant for effectiveness.

Format: Seven-point response

mode ranging from *definitely not true* to *extremely true.*

Reliability: Intercorrelations of the scales ranged from .33 to .53 except for the conflict and inconsistency scale which correlated from .52 to .62 with each of the other scales.

Author: Hill, M. A., and Morgan, C. P.

Article: Organizational climate as a predictor of organizational practices.

Journal: *Psychological Reports,* June 1977, *40*(3), 1191–1199.

Related Research: House, R. J., & Rizzo, J. R. (1972). Toward the measurement of organizational practices: Scale development and validation. *Journal of Applied Psychology, 56,* 388–396.

■ ■ ■

1973

Test Name: PEER COUNSELING OUTCOME MEASURE

Purpose: To measure the effectiveness of peer counseling.

Number of Items: 72

Format: Covers general self-concept, body image, decisiveness, academic adequacy, interpersonal adequacy, emotional control, equanimity, optimism, locus of control, school attitude, family relations, and mutual support using 5-point Likert scales.

Reliability: Scale test–retest reliabilities ranged from .18 to .76.

Author: Schweisheimer, W., and Walberg, H. J.

Article: A peer counseling experiment: High school students as small group leaders.

Journal: *Journal of Counseling Psychology,* July 1976, *23*(4), 398–401.

Related Research: Coopersmith, S. (1967). *The antecedents of self-esteem.* San Francisco: Freeman.

■ ■ ■

1974

Test Name: PILOT QUESTIONNAIRE

Purpose: To profile one's work situation as input (task to be performed and organizational characteristics), transform (manager's style and interpersonal skill), and output (effectiveness and satisfaction) factors.

Number of Items: 288

Format: Items are rated on 5- and 6-point Likert scales.

Validity: Of 93 eta coefficients, 71 are .50 or greater, indicating that respondents were describing the situation as they saw it.

Author: Bass, B. M., et al.

Article: Management styles associated with organizational, task, personal, and interpersonal contingencies.

Journal: *Journal of Applied Psychology,* December 1975, *60*(6), 720–729.

Related Research: Bass, B. M., et al. (1974). Magnitude estimations of expressions of frequency and amount. *Journal of Applied Psychology, 59,* 313–320.

■ ■ ■

1975

Test Name: POLITICAL CYNICISM SCALE

Purpose: To measure feelings of political distrust.

Number of Items: 6

Format: Example of items is given.

Reliability: Alpha coefficient was .61.

Author: Long, S.

Article: Explaining systemic failure: A two-dimensional analysis.

Journal: *Psychological Reports,* August 1977, *41*(1), 23–28.

Related Research: Agger, R., et al. (1961). Political cynicism: Measurement and meaning. *Journal of Politics, 23,* 477–506.

■ ■ ■

1976

Test Name: POLITICAL DISCONTENTMENT SCALE

Purpose: To measure dissatisfaction with policy outputs.

Number of Items: 4

Format: Example of items is given.

Reliability: Alpha coefficient was .66.

Author: Long, S.

Article: Explaining systemic failure: A two-dimensional analysis.

Journal: *Psychological Reports,* August 1977, *41*(1), 23–28.

Related Research: Olsen, M. (1969). Two categories of political alienation. *Social Forces, 47,* 288–299.

■ ■ ■

1977

Test Name: POLITICAL ESTRANGEMENT SCALE

Purpose: To measure feelings of political detachment.

Number of Items: 4

Format: Example of items is given.

Reliability: Alpha coefficient is .74.

Author: Long, S.

Article: Explaining systemic failure: A two-dimensional analysis.

Journal: *Psychological Reports,* August 1977, *41*(1), 23–28.

Related Research: Long, S. (1976). Political alienation among Black and White adolescents: A test of the social deprivation and political reality models. *American Politics Quarterly, 4,* 267–304.

■ ■ ■

1978

Test Name: SCHOOL ADMINISTRATOR MORALE MEASURE

Purpose: To isolate factors influencing subordinate administrator morale.

Number of Items: 53

Format: Likert scale with 34 positively worded and 19 negatively worded items.

Reliability: Test–retest reliability for a sample of 574 subordinate school administrators after a 2-week interval ranged from .62 to .83 with a median of .78.

Author: Bledsoe, J. C.

Article: Morale of curriculum directors as related to perceptions of leadership of superintendents.

Journal: *Psychological Reports,* December 1978, *43*(3), 1283–1288.

Related Research: *School administrator morale in selected Indiana school systems.* (1972). Unpublished doctoral dissertation, Purdue University. (University Microfilms No. 73–6073)

■ ■ ■

1979

Test Name: SOCIAL-ORGANIZATIONAL QUESTIONNAIRE

Purpose: To identify certain facets of the social environment of military units.

Number of Items: 251

Format: Includes background questions and 19 social-organizational scales.

Reliability: Correlation coefficients for the scales ranged from .19 to .95.

Validity: Biserial correlation with measures of level of drug use ranged from .346 to −.349.

Author: Cook, R., et al.

Article: Illicit drug use in the army: A social-organizational analysis.

Journal: *Journal of Applied Psychology,* June 1976, *61*(3), 262–272.

■ ■ ■

1980

Test Name: STUDENT PROBLEM AREAS SURVEY

Purpose: To determine broad problem areas within which relevant mental health programs may be developed.

Number of Items: 20 problem areas.

Format: Respondents rank how often they need assistance with the areas, from 1 (*never*) to 5 (*very often*).

Reliability: Pearson correlations over a 2-week interval ranged from the .30s to the .70s, with an average correlation around .55. A Spearman rho correlation between the item means of the two administrations of one reliability sample yielded a coefficient of .90.

Author: Westbrook, F. D., et al.

Article: Perceived problem areas of Black and White students and hints about comparative counseling needs.

Journal: *Journal of Counseling Psychology,* March 1978, *25*(2), 119–123.

Related Research: Westbrook, F. D., & Smith, J. B. (1976). Assisting Black resident students at a predominantly White institution: A paraprofessional

approach. *Journal of College Student Personnel, 17,* 205–210.

■ ■ ■

1981

Test Name: TASK CHARACTERISTICS QUESTIONNAIRE—MODIFIED

Purpose: To measure task challenge.

Number of Items: 10

Format: Items embrace job variety, autonomy, wholeness of work, feedback, visibility, learning growth, and interpersonal opportunities. Responses are made on a 7-point scale. An example is given.

Validity: With life stability, $r = .25$ ($N = 140$); personality match, $r = -.16$; supervisory success, $r = .34$.

Author: Vicino, F. L., and Bass, B. M.

Article: Lifespace variables and managerial success.

Journal: *Journal of Applied Psychology,* February 1978, *63*(1), 81–88.

Related Research: Hackman, J. R., & Lawler, E. E. (1971). Employee reactions to job characteristics [Monograph]. *Journal of Applied Psychology, 55,* 259–286.

■ ■ ■

1982

Test Name: TEACHER EDUCATION PROGRAM EVALUATION SCALE— REVISED

Purpose: To measure beginning teachers' perceptions of their pre-professional training.

Number of Items: 25

Format: Includes five factors: pre-professional skills and abilities, general education, sociological foundations, use of teaching materials, and personal development.

Reliability: Reliability coefficients for elementary teachers ($n = 161$) ranged from .79 to .91 and for secondary teachers ($n = 178$) ranged from .67 to .93.

Author: Bledsoe, J. C., and Flowers, J. D.

Article: Measuring beginning teachers' satisfaction with their pre-professional training.

Journal: *Perceptual and Motor Skills,* June 1977, *44*(3, Part 1), 779–782.

Related Research: Bledsoe, J. C., & Lightsey, R. (1966). Selected perceptions of beginning teachers in Georgia as related to certification status. *Journal of Teacher Education, 17*(4), 481–493.

■ ■ ■

1983

Test Name: TEXTBOOK APPRAISAL FORM

Purpose: To measure the impact of a textbook.

Number of Items: 13

Format: Subjects respond on a 5-point rating scale. Includes four items for appraising the textbook.

Reliability: Corrected split-half reliability was .92.

Author: Meredith, G. M.

Article: Brief scale for measuring the impact of a textbook.

Journal: *Perceptual and Motor Skills,* October 1980, *51*(2), 370.

Related Research: Kulik, J. A. (1976). *Student reactions to instruction* (Memo to the Faculty, No. 58). University of Michigan, Center for Research on Learning and Teaching.

CHAPTER 14
Motivation

1984

Test Name: ACADEMIC CURIOSITY SCALE

Purpose: To measure academic curiosity.

Number of Items: 80

Format: True–false self-report.

Reliability: Odd–even split-half reliability coefficient was .87, point-biserial correlations of scores on each item with the total score on the scale ranged from .05 to .48, with a median of .32.

Validity: Academic curiosity was shown to be positively correlated with academic performance ($p < .001$).

Author: Vidler, D. C., and Rawan, H. R.

Article: Further validation of a scale of academic curiosity.

Source: *Psychological Reports,* August 1975, *37*(1), 115–118.

Related Research: Vidler, D. C., & Rawan, H. R. (1974). Construct validation of a scale of academic curiosity. *Psychological Reports, 35,* 263–266.

■ ■ ■

1985

Test Name: ACADEMIC MOTIVATION INVENTORY

Purpose: To determine factors in academic motivation.

Number of Items: 75

Format: The inventory consists of 9 sections intended to measure 9 motivational factors. Each item consists of a declarative sentence responded to on a 5-point scale ranging from *not at all true of me* to *extremely true of me.*

Reliability: The reliability coefficients ranged from .52 to .87 for the nine scales with the size of the coefficients generally corresponding to the number of items in the scale.

Author: Doyle, K., and Vhoen, R.

Article: Toward the definition of a domain of academic motivation.

Journal: *Journal of Educational Psychology,* April 1978, *70*(2), 231–236.

Related Research: Vhoen, R., & Doyle, K. (1977). Construction and development of the Academic Motivation Inventory (AMI). *Educational and Psychological Measurement, 37,* 509–512.

■ ■ ■

1986

Test Name: ACHIEVEMENT MOTIVATION QUESTIONNAIRE

Purpose: To measure one's need to achieve.

Number of Items: 28

Format: Twenty-seven items were worded in the extreme positive direction and one in the extreme negative direction rated on 9-interval scales.

Validity: Fifteen of the 28 items had scale means significantly different ($p < .002$, two-tailed) from an expected neutral response mean.

Author: Reynolds, W. M.

Article: Social desirability of achievement motivation.

Journal: *Psychological Reports,* December 1976, *39*(3), 1182.

Related Research: Hermans, H. J. M. (1970). A questionnaire measure of achievement motivation. *Journal of Applied Psychology, 54,* 353–363.

■ ■ ■

1987

Test Name: ACHIEVEMENT MOTIVATION SCALE

Purpose: To measure academic achievement motivation.

Number of Items: 14

Format: Items common to both the male and female forms of the Mehrabian Scale of the Tendency to Achieve were used.

Reliability: Split-half reliabilities of .69 (male students, $N = 158$), and .55 (female students, $N = 160$). Test–retest reliability coefficients were .78 for a group of 110 male and .72 for 111 female students.

Author: Dixon, P. N., and Cameron, A. E.

Article: Personality and motivational factors on an intentional-incidental learning task.

Journal: *Psychological Reports,* December 1976, *39*(3), 1315–1320.

Related Research: Mehrabian, A. (1968). Male and female scales of tendency to achieve. *Educational and Psychological Measurement, 28,* 493–502.

1988

Test Name: ACHIEVEMENT MOTIVATION SCALE FOR MEN—REVISED

Purpose: To measure achievement motivation.

Number of Items: 26

Reliability: Test–retest ($n = 36$ for 2-week interval) was .81.

Validity: Correlation with Shy Venturesome Scale was .56 for men ($n = 114$), .44 for women ($n = 42$); Jackson's Achievement Motivation Scale was .62 for men ($n = 114$), .51 for women ($n = 42$); Neuroticism Scale was –.40 for men ($n = 114$), –.41 for women ($n = 42$); Crowne and Marlowe Social Desirability Scale was .24 for men ($n = 114$), .24 for women ($n = 42$)

Author: Dias, S., and Carifio, J.

Article: A note on sex differences in achievement motivation.

Journal: *Educational and Psychological Measurement,* Summer 1977, *37*(2), 513–517.

Related Research: Mehrabian, A. (1968). Male and female scales of the tendency to achieve. *Educational and Psychological Measurement, 28,* 493–502.

● ● ●

1989

Test Name: ACHIEVEMENT MOTIVATION TEST

Purpose: To measure achievement motivation in young adults.

Format: Three subscales measure achievement motivation and debilitating and facilitating anxiety.

Reliability: Kuder-Richardson formula 20 reliabilities were .82 for the achievement motivation and .86 for the debilitating anxiety.

Validity: Spearman rank

correlation of .52 ($p < .05$, two-tailed) between debilitating anxiety score and the order in which participants responded.

Author: Feij, J. A.

Article: Construct validation of a fear-of-failure measure using an operant type of behavior.

Source: *Psychological Reports,* December 1975, *37*(3), 1147–1151.

Related Research: Hermans, H. J. M. (1970). A questionnaire measure of achievement motivation. *Journal of Applied Psychology, 54,* 353–363.

● ● ●

1990

Test Name: ACHIEVEMENT MOTIVATION TEST

Purpose: To assess motivation to achieve.

Number of Items: 30

Format: Self-report, yes–no response; sample item: "Does it bother you if another student makes better grades than you do?"

Validity: Correlation with Math Achievement, .32; with Vocabulary, .33.

Author: Rowley, G.

Article: Which examinees are most favored by the use of multiple choice tests?

Journal: *Journal of Educational Measurement,* Spring 1974, *11*(1), 15–23.

Related Research: Marshall, J., & Christensen, D. L. (1973). Leniency in marking: Its effects on student motivation and achievement. *Education,* 93(3), 262–265.

Russell, I. (1969). Motivation for school achievement: Measurement and validation. *Journal of Educational Research, 62,* 261–266.

1991

Test Name: CHABASSOL ADOLESCENT STRUCTURE INVENTORY

Purpose: To measure structure needs and perceptions in adolescence.

Number of Items: 77

Reliability: Odd–even reliability coefficients for the Wants Structure and Has Structure scales are .92 and .91, respectively.

Validity: Wants Structure scale correlates –.41 ($p < .001$) with the Exhibitionism scale of the Adjective Check List.

Author: Chabassol, D. J.

Article: An attempt to validate a measure of structure in adolescence.

Source: *Journal of Experimental Education,* Spring 1975, *43*(3), 46–50.

Related Research: Chabassol, D. J. (1971, Fall). A scale for the evaluation of structure needs and perceptions in adolescence. *Journal of Experimental Education, 40,* 12–16.

● ● ●

1992

Test Name: CHANGE-SEEKER INDEX

Purpose: To measure the intensity of a person's need for varying stimulus input.

Number of Items: 95

Format: Consists of true–false items.

Reliability: Internal consistency and retest reliability estimates ranged from .77 to .91.

Validity: Correlation with the Sensation-seeking Scale was .63. Correlation with two art judgment tests was .30.

Author: Farley, F. H.

Article: Arousal and cognition: Creative performance, arousal, and the stimulation-seeking motive.

Journal: *Perceptual and Motor Skills,* December 1976, *43*(3, Part 1), 703–708.

Related Research: Garlington, W. K., & Shimota, H. E. (1964). The Change-Seeker Index: A measure of the need for variable sensory input. *Psychological Reports, 14,* 919–924.

See *DUEMM, 2,* 1978, 717.

■ ■ ■

1993

Test Name: CLASSROOM BEHAVIOR INVENTORY

Purpose: To measure achievement motivation.

Format: Requires each teacher to rate students on a continuum on a number of subjective items. Examples are presented.

Reliability: Concurrent reliability of interraters was .65; internal consistency (Kuder-Richardson formula 20) was .95.

Validity: With total reading achievement, .318; language achievement, .199; spelling achievement, .290; total math achievement, .257; self-concept, .206.

Author: Cole, J. L.

Article: The relationship of selected personality variables to academic achievement of average aptitude third graders.

Journal: *Journal of Educational Research,* March 1974, *67*(7), 329–333.

■ ■ ■

1994

Test Name: COMMUNITY COLLEGE MOTIVATION INVENTORY

Purpose: To measure intrinsic motivation, self-enhancement, person orientation, and goal deficiency.

Number of Items: 200

Format: True–false.

Reliability: Test–retest reliabilities over 6 weeks were as follows: Intrinsic motivation, .91; self-enhancement, .88; person orientation, .92; goal deficiency, .90.

Validity: Intrinsic motivation scale's association with the verbal scale of the School and College Aptitude Test was .54 for men, .44 for women.

Author: Caughren, H. J., Jr.

Article: An experimental measure of motivation for community college students.

Source: *Journal of College Student Personnel,* May 1975, *16*(3), 232–237.

Related Research: Caughren, H. J., Jr. (1965). The relationship of stimulus-structure and selected personality variables to the discomfort-relief quotient in autobiographies. *Journal of Counseling Psychology, 12,* 74–80.

■ ■ ■

1995

Test Name: DESIRE TO WORK SCALE

Purpose: To measure a woman's desire to work, with work motivation defined as a function of marital status, presence and age of children, number of children, adequacy of husband's salary, and husband's attitude toward a wife working.

Number of Items: 29 situations.

Format: Subjects rate their desire to work in the situations on a 7-point Likert scale.

Reliability: Retest correlations of

work commitment were .80 for an older sample and .45 for women tested as college seniors.

Author: Orcutt, M. A., and Walsh, W. B.

Article: Traditionality and congruence of career aspirations for college women.

Journal: *Journal of Vocational Behavior,* February 1979, *14*(1), 111.

Related Research: Miyahira, S. (1976). *Selected personal and background variables as discriminating variables of college women's career orientations.* Unpublished doctoral dissertation, The Ohio State University.

■ ■ ■

1996

Test Name: EMPLOYEE COMMITMENT QUESTIONNAIRE

Purpose: To measure one's commitment to the organization, profession, and community.

Number of Items: 16

Format: Five items related to the organization, five to the profession, and six to the community. Responses ranged from 1 (*strongly disagree*) to 7 (*strongly agree*). All items are given.

Reliability: Median interitem correlations corrected using the Spearman-Brown formula were .52 for commitment to the organization, .59 for commitment to the profession, and .70 for commitment to the community, all significant at the .01 level.

Author: London, M., and Howat, G.

Article: The relationship between employee commitment and conflict resolution behavior.

Journal: *Journal of Vocational*

Behavior, August 1978, *13*(1), 1–14.

Related Research: Gouldner, A. W. (1958). Cosmopolitans and locals: Toward an analysis of latent social roles—II. *Administrative Science Quarterly, 2,* 444–480.

■ ■ ■

1997

Test Name: ENVIRONMENTAL CONTROL SCALE

Purpose: To measure one's desire to control the environment.

Number of Items: 14

Format: Measures (a) verbal commitment to ecology or intention to behave in an ecologically appropriate manner, (b) actual commitment to ecology or reports of the frequency of behaving in an ecologically appropriate manner, (c) affect or the degree of emotionality about ecological issues, and (d) knowledge about ecological issues.

Reliability: Cronbach's alpha was .83 and homogeneity ratio was .28. Test–retest correlation over a 4-week period was .88.

Validity: Correlates –.36 ($p < .01$) with the Pastoralism Scale (McKechnie, 1974). Other similar validity data are presented.

Author: Jorgenson, D. O.

Article: Measure of desire for control of the physical environment.

Journal: *Psychological Reports,* April 1978, *42*(2), 603–608.

Related Research: McKechnie, G. E. (1974). *Manual for the Environmental Response Inventory.* Palo Alto, CA: Consulting Psychologists Press.

■ ■ ■

1998

Test Name: GROUP AROUSAL MEASURE

Purpose: To measure the degree to which group members feel activated or stimulated.

Number of Items: 4

Format: A semantic differential. Each bipolar pair of adjectives is presented.

Reliability: .68

Validity: Correlations with a variety of variables ranged from .12 to .66.

Author: Greene, C. N., and Schriesheim, C. A.

Article: Leader-group interactions: A longitudinal field investigation.

Journal: *Journal of Applied Psychology,* February 1980, *65*(1), 50–59.

Related Research: Scott, W. E. (1967). The development of semantic differential scales as measures of "morale." *Personnel Psychology, 20,* 179–188.

■ ■ ■

1999

Test Name: GROWTH NEED STRENGTH MEASURES

Purpose: To measure growth need strength defined as one's wishes for certain conditions in a job and the perception of the job's potential for providing growth need satisfaction.

Number of Items: 23

Format: Eleven items on a Would Like scale and 12 items on a Job Choice scale.

Reliability: Internal consistency reliabilities were .88 for the Would Like scale and .71 for the Job Choice scale.

Author: Stone, E. F., et al.

Article: Relationships between growth need strength and selected individual differences measures employed in job design research.

Journal: *Journal of Vocational*

Behavior, June 1979, *14*(3), 329–340.

Related Research: Hackman, J. R., & Oldham, G. R. (1975). Development of the job diagnostic survey. *Journal of Applied Psychology, 60,* 159–170.

■ ■ ■

2000

Test Name: HIGHER ORDER NEED STRENGTH INSTRUMENT

Purpose: To measure higher order need strength.

Number of Items: 12

Format: An ipsative instrument taken from an early version of the Job Diagnostic Survey.

Reliability: Internal consistency reliability was .75.

Validity: Correlations with task perceptions and employee responses ranged from –.20 to .28.

Author: Brief, A. P., and Aldag, R. J.

Article: Correlates of role indices.

Journal: *Journal of Applied Psychology,* August 1976, *61*(4), 468–472.

Related Research: Hackman, J. R., & Lawler, E. E. (1971). Employee reactions to job characteristics [Monograph]. *Journal of Applied Psychology, 55,* 259–286.

■ ■ ■

2001

Test Name: INTERNAL WORK MOTIVATION SCALE

Purpose: To measure the degree of an employee's self-motivation to perform effectively on the job.

Number of Items: 4

Format: Employs a 7-point response scale.

Reliability: Internal consistency

was .76. Coefficient alpha was .86.

Validity: Correlations with a variety of variables ranged from −.39 to .46.

Author: Ivancevich, J. M.

Article: A longitudinal study of behavioral expectation scales: Attitudes and performance.

Journal: *Journal of Applied Psychology*, April 1980, *65*(2), 139–146.

Related Research: Hackman, J. R., & Oldham, G. R. (1975). Development of the Job Diagnostic Survey. *Journal of Applied Psychology*, *60*, 159–170.

∎ ∎ ∎

2002

Test Name: JOB INVOLVEMENT SCALE

Purpose: To measure job involvement.

Number of Items: 6

Format: Items are rated on a Likert scale; a high score reflects high job involvement.

Reliability: Reliability estimated by applying the Spearman-Brown prophecy formula to the mean interitem correlation was .75.

Validity: Correlations with: Job Description Index ranged from .01 to .20; locus of control, −.04; salary, .16; age, .06; attitude toward collective bargaining, −.16 (N = 222).

Author: Bigoness, W. J.

Article: Correlates of faculty attitudes toward collective bargaining.

Journal: *Journal of Applied Psychology*, April 1978, *63*(2), 228–233.

Related Research: Batlis, N. (1978). Job involvement as a moderator of work

environment-job satisfaction relationships. *Psychological Reports*, *42*(1), 275–281.

Ben-Porat, A. (1980). Job involvement, central life interest and job satisfaction. *Psychological Reports*, *46*(2), 507–512.

Lodahl T. M., & Kejner, M. (1965). The definition and measurement of job involvement. *Journal of Applied Psychology*, *49*, 24–33.

Morris, J. H., & Snyder, R. A. (1979). A second look at need for achievement and need for autonomy as moderators of role perception–outcome relationships. *Journal of Applied Psychology*, *64*, 173–178.

∎ ∎ ∎

2003

Test Name: JOB INVOLVEMENT SCALE

Purpose: To measure job involvement.

Number of Items: 20

Reliability: Corrected odd–even reliability coefficients ranged from .72 to .89.

Validity: With personal-demographic characteristics, r ranged from −.19 to .34; with situational-job characteristics, r ranged from .20 to .30; with work outcomes, r ranged from −.24 to .52.

Author: Saal, F. E.

Article: Job involvement: A multivariate approach.

Journal: *Journal of Applied Psychology*, February 1978, *63*(1), 53–61.

Related Research: Lodahl, T. M., & Kejner, M. (1965). The definition and measurement of job involvement. *Journal of Applied Psychology*, *49*, 24–33.

2004

Test Name: JUNIOR INDEX OF MOTIVATION SCALE

Purpose: To assess young people's motivation to learn in school.

Number of Items: 80

Time Required: Untimed–approximately 30 minutes to complete.

Format: Paper-and-pencil questionnaire-type scale.

Author: Frymier, J. R., et al.

Article: A longitudinal study of academic motivation.

Source: *Journal of Educational Research*, October 1975, *69*(2), 63–66.

Related Research: Frymier, J. R. (1970). Development and validation of a motivation index. *Theory into Practice*, *9*, 56–85.

∎ ∎ ∎

2005

Test Name: MANIFEST NEEDS QUESTIONNAIRE

Purpose: To measure need for achievement.

Format: Subject responds on a 7-point Likert scale ranging from *always* to *never*.

Reliability: Test–retest reliability was .72.

Validity: Results are correlated with age (−.09), education (−.10), and tenure (.03; N = 115).

Author: Steers, R. M., and Spencer, D. G.

Article: The role of achievement motivation in job design.

Journal: *Journal of Applied Psychology*, August 1977, *62*(4), 472–479.

Related Research: Steers, R. M., & Braunstein, D. N. (1976). A behaviorally-based measure of manifest needs in work settings.

Journal of Vocational Behavior, 9, 251–266.

• • •

2006

Test Name: MEHRABIAN ACHIEVING-TENDENCY SCALE

Purpose: To measure the tendency to achieve.

Number of Items: 34

Format: Includes single statements with alternative responses ranging from +3 (*very strong agreement*) to –3 (*very strong disagreement*). The response to an item is assumed to reflect a behavioral disposition that differentiates high versus low achievers. Examples are given.

Validity: Correlations with subscales of the Sensation-seeking Scale ranged from –.31 to .41 (*n* ranged from 37 to 144).

Author: Blankstein, K. R., et al.

Article: A further correlate of sensation seeking: Achieving tendency.

Journal: *Perceptual and Motor Skills,* June 1976, *42*(3, Part 2), 1251–1255.

Related Research: Atkinson, J. W. (1957). Motivational determinants of risk-taking behavior. *Psychological Review, 64,* 359–372.

Mehrabian, A. (1968). Male and female scales of the tendency to achieve. *Educational and Psychological Measurement, 28,* 493–502.

• • •

2007

Test Name: NACH NAFF SCALE

Purpose: To measure one's need to achieve and one's need for affiliation.

Number of Items: 30 pairs of adjectives.

Format: Forced choice: half the adjectives are based on the Need for Achievement Scale and the other half on the Need for Affiliation scale of Gough's Adjective Check List.

Reliability: Split-half corrected reliability is .80, and test–retest with 13 subjects is .88.

Validity: Pearsonian correlation of bank tellers' scores with supervisors' ratings was .32 (*p* < .05; with educational level, .28 (*p* < .10).

Author: Lindgren, H. C.

Article: Measuring need to achieve by nAch–nAff Scale—A forced-choice questionnaire.

Journal: *Psychological Reports,* December 1976, *39*(3), 907–910.

Related Research: Gough, H. G. (1965). *The Adjective Check List.* Palo Alto, CA: Consulting Psychologists Press.

• • •

2008

Test Name: NEED-DESIRE INSTRUMENT

Purpose: To identify the desire for each of several needs.

Number of Items: 28

Format: Includes desire for such needs as existence, relatedness, and growth.

Reliability: Coefficient alpha for existence was .87; for relatedness was .86; and for growth was .80.

Author: Keller, R. T., and Holland, W. E.

Article: Individual characteristics of innovativeness and communication in research and development organizations.

Journal: *Journal of Applied Psychology,* December 1978, *63*(6), 759–762.

Related Research: Alderfer, C. P.

(1967). Convergent and discriminant validation of satisfaction and desire measures by interviews and questionnaires. *Journal of Applied Psychology, 51,* 509–520.

• • •

2009

Test Name: NEED FOR ACHIEVEMENT SCALE

Purpose: To measure manifest level of need for achievement in work-specific context.

Number of Items: 5

Format: A 7-point Likert response format was used.

Reliability: Spearman-Brown estimate of internal consistency was .63 (*N* = 262).

Validity: Correlations with other variables ranged from –.15 to .29 (*N* = 262).

Author: Morris, J. H., and Snyder, R. A.

Article: A second look at need for achievement and need for autonomy as moderators of role perception-outcome relationships.

Journal: *Journal of Applied Psychology,* April 1979, *64*(2), 173–178.

Related Research: Steers, R. M., & Braunstein, D. N. (1976). A behaviorally-based measure of manifest needs in work settings. *Journal of Vocational Behavior, 9,* 251–266.

• • •

2010

Test Name: NEED FOR AUTONOMY SCALE

Purpose: To measure manifest level of need for autonomy in work-specific context.

Number of Items: 5

Format: A 7-point Likert response format was used.

Reliability: Spearman-Brown estimate of internal consistency was .68 ($N = 262$).

Validity: Correlations with other variables ranged from −.30 to .26 ($N = 262$).

Author: Morris, J. H., and Snyder, R. A.

Article: A second look at need for achievement and need for autonomy as moderators of role perception–outcome relationships.

Journal: *Journal of Applied Psychology,* April 1979, *64*(2), 173–178.

Related Research: Steers, R. M., & Braunstein, D. N. (1976). A behaviorally based measure of manifest needs in work settings. *Journal of Vocational Behavior, 9,* 251–266.

■ ■ ■

2011

Test Name: NEED SATISFACTION SCALE

Purpose: To measure one's job related need satisfaction.

Number of Items: 23 job outcomes

Format: Subjects respond to each outcome by rating how much of the characteristic they would like (from 1 to 7) and how much of the characteristic is actually present on the job (also from 1 to 7).

Reliability: Internal consistency reliability was .80.

Author: Lopez, E. M., and Greenhaus, J. H.

Article: Self-esteem, race and job satisfaction.

Journal: *Journal of Vocational Behavior,* August 1978, *13*(1), 75–83.

Related Research: Wanous, J. P., & Lawler, E. E., III. (1972). Measurement and meaning of job satisfaction. *Journal of Applied Psychology, 56,* 95–105.

2012

Test Name: NEED SATISFACTION SCALE

Purpose: To measure how well the work setting satisfies an individual's needs according to Maslow's hierarchy.

Number of Items: 15

Format: Each item is a characteristic rated three times on 7-point scales according to how much of it is present, how much should be present, and how important it is.

Reliability: Test–retest (3-week interval) Spearman rank correlation coefficient was .84 ($n = .17$).

Author: Morrison, R. F.

Article: Career adaptivity: The effective adaptation of managers to changing role demands.

Journal: *Journal of Applied Psychology,* October 1977, *62*(5), 549–558.

Related Research: Porter, L. W., & Lawler, E. E. (1968). *Managerial attitudes and performance.* Homewood, IL: Irwin.

■ ■ ■

2013

Test Name: NEED SATISFACTION SCHEDULE

Purpose: To assess need satisfaction in lower SES subjects.

Number of Items: 32

Format: Subscales for physiological, physical safety, security, and affection.

Reliability: Stability (10 days) was .60 to .75; Cronbach's alphas were .56, .64, .78, .46, and .40 on subscales and total.

Validity: Significant relation with ratings of need levels by judges.

Author: Lollar, D.

Article: An operationalization and validation of the Maslow need hierarchy.

Journal: *Educational and Psychological Measurement,* Autumn 1974, *34*(3), 639–651.

■ ■ ■

2014

Test Name: ORGANIZATIONAL COMMITMENT QUESTIONNAIRE

Purpose: To measure organizational commitment.

Number of Items: 15

Format: Items are given. Responses are on a 7-point scale from 1 (*strongly disagree*) to 7 (*strongly agree*) with the midpoint being 4 (*neither disagree nor agree*).

Reliability: Internal consistency reliabilities (coefficient alpha) ranged from .82 to .93 with a median of .90. Test–retest reliabilities for retail management trainees were .72 over a 2-month period and .62 for 3 months.

Validity: Correlation with the Sources of Organizational Attachment Questionnaire (Mowday et al., 1974) gave convergent validities from .63 to .74, with a median of .70.

Author: Mowday, R. T., et al.

Article: The measurement of organizational commitment.

Journal: *Journal of Vocational Behavior,* April 1979, *14*(2), 224–247.

Related Research: Mowday, R. L., et al. (1974). Unit performance, situational factors and employee attitudes in spatially separated work units. *Organizational Behavior and Human Performance, 12,* 231–248.

Porter, L. W., et al. (1976). Organizational commitment and managerial turnover: A longitudinal study. *Organizational Behavior and Human Performance, 15,* 87–98.

■ ■ ■

2015

Test Name: ORGANIZATIONAL COMMITMENT SCALE

Purpose: To assess the degree to which employees feel committed to the organization.

Number of Items: 15

Format: Employs a 7-point Likert scale ranging from *strongly agree* to *strongly disagree.*

Reliability: Coefficient alphas ranged from .82 to .93.

Validity: Correlations with a variety of variables ranged from −.07 to .40.

Author: Ivancevich, J. M.

Article: A longitudinal study of behavioral expectation scales: Attitudes and performance.

Journal: *Journal of Applied Psychology,* April 1980, *65*(2), 139–146.

Related Research: Porter, L. W., et al. (1974). Organizational commitment, job satisfaction and turnover among psychiatric technicians. *Journal of Applied Psychology, 59,* 603–609.

Steers, R. M., & Spencer, D. G. (1977). The role of achievement motivation in job design. *Journal of Applied Psychology, 62,* 472–479.

■ ■ ■

2016

Test Name: ORGANIZATIONAL COMMITMENT SCALE

Purpose: To measure organizational commitment.

Number of Items: 9

Format: Includes: satisfaction with the organization, motivation, and

organization–employee value congruity. A 7-point Likert response format was used.

Reliability: Spearman-Brown estimate of internal consistency was .88 (*N* = 262).

Validity: Correlations with other variables ranged from −.41 to .58 (*N* = 262).

Author: Morris, J. H., and Snyder, R. A.

Article: A second look at need for achievement and need for autonomy as moderators of role perception–outcome relationships.

Journal: *Journal of Applied Psychology,* April 1979, *64*(2), 173–178.

Related Research: Porter, L. W., et al. (1974). Organizational commitment, job satisfaction, and turnover among psychiatric technicians. *Journal of Applied Psychology, 59,* 603–609.

■ ■ ■

2017

Test Name: PRESTATIE MOTIVATIE TEST

Purpose: To measure achievement motivation.

Number of Items: 29

Format: Guttman-scaled items with Likert format of stem responses.

Reliability: Kuder-Richardson formula 20 reliability was .85 in a neutral condition and .88 in the achievement-oriented condition.

Validity: In the achievement-oriented condition (in contrast to the neutral condition) significant Spearman correlations were obtained between the scores and various performance tasks (.32, .41, $p < .05$; .57, $p < .01$).

Author: Chandler, T. A., et al.

Article: Sex differences in self-reported achievement motivation.

Journal: *Psychological Reports,* April 1979, *44*(2), 575–581.

Related Research: Hermans, H. J. M. (1970). A questionnaire measure of achievement motivation. *Journal of Applied Psychology, 54,* 353–363.

Morris, J. H., et al. (1977). Influence of respondent sets on two objective measures of achievement motivation. *Educational and Psychological Measurement, 37,* 1051–1055.

O'Gorman, J. G. (1975). A note on the PMT as an objective test of achievement motivation. *Journal of Personality Assessment, 39,* 297–298.

Prawat, R. S. (1976). Mapping the affective domain in young adolescents. *Journal of Educational Psychology, 68,* 566–572.

Saal, F. E. (1978). Job involvement: A multivariate approach. *Journal of Applied Psychology, 63,* 53–61.

Schultz, C. B., & Pomerantz, M. (1974). Some problems in the application of achievement motivation to education: The assessment of motive to succeed and probability of success. *Journal of Educational Psychology, 66,* 599–608.

■ ■ ■

2018

Test Name: REINFORCEMENT SURVEY SCHEDULE

Purpose: To identify potential reinforcers for individuals.

Number of Items: 139

Format: Includes the areas "sports, reading, music, consumption, and human relations," which the subject rates on a 5-point scale; an overall potential reinforcement score reflects the total number of items that are potentially reinforcing.

Validity: Correlations between eight dimensions of emotion (Self Rating Index) and overall reinforcement index ranged .29 (*ns*) to .57 (*p* < .01).

Author: Plutchik, R., and Stein, S.

Article: Reinforced preferences and personality profiles of hospitalized schizophrenics.

Journal: *Psychological Reports,* October 1974, *35*(2), 695–700.

Related Research: Cautela, J., & Kastenbaum, A. (1967). Reinforcement Survey Schedule for use in therapy, training and research. *Psychological Reports, 20,* 1115–1130.

See *DUEMM, 2,* 1978, 735.

■ ■ ■

2019

Test Name: RESULTANT ACHIEVEMENT MOTIVATION TEST—SHORT FORM

Purpose: To measure motivation to succeed.

Number of Items: 22

Reliability: Internal consistency estimate of reliability was .55.

Validity: With Comprehensive Test of Basic Skills, *r* = .41; IQ, *r* = .29; Grade Point Average, *r* = .48.

Author: Schultz, C. B., and Pomerantz, M.

Article: Some problems in the application of achievement motivation to education: The assessment of motive to succeed and probability of success.

Journal: *Journal of Educational Psychology,* August 1974, *66*(4), 599–608.

Related Research: Mehrabian, A. (1969). Measures of achievement tendency. *Educational and Psychological Measurement, 29,* 445–451.

See *DUEMM, 2,* 1978, 728.

2020

Test Name: SELF-ANCHORING STRIVING SCALE

Purpose: To measure one's expectancy of future goal success.

Number of Items: 10

Format: Ladder format with the client's description of best and worst possible life as anchors for each end of the ladder (10 best, 0 worst).

Reliability: Test–retest correlations reportedly ranged from .43 to .70.

Author: Boone, S. E., et al.

Article: Hope and manifest anxiety: Motivational dynamics of acceptance of disability.

Journal: *Journal of Counseling Psychology,* November 1978, *25*(6), 551–556.

Related Research: Cantril, H. (1965). *The pattern of human concerns.* New Brunswick, NJ: Rutgers University Press.

■ ■ ■

2021

Test Name: SELF-APPRAISAL OF CURIOSITY INVENTORY

Purpose: To provide a self-appraisal of curiosity.

Number of Items: 39

Format: Each item is answered *yes* or *no.*

Reliability: Split-half reliability corrected by the Spearman-Brown formula was .68.

Author: Voss, H. G., and Keller, H.

Article: Critical evaluation of the Obscure Figures Test as an instrument for measuring "cognitive innovation."

Journal: *Perceptual and Motor Skills,* October 1977, *45*(2), 495–502.

Related Research: Maw, W. H., &

Maw, E. W. (1968). Self-appraisal of curiosity. *Journal of Educational Research, 61,* 462–465.

■ ■ ■

2022

Test Name: SELF DESCRIPTIVE QUESTIONNAIRE

Purpose: To measure need for achievement.

Number of Items: 20 paragraphs

Format: Respondents rank the paragraphs from most to least descriptive of themselves.

Reliability: Test–retest reliability of .64 for female freshmen (Stein, 1967).

Author: Marshall, S. J., and Wijting, J. P.

Article: Relationships of achievement motivation and sex-role identity to college women's career orientation.

Journal: *Journal of Vocational Behavior,* June 1980, *16*(3), 299–311.

Related Research: Stein, M. I. (1967). *Patterns of self description* (Progress Report No. 2). New York University.

■ ■ ■

2023

Test Name: SENSATION SEEKING SCALE

Purpose: To measure the need for arousal-seeking behavior.

Number of Items: 22

Time Required: 10 minutes.

Validity: Correlations with Barron's self-report measure of creativity and independence of judgment correlations ranged from .47 to .68. Correlations with ratings of creative class projects were .66 (men) and .37 (women).

Author: Davis, G. A., et al.

Article: Attitudes, motivation, sensation seeking, and belief in ESP as predictors of real creative behavior.

Journal: *Journal of Creative Behavior,* 1974, *8*(1), 31–39.

Related Research: Zuckerman, M., et al. (1964). Development of a sensation-seeking scale. *Journal of Consulting Psychology, 28,* 477–482.

See *DUEMM, 2* , 1978, 741.

■ ■ ■

2024

Test Name:
SENSATION-SEEKING SCALE

Purpose: To measure degree of sensation seeking.

Number of Items: 34

Format: Contains forced-choice item pairs describing a stimulating and less stimulating activity. Subject chooses the item of each pair which better expresses his or her preference for these activities.

Reliability: Kuder-Richardson formula 20 was .79 (*N* = 135).

Validity: With Novelty-Experiencing scale, *r* = .44 (*N* = 135); with Unusual Meaning Vocabulary, *r* = .10 (*N* = 135); with Stroop Color-Word Test, *r* = –.06 (*N* = 54).

Author: Gaines, L. S., and Coursey, R. D.

Article: Novelty-experiencing, internal scanning, and cognitive control.

Journal: *Perceptual and Motor Skills,* June 1974, *38*(3, Part I), 891–898.

Related Research: Farley, F. J. (1976). Arousal and cognition: Creative performance, arousal and the stimulation-seeking motive. *Perceptual and Motor Skills, 43,* 703–708.

Kurtz, J. P., & Zuckerman, M.

(1978). Race and sex differences on the Sensation-Seeking Scales. *Psychological Reports, 43,* 529–530.

Zuckerman, M. (1964). Development of a sensation-seeking scale. *Journal of Consulting Psychology, 28,* 477–482.

See *DUEMM, 2,* 1978, 741.

■ ■ ■

2025

Test Name:
SENSATION-SEEKING SCALE IV

Purpose: To assess tendency to seek out sensation.

Number of Items: 22

Time Required: 10 minutes.

Format: Consists of five scales: General, Thrill, and Adventure Seeking, Experience Seeking, Disinhibition, and Boredom Susceptibility.

Validity: Scales were relatively independent of SAT measured ability; male participants were significantly higher (*p* < .05) on Thrill and Adventure Seeking, and Disinhibition scales than female participants: correlations with Barrons self-report measure of creativity ranged .47 to .68 (Davis, 1974); correlations with ratings of creative class projects were .66 (male students) and .37 (female students; Davis, 1974).

Author: Waters, C.

Article: Multidimensional measures of novelty experiencing, sensation seeking, and ability: Correlational analysis for male and female college samples.

Journal: *Psychological Reports,* 1974, *34*(1), 43–46.

Related Research: Blankenstein, K. R., et al. (1976). A further correlate of sensation seeking: Achieving tendency. *Perceptual*

and Motor Skills, 42(3), Part 2, 1251–1255.

Davis, G. A., et al. (1974). Attitudes, motivation, sensation seeking, and belief in ESP as predictors of real creative behavior. *Journal of Creative Behavior, 8*(1), 31–39.

Farley, F. (1974). Measuring the stimulation-seeking motive by global self rating. *Perceptual and Motor Skills, 39*(1), Part I, 101–102.

Kymbaugh, K., & Garrett, J. (1974). Sensation seeking among skydivers. *Perceptual and Motor Skills, 38*(1), 118.

Zuckerman, M. (1972). *Manual and research report on the sensation seeking scale.* Newark: University of Delaware.

See *DUEMM, 2,* 1978, 741.

■ ■ ■

2026

Test Name: SENTENCE COMPLETION TEST OF ACHIEVEMENT MOTIVATION

Purpose: To measure achievement motivation.

Number of Items: 14

Format: Each item is an incomplete sentence with farming as a key word.

Validity: Correlation with an adapted version of McClelland's Thematic Apperception Test of Need Achievement was –.04 and with the Graphic Expression Method of Achievement Motivation was –.16.

Author: Singh, S.

Article: Relationships among projective and direct verbal measures of achievement motivation.

Journal: *Journal of Personality Assessment,* February 1979, *43*(1), 45–49.

Related Research: Rogers, E. M., & Neill, R. E. (1966). *Achievement motivation among Colombian peasants.* Unpublished paper, Department of Communication, Michigan State University.

■ ■ ■

2027

Test Name: STUDENT ASPIRATION SCALE

Purpose: To measure aspirations in the areas of wealth, fame, occupational status, and educational goals.

Number of Items: 11

Format: In responding to each question the student chooses from two or three alternatives. Examples are given.

Reliability: Alpha reliabilities were .65 (pretest) and .62 (posttest).

Author: Sheehan, D. S.

Article: A study of attitude change in desegregated intermediate schools.

Journal: *Sociology of Education,* January 1980, *53*(1), 51–59.

Related Research: Rosenberg, M., & Simmons, R. (1971). *Black and White self-esteem: The urban*

school child. Washington, DC: Arnold M. and Caroline Rose Monograph Series.

■ ■ ■

2028

Test Name: STUDENT ATTITUDE INVENTORY

Purpose: To assess academic achievement motivation in junior high school students.

Number of Items: 159

Format: Three parts: Part I, seven identifying biographical questions; Part II, 59 questions from the Academic Achievement Motivation Scale; Part III, 93 questions from the Children's Report of Parental Behavior Inventory.

Validity: Each item was judged by a panel of educators and psychologists in terms of academic achievement motivation. Each item used had a mean rating of 3.6 or greater on the 5-point rating scale.

Author: Lehrer, B., and Hieronymous, A.

Article: Predicting achievement using intellectual academic-motivational and selected non-intellectual factors.

Journal: *Journal of Experimental*

Education, Summer 1977, *45*(4), 44–51.

Related Research: Schaefer, E. (1965). Children's reports of parental behaviors: An inventory. *Child Development, 36,* 413–424.

■ ■ ■

2029

Test Name: WORK PREFERENCE QUESTIONNAIRE

Purpose: To measure the need for achievement of British managerial populations.

Number of Items: 24

Format: Forced-choice comprising 24 pairs of statements each pair matched for social desirability, and logically related.

Reliability: Test–retest reliability over 1-year was .58

Validity: Correlation with the achievement motive scale of the Ghiselli Self-Description Inventory was .42

Author: Fineman, S.

Article: The work preference questionnaire: A measure of managerial need for achievement.

Source: *Journal of Occupational Psychology,* 1975, *48*(1), 11–32.

CHAPTER 15
Perception

2030

Test Name: ACADEMIC SELF-CONCEPT SCALE

Purpose: To serve as a measure of an academic facet of generalized self-concept.

Number of Items: 40

Format: Includes a 4-point Likert response format.

Reliability: Cronbach's coefficient alpha was .91.

Validity: Correlation with grade point average was .40. Correlation with the Rosenberg Self-Esteem Scale was .45.

Author: Reynolds, W. M.

Article: Initial development and validation of the Academic Self-Concept Scale.

Journal: *Educational and Psychological Measurement,* Winter 1980, *40*(4), 1013–1016.

...

2031

Test Name: ACADEMIC SELF-ESTEEM SCALE

Purpose: To measure a student's perception of his or her capabilities in an academic setting.

Number of Items: 11

Format: Student responds either *yes* or *no* to each item. Examples are presented.

Reliability: Alpha reliabilities were .66 (pretest) and .71 (posttest).

Author: Sheehan, D. S.

Article: A study of attitude change in desegregated intermediate schools.

Journal: *Sociology of Education,* January 1980, *53*(1), 51–59.

Related Research: Vitale, M. (1974). *Evaluation of the Title III Dallas Junior High School Career Education Project: 1973–1974* (Research Report No. 74–291). Dallas, TX: Dallas Independent School District, Department of Research, Evaluation, and Information Systems.

...

2032

Test Name: ACTIVITY-STEREOTYPES SCALE

Purpose: To assess stereotyping of girls.

Number of Items: 50

Format: Each item was identified by the child as to whether it is done by ladies, by men, or by both.

Reliability: Split-half corrected $r = .96$.

Validity: Correlation with Quality-Stereotypes measure was .60.

Author: Marantz, S. A., and Mansfield, A. F.

Article: Maternal employment and the development of sex-role stereotyping in five-to eleven-year-old girls.

Journal: *Child Development,* June 1977, *48*(2), 668–673.

2033

Test Name: ADULT NOWICKI-STRICKLAND I-E SCALE

Purpose: To measure adult locus of control.

Number of Items: 40

Format: Each item is answered *yes* or *no* and poses an internal or external belief.

Reliability: Internal consistency coefficients ranged from .74 to .86 and a stability coefficient of .83 was reported.

Validity: Correlations with the Pleasant Events Schedule ranged from −.24 to −.42 ($N = 32$, men) and from −.03 to −.13 ($N = 42$, women).

Author: Cash, T. F., and Burns, D. S.

Article: The occurrence of reinforcing activities in relation to locus of control, success-failure expectancies, and physical attractiveness.

Journal: *Journal of Personality Assessment,* August 1977, *41*(4), 387–391.

Related Research: Dixon, D. N., et al. (1976). Dimensionality of three adult, objective locus of control scales. *Journal of Personality Assessment, 40,* 310–319.

Marecek, J., & Frasch, C. (1977). Locus of control and college women's role expectations. *Journal of Counseling Psychology, 24,* 132–136.

Nowicki, S., Jr., & Duke, M. P. (1974). A locus of control scale for noncollege as well as college adults.

Journal of Personality Assessment, 38, 136–137.

■ ■ ■

2034

Test Name: AESTHETIC SENSITIVITY SCALE

Purpose: To measure visual aesthetic sensitivity.

Number of Items: 42

Format: Each item contains two non-representational pictures, one of which has intentional design faults. The subject is to identify the correct picture in each pair. Examples are provided.

Reliability: Split-half corrected reliability was .84.

Validity: Correlations with the Eysenck Personality Questionnaire ranged from –.21 to .16.

Author: Götz, K. O., et al.

Article: A new visual aesthetic sensitivity test: I. Construction and psychometric properties.

Journal: *Perceptual and Motor Skills,* December 1979, *49*(3), 795–802.

Related Research: Eysenck, H. J., & Eysenck, S. B. G. (1976). *Psychoticism as a dimension of personality.* London: Hodder and Stoughton.

■ ■ ■

2035

Test Name: ALTERNATE FORM SELF-CONCEPT INVENTORY

Purpose: To assess the global self-concept of college students.

Number of Items: 26

Format: Subjects rate themselves on a 5-point scale ranging from *stand very high* to *stand very low* for each trait listed.

Validity: Pearson product–moment correlations between Brownfain Self-Rating Inventory and alternate form ranged from .85 to .88.

Author: Hamm, R. J.

Article: Alternate forms for global self-concept and an achievement-related subscale using the Brownfain Self-rating Inventory.

Journal: *Psychological Reports,* December 1976, *39*(3), 1196–1198.

Related Research: Brownfain, J. J. (1952). Stability of the self-concept as a dimension of personality. *Journal of Abnormal and Social Psychology, 47,* 597–606.

■ ■ ■

2036

Test Name: APPRAISAL INTERVIEW AND SUPERVISION SCALE

Purpose: To assess workers' perceptions of their appraisal interview and supervisors.

Number of Items: 7

Format: Four items using a 7-point continuum are used to describe the appraisal interview. Three-items using a 7-point continuum are used to indicate degree of satisfaction with the supervision on the job.

Reliability: Interitem reliability for the job satisfaction items is .72.

Validity: Measure of satisfaction with the supervisor is not independent from the measure of reaction to the appraisal ($r = .44$, $p < .001$).

Author: Greiler, M. M.

Article: Subordinate participation and reactions to the appraisal interview.

Journal: *Journal of Applied Psychology,* October 1975, *60*(5), 544–549.

Related Research: Hackman, J. R., & Lawler, E. E. (1971). Employee reactions to job characteristics. *Journal of Applied Psychology, 55,* 259–286.

Wexley, K. N., et al. (1973). Subordinate personality as a moderator of the effects of participation in three types of appraisal interviews. *Journal of Applied Psychology, 58,* 54–59.

■ ■ ■

2037

Test Name: BARRETT-LENNARD RELATIONSHIP INVENTORY

Purpose: To measure one's perceptions of the counseling relationship.

Number of Items: 36

Format: Subjects indicate their degree of agreement with each item on a 7-point scale from *mostly disagree* to *mostly agree.* A four-item scale is used to measure resistance to the interviewer's statement.

Reliability: Cronbach's alpha internal consistency reliabilities for Emphatic Understanding, $r = .61$; Unconditionality of Regard, $r = .56$; Level of Regard, $r = .81$; Congruence, $r = .82$ and Resistance, $r = .53$.

Author: Strong, S. R., et al.

Article: Motivational and equipping functions of interpretation in counseling.

Journal: *Journal of Counseling Psychology,* March 1979, *26*(2), 98–107.

Related Research: Mann, B., & Murphy, K. C. (1975). Timing of self-disclosure, reciprocity of self-disclosure and reactions to an initial interview. *Journal of Counseling Psychology, 22,* 304–308.

2038

Test Name: BARTH SCALE

Purpose: To describe how teachers view their role and the process of children's learning.

Number of Items: 28

Format: Likert items using a 5-point scale ranging from *strongly agree* to *strongly disagree*. Includes seven factors: curricular flexibility, intellectual development, evaluating the child, learning through involvement, learning facilitators, evaluating the child's work, and learning through exploration. Items are presented.

Reliability: Alpha internal consistency reliabilities of the derived factors ranged from .62 to .76.

Author: Coletta, A. J., and Gable, R. K.

Article: The content and construct validity of the Barth Scale: Assumptions of open education.

Journal: *Educational and Psychological Measurement,* Summer 1975, *35*(2), 415–425.

Related Research: Barth, R. S. (1971). So you want to change to an open classroom. *Phi Delta Kappan, 53,* 97–99.

■ ■ ■

2039

Test Name: BEHAVIOR RATING FORM

Purpose: To measure a child's self-esteem.

Number of Items: 13

Format: Observer-report instrument. Child is rated on a 5-point Likert scale with respect to 13 behaviors assumed to be external manifestations of the child's self-esteem.

Reliability: Test–retest reliability

by one teacher-observer after an 8-week interval was .96.

Author: Zirkel, P., and Gable, R. K.

Article: The reliability and validity of various measures of self-concept among ethnically different adolescents.

Journal: *Measurement and Evaluation in Guidance,* April 1977, *10*(1), 48–54.

Related Research: Coopersmith, S. (1967). *The antecedents of self-esteem.* San Francisco: Freeman.

Cowan, R., et al. (1978). A validity study of selected self-concept instruments. *Measurement and Evaluation in Guidance, 10,* 211–221.

■ ■ ■

2040

Test Name: BETTS-SHEEHAN QUESTIONNAIRE UPON MENTAL IMAGERY

Purpose: To assess imagery vividness.

Number of Items: 35

Time Required: 10 minutes.

Format: The subject is asked to imagine various objects and scenes in seven sensory modalities and to rate the degree of clarity of the mental image compared to the clarity of the real object or scene on a 7-point scale. Total score ranges from 35 to 245.

Author: Tedford, W. H., Jr., and Penk, M. L.

Article: Intelligence and imagery in personality.

Journal: *Journal of Personality Assessment,* August 1977, *41*(4), 405–413.

Related Research: Sheehan, P. W. (1967). A shortened form of the Betts questionnaire upon mental

imagery. *Journal of Consulting Psychology, 23,* 386–389.

■ ■ ■

2041

Test Name: BIALER SCALE FOR CHILDREN

Purpose: To measure children's locus of control.

Number of Items: 23

Format: Subjects respond with *yes–no* answer.

Reliability: Overall test–retest reliability was .68 (2–3 week interval). Test–retest was .88 for girls and .39 for boys.

Validity: Correlation with the Stanford Preschool I-E Scale (N= 130) was .18.

Author: Bachrach, R., and Peterson, R. A.

Article: Test–retest reliability and interrelation among three locus of control measures for children.

Journal: *Perceptual and Motor Skills,* August 1976, *43*(1), 260–262.

Related Research: Bialer, I. (1961). Conceptualization of success and failure in mentally retarded and normal children. *Journal of Personality, 29,* 303–320.

Guttentag, M., & Klein, I. (1976). The relationship between inner versus outer locus of control and achievement in Black middle school children. *Educational and Psychological Measurement, 36,* 1101–1109.

■ ■ ■

2042

Test Name: BLOCK COUNTING TEST

Purpose: To assess spatial orientation and visualization.

Number of Items: 30

Time Required: 3.6 minutes.

Format: Subjects count the number of blocks in a pictured pile.

Reliability: .63 (Kuder-Richardson coefficient).

Author: Undheim, J.

Article: Broad ability in 12 to 13 year old children, the theory of fluid and crystallized intelligence, and the differentiation hypothesis.

Journal: *Journal of Educational Psychology*, June 1978, *70*(3), 433–443.

Related Research: Guilford, J., & Hoepfner, R. (1971). *The analysis of intelligence.* New York: McGraw-Hill.

• • •

2043

Test Name: BODY CATHEXIS

Purpose: To measure feelings of satisfaction or dissatisfaction with different parts or processes of the body.

Number of Items: 46

Format: Items identify parts of the body or their functions and are rated on a 5-point scale.

Reliability: Coefficient of reliability was .78 and .83.

Author: Kernaleguen, A., and Conrad, Sister G.

Article: Analysis of five measures of self-concept.

Journal: *Perceptual and Motor Skills,* December 1980, *51*(3, Part 1), 855–861.

Related Research: Secord, P. J., & Jourard, S. M. (1953). The appraisal of body cathexis: Body cathexis dnd the self. *Journal of Consulting Psychology, 17,* 343–347.

2044

Test Name: BODY IMAGE SATISFACTION SCALE

Purpose: To measure body appearance satisfaction.

Number of Items: 24

Format: The subject rates on a 7-point scale (from 3 to –3) degree of satisfaction with the appearance of each of 24 body parts.

Reliability: Test–retest reliability of .84 and .73. Internal consistency reliability of .83.

Validity: Correlations with Self-Cathexis Scale, .39; Janis-Field-Eagly Scale, .45; Job Interview Expectations, .24; Interview Self-ratings, .14; judges' ratings, .08; self-rating discrepancy scores, .06 (*N* = 87).

Author: King, M. R., and Manaster, G. J.

Article: Body image, self-esteem, expectations, self-assessments, and actual success in a simulated job interview.

Journal: *Journal of Applied Psychology,* October 1977, *62*(5), 589–594.

Related Research: Rosen, G. M., & Ross, A. O. (1968). Relationship of body image to self-concept. *Journal of Consulting and Clinical Psychology, 32,* 100.

• • •

2045

Test Name: CANADIAN SELF-ESTEEM INVENTORY

Purpose: To measure an individual's perception in four areas: self, peers, parents, and school.

Number of Items: 60

Format: Five sub-scales, one of which is a lie scale designed to measure defensiveness.

Validity: Correlations with the

Coopersmith Self-Esteem Inventory ranged from .71 to .80 for all subjects; values for boys ranged from .72 to .84, and for girls from .66 to .91.

Author: Battle, J.

Article: Comparison of the self-report inventories.

Journal: *Psychological Reports,* August 1977, *41*(1), 159–160.

Related Research: Battle, J. (1979). Self-esteem of students in regular and special classes. *Psychological Reports, 44*(1), 212–214.

Coopersmith, S. (1967). *The antecedents of self-esteem.* San Francisco: Freeman.

• • •

2046

Test Name: CANADIAN SELF-ESTEEM INVENTORY FOR ADULTS

Purpose: To measure self-esteem of adults.

Number of Items: 50

Format: Includes three areas of perception: self, personal, and social. Also includes a lie scale.

Reliability: Test–retest reliability was .81. Alpha (Kuder-Richardson formula 20) analysis of internal consistency ranged from .57 to .78.

Validity: Correlations with measure of depression ranged from –.34 to –.78.

Author: Battle, J.

Article: Relationship between self-esteem and depression among high school students.

Journal: *Perceptual and Motor Skills,* August 1980, *51*(1), 157–158.

Related Research: Battle, J. (1971). Test–retest reliability of the Canadian Self-esteem

Inventory for Adults. *Perceptual and Motor Skills, 44*(1), 38.

Battle, J. (1978). Relationship between self-esteem and depression. *Psychological Reports, 42*, 745–746.

■ ■ ■

2047

Test Name: CANTRIL'S SELF-ANCHORING STRIVING SCALE

Purpose: A measure of life perspective, including one's perception of current, future, and past life statuses relative to each person's expressed best possible and worst possible life.

Format: An 11-point ladder with Point 1 representing worst possible life and Point 11, best possible life.

Reliability: Test–retest reliability coefficients ranged from .43 to .70.

Author: Roessler, R., et al.

Article: Effects of systematic group counseling on work adjustment clients.

Journal: *Journal of Counseling Psychology*, July 1977, *54*(4), 313–317.

Related Research: Cantril, H. (1965). *The pattern of human concerns.* New Brunswick, NJ: Rutgers University Press.

■ ■ ■

2048

Test Name: CARD ROTATION TEST

Purpose: To assess spatial orientation and visualization.

Number of Items: 168

Time Required: 6 minutes.

Format: Subjects indicate whether or not each of eight figures is identical to a standard figure when rotated in a plane.

Reliability: 72 (Kuder-Richardson coefficient).

Author: Undheim, J.

Article: Broad ability factors in 12 to 13 year old children, the theory of fluid and crystallized intelligence, and the differentiation hypothesis.

Journal: *Journal of Educational Psychology*, June 1978, *70*(3), 433–443.

Related Research: Guilford, J., & Hoepfner, R. (1971). *The analysis of intelligence.* New York: McGraw-Hill.

■ ■ ■

2049

Test Name: CHILDREN'S LOCUS OF EVALUATION AND CONTROL SCALE

Purpose: To assess internal–external locus of control.

Number of Items: 48

Format: Includes two subscales to gauge locus of evaluation and locus of control.

Reliability: Split-half reliability coefficient was .74 ($n = 148$).

Author: Shavit, H., and Rabinowitz, A.

Article: Locus of control and effects of failure on performance and perceived competence.

Journal: *Journal of Personality Assessment*, June 1978, *42*(3), 265–271.

Related Research: Miller, J. O. (1963). *CLOEC Scale.* Unpublished test, George Peabody College, Nashville, TN.

■ ■ ■

2050

Test Name: CLASS ATMOSPHERE SCALE

Purpose: Measures perceived

environment in order to specify degree of consensus and inferentially, the strength of behavioral press along several dimensions.

Number of Items: 120

Time Required: 30 minutes.

Format: 12 subscales, including: Aggression, Submission, Autonomy, Order, Affiliation, Involvement, Insight, Practicality, Spontaneity, Support, Variety, and Clarity. True–false items.

Author: Silbergeld, S., et al.

Article: Classroom psychosocial environment.

Journal: *Journal of Educational Research*, December 1975, *69*(4), 151–155.

Related Research: Silbergeld, S., et al. (1976). Assessment of the psychosocial environment of the classroom: The Class Atmosphere Scale. *Journal of Social Psychology, 100*, 65–76.

■ ■ ■

2051

Test Name: CONFIDENCE IN CHILD MANAGEMENT SCALE

Purpose: To enable practitioners to rate their confidence in managing children's problem behaviors.

Number of Items: 20

Format: Subject responds to each item on a 10-point behaviorally anchored scale. Sample items are presented.

Reliability: Intrarater reliability coefficient was .93. Interrater reliability coefficient was .89.

Author: Wurster, C. A., et al.

Article: Communication patterns in pedodontics.

Journal: *Perceptual and Motor Skills,* February 1979, *48*(1), 159–166.

Related Research: Wright, G. Z. (1975). *Behavior management in dentistry for children.* Philadelphia, PA: Saunders.

■ ■ ■

2052

Test Name: CONTROL OF IMAGERY QUESTIONNAIRE

Purpose: To assess a subject's ability voluntarily to control various aspects of imagery.

Number of Items: 35

Format: Each item first directs the subject to have a specific image and then to change the initial image in a specific way. The subject then responds on a 0 to 4 rating scale the ease with which he or she is able to make the change. Examples are provided.

Reliability: Total score reliability was .85.

Validity: Correlation with Gordon Test of Visual Imagery Control was .53; with Betts Questionnaire Upon Mental Imagery was .57.

Author: Lane, J. B.

Article: Problems in assessment of vividness and control of imagery.

Journal: *Perceptual and Motor Skills,* October 1977, *45*(2), 363–368.

■ ■ ■

2053

Test Name: COOPERSMITH SELF-ESTEEM INVENTORY

Purpose: To measure self-esteem.

Number of Items: 25

Format: Subjects respond to each item by indicating whether it is *like me* or *unlike me.*

Reliability: Coefficient alpha was .67.

Author: Adler, S.

Article: Self-esteem and causal attributions for job satisfaction

and dissatisfaction.

Journal: *Journal of Applied Psychology,* June 1980, *65*(3), 327–332.

Related Research: Coopersmith, S. (1967). *The antecedents of self-esteem.* San Francisco: Freeman.

■ ■ ■

2054

Test Name: COOPERSMITH SELF-ESTEEM INVENTORY

Purpose: Revised to measure evaluative attitudes of adults toward the self.

Number of Items: 58

Format: Self-report. Test–retest reliability of .78 and .80 for 32 adult women after 6 to 58 weeks.

Validity: Correlates .47 with the Marlowe-Crowne Social Desirability Scale for a group of 51 college students.

Author: Ryden, M. B.

Article: An adult version of the Coopersmith Self-Esteem Inventory: Test–retest reliability and social desirability.

Journal: *Psychological Reports,* December 1978, *43*(3), 1189–1190.

Related Research: Battle, J. (1977). Comparison of two self-report inventories. *Psychological Reports,* August, *41*(1), 159–160.

Coopersmith, S. (1967). *The antecedents of self-esteem.* San Francisco: Freeman.

Drummond, R. J., et al. (1977). Stability and sex differences on the Coopersmith Self-Esteem Inventory for students in grades two to twelve. *Psychological Reports, 40*(3), 943–946.

McIntire, W. G., & Drummond, R. J. (1976). The structure of self-concept in second and fourth

grade children. *Educational and Psychological Measurement,* Summer, *36*(2), 529–536.

■ ■ ■

2055

Test Name: DEMOCRATIC DEFICIENCY SCALE

Purpose: To measure perceptions of unmet democratic values.

Number of Items: 9

Format: Example of items is given.

Reliability: Alpha coefficient of .70.

Author: Long, S.

Article: Explaining systemic failure: A two-dimensional analysis.

Journal: *Psychological Reports,* August 1977, *41*(1), 23–28.

Related Research: Long, S. (1976). *Cognitive-perceptual factors in the political alienation process: A test of six models.* Paper presented at the meeting of the Midwest Political Science Association, Chicago.

■ ■ ■

2056

Test Name: DIMENSIONS OF SELF-CONCEPT

Purpose: To measure self-concept that emphasizes school-related activities.

Number of Items: 70

Format: Includes five dimensions of self-concept: level of aspiration, anxiety, academic interest and satisfaction, leadership and initiative, and identification versus alienation. Two forms are available.

Reliability: Internal consistency estimates or reliability for each of the five dimensions ranged from .70 to .90.

Validity: Correlations of each of the five dimensions with Comprehensive Test of Basic Skills ranged from –.45 to .47; with Gates-MacGinitie Reading Tests, Sur E ranged from –.11 to .08.

Author: Michael, W. B., et al.

Article: Further development and validation of a self-concept measure involving school-related activities.

Journal: *Educational and Psychological Measurement,* Summer 1978, *38*(2), 527–535.

Related Research: Fernandes, L. M., et al. (1978). The factorial validity of three forms of the dimensions of self-concept measure. *Educational and Psychological Measurement, 38,* 537–545.

Michael, W. B., & Smith, R. A. (1976). The development and preliminary validation of three forms of a self-concept measure emphasizing school-related activities. *Educational and Psychological Measurement, 36,* 521–528.

. . .

2057

Test Name: EDUCATIONAL FORCES INVENTORY

Purpose: To assess the constellation of forces in the teacher's social-psychological field.

Number of Items: 39; 13 forces evaluated 3 ways.

Format: Respondents evaluate the forces by ranking their importance in influencing teaching, assigning a weight for relative importance in influencing teaching, and rating the forces on a scale of 1 to 5 according to the positive/negative effect on teaching.

Reliability: Over a 1-year interval, reliability/stability correlation

ratios range from .65 to .93.

Validity: Correlations between the Purdue Teacher Opinionaire and the Educational Forces Inventory ranged from .20 to .68.

Author: Rayder, N. F., and Bödy, B.

Article: The Educational Forces Inventory: A new technique for measuring influences on the classroom.

Journal: *Journal of Experimental Education,* Winter 1975, *44*(2), 26–34.

Related Research: Rayder, N. F., & Bödy, B. (1975). The Educational Forces Inventory: Psychometric properties. *Journal of Experimental Education, 44,* 35–44.

. . .

2058

Test Name: EXPECTATIONS ABOUT COUNSELING

Purpose: To measure student expectancies about counseling.

Number of Items: 141

Format: Likert format with 7 response options ranging from 1 (*not true*) to 7 (*definitely true*).

Reliability: Alpha reliabilities of the scales ranged from .75 to .92.

Author: Parham, W. D., and Tinsley, H. E. A.

Article: What are friends for? Students' expectations of the friendship encounter.

Journal: *Journal of Counseling Psychology,* September 1980, *27*(5), 524–527.

Related Research: Tinsley, H. E. A., et al. (1980). Factor analysis of the domain of client expectancies about counseling. *Journal of Counseling Psychology, 27,* 561–570.

2059

Test Name: FIGURE ANALOGIES TEST

Purpose: To assess ability at recognizing figural relations.

Number of Items: 16

Time Required: 6.5 minutes.

Format: Subjects select one of five figures to complete an analogy.

Reliability: .88 (Kuder-Richardson coefficient).

Author: Undheim, J.

Article: Broad ability factors in 12 to 13 year old children, the theory of fluid and crystallized intelligence, and the differentiation hypothesis.

Journal: *Journal of Educational Psychology,* June 1978, *70*(3), 433–443.

Related Research: Guilford, J., & Hoepfner, R. (1971). *The analysis of intelligence.* New York: McGraw-Hill.

. . .

2060

Test Name: FOLDING BLOCKS TEST

Purpose: To measure spatial relations ability.

Number of Items: 10

Format: The child visually examines each two-dimensional layout to determine which geometric shape it would form when folded up.

Validity: Correlations with the Children's Embedded Figures Test ranged from –.139 to .676.

Author: Connor, J. M., et al.

Article: Sex-related differences in response to practice on a visual-spatial test and generalization to a related test.

Journal: *Child Development,* March 1978, *49*(1), 24–29.

Related Research: Lifschitz, S. (1977, March). *A study of sex and age differences on a spatial relations test in elementary school children.* Paper presented at the meeting of the Society for Research in Child Development, New Orleans.

■ ■ ■

2061

Test Name: GENERAL SELF-ESTEEM SCALE

Purpose: To measure whether students have a favorable view toward themselves.

Number of Items: 6

Format: Response to each question is either *a lot, a little,* or *never.* Examples are given.

Reliability: Alpha reliabilities were .65 (pretest) and (posttest).

Author: Sheehan, D. S.

Article: A study of attitude change in desegregated intermediate schools.

Journal: *Sociology of Education,* January 1980, *53*(1), 51–59.

Related Research: Rosenberg, M., & Simmons, R. (1971). *Black and White self-esteem: The urban school child.* Washington, DC: Arnold M. and Caroline Rose Monograph Series.

■ ■ ■

2062

Test Name: GRADUATE ENVIRONMENTAL PERCEPTION SCALES

Purpose: To measure graduate students' expectations and perceptions of the college environment.

Number of Items: 100

Format: Five scales with 20 items each, including Conventionality, Academic, Camaraderie, Cosmopolitanism, and Decorum.

Reliability: Two-week test–retest reliability estimates ranged from .64 to .85 for students and .63 to .86 for faculty. Modified Hoyt reliability estimates ranged from .88 to .95 for entering graduate students, from .92 to .96 for established graduate students, and from .85 to .93 for faculty.

Author: Winston, R. B., Jr.

Article: Graduate school environments: Expectations and perceptions.

Journal: *Journal of College Student Personnel,* January 1976, *17*(1), 43–49.

Related Research: Pace, C. R. (1969). *College and University Environment Scales, technical manual* (2nd ed.). Princeton, NJ: Educational Testing Service.

■ ■ ■

2063

Test Name: GUY EMOTIVE IMAGING SCALE

Purpose: To measure the vividness of one's emotive images.

Number of Items: 36

Format: Includes six emotions: shame, surprise, interest, distress, fear, and anger. The subject rates on a 7-point scale the clarity of each emotion as experienced in each of six situations. An example is given.

Reliability: Alpha coefficient was .87.

Validity: Correlation with the Betts Questionnaire Upon Mental Imagery was .50.

Author: Guy, M. E., and McCarter, R. E.

Article: A scale to measure emotive imagery.

Journal: *Perceptual and Motor Skills,* June 1978, *46*(3, Part 2), 1267–1274.

2064

Test Name: HARE SELF-ESTEEM SCALE

Purpose: To measure home, peer, and school self-esteem.

Number of Items: 30

Format: Subscales include peer, home, and school. Subjects respond to each item by indicating *strongly disagree, disagree, agree,* or *strongly agree.*

Validity: Correlation with Coopersmith's Self-Esteem Inventory was .83; with Rosenberg's general self-esteem measure was .74.

Author: Shoemaker, A. L.

Article: Construct validity of area specific self-esteem: The Hare Self-Esteem Scale.

Journal: *Educational and Psychological Measurement,* Summer 1980, *40*(2), 495–501.

Related Research: Hare, B. R. (1975). *The relationship of social background to the dimensions of self-concept.* Unpublished doctoral dissertation, University of Chicago.

■ ■ ■

2065

Test Name: HAZARD PERCEPTION TEST

Purpose: To assess hazard perception in automobile drivers.

Number of Items: 60

Time Required: 5 to 10 minutes.

Format: The subject rates for danger of an accident on a 7-point rating scale one- or two-sentence descriptions of commonly encountered driving situations. Examples are provided.

Reliability: Spearman rhos for odd/even split-half correlations were .73 and .91.

Validity: Tetrachoric coefficients between test scores and occurrence of violations ranged from .17 to .33.

Author: Soliday, S. M.

Article: Development and preliminary testing of a driving hazard questionnaire.

Journal: *Perceptual and Motor Skills,* December 1975, *41*(3), 763–770.

■ ■ ■

2066

Test Name: HEALTH LOCUS OF CONTROL SCALE

Purpose: To measure the degree to which an individual perceives that he or she has control over his or her health.

Format: High scores are related to an external expectancy.

Validity: Health Scale correlated .33 with Rotter's I-E Scale.

Author: Tolor, A.

Article: Some antecedents and personality correlates of health locus of control.

Journal: *Psychological Reports,* December 1978, *43*(3), 1159–1165.

Related Research: Wallston, B. S., et al. (1976). Development and validation of the Health Locus of Control (HLC) Scale. *Journal of Consulting and Clinical Psychology, 44,* 580–585.

■ ■ ■

2067

Test Name: HEALTH OPINION SURVEY

Purpose: To measure one's view of own's own health.

Number of Items: 18

Format: Five-point Likert format from *never* to *almost always.*

Reliability: Alpha reliability

coefficient was .84.

Author: Butler, M. C., and Burr, R. G.

Article: Unity of a multidimensional locus of control scale in predicting health and job-related outcomes in military environments.

Journal: *Psychological Reports,* December 1980, *47*(3), 719–728.

Related Research: Macmillan, A. M. (1957). The Health Opinion Survey: Technique for estimating prevalence of psychoneurotic and related types of disorder in communities. *Psychological Reports, 3,* 325–339.

■ ■ ■

2068

Test Name: I-E SCALE

Purpose: To measure locus of control.

Number of Items: 29

Format: Forced-choice scale.

Reliability: Split-half and test–retest reliabilities ranged from .65 to .70.

Validity: Correlation with perceived stress was .61 ($N = 90$).

Author: Anderson, C. R.

Article: Locus of control, coping behaviors, and performance in a stress setting: A longitudinal study.

Journal: *Journal of Applied Psychology,* August 1977, *62*(4), 446–451.

Related Research: Rotter, J. B. (1966). Generalized expectancies for internal vs. external control of reinforcement. *Psychological Monographs, 80* (1 Whole No. 609).

■ ■ ■

2069

Test Name: I FEEL-ME FEEL INVENTORY

Purpose: To measure five dimensions of self concepts.

Number of Items: 40

Format: Includes five dimensions of self concepts: general adequacy, peer, teacher-school, academic, and physical. Each item is a black and white picture of an event related to a young child's life experiences. Five faces graphically representing sadness to happiness are painted below each picture. The respondent is asked to put an X on the picture that shows how he or she feels about the picture.

Reliability: Test–retest reliability ($N = 4,000$) was .82 for kindergarten, .81 for first grade, .78 for second grade, .79 for third grade.

Validity: With Metropolitan Readiness, $r = .68, .24$; with California Achievement Test, $r = .73, .79$; with Behavorial Maturity Scale, $r = .24$.

Author: White, W. F., and Simmons, M.

Article: First-grade readiness predicted by teachers' perception of students' maturity and students' perception of self.

Journal: *Perceptual and Motor Skills,* August 1974, *39*(1 Part 2), 395–399.

Related Research: Montague, J. C., Jr., & Cage, B. N. (1974). Self-concepts of institutional and non-institutional educable mentally retarded children. *Perceptual and Motor Skills, 38* (3), Part 1, 977–978.

Yeatts, P., & Bentley, E. L. (1971). *The development of a nonverbal measure to assess the self-concept of young and low-verbal children.* Paper presented to the American Educational Research Association Meeting, New York.

2070

Test Name: INDIVIDUAL SENSE OF COMPETENCE TEST

Purpose: To measure one's sense of competence.

Number of Items: 23

Format: Likert agreement–disagreement scale from +4 (*very strong agreement*) to –4 (*very strong disagreement*).

Reliability: Internal reliability, .96; test–retest was .84 over a 2-month period.

Validity: Predictive validity between high and low performer groups $p < .001$.

Author: Wagner, F. R., and Morse, J. J.

Article: A measure of individual sense of competence.

Journal: *Psychological Reports*, April 1975, *36*(2), 451–459.

■ ■ ■

2071

Test Name: INTELLECTUAL ACHIEVEMENT RESPONSIBILITY QUESTIONNAIRE

Purpose: To assess locus-of-control.

Number of Items: 34

Format: The test provides a total I score representing the overall degree of internality which includes two subscores: belief in internal responsibility for successes (I+) and belief in internal responsibility for failures (I–).

Reliability: For I+, $r = .66$; for I–, $r = .74$; test–retest (3 weeks), I+, $r = .55$; I–, $r = .60$; I total, $r = .62$.

Author: Wolk, S., and Eliot, J.

Article: Information-generated influence as a function of locus-of-control patterns in children.

Journal: *Child Development*, December 1974, *45*(4), 928–934.

Related Research: Bauer, D. H. (1975). The effect of instructions, anxiety, and locus of control on intelligence test scores. *Measurement and Evaluation in Guidance, 8*(1), 13–19.

Crandall, V., et al. (1962). Motivational and ability determinants of young children's intellectual achievement behaviors. *Child Development, 33*(3), 643–648.

Crandall, V. C., et al. (1965). Children's beliefs in their own control of reinforcements in intellectual-academic achievement situations. *Child Development, 36,* 91–109.

Lifshitz, M. (1973). Internal–external locus-of-control dimension as a function of age and the socialization milieu. *Child Development, 44*(3), 538–546.

Murray, H., & Staebler, B. (1974). Teacher's locus of control and student achievement gains. *Journal of School Psychology,* Winter, *12*(4), 305–309.

See *DUEMM, 2,* 1978, 786.

■ ■ ■

2072

Test Name: INTELLECTUAL ACHIEVEMENT RESPONSIBILITY SCALE/ MODIFIED

Purpose: To assess adolescents' locus of control.

Number of Items: 34

Format: Includes three clusters: intellectual achievement, social interactions, and work. A few items are presented.

Validity: Correlations with parental locus of control measures ranged from –.48 to .58.

Author: Lifshitz, M., and Ramot, L.

Article: Toward a framework for developing children's locus-of-control orientation: Implication from the Kibbutz system.

Journal: *Child Development,* March 1978, *49*(1), 85–95.

Related Research: Crandall, V. C., et al. (1965). Children's beliefs in their own control of reinforcements in intellectual-academic achievement situations. *Child Development, 36,* 91–109.

■ ■ ■

2073

Test Name: INTELLECTUAL SELF-CONFIDENCE SCALE

Purpose: To measure intellectual self-confidence.

Number of Items: 33

Format: A nonreactive measure of three behavioral tendencies: expectation of success, attraction to intellectual tasks, and self-reliance.

Reliability: .75

Validity: With Achievement Test Anxiety, Debilitating subscales, $r = .37$; with Achievement Test Anxiety, Facilitating Subscale, $r = .23$; with American College Test, $r = .31$.

Author: Hiller, J. H.

Article: Learning from prose text: Effects of readability level, inserted question difficulty, and individual differences.

Journal: *Journal of Educational Psychology,* April 1974, *66*(2), 202–211.

Related Research: Kirby, E. A., & Hiller, J. H. (1973, February). *Comparative validation of a direct and an indirect measure of academic self-confidence.* Paper presented at the meeting of the American Educational Research Association, New Orleans.

2074

Test Name: INTERNAL–EXTERNAL LOCUS OF CONTROL SCALE

Purpose: To measure locus of control.

Number of Items: 29

Format: A self-administering, forced choice instrument.

Reliability: Test–retest reliability coefficients of .60 ($N = 30$), .78 ($N = 28$), and .49 ($N = 63$) were reported for men.

Validity: Correlations with scale scores of the California Personality Inventory ranged from –.01 to –.45 ($N = 100$). Correlations with MMPI scale scores ranged from .49 to –.46 ($N = 100$). Correlation with Taylor's Manifest Anxiety (MAs) was .44 ($N = 100$).

Author: Scott, D. P., and Severance, L. J.

Article: Relationships between the CPI, MMPI, and locus of control in a nonacademic environment.

Journal: *Journal of Personality Assessment*, April 1975, *39*(2), 141–145.

Related Research: Andrisani, P. J., & Nestel, G. (1976). Internal–external control as contributor to and outcome of work experience. *Journal of Applied Psychology, 61*, 156–165.

Dixon, D. N., et al. (1976). Dimensionality of three adult, objective locus of control scales. *Journal of Personality Assessment, 40*, 310–319.

Horne, A. M., et al. (1976). Institutional males' perceptions of three counseling techniques. *Perceptual and Motor Skills, 43*, 383–387.

Klockars, A. J., & Varnum, S. W. (1975). A test of the dimensionality assumptions of Rotter's Internal–External Scale. *Journal of Personality Assessment, 39*, 397–404.

Rotter, J. B. (1966). Generalized expectancies for internal versus external control reinforcement. *Psychological Monographs, 80*(1, Whole No. 609).

Sanders, M. G., et al. (1976). Internal–external locus of control and performance on a vigilance task. *Perceptual and Motor Skills, 42*, 939–943.

Strahan, R., & Huth, H. (1975). Relations between embedded figures test performance and dimensions of the I-E Scale. *Journal of Personality Assessment, 39*, 523–524.

Zerega, W. D., Jr., et al. (1976). Stability and concurrent validity of the Rotter Internal–External Locus of Control Scale. *Educational and Psychological Measurement, 36*, 473–475.

■ ■ ■

2075

Test Name: INTERPERSONAL CONTROL SCALE

Purpose: To measure the expectancy for control or influence of interpersonal outcomes.

Number of Items: 40

Format: Twenty-four items with 16 filler items.

Reliability: Internal consistency alpha reliability coefficient was .87.

Validity: Over-all scores correlated .48 with Rotter's Introversion–Extraversion Scale (1966).

Author: Dudley, G. E.

Article: Predicting interpersonal behavior from a measure of expectancy for interpersonal control.

Journal: *Psychological Reports*, December 1977, *41*(3), 1223–1230.

Related Research: Rotter, J. B. (1966). Generalized expectancies for internal versus external control of reinforcement. *Psychological Monographs, 80*(1 Whole No. 609).

■ ■ ■

2076

Test Name: INTERPERSONAL PERCEPTION METHOD—MODIFIED

Purpose: To identify interpersonal perceptions between teacher and child.

Number of Items: 49

Time Required: 60–75 minutes.

Format: Around each of 49 dyadic issues, 12 questions are asked. Each issue is used to view four relationships and three perspectives. An example of one issue is given.

Author: Bryant, B. K.

Article: Locus of control related to teacher–child interperceptual experiences.

Journal: *Child Development*, March 1974, *45*(1), 157–164.

Related Research: Bryant, B. (1971). *Student-teacher relationships as related to internal–external locus of control.* Unpublished doctoral dissertation, University of Minnesota.

■ ■ ■

2077

Test Name: INTOLERANCE OF AMBIGUITY SCALE

Purpose: To measure the level of threat perceived in ambiguous situations.

Number of Items: 16

Format: Responses are made on a 7-point Likert scale.

Reliability: Test–retest 3-week interval, Spearman rank order correlation coefficient was .72 (n = 25).

Author: Morrison, R. F.

Article: Career adaptivity: The effective adaptation of managers to changing role demands.

Journal: *Journal of Applied Psychology,* October 1977, *62*(5), 549–558.

Related Research: Budner, S. (1973). Intolerance of ambiguity. In J. P. Robinson & P. R. Shaver (Eds.), *Measures of social psychological attitudes* (rev. ed.). Ann Arbor, MI: Survey Research Center.

Lichtenberg, J. W., & Heck, E. J. (1979). Interactional structure of interviews conducted by counselors of different levels of cognitive complexity. *Journal of Counseling Psychology, 26,* 15–22.

• • •

2078

Test Name: INTOLERANCE OF TRAIT INCONSISTENCY

Purpose: To measure intolerance of trait inconsistency.

Number of Items: 15

Format: Subjects choose which of two pairs of traits (one pair equally good, the other unequally good) are more likely to occur together in people.

Validity: A loading of .56 on Vannoy's (1965) Factor IV.

Author: Lichtenberg, J. W., and Heck, E. J.

Article: Interactional structure of interviews conducted by counselors of different levels of cognitive complexity.

Journal: *Journal of Counseling Psychology,* January 1979, *26*(1), 15–22.

Related Research: Laing, R. D., et al. (1966). *Interpersonal perception.* New York: Springer.

Vannoy, J. S. (1965). Generality of cognitive complexity–simplicity as a personality construct. *Journal of Personality and Social Psychology, 2,* 385–396.

• • •

2079

Test Name: INVASION OF PRIVACY QUESTIONNAIRE

Purpose: To measure the degree to which subjects think their privacy is being invaded.

Number of Items: 66

Format: Includes five factors: family background and influences, personal history data, interests and values, financial management data, and social adjustment.

Reliability: Internal consistency for each factor ranged from .78 to .93.

Author: Wade, M.

Article: Personnel research.

Journal: *Personnel Journal,* April 1974, *53*(4), 306–308.

Related Research: Rosenbaum, B. L. (1973). Attitude toward invasion of privacy in the personnel selection process and job applicant demographic and personality correlates. *Journal of Applied Psychology, 58,* 333–338.

• • •

2080

Test Name: INVENTORY OF TEMPORAL EXPERIENCES

Purpose: To provide a means for self-reporting temporal experiences.

Number of Items: 101

Format: Includes four scales: human time, animal time, vital time, and physical time.

Reliability: Corrected split-half reliability coefficients for each of the four scales were .85 (human time), .82 (animal time), .82 (vital time), and .84 (physical time).

Validity: Correlations of the four scales with the Scales of the Personal Orientation Inventory ranged from –.48 to .53.

Author: Yonge, G. D.

Article: Time experiences, self-actualizing values, and creativity.

Journal: *Journal of Personality Assessment,* December 1975, *39*(6), 601–606.

Related Research: Yonge, G. D. (1973). Time experiences as measures of personality. *Measurement and Evaluation in Guidance, 5,* 475–482.

• • •

2081

Test Name: JAMES I-E SCALE

Purpose: To measure internal–external locus of control.

Number of Items: 60

Format: Likert scale with all items worded in the external direction. The four response choices ranged from 3 (*strongly agree*) to 0 (*strongly disagree*). Scores ranged from 0 to 90.

Reliability: Split-half adjusted reliability was .89 (men) and .94 (women). Test–retest reliability for a 3–month period was .79 (men) and .82 (women) and for a 6–month period was .76 (men) and .78 (women).

Validity: Correlations with Rotter I-E were .57 (men, n = 98) and .60 (women, n = 123); with Adult Nowicki Strickland I-E the correlations were .50 (men) and .51 (women).

Author: Dixon, D. N., et al.

Article: Dimensionality of three adult, objective locus of control scales.

Journal: *Journal of Personality Assessment,* June 1976, *40*(3), 310–319.

Related Research: MacDonald, A. P., Jr. (1973). Measures of internal–external control. In J. P. Robinson & P. R. Shaver (Eds.), *Measures of social psychological attitudes.* Ann Arbor: The University of Michigan, Institute for Social Research.

■ ■ ■

2082

Test Name: JANIS-FIELD-EAGLY SELF-ESTEEM SCALE

Purpose: To measure self-esteem.

Number of Items: 10

Format: Focuses directly on reported feelings of self-esteem and confidence in interpersonal interactions.

Reliability: Internal consistency reliabilities were .84 and .79.

Validity: With Body Satisfaction, r = .45; Self-Cathexis Scale, r = .57; Job interview expectations, r = .52; Interview self-ratings, r = .47; Judges' ratings, r = .19; Self-rating discrepancy scores, r = .25 (N = 87).

Author: King, M. R., and Manaster, G. J.

Article: Body image, self-esteem, expectations, self-assessments, and actual success in a simulated job interview.

Journal: *Journal of Applied Psychology,* October 1977, *62*(5), 589–594.

Related Research: Berscheid, E., et al. (1973, March). *Body image, physical appearance, and self-esteem.* Paper presented at the meeting of the American Sociological Association, New York.

■ ■ ■

2083

Test Name: JOB COMPLEXITY SCALE

Purpose: To measure one's perception of job complexity.

Number of Items: 5

Format: Items are given.

Validity: Pearson correlations of self-reported complexity with various factors were .36 ($p < .001$) for salary; .45 ($p < .001$) for occupational class; and .37 ($p < .001$) for level of occupation. Correlations with observer-reported complexity were .7 ($p < .001$) for salary; .80 ($p < .001$) for occupational class; and .73 ($p < .001$) for level.

Author: Gould, S.

Article: Age, job complexity, satisfaction, and performance.

Journal: *Journal of Vocational Behavior,* April 1979, *14*(2), 209–223.

Related Research: Beach, D. S. (1975). *Personnel: The management of people at work* (3rd ed.). New York: Macmillan.

■ ■ ■

2084

Test Name: LEADERSHIP BEHAVIOR AND DESCRIPTION QUESTIONNAIRE

Purpose: To measure perceptions of leadership behavior.

Format: Included are the scales of initiating structure and consideration.

Reliability: Coefficient alphas were .81 for initiating structure, .76 for consideration.

Validity: Correlations with such variables as trust, influence, promotion in organization, and job problems ranged from –.56 to .40.

Author: Adams, E. F.

Article: A multivariate study of subordinate perceptions of and attitudes toward minority and majority managers.

Journal: *Journal of Applied Psychology,* June 1978, *63*(3), 277–288.

Related Research: Stogdill, R. M., et al. (1962). The leader behavior description subscale. *Journal of Psychology,* 56, 3–8.

■ ■ ■

2085

Test Name: LOCUS OF CONFLICT RATING SCALE

Purpose: To provide a measure of internalization and externalization of conflict.

Number of Items: 30

Format: Four-point rating scales for short behavioral descriptions.

Reliability: Test–retest reliability of about .90 for each portion of the scale.

Author: Nelson, W. M., et al.

Article: Anxiety and locus of control in normal children.

Journal: *Psychological Reports,* October 1977, *41*(2), 375–378.

Related Research: Armentrout, J. A. (1971). Parental child-rearing attitudes and preadolescents' problem behaviors. *Journal of Consulting and Clinical Psychology,* 37, 278–285.

■ ■ ■

2086

Test Name: LOCUS OF CONTROL INVENTORY FOR THREE ACHIEVEMENT DOMAINS

Purpose: To assess locus of control orientation in three achievement domains: intellectual, social, and physical.

Number of Items: 48

Format: Items are answered *yes* or *no.*

Reliability: Kuder-Richardson

formula 20 reliability coefficients for 373 students aged 12 to 18 years: Social subscale ($r = .54$), Physical subscale ($r = .52$), Intellectual subscale ($r = .53$), and total scale ($r = .75$).

Validity: Correlation between the Intellectual subscale and Crandall's Intellectual Achievement Responsibility scale, $r(58) = .78$, $p < .01$. Correlations for Social and Physical subscales were .45 and .54. Correlations between the subscales and the Children's Scale ranged from .43 to .49.

Author: Bradley, R. H., et al.

Article: A new scale to assess locus of control in three achievement domains.

Journal: *Psychological Reports,* October 1977, *41*(2), 656.

Related Research: Bradley, R. H., & Webb, R. (1976). Age-related differences in locus of control orientation in three behavior domains. *Human Development, 19*(1), 49–55.

Crandall, C. V., et al. (1965). Children's beliefs in their own control of reinforcements in intellectual-academic achievement situations. *Child Development, 36,* 91–109.

Nowicki, S., & Strickland, B. (1973). A locus of control scale for children. *Journal of Consulting and Clinical Psychology, 40,* 148–155.

■ ■ ■

2087

Test Name: LOCUS OF CONTROL OF INTERPERSONAL RELATIONSHIPS QUESTIONNAIRE

Purpose: To measure one's belief in personal or internal control of social outcomes.

Number of Items: 23

Format: Subjects indicate whether they "most agree" with a statement reflecting a belief in personal or internal control of social outcomes or one reflecting a belief in external control of those outcomes.

Reliability: Cronbach's alpha was .76 and test–retest reliability after 8 weeks for 49 volunteers was .67.

Validity: Correlated .37 with scores on the Marlowe-Crowne Social Desirability Scale and .38 with scores on Rotter's I-E Scale.

Author: Lewis, P., et al.

Article: Locus of control of interpersonal relationships questionnaire.

Journal: *Psychological Reports,* October 1977, *41*(2), 507–510.

■ ■ ■

2088

Test Name: LOCUS OF CONTROL SCALE

Purpose: To measure locus of control.

Number of Items: 11

Format: The items represent adult work-oriented perceptions and the lower the score, the greater the degree of internal control.

Reliability: Kuder-Richardson internal consistency reliability estimates of .746 and .749 for two administrations of the scale in 1969 and 1971.

Author: Dailey, R. C.

Article: Relationship between locus of control, perceived group cohesiveness, and satisfaction with coworkers.

Journal: *Psychological Reports,* February 1978, *42*(1), 311–316.

Related Research: Andrisani, P., & Nestle, G. (1976). Internal–external control as contributor to and outcome of work experience. *Journal of Applied Psychology, 61,* 156–165.

2089

Test Name: LOCUS OF CONTROL SCALE

Purpose: To assess subjects' personal control beliefs.

Number of Items: 50

Format: Items are rated on a 6-point Likert scale. Scale includes a 12-item Internal–External scale, a 7-item Perceived Competence scale, and an 11–item Origin–Pawn scale.

Reliability: Alpha reliability coefficients: Internal–External, .81; Perceived Competence, .72; Origin–Pawn, .56.

Validity: Correlation between Internal–External and Origin–Pawn scales was .48 ($df = 98$, $p < .001$).

Author: Graybill, D.

Article: Effects of perceived freedom on the relationship of locus of control beliefs to typical shifts in expectancy.

Journal: *Psychological Reports,* December 1978, *43*(3), 815–820.

■ ■ ■

2090

Test Name: LOCUS OF CONTROL SCALE

Purpose: To measure the extent to which an individual perceives herself or himself in control of his or her life.

Number of Items: 24

Format: Likert scaled items yielding three scores: Internal (I), Powerful Others (P), and Chance (C).

Reliability: Kuder-Richardson reliabilites were .64 (I Scale), .74 (P Scale), and .78 (C Scale). One-week test–retest reliabilities were .64, .74, and .78, respectively.

Author: Spokane, A. R., and Derby, D. P.

Article: Congruence, personality pattern and satisfaction in college women.

Journal: *Journal of Vocational Behavior,* August 1979, *15*(1), 36–42.

Related Research: Levenson, H. (1972). Distinctions within the concept of internal–external control: Development of a new scale. In *Proceedings of the American Psychological Association,* 259–260.

■ ■ ■

2091

Test Name: LOCUS OF CONTROL SCALE ADAPTED

Purpose: To measure locus of control.

Number of Items: 46

Format: Responses are made on a 5-point scale ranging from *agree strongly* to *disagree strongly.*

Validity: Correlation with Much IV Scale was –.31.

Author: Duffy, P. J., et al.

Article: Locus of control: Dimensionality and predictability using Likert scales.

Journal: *Journal of Applied Psychology,* April 1977, *62*(2), 214–219.

Related Research: Collins, B. E. (1974). Four components of the Rotter Internal–External Scale: Belief in a difficult world, the just world, a predictable world, and a politically responsive world. *Journal of Personality and Social Psychology, 29,* 381–391.

Rotter, J. B. (1966). Generalized expectancies for internal versus external control of reinforcement. *Psychological Monographs, 80* (1, Whole No. 609).

2092

Test Name: LOCUS OF CONTROL SCALE FOR CHILDREN

Purpose: To measure locus of control orientation.

Number of Items: 40

Format: A paper and pencil format on which each item is answered *yes* or *no.*

Validity: Correlations were with Self-concept, –.26; Grade point average, –.20; Language achievement, –.23; Math achievement, –.21; and Effort, –.13 (*N* = 113).

Author: Gordon, D. A.

Article: Children's beliefs in internal–external control and self-esteem as related to academic achievement.

Journal: *Journal of Personality Assessment,* August 1977, *41*(4), 383–386.

Related Research: Nowicki, S., & Strickland, B. (1973). A locus of control scale for children. *Journal of Consulting and Clinical Psychology, 40,* 148–154.

■ ■ ■

2093

Test Name: LOCUS OF CONTROL TEST

Purpose: To measure locus of control in high school students.

Number of Items: 23

Format: Yes–no response.

Reliability: Test–retest for a heterogeneous sample of retardates was .84.

Author: Prawat, R. S.

Article: Mapping the affective domain in young adolescents.

Journal: *Journal of Educational Psychology,* October 1976, *68*(5), 566–572.

Related Research: Bialer, L. (1961). Conceptualization of success and failure in mentally retarded and normal children. *Journal of Personality, 29,* 303–320.

■ ■ ■

2094

Test Name: MACDONALD-TSENG INTERNAL–EXTERNAL LOCUS OF CONTROL SCALE

Purpose: To measure locus of control.

Number of Items: 12

Format: A forced-choice format.

Validity: Correlation with the Rotter internal–external Locus of Control Scale was *r* = .42 (*N* = 541).

Author: Zerega, W. D., Jr., et al.

Article: Stability and concurrent validity of the Rotter Internal–External Locus of Control Scale.

Journal: *Educational and Psychological Measurement,* Summer 1976, *36*(2), 473–475.

Related Research: MacDonald, A. P., & Tseng, M. S. (1971). *Dimensions of internal versus external control revisited.* Unpublished paper, West Virginia University.

■ ■ ■

2095

Test Name: MELBOURNE PAIN APPERCEPTION TEST

Purpose: To measure pain reactivity.

Number of Items: 10

Format: Subjects respond to 10 film segments.

Reliability: Spearman-Brown split-half reliability was .86.

Validity: Correlation with pain threshold was .21 and with pain tolerance was .45.

Author: Elton, D., et al.

Article: A new test of pain reactivity.

Journal: *Perceptual and Motor Skills,* August 1978, *47*(1), 125–126.

Related Research: Elton, D., et al. (1978). The Melbourne Pain Apperception Test. *Melbourne Psychology Reports, 45,* 1–12.

● ● ●

2096

Test Name: MENTAL HEALTH LOCUS OF CONTROL SCALE

Purpose: To provide an area-specific measure of locus of control expectancies.

Number of Items: 22

Format: Includes 14 external and 8 internal items. Employs 6-point Likert format. All items are presented.

Reliability: Coefficient alpha was .84.

Validity: Correlation with the Mental Health Locus of Origin Scale was .40.

Author: Hill, D. J., and Bale, R. M.

Article: Development of the Mental Health Locus of Control and Mental Health Locus of Origin Scales.

Journal: *Journal of Personality Assessment,* April 1980, *44*(2), 148–156.

Related Research: Wallston, B. S., et al. (1976). Development and validation of the Health Locus of Control Scale. *Journal of Consulting and Clinical Psychology, 44,* 580–585.

2097

Test Name: MENTAL ROTATIONS TEST

Purpose: To measure spatial visualization.

Number of Items: 20

Format: Each item consists of four views of two-dimensional drawings of three-dimensional clusters of blocks. Two views are correct and two are incorrect versions of the stimulus drawing. Examples are presented.

Reliability: Kuder-Richardson formula 20 was .88 (n = 3,268 adults and adolescents). Test–retest correlations were .83 (n = 336, 1 year or more interval); and .70 (n = 456, 1 year or more interval).

Validity: Correlations with other spatial ability tests ranged from .31 to .68 (ns were either 456 or 3,435).

Author: Vandenberg, S. G., and Kuse, A. R.

Article: Mental rotations, a group test of three-dimensional spatial visualization.

Journal: *Perceptual and Motor Skills,* October 1978, *47*(2), 599–604.

Related Research: McGee, M. G. (1978). Handedness and mental rotation. *Perceptual and Motor Skills, 47,* 641–642.

Shepard, R. N., & Metzler, J. (1971). Mental rotation of three-dimensional objects. *Science, 171,* 701–703.

● ● ●

2098

Test Name: MOTION PICTURE TEST OF PERCEPTUAL ABILITIES

Purpose: To assess perceptual abilities of elementary school children.

Number of Items: 50

Time Required: Approximately 30 minutes.

Format: A self-administering 16 mm sound film that includes two parts: Part I requires the child to identify a hidden stimulus figure within one of four designs and Part 2 requires the child to identify from four alternatives a figure formed by separate lines that have been presented successively.

Reliability: Kuder-Richardson formula 20 coefficients were .74 for Part 1, .75 for Part 2, and .84 for the total score (N = 300).

Validity: With reading test scores and Part I, r = .34; for Part 2, r = .28; and for total score, r = .36 (N = 205). With Otis Lennon Intelligence Test and total score, r = .36 (N = 205); and r = .48 (N = 91 fourth and fifth graders). In addition, r = .44 with Stanford Achievement Word Meaning, and r = .48 with Stanford Achievement Paragraph Meaning (N = 91).

Author: McDaniel, E. D.

Article: Development of a group test for assessing perceptual abilities.

Journal: *Perceptual and Motor Skills,* August 1974, *39*(1, Part 2), 669–670.

Related Research: McDaniel, E. (1973). Ten motion picture tests of perceptual abilities. *Perceptual and Motor Skills, 36,* 755–759.

● ● ●

2099

Test Name: NOISE SENSITIVITY SCALE

Purpose: To assess self-reported sensitivity to noise.

Number of Items: 21

Format: Most items are answered on a 6-point scale ranging from 1 (*agree strongly*) to 6 (*disagree strongly*). All items are presented.

Reliability: Kuder-Richardson reliability ranged from .84 to .87. Test–retest reliability (9 weeks) was .75 (*n* = 72).

Validity: With percentile rank in high school class, *r* = .30 (*n* = 62), *r* = .28 (*n* = 54); Scholastic Aptitude Test total, *r* = –.26 (*n* = 62), *r* = –.43 (*n* = 54); First year college grade point average, *r* = –.07 (*n* = 62), *r* = –.18 (*n* = 54); General Scholastic ability, *r* = –.33 (*n* = 62), *r* = –.43 (*n* = 54).

Author: Weinstein, N. D.

Article: Individual differences in reactions to noise: A longitudinal study in a college dormitory.

Journal: *Journal of Applied Psychology*, August 1978, *63*(4), 458–466.

■ ■ ■

2100

Test Name: NOWICKI-STRICKLAND LOCUS OF CONTROL SCALE FOR ADULTS

Purpose: To assess locus of control.

Number of Items: 40

Format: Yes–no response. Sample item: "Do you believe it is better to be smarter than lucky?"

Validity: Correlations with 16 Adjective Checklist Scales: 6/16 were significant ranging from .25 to .46 for 36 undergraduate men and women.

Author: Duke, M., and Nowicki, S.

Article: Personality correlates of the Nowicki-Strickland locus of control scale for adults.

Journal: *Psychological Reports,* August 1973, *33*(1), 267–270.

Related Research: Chandler, T. A., & Dugovics, D. A. (1977). Sex differences in research on

locus of control. *Psychological Reports,* August, *41*(1), 47–53.

Nowicki, S., & Duke, M. (1973). A locus of control scale for college as well as non-college adults. *Journal of Personality Assessment.*

See *DUEMM, 2,* 1978, 799.

■ ■ ■

2101

Test Name: NOWICKI-STRICKLAND CHILDREN'S LOCUS OF CONTROL—MODIFIED SCALE

Purpose: To evaluate each students' perception of parents' perceived locus of control.

Number of Items: 40

Format: Paper and pencil test in which subject answers each item *yes* or *no.*

Reliability: With 150 college students internal consistency estimates ranged from .75 to .81; Test–retest reliability for 58 students over four weeks was .86.

Validity: Locus of control with Perceived for Father: grade point average, –.22 (male), –.17 (female); extracurricular activities, .14 (male), –.21 (female); number offices held, .04 (male), –.20 (female); Iowa Test of Basic Skills Composition, –.03 (male), –.35 (female); Reading, .03 (male), –.25 (female); Math, .05 (male), –.28 (female). Locus of control with Perceived for Mother: grade point average, –.27 (male), –.16 (female); extracurricular activities, –.02 (male), .03 (female); number offices held, –.03 (male), –.19 (female); Iowa Test of Basic Skills Composition, –.19 (male), –.29 (female); Reading, –.06 (male), –.19 (female); Math, –.10 (male), –.13 (female). Correlation with reverse locus of control was .37 (*p* < .005; Finch & Nelson, 1974).

Author: Nowicki, S., and Segal, W.

Article: Perceived parental characteristics, locus of control orientation, and behavioral correlates of locus of control.

Journal: *Developmental Psychology,* January 1974, *10*(1), 33–37.

Related Research: Finch, A., & Nelson, W. (1974). Locus of control and anxiety in emotionally disturbed children. *Psychological Reports, 35*(1), 469–470.

Nowicki, S., & Strickland, B. (1973). A locus of control scale for children. *Journal of Consulting and Clinical Psychology, 40,* 148–154.

See *DUEMM, 2,* 1978, 799.

■ ■ ■

2102

Test Name: NOWICKI-STRICKLAND PERSONAL REACTION SURVEY

Purpose: To measure locus of control.

Number of Items: 40

Format: Paper and pencil test in which the subject answers *yes* or *no* to each item. A generalized expectancy of reinforcement score is produced with a high score associated with externality.

Reliability: Test–retest reliability ranged from .63 to .82; internal consistency from .63 to .79.

Validity: Correlations with grade point average, –.28 (male), –.29 (female); extracurricular activities, –.12 (male), .37 (female); number offices held, –.18 (male), .16 (female); Iowa Test of Basic Skills Composition, .35 (male), .01 (female); Reading, .32 (male), .12 (female); Math, .32 (male), –.10 (female).

Author: Nowicki, S., and Segal, W.

Article: Perceived parental characteristics, locus of control orientation, behavioral correlates of locus of control.

Journal: *Developmental Psychology*, January 1974, *10*(1), 33–37.

Related Research: See *DUEMM, 2,* 1978, 799.

■ ■ ■

2103

Test Name: OFFER'S SELF IMAGE QUESTIONNAIRE

Purpose: To assess adolescent self concept.

Format: 11 scales include factor.

Reliability: Internal consistency reliability was .86 for Parent–Teenager Relations (Offer, 1966).

Author: Bledsoe, J., and Wiggins, R.

Article: Self concepts and academic aspirations of "understood" and "misunderstood" boys and girls in ninth grade.

Journal: *Psychological Reports,* August 1974, *35*(1), 57–58.

Related Research: Offer, D. (1969). *The psychological world of the teenager.* New York: Basic Books.

■ ■ ■

2104

Test Name: OPINION LEADERSHIP SCALE

Purpose: To elicit self-identified position on a continuum of opinion leadership.

Number of Items: 7

Format: A high score suggests a high degree of leadership.

Reliability: Split-half reliability was .703.

Validity: Comparison with a sociometric technique of asking group members to identify

members of whom they ask advice and using key informants to indicate opinion leaders produced correlations from .225 to .640.

Author: Brett, J. E., and Kernalequen, A.

Article: Perceptual and personality variables related to opinion leadership in fashion.

Source: *Perceptual and Motor Skills,* June 1975, *40*(3), 775–779.

Related Research: Rogers, E. M. (1958). Categorizing the adopters of agricultural practices. *Rural Sociology, 23,* 345–354.

■ ■ ■

2105

Test Name: ORGANIZATIONAL CHOICE SCALE

Purpose: To measure the desirability of job outcomes and the person's perceptions that the organization can provide certain outcomes or rewards.

Number of Items: 18 job outcomes.

Format: Subjects rate how desirable each outcome is on a 5-point scale from +2 (*extremely desirable*) through 0 (*doesn't matter*) to –2 (*extremely undesirable*). Subjects also rate how readily attainable they think the outcomes are in big or small companies on a 5-point scale from +2 (*much more likely in a big company*) through 0 (*equally likely*) to –2 (*much more likely in a small company*).

Reliability: The reliability alpha of the ratings for each outcome multiplied together and the product terms summed across all 18 outcomes was .76.

Author: Greenhaus, J. H., et al.

Article: Relationships between perceptions of organizational size and the organizational choice process.

Journal: *Journal of Vocational Behavior,* August 1978, *13*(1), 113–125.

■ ■ ■

2106

Test Name: PAPER FORM BOARD TEST

Purpose: To assess spatial orientation and visualization.

Number of Items: 29

Time Required: 6 minutes.

Format: Subjects indicate what pieces may be put together to make a certain figure.

Reliability: .61 (Kuder-Richardson coefficient).

Author: Undheim, J.

Article: Broad ability factors in 12 to 13 year old children, the theory of fluid and crystallized intelligence and the differentiation hypothesis.

Journal: *Journal of Educational Psychology,* June 1978, *70*(3), 433–443.

Related Research: Guilford, J., & Hoepfner, K. *The analysis of intelligence.* New York: McGraw-Hill.

■ ■ ■

2107

Test Name: PERSONAL ANTICIPATIONS QUESTIONNAIRE

Purpose: To measure how much group participants expect a growth group experience will result in personal change and offer new opportunities for positive emotional experiences.

Number of Items: 15

Format: Nine-point scales.

Reliability: Split-half reliabilities for two samples were .87 and .85; coefficients alpha were .84 and .82.

Author: Peteroy, E. T.

Article: Expectational composition and development of group cohesiveness across time periods.

Journal: *Psychological Reports,* August 1980, *47*(3), 243–249.

Related Research: Liebarman, M. A., et al. (1973). *Encounter groups: First facts.* New York: Basic Books.

Peteroy, E. T. (1979). Effect of number and leader expectations on group outcome. *Journal of Counseling Psychology, 26,* 534–537.

■■■

2108

Test Name: PERSONAL ATTRIBUTE INVENTORY

Purpose: To measure self-concept.

Number of Items: 100

Format: Subject selects 30 adjectives from the list of 100 that apply to the subject.

Reliability: Selected correlations with Gough's Adjective Check List ranged from −.73 to .80. Correlations with the self-concept factor of the 16PF test ranged from .29 to .47.

Author: Kappes, B. M.

Article: Concurrent validity of the Personal Attribute Inventory as a self-concept scale.

Journal: *Perceptual and Motor Skills,* December 1980, *51*(3, Part 1), 752–754.

Related Research: Parish, T., et al. (1976). Further report on the validation of the Personal Attribute Inventory. *Perceptual and Motor Skills, 42,* 1257–1258.

■■■

2109

Test Name: PERSONAL ATTRIBUTE INVENTORY FOR CHILDREN

Purpose: To measure self-concept.

Number of Items: 48

Format: Consists of half a list of positive and half a list of negative words. The child identifies 15 of the words that best describe him or her.

Reliability: Test–retest correlations over grades 3 through 8 with *n*s varying from 44 to 77 ranged from .61 to .98 (1 month interval).

Validity: Correlations with the Piers-Harris Children's Self-Concept Scale over grades 3 through 8 with *n*s ranging from 48 to 77 ranged from −.06 to .71.

Author: Parish, T. S., and Taylor, J. C.

Article: A further report on the validity and reliability of the personal attribute inventory for children as a self-concept scale.

Journal: *Educational and Psychological Measurement,* Winter 1978, *38*(4), 1225–1228.

Related Research: Parish, T., & Taylor, J. (1978). The Personal Attribute Inventory for Children: A report on its validity and reliability as a self-concept scale. *Educational and Psychological Measurement, 38,* 565–569.

Parish, T. S., & Taylor, J. C. (1978). The Personal Attribute Inventory for Children: A report on its validity and reliability as a serf-concept scale. *Educational and Psychological Measurement,* Summer, *38*(2), 565–569.

■■■

2110

Test Name: PERSONAL ATTRIBUTES QUESTIONNAIRE—SHORT FORM

Purpose: To measure sex role perceptions.

Format: First, subjects rate themselves on bipolar items to determine their sex role perception. Then the subjects compare typical male and female behavior on a 5-point scale that yields a measure of each subject's perception of male–female sex role differences.

Reliability: Alpha coefficients ranged from .73 to .91 for men and women, respectively.

Validity: Correlations with other variables ranged from −.22 to .57 (men). Correlations with other variables ranged from −.43 to .35 (women).

Author: Muldrow, T. W., and Beyton, J. A.

Article: Men and women executives and processes related to decision accuracy.

Journal: *Journal of Applied Psychology,* April 1979, *64*(2), 99–106.

Related Research: Spence, J. T., et al. (1974). The Personal Attributes Questionnaire: A measure of sex role stereotypes and masculinity-feminity. *JSAS Catalog of Selected Documents in Psychology, 4,* 617.

■■■

2111

Test Name: POLITICAL INCAPABILITY SCALE

Purpose: To measure feelings of political powerlessness.

Number of Items: 4

Format: Example of items is given.

Reliability: Alpha coefficient was .62.

Author: Long, S.

Article: Explaining system failure: A two-dimensional analysis.

Journal: *Psychological Reports,* August 1977, *41*(1), 23–28.

Related Research: Olsen, M. (1969). Two categories of political alienation. *Social Forces, 47,* 288–299.

• • •

2112

Test Name: POWERLESSNESS SCALE

Purpose: To measure feelings of powerlessness.

Number of Items: 18

Format: Scored on a 6-point scale from *strongly agree* to *strongly disagree.*

Reliability: Kuder-Richardson formula 20, *r* = .82.

Validity: With Barron's independence of judgment scale Pearson product–moment correlation was .41.

Author: Garrahan, D. Q.

Article: The relationship between social activism and feelings of powerlessness among low socioeconomic college students.

Journal: *Journal of College Student Personnel,* March 1974, *15*(2), 120–124.

Related Research: Coleman, J. (1966). *Equality of educational opportunity.* Washington, DC: U.S. Government Printing Office.

Rotter, J. (1966). Generalized expectancies for internal versus external control of reinforcement. *Psychological Monographs: General and Applied, 80,* 1–28.

• • •

2113

Test Name: PRESCHOOL AND PRIMARY NOWICKI-STRICKLAND INTERNAL–EXTERNAL CONTROL SCALE

Purpose: To measure locus of control for preschool and primary age children.

Number of Items: 34

Format: Each item is in cartoon form and the subject draws a line through or circles around *yes* or *no* in answer to each question. The questions for each item are presented.

Reliability: Six-week test–retest reliability for 7-year-olds (*N* = 60) was .79.

Validity: With Iowa Basic Skills for males (*N* = 66) correlations ranged from –.20 to .85 and for females (*N* = 67) correlations ranged from –.45 to .84.

Author: Nowicki, S., Jr., and Duke, M. P.

Article: A preschool and primary internal–external control scale.

Journal: *Developmental Psychology,* November 1974, *10*(6), 874–880.

Related Research: Nowicki, S., & Strickland, B. R. (1973). A locus of control scale for children. *Journal of Consulting and Clinical Psychology, 40,* 148–155.

See *D. U. E. M. M., 2,* 1978, 799.

• • •

2114

Test Name: PRIMARY SELF-CONCEPT INVENTORY

Purpose: To identify children with adequate and those with undesirably low self-concepts.

Number of Items: 18

Format: Includes personal, social, and intellectual domains of self-concept.

Reliability: Test–retest correlation coefficient was .91.

Validity: Correlation with age (1st grade) was .29.

Author: Husak, W. S., and Magill, R. A.

Article: Correlations among perceptual-motor ability, self-concept and reading achievement in early elementary grades.

Journal: *Perceptual and Motor Skills,* April 1979, *48*(2), 447–450.

• • •

2115

Test Name: PRIMARY SELF-CONCEPT SCALE

Purpose: To evaluate characteristics of self-concept relevant to school success.

Number of Items: 24

Format: Includes eight factors: peer aggressiveness, peer ostracism, intellectual self-image, helpfulness, physiological self, adult acceptance or rejection, emotional self, and success or nonsuccess.

Reliability: Test–retest (phi) coefficients ranged from .25 to .69 (*n* = 83) for the eight factor scales.

Validity: Correlations with a Teacher Questionnaire produced (phi) coefficients for the eight factor scales ranging from .49 to –.19 (*n* = 62).

Author: Jensen, J. M., and Michael, J. J.

Article: The concurrent validity of the primary self-concept scale for a sample of third-grade children.

Journal: *Educational and Psychological Measurement,* Winter 1975, *35*(4), 1011–1016.

Related Research: Muller, D. G., & Leonetti, R. (1972). *Primary self-concept scale, study for the National Consortia for Bilingual Education.* Washington, DC: Office of Education (DHEW). (ERIC Document Reproduction Service No. ED062847)

• • •

2116

Test Name: PUNCHED HOLES TEST

Purpose: To assess spatial orientation and visualization.

Number of Items: 24

Time Required: 3 minutes.

Format: Multiple-choice test with five alternatives in which subjects imagine the folding and unfolding of pieces of paper.

Reliability: .68 (Kuder-Richardson coefficient).

Author: Undheim, J.

Article: Broad ability factors in 12 to 13 year old children, the theory of fluid and crystallized intelligence, and the differentiation hypothesis.

Journal: *Journal of Educational Psychology,* June 1978, *70*(3), 433–443.

Related Research: Guilford, J., & Hoepfner, R. (1971). *The analysis of intelligence.* New York: McGraw-Hill.

■ ■ ■

2117

Test Name: PUPIL CONTROL IDEOLOGY FORM

Purpose: To assess pupil control ideology.

Number of Items: 20

Format: Likert format with range from 1 (*strongly disagree*) to 5 (*strongly agree*); higher scores were associated with a greater custodial orientation.

Reliability: Split-half reliabilities ranged .91–.95.

Validity: "Supported by the method of know groups" and reference is given to Willower et al. (1967) in this study. The study reports significant differences in pupil control ideology when teachers differing in degree of openmindedness were compared.

Author: Lunenburg, F., and O'Reilly, R.

Article: Personal and organizational influence on pupil control ideology.

Journal: *Journal of Experimental Education,* Spring 1974, *42*(3), 31–35.

Related Research: Barfield, V., & Burlingame, M. (1974). The pupil control ideology of teachers in selected schools. *Journal of Experimental Education, 42*(4), 6–11.

Willower, D., et al. (1967). *The school and pupil control ideology* (Penn State Studies Monograph, No. 24). University Park: Pennsylvania State University.

See *D. U. E. M. M., 2,* 1978, 810.

■ ■ ■

2118

Test Name: QUESTIONNAIRE UPON MENTAL IMAGERY— REVISED

Purpose: To measure vividness of self-reported imagery.

Format: 35

Reliability: Test–retest reliability was .78.

Validity: With the original 150 item test, $r = .92$; With the Stanford Hypnotic Susceptibility Scale, Form C, $r = .58$ (males), $r = .20$ (females).

Author: Wagman, R., and Stewart, C. G.

Article: Visual imagery and hypnotic susceptibility.

Journal: *Perceptual and Motor Skills,* June 1974, *38*(3, Part 1), 815–822.

Related Research: Betts, G. H. (1909). The distribution and functions of mental imagery. *Teachers College Contributions to Education, 26.*

Richardson, A. (1969). *Mental imagery.* London: Routledge & Kegan Paul.

Rossi, J. S., & Fingeret, A. L. (1977). Individual differences in verbal and imagery abilities: Paired-associate recall as a function of stimulus and response concreteness. *Perceptual and Motor Skills, 44*(3), Part 2, 1043–1049.

■ ■ ■

2119

Test Name: REFERRAL PROCESS INVENTORY

Purpose: To measure one's perceptions of how to make a referral, to whom to make a referral, the kinds of problems to refer, and one's desire to improve one's knowledge of the referral process.

Number of Items: 22

Format: Likert scale ranging from 1 (*strongly disagree*) to 5 (*strongly agree*).

Reliability: Hoyt reliabilities for internal consistency were all greater than .73 (given in the article).

Author: O'Neil, J. M., et al.

Article: An empirical investigation of the counseling referral process.

Journal: *Journal of College Student Personnel,* July 1978, *19*(4), 306–308.

Related Research: O'Neil, J. M., et al. (1975). *The Referral Process Inventory.* Lawrence: University of Kansas, University Counseling Center.

■ ■ ■

2120

Test Name: REWARD CONTINGENCY SCALE

Purpose: To measure the degree to which the subordinate perceives that the rewards or outcomes (positive and punitive) received through a supervisor were contingent or reflected their performance or accomplishments on the job.

Number of Items: 22

Format: Five-point Likert scale ranging from *very false* to *very true.*

Reliability: Reliabilities (coefficient alpha) were .91 for positive reward behavior and .92 for punitive reward behavior.

Author: Szilagyi, A. D.

Article: Reward behavior by male and female leaders: A causal inference analysis.

Journal: *Journal of Vocational Behavior*, February 1980, *16*(1), 59–72.

Related Research: Sims, H. P., & Szilagyi, A. D. (1975). Leader reward behavior and subordinate satisfaction and performance. *Organizational Behavior and Human Performance, 14*, 426–438.

■ ■ ■

2121

Test Name: ROLE CONFLICT AND AMBIGUITY SCALE

Purpose: To measure subjects' perceptions of role conflict and role ambiguity.

Number of Items: 10

Format: Role conflict items emphasized the incompatibilities or incongruities arising out of perceptions or performance of role requirements. Role ambiguity items stressed the clarity of behavioral requirements.

Reliability: Role ambiguity internal consistency was about .80; role conflict internal consistency was .82.

Validity: Role conflict correlated with job satisfaction, $r = .13$; with propensity to leave the organization, $r = .07$; with reported influence, $r = -.19$; with

perceived threat and anxiety, $r = .27$. Role ambiguity correlated with job satisfaction, $r = -.25$; with job threat and anxiety, $r = .33$; with propensity to leave the organization, $r = .97$.

Author: Hamner, W. C., and Tosi, H. L.

Article: Relationship of role conflict and role ambiguity to job involvement measures.

Journal: *Journal of Applied Psychology*, August 1974, *59*(4), 497–499.

Related Research: Rizzo, J. R., et al. (1970). Role conflict and ambiguity in complex organizations. *Administrative Science Quarterly, 15*, 150–163.

■ ■ ■

2122

Test Name: ROLE CONFLICT AND AMBIGUITY SCALE

Purpose: To measure role conflict and ambiguity.

Number of Items: 14

Format: Role conflict included three dimensions: person–role, intersender, and resource-related. Role ambiguity consisted of uncertainty about behavioral expectations and uncertainty about the outcomes of behavior. A 7-point Likert response format was used.

Reliability: Spearman-Brown estimates of internal consistency ranged from .65 to .77 ($N = 262$).

Validity: Correlations with other variables ranged from $-.38$ to .59 ($N = 262$).

Author: Morris, J. H., and Snyder, R. A.

Article: A second look at need for achievement and need for autonomy as moderators of role perception-outcome relationships.

Journal: *Journal of Applied*

Psychology, April 1979, *64*(2), 173–178.

Related Research: Rizzo, J., et al. (1970). Role conflict and ambiguity in complex organizations. *Administrative Science Quarterly, 15*, 150–163.

■ ■ ■

2123

Test Name: ROLE PERCEPTION SCALE

Purpose: To measure the individual's impression that personal behavior is due to personal values and ideas rather than external factors.

Number of Items: 12

Format: Items are personality-type traits that the respondent ranks in order of importance.

Reliability: Inner directedness scale: test–retest (3-week interval) Spearman rank order correlation coefficient was .75 ($n = 15$). Other directedness scale: test–retest (3-week interval) Spearman rank order correlation coefficient was .74 ($n = 15$).

Author: Morrison, R. F.

Article: Career adaptivity: The effective adaptation of managers to changing role demands.

Journal: *Journal of Applied Psychology*, October 1977, *62*(5), 549–558.

Related Research: Porter, L. W., & Lawler, E. E. (1968). *Managerial attitudes and performance.* Homewood, IL: Irwin.

■ ■ ■

2124

Test Name: ROSENBERG SELF-ESTEEM SCALE

Purpose: To measure self-esteem.

Number of Items: 10

Format: Subjects indicate their agreement with statements about their own perceived worth and competence.

Reliability: Coefficient alpha reliability was .75.

Validity: Correlations with value similarity ranged from −.34 to .40.

Author: Weiss, H. M.

Article: Social learning of work values in organizations.

Journal: *Journal of Applied Psychology,* December 1978, *63*(6), 711–718.

Related Research: Keller, R. T., & Holland, W. E. (1978). Individual characteristics of innovativeness and communication in research and development organizations. *Journal of Applied Psychology, 63,* 759–762.

Kernaleguen, A., & Conrad, Sister G. (1980). Analysis of five measures of self-concept. *Perceptual and Motor Skills, 51*(3, Part 1), 855–861.

Rosenberg, M. (1965). *Society and the adolescent self image.* Princeton, NJ: Princeton University Press.

Whiteman, V. L., & Shorkey, C. T. (1978). Validation testing of the Rational Behavior Inventory. *Educational and Psychological Measurement, 38*(4), 1143–1149.

■ ■ ■

2125

Test Name: SELF-ACCEPTANCE SCALE

Purpose: To measure self-acceptance.

Number of Items: 36

Format: Likert items. Respondents rate the applicability to themselves of each self-descriptive statement on a 5-point scale ranging from *not at all true of myself* to *true of myself.*

Reliability: Berger (1952) found split-half reliability coefficients of .894 or greater with groups of college students, prisoners, and stutterers.

Author: Karmos, A. H., and Karmos, J. S.

Article: Construct validity analysis of a "nonverbal" measure of self-esteem: The Sliding Person Test.

Journal: *Psychological Reports,* June 1979, *44*(3), 895–910.

Related Research: Berger, E. M. (1952). The relation between expressed acceptance of self and expressed acceptance of others. *Journal of Abnormal and Social Psychology, 47,* 778–782.

Chiappone, D. I., & Kroes, W. H. (1979). Fatalism in coal miners. *Psychological Reports, 44*(3), 1175–1180.

■ ■ ■

2126

Test Name: SELF-CATHEXIS SCALE

Purpose: To measure self-esteem.

Number of Items: 55

Format: Subject indicates on a 5-point scale the degree of satisfaction with a list of items considered to represent a global sampling of various conceptual aspects of self.

Reliability: Split-half reliability was .88 for men and .92 for women. Test–retest reliability was .74. Internal consistency was .87.

Validity: Correlations with Body Satisfaction, .39; Janis-Field-Eagly Scale, .57; Job interview expectations, .30; Interview self-ratings, .31; Judges' ratings, .08; Self-rating discrepancy scores, .18 (*N*= 87).

Author: King, M. R., and Manaster, G. J.

Article: Body image, self-esteem, expectations, self-assessments, and actual success in a simulated job interview.

Journal: *Journal of Applied Psychology,* October 1977, *62*(5), 589–594.

Related Research: Secord, P. F., & Jourard, S. M. (1953). The appraisal of body-cathexis: Body-cathexis and the self. *Journal of Consulting Psychology, 17,* 343–347.

■ ■ ■

2127

Test Name: SELF-CONCEPT INVENTORY

Purpose: To measure self-concept.

Number of Items: 26

Format: A semantic differential in which the approach to self-concept is based on the difference between the subject's present self-evaluation and aspired self-evaluation. The lower the score the higher the self-concept.

Validity: With career certainty factors, *r* = .21 (men), *r* = .22 (women); With esteem, *r* = .37.

Author: Wigent, P. A.

Article: Personality variables related to career decision-making abilities of community college students.

Journal: *Journal of College Student Personnel,* March 1974, *15*(2), 105–108.

Related Research: Sherwood, J. J. (1963). *Self-identity and self-actualization: A theory and research.* Unpublished doctoral dissertation, University of Michigan.

■ ■ ■

2128

Test Name: SELF-CONCEPT OF ACADEMIC ABILITY

Purpose: To measure the specific aspects of self-concept concerning school ability.

Number of Items: 8

Format: Responses are made along a 5-point continuum on eight Guttman scales.

Reliability: .95 for male and .96 for female students.

Author: Carter, D. E., et al.

Article: Peer acceptance and school-related variables in an integrated junior high school.

Journal: *Journal of Educational Psychology*, April 1975, *67*(2), 267–273.

Related Research: Brookover, W. B., et al. (1965). *Self concept of ability and school achievement, II* (Educational Research Series No. 31). East Lansing: Michigan State University, College of Education.

■ ■ ■

2129

Test Name: SELF-CONCEPT SEMANTIC DIFFERENTIAL

Purpose: To measure self-concept.

Number of Items: 18

Format: Each item includes two bipolar adjectives spaced 10 equal sections apart.

Reliability: Test–retest (2 months) correlation was .76 ($n = 196$).

Validity: Correlations with: anxiety ranged from –.54 to .69. Anxiety Test for Children was –.61 ($n = 146$). Positive sociometric status was .48.

Author: Ziv, A., et al.

Article: Parental perception and self-concept of gifted and average underachievers.

Journal: *Perceptual and Motor Skills*, April 1977, *44*(2), 563–568.

2130

Test Name: SELF-CONCEPT SEMANTIC DIFFERENTIAL RATING SCALE

Purpose: To assess self-concept.

Number of Items: 44

Format: Semantic differential rating scale.

Reliability: Test–retest reliability was .82. Internal consistency was .96.

Validity: Correlations with perceived physical performance were .53 (pretest) and .57 (posttest). Correlation with actual physical performance was .01.

Author: Leonardson, G. R., and Garguilo, R. M.

Article: Self-perception and physical fitness.

Journal: *Perceptual and Motor Skills*, February 1978, *46*(1), 338.

■ ■ ■

2131

Test Name: SELF-DEROGATION SCALE

Purpose: To measure actual feelings toward one's self.

Number of Items: 10

Format: Subject indicates agreement or disagreement with each item on a 4-point scale ranging from *strongly agree* to *strongly disagree*.

Reliability: Test–retest reliability coefficient was .79.

Validity: Correlations with Repression-Sensitization Scale, .64; MMPI K Scale, –.38; Ego-control Scale, .22; A-Trait Scale, .69 ($N = 158$).

Author: Rios-Garcia, L. R., and Cook, P. E.

Article: Self-derogation and

defense style in college students.

Journal: *Journal of Personality Assessment,* June 1975, *39*(3), 273–281.

Related Research: Kaplan, H. B., & Pokorny, A. D. (1969). Self-derogation and psychosocial adjustment. *Journal of Nervous and Mental Disease, 149,* 421–434.

■ ■ ■

2132

Test Name: SELF-DESCRIPTIVE LIST

Purpose: To measure adult stereotypic sex-role concepts of masculinity.

Number of Items: 12

Time Required: 2 to 6 minutes.

Format: Subject responds *very much unlike me, unlike me, not like or unlike me, like me,* or *very much like me.*

Reliability: Test–retest reliability using Pearson product–moment correlations over 7 days: men, $r = .759$ ($p < .001$), and women, $r = .834$ ($p < .001$).

Author: Newman, R. C., II

Article: Development and standardization of measures of stereotypic sex-role concepts and of sex-role adoption in adults.

Journal: *Psychological Reports,* October 1976, *39*(2), 623–638.

Related Research: Bem, S. L. (1974). The measurement of psychological androgyny. *Journal of Consulting and Clinical Psychology, 42,* 155–162.

■ ■ ■

2133

Test Name: SELF-ESTEEM INVENTORY

Purpose: To measure self-concept.

Number of Items: 42

Format: Verbal self-report covering three categories: self (26 items), social self (8 items), and school self (8 items).

Reliability: Test–retest reliability after a 5-week interval with a sample of 30 fifth-grade students of .88 and of .70 with a different sample of 56 children over a 3-year interval.

Author: Zirkel, P., and Gable, R. K.

Article: The reliability and validity of various measures of self-concept among ethnically different adolescents.

Journal: *Measurement and Evaluation in Guidance,* April 1977, *10*(1), 48–54.

Related Research: Coopersmith, S. (1967). *The antecedents of self-esteem.* San Francisco: Freeman.

■ ■ ■

2134

Test Name: SELF-ESTEEM MEASURE

Purpose: To measure student's global self-esteem.

Number of Items: 6

Format: Guttman scale.

Reliability: Coefficient of reproducibility was .931. Coefficient of scalability was .764.

Author: Blyth, D. A., et al.

Article: The transition into early adolescence: A longitudinal comparison of youth in two educational contexts.

Journal: *Sociology of Education,* July 1978, *51*(3), 149–162.

Related Research: Simmons, R. G., et al. (1973). Disturbance in the self-image at adolescence. *American Sociological Review, 38,* 553–568.

2135

Test Name: SELF-ESTEEM QUESTIONNAIRE

Purpose: To measure self-esteem.

Number of Items: 18

Format: Subjects respond to each item by answering either *T* or *F*. All items are given.

Reliability: Coefficient alpha was .64 ($N = 235$). Test–retest (3 weeks) was .86 ($N = 235$).

Validity: Correlation with Edwards Social Desirability Scale was .50 and with Marlowe-Crown Social Desirability Scale was .29. Bill's Self-Construct Measures ranged from –.36 to .52. Heron and Eysenck Neuroticism Measures were each –.44. Heron Introversions Scale was .05. Eysenck Extroversion Scale was –.22.

Author: Watkins, D.

Article: The development and evaluation of self-esteem measuring instruments.

Journal: *Journal of Personality Assessment,* April 1978, *42*(2), 171–182.

■ ■ ■

2136

Test Name: SELF ESTEEM SCALE

Purpose: To assess "feelings of generalized self esteem."

Number of Items: 10

Format: Modification of Rosenberg Self Esteem Scale; Likert items.

Reliability: Design not specified, .89.

Author: Abramowitz, S., and Jackson, C.

Article: Comparative effectiveness of there-and-then versus here-and-now therapist interpretations in group psychotherapy.

Journal: *Journal of Counseling Psychology,* July 1974, *21*(4), 288–293.

Related Research: Rosenberg, M. (1965). *Society and the adolescent self image.* Princeton, NJ: Princeton University Press.

■ ■ ■

2137

Test Name: SELF-ESTEEM INVENTORY

Purpose: To measure the perceptions of children aged 8 to 10 years in the areas of peers, parents, school, and self.

Number of Items: 50

Format: Declarative statements (18 positive and 32 negative) that the subject checks.

Reliability: Test–retest reliability for a sample of 56 children over a period of 3 years was .70.

Author: Cowan, R., et al.

Article: A validity study of selected self-concept instruments.

Journal: *Measurement and Evaluation in Guidance,* January 1978, *10*(4), 211–221.

Related Research: Rogers, C., & Dymond, R. (1954). *Psychotherapy and personality change.* Chicago: University of Chicago Press.

■ ■ ■

2138

Test Name: SELF-ESTEEM SCALE

Purpose: To assess subject self-esteem.

Number of Items: 9

Format: A Guttman-type scale with a range from 1 *(low self-esteem)* to 9 *(high self-esteem).*

Reliability: Coefficient of

reproducibility was .90.

Author: Giacquinta, J. B.

Article: Status, risk, and receptivity to innovations in complex organizations: A study of the responses of four groups of educators to the proposed introduction of sex education in elementary school.

Journal: *Sociology of Education,* Winter 1975, *48*(1), 38–58.

Related Research: Hensley, W. E., & Roberts, M. K. (1976). Dimensions of Rosenberg's self-esteem scale. *Psychological Reports, 38,* 583–584.

Rosenberg, M. (1965). *Society and the adolescent self-image.* Princeton, NJ: Princeton University Press.

Youngblood, R. L. (1976). Self-esteem and academic achievement of Filipino high school students. *Educational Research Quarterly, 1,* 27–36.

● ● ●

2139

Test Name: SELF-ESTEEM SCALE

Purpose: To measure college student self-esteem.

Number of Items: 10

Reliability: Cronbach's alpha was .85.

Validity: Correlations with 16 characteristics ranged from –.103 to .342.

Author: Reitzes, D. C., and Mutran, E.

Article: Significant others and self conceptions: Factors influencing educational expectations and academic performance.

Journal: *Sociology of Education,* January 1980, *53*(1), 21–32.

Related Research: Lopez, E. M., & Greenhaus, J. H. (1978).

Self-esteem, race and job satisfaction. *Journal of Vocational Behavior,* August, *13*(1), 75–83.

Peteroy, E. T. (1979). Effects of number and leader expectations on group outcome. *Journal of Counseling Psychology, 26,* 534–537.

Rosenberg, M. (1965). *Society and the adolescent self-image.* Princeton, NJ: Princeton University Press.

Simpson, C. K., & Boyle, D. (1975). Esteem construct generality and academic performance. *Educational and Psychological Measurement, 35,* 897–904.

● ● ●

2140

Test Name: SELF-ESTEEM SCALES

Purpose: To assess one's self-esteem along the dimensions of friendliness, independence, physical attractiveness, intelligence, openness, leadership ability, insightfulness, and emotional stability.

Format: Response alternatives are labeled *high*, *above average*, *below average*, and *low*.

Reliability: Internal consistency coefficient alphas were .69 (close authority), .77 (distant authority), .74 (close peer), and .64 (distant peer). Coefficient alpha for the self-esteem scale was .56.

Author: Schwab, M. R., and Lundgren, D. C.

Article: Birth order, perceived appraisals by significant others, and self-esteem.

Journal: *Psychological Reports,* October 1978, *43*(2), 443–454.

● ● ●

2141

Test Name: SELF-EVALUATIVE INVENTORY

Purpose: To assess self-esteem.

Number of Items: 80

Format: Forty body-cathexis items and 40 self-cathexis items arranged in an intermixed random order. Subjects evaluate "How much you are satisfied with each of these characteristics as you perceive them in yourself" along a 5-point scale.

Validity: Correlations of .57 between scores obtained for men and women.

Author: Sappenfield, B. R., and Harris, C. L.

Article: Self-reported masculinity-femininity as related to self-esteem.

Journal: *Psychological Reports,* October 1975, *37*(2), 669–670.

Related Research: Second, P. F., & Jourard, S. M. (1953). An appraisal of body-cathexis: Body-cathexis and the self. *Journal of Consulting Psychology, 17,* 343–347.

● ● ●

2142

Test Name: SELF-RATING DEPRESSION INVENTORY

Purpose: To measure self-esteem.

Number of Items: 10

Format: Consists of Likert items with five alternative responses per item.

Validity: Correlations with Job Descriptive Index: ranged from .07 to .34 ($n = 50$), ranged from –.05 to .33 ($n = 43$).

Author: Inkson, J. H. K.

Article: Self-esteem as a moderator of the relationship between job performance and job satisfaction.

Journal: *Journal of Applied Psychology,* April 1978, *63*(2), 243–247.

Related Research: Hunt, S., et al. (1967). Components of depression: Identified from a self-rating inventory for survey use. *Archives of General Psychiatry, 16,* 441–447.

Robinson, J. P., & Shaver, P. R. (1969). *Measures of social psychological attitudes.* Ann Arbor: University of Michigan, Institute for Social Research.

■ ■ ■

2143

Test Name: SHAPE-O BALL TEST

Purpose: To measure three aspects of perceptual-motor skill.

Format: Consists of a hollow plastic sphere, 6 inches in diameter, with differently shaped geometric holes in the surface. Plastic geometric pieces matching the holes are inserted into the sphere's holes as rapidly as possible. The test appears to measure form discrimination, fine eye-hand coordination, and visual-motor match.

Reliability: .88

Validity: Correlation with Frostig Test, –.78; with Oseretsky Test, –.09; with Otis-Lennon, –.63; with Teachers' Rating, –.77.

Author: Chissom, B. S., et al.

Article: Relationships among perceptual-motor measures and their correlations with academic readiness for preschool children.

Journal: *Perceptual and Motor Skills,* August 1974, *39*(1, Part 2), 467–473.

Related Research: Chissom, B. S., et al. (1972). Canonical validity of perceptual-motor skills for predicting an academic criterion. *Educational and Psychological Measurement, 32,* 1095–1098.

See *DUEMM, 2,* 1978, 477.

2144

Test Name: SURFACE DEVELOPMENT TEST

Purpose: To assess spatial orientation and visualizations.

Number of Items: 18

Time Required: 6 minutes.

Format: Subjects indicate among four figures the one that can be made by folding a piece of paper along dotted lines.

Reliability: 84 (Kuder-Richardson coefficient).

Author: Undheim, J.

Article: Broad ability factors in 12 to 13 year old children, the theory of fluid and crystallized intelligence, and the differentiation hypothesis.

Journal: *Journal of Educational Psychology,* June 1978, *70*(3), 433–443.

Related Research: Guilford, J., & Hoepfner, R. (1971). *The analysis of intelligence.* New York: McGraw-Hill.

■ ■ ■

2145

Test Name: STABILITY OF SELF SCALE

Purpose: To measure the stability of the self-concept.

Number of Items: 5

Format: Nine-point Likert scale.

Reliability: Coefficient of reproducibility was 94% and a coefficient of scalability was 77%.

Author: Franzoni, S. L., et al.

Article: Factor analysis of the stability of self scale.

Journal: *Psychological Reports,* December 1980, *47*(3), 1160–1162.

Related Research: Rosenberg, M. (1979). *Conceiving the self.* New York: Basic Books.

2146

Test Name: STANFORD PRESCHOOL I-E SCALE

Purpose: To measure children's locus of control.

Number of Items: 14

Format: Forced-choice format provides scores for expectancies for internal control of positive events, negative events, and a sum of the two.

Reliability: Test–retest reliability was .59 (2–3 week interval).

Validity: Correlation with the Bialer Scale for Children was .18 (N = 130).

Author: Bachrach, R., and Peterson, R. A.

Article: Test–retest reliability and interrelation among three locus of control measures for children.

Journal: *Perceptual and Motor Skills,* August 1976, *43*(1), 260–262.

Related Research: Chartier, G. M., et al. (1976). The Stanford Preschool Internal–External Scale: Extension for Kindergarteners. *Journal of Personality Assessment, 40,* 431–435.

Mischel, W., et al. (1974). Internal–external control and persistance: Validation and implications of the Stanford Pre-School Internal–External Scale. *Journal of Personality and Social Psychology, 29,* 265–278.

■ ■ ■

2147

Test Name: STUDENT'S PERCEPTION OF ABILITY SCALE

Purpose: To assess academic self-concept in elementary school children in grades 2 to 6.

Number of Items: 70

Format: Includes six subscales: perception of general ability, perception of arithmetic ability, general school satisfaction, perception of reading and spelling ability, perception of penmanship and neatness, and confidence in academic ability.

Reliability: Full Scale Cronbach's alpha was .914.

Author: Chapman, J. W., and Boersma, F. J.

Article: Comments on discriminant validity of self-concept constructs.

Journal: *Perceptual and Motor Skills,* June 1979, *48*(3, Part 2), 1255–1258.

Related Research: Boersma, F. J., et al. (1979). *Technical data on the Student's Perception of Ability Scale.* Edmonton: University of Alberta. (ERIC Documents Reproduction Service No. TM 008213)

■ ■ ■

2148

Test Name: TEL AVIV LOCUS OF CONTROL

Purpose: To measure locus of control in children grades 4 through 8.

Number of item: 48

Format: Includes the positive–negative dimension of the Intellectual Achievement Responsibility Questionnaire (Crandall, et al., 1965), and content and time scales (Past and Future).

Reliability: Split–half reliabilities for the Past scale ranged from .31 to .67; for the Future scale from .74 to .93.

Validity: Significant differences (*p* < .01) between Past and Future scales and subjects by age, sex, and intelligence level.

Author: Milgram, N. A., and Milgram, R. M.

Article: Dimensions of locus of control in children.

Journal: *Psychological Reports,* October 1975, *37*(2), 523–538.

Related Research: Crandall, V. C., et al. (1965). Children's beliefs in their own control of reinforcements in intellectual-academic achievement situations. *Child Development, 36,* 91–109.

■ ■ ■

2149

Test Name: TEXAS SOCIAL BEHAVIOR INVENTORY

Purpose: To measure self-esteem.

Number of Items: 16

Format: Five-point Likert scales from 0 (*not at all*) to 4 (*very characteristic*) with higher scores indicating higher self-esteem (from 0 to 64).

Reliability: Coefficient alphas derived from college student samples ranged from .87 to .92.

Author: Gilbert, L. A., and Mangelsdorff, D.

Article: Influence of perceptions of personal control on reactions to stressful events.

Journal: *Journal of Counseling Psychology,* November 1979, *26*(6), 473–480.

Related Research: Helmreich, R., & Stapp, J. (1974). Short form of the Texas Social Behavior Inventory, an objective measure of self-esteem. *Bulletin of the Psychonomic Society, 4,* 473–475.

■ ■ ■

2150

Test Name: TRENT ATTRIBUTION PROFILE

Purpose: To measure locus of control.

Number of Items: 12

Format: Each item is followed by four possible explanations and the respondent rates the importance of each on a 5-point scale from 1 (*not at all important*) to 5 (*very important*). Provides separate measures of internality externality, stability, and unstability. An example is presented.

Reliability: Test–retest reliability coefficients (Pearson *r*s) ranged from .279 to .753.

Validity: Correlations with the I-E Scale ranged from .37 to .51.

Author: Wong, P. T. P., et al.

Article: Initial validity and reliability of the Trent Attribution Profile (TAP) as a measure of attribution schema and locus of control.

Journal: *Educational and Psychological Measurement,* Winter 1978, *38*(4), 1129–1134.

■ ■ ■

2151

Test Name: TRUSTWORTHY SCALE

Purpose: To assess the extent to which people are seen as moral, honest, and reliable.

Number of Items: 14

Format: Five-point Likert scales from *strongly agree* to *strongly disagree.*

Validity: Correlation with Rotter Interpersonal Trust Scale is .76.

Author: Chun, K-T., and Campbell, J. B.

Article: Notes on the internal structure of Wrightsman's Measure of Trustworthiness.

Journal: *Psychological Reports,* August 1975, *37*(1), 323–330.

Related Research: Wrightsman, L. S. (1974). *Assumptions about human nature: A*

social-psychological approach.
Monterey, CA: Brooks/Cole.

■ ■ ■

2152

Test Name: VISUO-SPATIAL
MEMORY TEST

Purpose: To assess year-to-year
children's immediate visual
memory for designs independently
of motor activity.

Number of Items: 15

Format: The separate designs are
individually presented in a booklet
for 5 seconds each.

Reliability: Test–retest ($N = 69$ with
interval of 4 months): correlations
ranged from .06 to .44; Test–retest
($N = 20$ with interval of 3 weeks): r
= .72; Kuder-Richardson formula
21 ranged from .32 to .68.

Validity: With Memory-for-
Designs, $r = .47$; With Bender
Koppity, $r = -.40$; With Bender
number correct, $r = .34$; With
Memory-for-Designs error score, r
= −.39; With Rutgers Drawing Test
number correct, $r = .33$.

Author: Aliotti, N. C.

Article: Note on validity and
reliability of the Bannatyne
visuo-spatial memory test.

Journal: *Perceptual and Motor
Skills,* June 1974, *38*(3, Part I),
963–966.

Related Research: Bannatyne,
A. D. (1968). *Visuo-spatial
Memory Test.* South Miami, FL:
Author (P.O. Box 90).

■ ■ ■

2153

Test Name: VIVIDNESS OF
IMAGERY SCALE

Purpose: To measure vividness of
imagery production.

Number of Items: 35

Format: Subject is asked to rate
the vividness of the image

produced to each item using a 5-
point scale. Ratings on all items
are averaged to give a mean
vividness of imagery index. Some
examples are given.

Validity: Correlations with What
Kind of Person Are You? Test
ranged from .01 to .20 ($N = 107$).
Correlations with Something
About Myself ranged from .04 to
.24 ($N = 107$).

Author: Khatena, J.

Article: Vividness of imagery and
creative self perception.

Journal: *The Gifted Child
Quarterly,* Spring 1975, *19*(1), 33–
37.

Related Research: Sheehan, P. W.
(1967). A shortened form of Betts'
Questionnaire upon mental
imagery. *Journal of Clinical
Psychology, 23,* 386–389.

■ ■ ■

2154

Test Name: VIVIDNESS OF
VISUAL IMAGERY
QUESTIONNAIRE

Purpose: To measure visual
imagery.

Number of Items: 16

Format: A questionnaire based on
the visual section of the shortened
form of the Betts' Questionnaire
on Mental Imagery.

Reliability: Test–retest reliability
was .67 ($N = 33$); split-half was .93
($N = 87$); Parallel form was .54 ($N
= 45$).

Author: McKelvie, S. J., and
Gingras, P. P.

Article: Reliability of two measures
of visual imagery.

Journal: *Perceptual and Motor
Skills,* August 1974, *39*(1, Part 2),
417–418.

Related Research: Marks, D. F.
(1973). Visual imagery differences
in the recall of pictures. *British*

Journal of Psychology, 64, 17–24.

Rossi, J. S., & Fingeret, A. L.
(1977). Individual differences in
verbal and imagery abilities:
Paired-associate recall as a
function of stimulus and response
concreteness. *Perceptual and
Motor Skills,* June, *44*(3, Part 2),
1043–1049.

■ ■ ■

2155

Test Name: VOCATIONAL
RATING SCALE

Purpose: To measure vocational
self-concept crystallization.

Number of Items: 40

Format: Each item is rated on a 5-
point Likert scale in terms of how
true the respondent perceives the
statement as being for him or her
at the time of testing.

Reliability: Cronbach's alpha
coefficient for internal consistency
was .94. Test–retest product–
moment correlation over 2 weeks
for 20 students was .76.

Validity: Mean score of the high
group significantly exceeded that
of the low group ($p < .01$).

Author: Barrett, T. C., and
Tinsley, H. E. A.

Article: Measuring vocational
self-concept crystallization.

Journal: *Journal of Vocational
Behavior,* October 1977, *11*(3),
305–313.

■ ■ ■

2156

Test Name: WHEN I WAS BORN

Purpose: To measure adolescents'
perceptions of parental reactions
at the time of their births.

Number of Items: 32

Format: A multiple choice test.
Includes four factors: parental
emotion, parental apprehension,
parental pride, and parental

nurturance. An example is presented.

Reliability: Test–retest reliability was .95 ($N = 29$ with 9.8-month interval).

Validity: Correlations with the: Self-Satisfaction Scale ranged from −.012 to .274; Self-Rating Scale ranged from .085 to .461.

Author: Clifford, E., and Brantley, H. T.

Article: When I was born: Perceived parental reactions of adolescents.

Journal: *Journal of Personality Assessment,* December 1977, *41,* 604–609.

Related Research: Clifford, E. (1969). The impact of symptom: A preliminary comparison of cleft lip-palate and asthmatic children. *Cleft Palate Journal, 6,* 221–227.

■ ■ ■

2157

Test Name: WHITE PREJUDICE SCALE

Purpose: To assess a student's feelings toward Whites.

Number of Items: 4

Format: Response to each question is either *yes* or *no.* Examples are provided. May be adapted for use as a Black or Mexican-American Prejudice Scale.

Reliability: Alpha reliabilities were .55 (pretest) and .60 (posttest). Alpha reliabilities were .56 (pretest) and .65 (posttest) when used as a Black Prejudice Scale.

Alpha reliabilities were .55 (pretest) and .63 (posttest) when used as a Mexican-American Prejudice Scale.

Author: Sheehan, D. S.

Article: A study of attitude change in desegregated intermediate schools.

Journal: *Sociology of Education,* January 1980, *53*(1), 51–59.

Related Research: Sheehan, D., & Marcus, M. (1977). *Desegregation report No. 1: The effects of busing status and student ethnicity on achievement test scores* (Research Report No. IR77–024). Dallas, TX: Department of Research, Evaluation, and Information Systems, Dallas Independent School District.

CHAPTER 16
Personality

2158

Test Name: ARROW-DOT TASK

Purpose: To measure rule-orientation behavior.

Number of Items: 23

Format: One of four subtests of the Id-Ego-Superego Test. An untimed perceptual motor task requiring the solution of graphic problems. Requires direct problem-solving behaviors under specific instructions centering around simple rules.

Reliability: Test–retest reliability coefficients ranged from .59 to .83.

Author: Phillips, V. K., and Hudgins, A. L.

Article: Relationship between creativity, sex, and rule-orientation behavior.

Journal: *Perceptual and Motor Skills,* June 1974, *38*(3, Part 2), 1163–1171.

Related Research: Dombrose, L. A., & Slobin, M. S. (1958). The IES Test. *Perceptual and Motor Skills, 8,* 347–389 (Monograph Supplement 3–V8).

Goldberg, L. S., & Meltzer, G. (1974). IES Arrow-Dot comparisons for drug addicts with neurotic and delinquent personalities. *Perceptual and Motor Skills,* April, *38* (2), 636–638.

Herron, W. G. (1966). The IES experiment. *Perceptual and Motor Skills, 23,* 279 290.

Roll, S., & Hertel, P. (1974). Arrow-dot measures of impulse, ego, and superego functions in

noncheaters, cheaters, and supercheaters. *Perceptual and Motor Skills, 39*(3), 1035–1038.

2159

Test Name: BIOGRAPHICAL INVENTORY FOR THE ARTS

Purpose: To predict an art versus nonart dichotomous criterion as well as several different performance criteria for art students in four art areas (music, dance, theater, and the visual arts).

Number of Items: 249

Format: Contains general biographical items and biographical items specific to the arts.

Validity: Average cross-validity for predicting the art versus nonart criterion was .67.

Author: James, L. R., et al.

Article: Prediction of artistic performance from biographical data.

Journal: *Journal of Applied Psychology,* February 1974, *59*(1), 84–86.

Related Research: Taylor, C. W., & Ellison, R. L. (1967). Predictors of scientific performance. *Science, 155,* 1075–1079.

2160

Test Name: CHOICE DILEMMA QUESTIONNAIRE

Purpose: To measure risk-taking.

Number of Items: 12

Format: Hypothetical situations are described and the subject chooses the minimum level of certainty before he would choose a risky but desirable alternative.

Validity: Correlation with need for information was .15; confidence in decisions was .14; tendency to defer decisions was .09; self appraisal of derisiveness was .02; peer rating of decisiveness was .03.

Author: Weissman, M. S.

Article: Decisiveness and psychological adjustment.

Journal: *Journal of Personality Assessment,* August 1976, *40*(4), 403–412.

Related Research: Kogan, N., & Wallach, M. A. (1961). The effect of anxiety on relations between subjective age and caution in an older sample. In P. H. Hack & J. Zubin (Eds.), *Psychopathology of aging* (pp. 123–135). New York: Grune & Stratton.

2161

Test Name: CHOICE DILEMMAS QUESTIONNAIRE REVISED

Purpose: To provide a measure of risk-taking propensity.

Number of Items: 10

Format: For each of 10 situations the subjects indicate the highest risk they are willing to take.

Reliability: Odd–even (Spearman-Brown) reliability coefficients were .53 (men), and .62 (women).

Validity: Correlations with other

variables (men) ranged from −.13 to .18. Correlations with other variables (women) ranged from −.14 to .18.

Author: Muldrow, T. W., and Bayton, J. A.

Article: Men and women executives and processes related to decision accuracy.

Journal: *Journal of Applied Psychology*, April 1979, *64*(2), 99–106.

Related Research: Kogan, N., & Dorros, K. (1975). *Sex differences in risk taking and its attribution.* Unpublished manuscript, New School for Social Research, New York.

■ ■ ■

2162

Test Name: COAN EXPERIENCE INVENTORY

Purpose: To measure a subject's openness to experiences.

Number of Items: 83

Format: Includes the following components: aesthetic sensitivity, unusual perceptions and associations, openness to theoretical or hypothetical ideas, constructive utilization of fantasy and dreams, openness to unconventional views of reality, indulgence of fantasy, and deliberate and systematic thought.

Validity: Correlations with the Conservatism Scale ranged from −.39 to .27 for men and from −.50 to .81 for women.

Author: Joe, V. C., et al.

Article: Conservatism, openness to experience and sample bias.

Journal: *Journal of Personality Assessment*, October 1977, *41*(5), 527–531.

Related Research: Coan, R. W. (1972). Measurable components of

openness to experience. *Journal of Consulting and Clinical Psychology, 39,* 346 (Extended Report).

■ ■ ■

2163

Test Name: COUNSELOR R SCALE

Purpose: To measure a restrictive–nonrestrictive dimension of counselor functioning.

Format: Includes Likert scale in which high scores are indicative of restrictiveness and low scores reflect nonrestrictiveness.

Reliability: Test–retest reliability was .84 (n = 64 over 2-week period) and .76 (n = 60 over 1 to 4 month period).

Validity: Coefficient alpha produced an internal consistency index of .84 (n = 107). Correlation with Rokeach Dogmatism Scale was .31.

Author: Seay, T. A., and Riley, F. T.

Article: A preliminary validation of an instrument to measure the degree of counselor restrictive–nonrestrictive cognitive orientation.

Journal: *Educational and Psychological Measurement,* Winter 1975, *35*(4), 921–928.

■ ■ ■

2164

Test Name: EGO STRENGTH SCALE

Purpose: To measure various aspects of effective personal functioning usually considered descriptive of ego strength.

Number of Items: 68

Format: Includes true or false descriptions of the subject.

Reliability: Odd–even reliability was .76 (n = 126 patients). Test–retest reliability (3 months) was .71 (n = 30).

Validity: Pearson product–moment correlation with the Dogmatism Scale was −.42.

Author: Martin, J. D., et al.

Article: A correlation of Barron's Ego Strength Scale and Rokeach's Dogmatism Scale.

Journal: *Educational and Psychological Measurement,* Summer 1978, *38*(2), 583–586.

Related Research: Barron, F. (1953). Some test correlates of response to therapy. *Journal of Consulting Psychology, 17,* 235–241.

■ ■ ■

2165

Test Name: EMOTIONS PROFILE INDEX

Purpose: To provide self assessment of importance of various emotions to an individual.

Number of Items: 24

Format: Subject rates, on 5-point scale, how important specific emotions are to him or her.

Validity: Correlations of eight scales with Reinforcement Potential ranged from .29 (NS) to .57 (p < .01) for schizophrenic patients.

Author: Plutchik, R., and Stein, S.

Article: Reinforcement preferences and personality profiles of hospitalized schizophrenics.

Journal: *Psychological Reports,* October 1974, *35*(2), 695–700.

Related Research: Kellerman, H., & Plutchik, R. (1968). Emotion-trait interrelations and the measurement of personality. *Psychological Reports, 55,* 91–95.

2166

Test Name: ERIKSONIAN INVENTORY

Purpose: To measure the extent of identity resolution of diffusion among young adults.

Number of Items: 60

Format: Items are distributed equally among 12 subtests that measure the outcome of the first six psychosocial crises of the Eriksonian life cycle theory. Half of these subtests measure the positive aspects of the first six psychosocial dilemmas and the other half measure the negative aspects of these dilemmas.

Validity: Pearsonian intercorrelations with the Runner Studies of Attitude Patterns (Runner, 1973) resulted in 87 or 52% of 168 possible intercorrelations that are statistically significant ($p < .05$).

Author: Varghese, R.

Article: Personality factor structure underlying two psychoanalytic measures of personality.

Journal: *Psychological Reports,* December 1978, *53*(3), 1239–1244.

Related Research: Runner, K. (1973). *A theory of persons.* San Diego, CA: Runner Associates.

● ● ●

2167

Test Name: FELT FIGURE REPLACEMENT TECHNIQUE

Purpose: To assess personality.

Format: The subject views two different colored felt figures that have been placed on a felt covered board. The figures are removed and the subject is asked to replace them as they were.

Reliability: Test–retest ($N = 52$ women) reliability ranged from .10 to .54. Test–retest ($N = 47$ men) reliability ranged from –.09 to .43.

Validity: Correlations with the Eysenck Personality Inventory ranged from .27 to .37 ($N = 52$ women) and from .15 to .20 ($N = 47$ men).

Author: Klopfer, F. J., et al.

Article: The Felt Figure Replacement Technique as a personality assessment device: Validity reconsidered.

Journal: *Journal of Personality Assessment,* August 1977, *41*(4), 392–395.

Related Research: Kuethe, J. L. (1962). Social schemas and the reconstruction of social object displays from memory. *Journal of Abnormal and Social Psychology, 65,* 71–74.

● ● ●

2168

Test Name: HOW DO YOU THINK INVENTORY

Purpose: To assess attitudes, motivations, interests, values, beliefs, and other personality and biographical matters strongly suspected to underlie creative behavior.

Number of Items: 102

Format: Each item is answered on a 5-point rating scale from *disagree* to *agree.*

Reliability: Hoyt internal reliability was .94 ($n = 68$).

Validity: Correlation with creativity ratings was .64 (for 15 men), .36 (for 47 women), and .42 (for the total 62).

Author: Davis, G. A.

Article: In frumious pursuit of the creative person.

Journal: *Journal of Creative Behavior,* 1975, *9*(2), 75–87.

2169

Test Name: LORR INTERPERSONAL STYLE INVENTORY

Purpose: To measure personality style.

Number of Items: 430

Format: Measures 16 bipolar dimensions (e.g., directive, achieving, attention seeking, trusting, etc.).

Reliability: Kuder-Richardson formula 20 ranged .71 to .89. Test–retest ranged from .81 to .91 (2 weeks).

Validity: Sex variables significantly differentiated between men and women.

Author: Stefic, E., and Lorr, M.

Article: Age and sex differences in personality during adolescence.

Journal: *Psychological Reports,* December 1974, *35*(3), 1123–1126.

Related Research: Lorr, M., & Younis, R. (1973). An inventory of personal style. *Journal of Personality Assessment, 37,* 165–173.

● ● ●

2170

Test Name: MATCHING FAMILIAR FIGURES TEST— REVISED

Purpose: To measure reflection-impulsivity.

Number of Items: 9

Format: Includes six randomly selected items from the adult test plus three from the children's test. Forms A and B.

Reliability: Coefficient alpha for errors was .44 for Form A and .48 for Form B. Latency measure was .80 for Form A and .83 for Form B.

Author: Brodzinsky, D. M., and Dein, P.

Article: Short-term stability of adult reflection-impulsivity.

Journal: *Perceptual and Motor Skills,* December 1976, *43*(3, Part 1), 1012–1014.

Related Research: Messer, S. B. (1976). Reflection–impulsivity a review. *Psychological Bulletin, 83*(6), 1026–1052.

■ ■ ■

2171

Test Name: PERSONAL ATTRIBUTE INVENTORY

Purpose: To serve as a personality assessment instrument and as a self-concept scale.

Number of Items: 100

Format: Subject indicates which 30 of the positive and negative adjectives are most descriptive of a target individual or group.

Validity: Correlations with the factors of the 16PF ranged from –.47 to .35.

Author: Kappes, B. M., and Parish, T. S.

Article: The Personal Attribute Inventory: A measure of self-concepts and personality profiles.

Journal: *Educational and Psychological Measurement,* Winter 1979, *39*(4), 955–958.

Related Research: Parish, T., et al. (1977). The Personal Attribute Inventory as a self concept scale: A preliminary report. *Psychological Reports, 41,* 1141–1142.

■ ■ ■

2172

Test Name: SENSATIONS SEEKING SCALE

Purpose: To determine risk-taking propensity.

Number of Items: 72

Format: Paired items covering: thrill and adventure, experience seeking, disinhibition, boredom susceptibility and general.

Reliability: Test–retest reliabilities ranged from .72 to .93 over 1 hour, 1 week, and 3 months. All were significant at the .01 level.

Author: Musolino, R. F., and Hershenson, D. B.

Article: Avocational sensation seeking in high and low risk-taking occupations.

Journal: *Journal of Vocational Behavior,* June 1977, *10*(3), 358–365.

Related Research: Zuckerman, M., et al. (1964). Development of a Sensation Seeking Scale. *Journal of Consulting Psychology, 28,* 477–482.

■ ■ ■

2173

Test Name: SOCIAL, PERSONALITY, AND DEMOGRAPHIC QUESTIONNAIRE

Purpose: To measure social, personality, and demographic data.

Number of Items: 80

Format: Includes 13 scales: morale, perceived lifespace, social lifespace, education, occupation, age, frequency of attending church, number of groups in which there is membership, number of leisure activities, number of items read, change in number of leisure activities, conformity versus alienation, and

modified F or authoritarian personality scale.

Reliability: Pearson product–moment reliability coefficient was .83 with 1-week interval ($N = 10$) and .95 with a 2-day interval.

Author: Fleishman, J. J.

Article: Social relatedness and perceptual performance among the aged.

Journal: *Perceptual and Motor Skills,* December 1976, *43*(3, Part 2), 1243–1247.

Related Research: Cumming, E., & Henry, W. (1961). *Growing old.* New York: Basic Books.

■ ■ ■

2174

Test Name: ZAX INFORMATION PROFILE

Purpose: To assess personality through the measurement of knowledge of general information.

Number of Items: 195

Format: 24 Content Areas (given in article).

Reliability: Kuder-Richardson formula 20 for the 24 subtests are given and are generally rather low.

Validity: Principal component factor analysis revealed six factors; authors predicted and found significant sex and subject major differences in college students.

Author: Zax, M., et al.

Article: Development of a personality test based on general fund of information.

Journal: *Journal of Personality Assessment,* June 1974, *38*(3), 215–222.

CHAPTER 17
Preference

2175

Test Name: ADOLESCENT STRUCTURE INVENTORY

Purpose: To measure structure in adolescence.

Number of Items: 40

Format: Twenty items that determine whether the youth wants guidance, advice, information, clarity, or direction offered by an adult figure of authority and 20 items that determine whether the person has such structure.

Reliability: Odd–even coefficients of reliability of .93 for the wants-structure scale and .91 for the has-structure scale.

Author: Chabassol, D. J., and Thomas, D.

Article: Needs for structure, tolerance of ambiguity, and dogmatism in adolescents.

Journal: *Psychological Reports,* October 1975, *37*(2), 507–510.

Related Research: Chabassol, D. J. (1971). A scale for the evaluation of structure needs and perceptions in adolescence. *Journal of Experimental Education, 40,* 12–16.

• • •

2176

Test Name: BEM SEX ROLE INVENTORY

Purpose: To measure the concept of psychological androgyny.

Number of Items: 20

Format: Items consist of masculine, feminine, and neutral adjectives on which subjects rate themselves on a 7-point scale.

Validity: Correlation with PRF Andro Scale (Masculinity) was .65 for males and .62 for females and (Femininity) was .57 for males, .55 for females.

Author: Gayton, W. F., et al.

Article: A comparison of the Bem Sex Role Inventory and the PRF Andro Scale.

Journal: *Journal of Personality Assessment,* December 1977, *41*(6), 619–621.

Related Research: Bem, D. J., & Allen, A. (1974). On predicting some of the people some of the time: The search for cross-situational consistencies in behavior. *Psychological Review, 81,* 506–520.

Bem, S. L. (1974). The measurement of psychological androgyny (SIC). *Journal of Consulting and Clinical Psychology, 42,* 155–162.

Bem, S. L., & Watson, C. (1976). *Scoring packet: Bem Sex Role Inventory.* Unpublished manuscript. (Available from S. L. Bem, Department of Psychology, Stanford University, Stanford, California, 94305)

Bernard, L. C., & Epstein, D. J. (1978). Sex role conformity in homosexual and heterosexual males. *Journal of Personality Assessment, 42,* 505–511.

Cohen, D., & Schmidt, J. P. (1979). Ambiversion: Characteristics of midrange responders on the introversion–extraversion continuum. *Journal of Personality Assessment, 43,* 514–516.

Conley, J. J. (1978). Sex differences and androgyny in fantasy content. *Journal of Personality Assessment, 42,* 604–610.

Feldman, S. S., & Nash, S. C. (1979). Changes in responsiveness to babies during adolescence. *Child Development, 50,* 942–949.

Forisha, B. L. (1978). Creativity and imagery in men and women. *Perceptual and Motor Skills, 47,* 1255–1264.

Hinrichsen, J. J., & Stone, L. (1978). Effects of three conditions of administration on Bem Sex Role Inventory scores. *Journal of Personality Assessment, 42,* 512.

Milgram, R. M., et al. (1977). Creativity and sex-role identity in elementary school children. *Perceptual and Motor Skills, 45,* 371–376.

Millimet, C. R., & Votta, R. P. (1979). Acquiescence and the Bem Sex-Role Inventory. *Journal of Personality Assessment, 43,* 164–165.

Paludi, M. A. (1978). Machover revisited: Impact of sex-role orientation on sex sequence on the Draw-A Person Test. *Perceptual and Motor Skills, 47,* 713–714.

Puglisi, J. T. (1980). Equating the social desirability of Bem Sex-Role Inventory masculinity and femininity subscales. *Journal of Personality Assessment, 44,* 272–276.

Small, A. C., et al. (1979). A comparison of the Bem Sex-Role

Inventory and the Heilbrun Masculinity and Femininity Scales. *Journal of Personality Assessment, 43,* 393–395.

■ ■ ■

2177

Test Name: CAUSAL CONSTRUCT SCALE

Purpose: To identify causal preference.

Number of Items: 36

Format: Includes 18 sayings for each of four causal meanings. Each item consists of a pair of causal meanings. Samples are presented.

Reliability: One week test–retest stability coefficients (80 junior and senior high school students) were in the .50s and .60s. One week reliability check (37 male laborers) produced Pearson correlational values that exceeded .70.

Validity: Correlations with the MMPI ($N = 77$) ranged from −.400 to .343. Correlations with the Shipley Institute of Living Scale for Measuring Intellectual Impairment ($N = 77$) ranged from −.219 to .270.

Author: Rychlak, J. F., and Ingwell, R. H.

Article: Causal orientation and personal adjustment of hospitalized veterans.

Journal: *Journal of Personality Assessment,* June 1977, *41*(3), 299–303.

Related Research: Rychlak, J. F., & Barna, J. D. (1971). Causality and the proper image of man in scientific psychology. *Journal of Personality Assessment, 34,* 403–419.

■ ■ ■

2178

Test Name: CLERICAL JOB CONDITION AND TASK PREFERENCE SCHEDULE

Purpose: To identify task and working condition preferences of clerical applicants.

Number of Items: 28

Format: Subjects indicate which job conditions and job tasks they like most and which they like least. All items are presented.

Reliability: Correlations ranged from −.333 to .833. Kappa ranged from .119 to. 377.

Validity: Correlations with ethnicity ranged from −.767 to .833.

Author: Ash, R. A., et al.

Article: Exploratory study of a matching approach to personnel selection: The impact of ethnicity.

Journal: *Journal of Applied Psychology,* February 1979, *64*(1), 35–41.

■ ■ ■

2179

Test Name: COGNITIVE PREFERENCE TEST

Purpose: To measure one's cognitive preference in three areas: science, social-studies, and mathematics.

Number of Items: 60-item triads

Format: Includes 20 item triads for each subject, and scores for preference for facts or terms, principles or generalizations, and practical application.

Reliability: Item total correlations ranged from .1068 to .7438 with a mean of .5163. Odd–even correlations ranged from .789 to .900, and test–retest correlations over 9 days ranged from .807 to .893.

Author: Williams, C.

Article: A study of cognitive preferences.

Journal: *Journal of Experimental*

Education, Spring 1975, *43*(3), 61–77.

Related Research: Heath, R. W. (1964). Curriculum, cognition, and educational measurement. *Educational and Psychological Measurement, 24,* 239–253.

■ ■ ■

2180

Test Name: DECISION-DIFFICULTY CHECKLIST

Purpose: To measure the degree of difficulty experienced with commonly encountered decisions.

Number of Items: 61

Format: Four decision areas include school, dating-marriage, career, and interpersonal.

Reliability: Total scale coefficient alpha reliability was .94, with subscale reliabilities ranging from .80 to .84.

Author: Mendonca, J. D., and Siess, T. F.

Article: Counseling for indecisiveness: Problem-solving and anxiety-management training.

Journal: *Journal of Counseling Psychology,* July 1976, *23*(4), 339–347.

Related Research: Mendonca, J. D. (1974). *Effectiveness of problem-solving and anxiety-management training in modifying vocational indecision.* Unpublished doctoral dissertation, University of Western Ontario.

■ ■ ■

2181

Test Name: GROUP TOY PREFERENCE TEST

Purpose: To measure current sex-role preference.

Number of Items: 10

Format: Includes pictures of masculine and feminine objects.

Reliability: .81 and .96.

Author: Garrett, C. S., and Cunningham, D. J.

Article: Effects of vicarious consequences and model and experimenter sex on imitative behavior in first-grade children.

Journal: *Journal of Educational Psychology,* December 1974, *66*(6), 940–947.

■ ■ ■

2182

Test Name: HIGHER ORDER NEED STRENGTH QUESTIONNAIRE

Purpose: To measure preferences for specific amounts of various job characteristics.

Number of Items: 8

Format: Items were concerned with: variety, task identity, task feedback, management feedback, challenge, meaningfulness, and use of valued skills.

Reliability: Internal consistency with Spearman-Brown formula applied to average item intercorrelation was .78.

Author: Wanous, J. P.

Article: Individual differences and reactions to job characteristics.

Journal: *Journal of Applied Psychology,* October 1974, *59*(5), 616–622.

Related Research: Hackman, J. R., & Lawler, E. E., III. (1971). Employee reactions to job characteristics. *Journal of Applied Psychology, 55,* 259–286.

■ ■ ■

2183

Test Name: JUDGMENT ANALYSIS

Purpose: To assess policies used in judging the beauty of paintings.

Format: Judges rated 19 paintings for beauty on a 1–7 scale and noted 11 characteristics attended to, for example, color, realism, depth.

Validity: It was reported that five different judgment policies were used.

Author: Holmes, G., and Zedeck, S.

Article: Judgment analysis for assessing paintings.

Journal: *Journal of Experimental Education,* Summer 1973, *41*(4), 26–30.

■ ■ ■

2184

Test Name: LEAST-PREFERRED CO-WORKER SCALE

Purpose: To identify the leader's motivational style.

Number of Items: 22

Format: Items form a bipolar adjective scale on which the respondent is able to describe the one person with whom he or she could work least well. A high score indicates a basic motivation to relate to others while a low score indicates a task-motivation.

Validity: Spearman rank-order correlations with performance ranged from –.70 to .80.

Author: Csoka, L. S.

Article: A relationship between leader intelligence and leader rated effectiveness.

Journal: *Journal of Applied Psychology,* February 1974, *59*(1), 43–47.

Related Research: Fiedler, F. E. (1967). *A theory of leadership effectiveness.* New York: McGraw-Hill.

2185

Test Name: LEISURE ACTIVITIES QUESTIONNAIRE

Purpose: To measure the need-satisfying properties of leisure activities.

Number of Items: 334

Format: Includes 45 need-satisfier dimensions employing a Likert format.

Reliability: Split-group reliabilities ranged from .86 to .97.

Author: Tinsley, H. E. A., and Kass, R. A.

Article: The construct validity of the Leisure Activities Questionnaire and of the Paragraphs about Leisure.

Journal: *Educational and Psychological Measurement,* Spring 1980, *40*(1), 219–226.

Related Research: Tinsley, H. E. A., & Kass, R. A. (1978). Leisure activities and need satisfaction: A replication and extension. *Journal of Leisure Research, 10,* 191–202.

■ ■ ■

2186

Test Name: LIFE STYLE ORIENTATION QUESTIONNAIRE

Purpose: To measure lifestyle orientation.

Number of Items: 24

Format: Three dimensions assessed: formalistic, sociocentric, and personalistic.

Validity: Correlations with attitude toward teacher and classroom measures are given.

Author: DiMarco, N.

Article: Lifestyle, learning structure, congruence and student attitudes.

Journal: *American Educational Research Journal*, Spring 1974, *11*(2), 203–209.

Related Research: Friedlander, F. (1971). *Generational lifestyles and organization structure* (U.S. Department of Health, Education and Welfare Grant MH 20719–01). Washington, DC: U.S. Public Health Service.

■ ■ ■

2187

Test Name: NOVELTY-EXPERIENCING SCALE

Purpose: To measure novelty-experiencing.

Number of Items: 80

Format: Includes four subscales: internal cognition, internal sensation, external cognition, external sensation. Subjects indicate whether they like or dislike the activities described in the item. The test provides for subscale and total scores.

Reliability: Kuder-Richardson formula 20 internal consistency (N = 135) for the four subscales ranged from .74 to .83; Kuder-Richardson formula 20 internal consistency (N = 135) for the full scale was .85; test–retest (6 to 8 weeks, N = 54) reliability for the four subscales ranged from .69 to .84; test–retest (6 to 8 weeks, N = 54) for the full scale was .76.

Validity: Subscales with sensation-seeking scale (N = 135) ranged from .02 to .55; subscales with Willner Unusual Meanings Vocabulary Test (N = 135) ranged from .0 to .22; subscales with the Stroop Color-Word Test (N = 54) ranged –.19 to .02; full scale with sensation-seeking scale (N = 135) was .44; full scale with Willner Unusual Meanings Vocabulary Test (N = 135) was .19; Full scale with Stroop Color-Word Test (N = 54) was –.10.

Author: Gaines, L. S., and Coursey, R. D.

Article: Novelty-experiencing, internal scanning, and cognitive control.

Journal: *Perceptual and Motor Skills*, June 1974, *38*(3, Part I), 891–898.

Related Research: Pearson, P. (1970). Relationships between global and specified measures of novelty seeking. *Journal of Consulting and Clinical Psychology, 34*, 199–204.

Waters, C. (1974). Multidimensional measures of novelty experiencing, sensation seeking, and ability: Correlational analysis for male and female college samples. *Psychological Reports, 34*, 43–46.

■ ■ ■

2188

Test Name: PLEASANT EVENTS SCHEDULE

Purpose: To measure the retrospective frequency and value of positive reinforcement.

Number of Items: 320

Format: Subject rates each item for frequency of occurrence during the past month on a 3-point rating scale from *did not occur* to *occurred seven or more times* and then rates the subjective enjoyability of each activity on a 3-point scale (from *not pleasurable* to *extremely pleasurable*).

Validity: Correlations with Adult Nowicki-Strickland I-E Scale ranged from –.24 to –.42 (N = 32, men) and from –.01 to –.13 (N = 42, women); Success-Failure Inventory ranged from .29 to .55 (N = 32, men) and from .01 to .49 (N = 42, women); Physical Attractiveness Ratings ranged from .20 to .52 (N = 32, men) and from –.09 to .36 (N = 42, women).

Author: Cash, T. F., and Burns, D. S.

Article: The occurrence of reinforcing activities in relation to locus of control, success-failure expectancies, and physical attractiveness.

Journal: *Journal of Personality Assessment*, August 1977, *41*(4), 387–391.

Related Research: MacPhillamy, D. J., & Lewinsohn, P. M. (1971). The pleasant events schedule (mimeo). Eugene: University of Oregon.

■ ■ ■

2189

Test Name: POSITIVE REINFORCEMENT OBSERVATION SCHEDULE

Purpose: To obtain data concerning expressed preference for and observed use of positive reinforcement in integrated classrooms.

Number of Items: 10

Format: Includes 10 categories of behaviors that may be emitted by mediators, that is, teachers or parents. All items are presented.

Reliability: Correlation between observers ranged from .88 to .99.

Author: Byalick, R., and Bersoff, D. N.

Article: Reinforcement practices of Black and White teachers in integrated classrooms.

Journal: *Journal of Educational Psychology*, August 1974, *66*(4), 473–480.

Related Research: Bersoff, D. N., & Moyer, D. (1973). Positive Reinforcement Observation Schedule (PROS): Development and applications to educational settings [Summary]. *Proceedings of the 81st Annual Convention of the American Psychological Association, 8*, 713–714.

2190

Test Name: PREFERENCE FOR AGGRESSION-CONDUCIVE ACTIVITIES ASSESSMENT SCALE

Purpose: To determine the degree of preference for aggression-conducive activities.

Number of Items: 20

Format: The child selects from each pair of line drawings the childhood activity preferred. All items are presented.

Reliability: Temporal stability was $r = .58$ (girls) and $r = .51$ (boys).

Validity: Correlations with assessed aggression ranged from .17 to .36.

Author: Bullock, D., and Merrill, L.

Article: The impact of personal preference on consistency through time: The case of childhood aggression.

Journal: *Child Development,* September 1980, *51*(3), 808–*814.*

■ ■ ■

2191

Test Name: PUPIL PROBLEM BEHAVIOR INVENTORY

Purpose: To measure teachers' preferences for consultation or referral approaches for working with problem students.

Number of Items: 48

Format: Preference for Consultation Scale and Problem Severity Scale each divided into three subscales: Acting Out, Withdrawal, and Academic. Ratings on all scales are from 1 to 5.

Reliability: Alpha coefficients of reliability for all the subscales ranged from .55 to .80 with a median coefficient of .75. The overall alpha for all items was .87.

Author: Gutkin, T. B., et al.

Article: Teacher reactions to school-based consultation services: A multivariate analysis.

Journal: *Journal of School Psychology,* 1980, *18*(2), 126–134.

Related Research: Stott, D. H. (1972). *Bristol Social Adjustment Guides.* San Diego: Educational and Industrial Testing Service.

Quay, H. C., & Peterson, D. R. (1967). *Behavior Problem Checklist.* Champaign, IL: Children's Research Center, University of Illinois.

■ ■ ■

2192

Test Name: RATING SCALE FOR ADULTS

Purpose: A measure of sex-role adoption.

Time Required: 3 to 8 minutes.

Format: Taps sex-typed behaviors that could be abstracted as degrees of activity.

Reliability: Test–retest reliability over 7 days using Pearson product–moment correlations: men, .627 ($p < .001$), women, .709 ($p < .001$).

Author: Newman, R. C., II

Article: Development and standardization of measures of stereotypic sex-role concepts and of sex-role adoption in adults.

Journal: *Psychological Reports,* October 1976, *39*(2), 623–630.

Related Research: Biller, H. B. (1973). Sex-role uncertainty and psychopathology. *Journal of Individual Psychology, 29,* 24–25.

■ ■ ■

2193

Test Name: SELF-DIRECTED LEARNING READINESS SCALE

Purpose: To gather data on learning preferences and attitudes toward learning.

Number of Items: 58

Format: Self-report questionnaire, Likert items.

Reliability: Reliability coefficient of .87 (Guglielmino, 1977).

Validity: Statistically significant correlations with originality measures ($rs = .52, .38, .52$), a measure of the ability to produce analogies ($r = .48$), creative achievements and experiences ($r = .71$), and the right and left hemisphere styles of learning ($rs = .43$ and $-.34$, respectively).

Author: Torrance, E. P., and Mourad, S.

Article: Some creativity and style of learning and thinking correlates of Guglielmino's Self-directed Learning Readiness Scale.

Journal: *Psychological Reports,* December 1978, *43*(3), 1167–1171.

Related Research: Guglielmino, L. M. (1977). *Development of the Self-directed Learning Readiness Scale.* Doctoral Dissertation, University of Georgia.

■ ■ ■

2194

Test Name: SEX ROLE DISAPPROVAL MEASURE

Purpose: To assess extent of approval of cross-sex roles of boys and girls.

Number of Items: 10

Format: Ten descriptions of girls and boys engaging in cross sex behavior (e.g., a girl helping her father repair a car) were rated by subjects on a 7-point scale 1 (*extreme approval*) to 7 (*extreme disapproval*).

Reliability: Cronbach's alphas were .73, .63, and .67 for total, male, and female scores, respectively.

Validity: Male subjects were more disapproving than female subjects; disapproval for cross sex behavior of boys was greater than girls' cross sex behavior.

Author: Feinman, S.

Article: Approval of cross-sex-role behavior.

Journal: *Psychological Reports,* August 1974, *35*(1), 643–648.

• • •

2195

Test Name: SEX ROLE LEARNING INDEX

Purpose: To measure early sex role acquisition in preschool-aged children.

Number of Items: 30

Format: Black-and-white line drawings organized into three sections (a) the child figures section, (b) the adult figures section, and (c) the objects section. Subjects indicate which they think are for boys, girls, or both boys and girls.

Reliability: Test–retest reliabilities ranged from –.17 to .90. Of the 12 product–moment correlations, 9 are significant at the .05 level or better.

Author: Edelbrock, C., and Sugawara, A. I.

Article: Acquisition of sex-typed preferences in preschool-aged children.

Journal: *Developmental Psychology,* November 1978, *14*(6), 614–623.

• • •

2196

Test Name: SEX ROLE QUESTIONNAIRE

Purpose: To measure sex-role stereotypes.

Number of Items: 45

Format: Subjects rate a target person along 9-point semantic differential type scales appearing between the pairs of bipolar items.

Reliability: Overall reliability alpha of .83. Alpha coefficients of .89 for the Assertiveness Scale, .88 for the Sensitivity Scale, and .87 for the Rationality Scale were also obtained.

Author: Smith, R. L., and Bradley, D. W.

Article: Factor validation and refinement of the Sex-role Questionnaire and its relationship to the Attitudes Toward Women Scale.

Journal: *Psychological Reports,* June 1979, *44*(3), 1155–1174.

Related Research: Rosenkrantz, P., et al. (1968). Sex-role stereotypes and self-concepts in college students. *Journal of Consulting and Clinical Psychology, 32,* 287–295.

• • •

2197

Test Name: THERAPIST'S BEHAVIOR SCALE

Purpose: To measure one's preferences for more or less directive therapist's behavior.

Number of Items: 40

Format: Items are answered *preferred* or *not preferred* on a 5-point scale.

Reliability: Test–retest reliability of .79 over a 3-week period.

Author: Duckro, P., et al.

Article: Malleability of preference for therapists' response style.

Journal: *Psychological Reports,* August 1978, *43*(1), 299–304.

Related Research: Reiter, M. (1967). Variables associated with

the degree of preferred directiveness in therapy. *Dissertation Abstracts, 27,* 3679B.

• • •

2198

Test Name: VOCATIONAL ORIENTATION OF WOMEN QUESTIONNAIRE

Purpose: To determine women's identification with a career outside the home and/or the homemaker role.

Number of Items: 52

Format: Five-response liken scale from *stongly agree* to *strongly disagree.*

Reliability: Test–retest reliability coefficients of .90 and .91 were obtained for 22 undergraduate students over a 2-week period on two factors.

Author: Bledsoe, J. C.

Article: Vocational orientation of college women as related to selected personality characteristics.

Journal: *Psychological Reports,* June 1978, *42*(3), 835–841.

Related Research: Dunn, M. S. (1960). Marriage role expectations of asolescents. *Marriage and Family Living, 22,* 99–111.

• • •

2199

Test Name: YOUR STYLE OF LEARNING AND THINKING

Purpose: To estimate the relative psychological dependence of an individual on the right or left hemisphere of the brain.

Number of Items: 36 (Form A), 40 (Form B)

Format: The subject chooses one of three responses to each item. All items of Forms A and B are presented.

Reliability: Equivalent forms reliability coefficients ranged from .54 to .97.

Author: Reynolds, C. R., et al.

Article: A children's form of Your Style of Learning and Thinking: Preliminary norms and technical data.

Journal: *The Gifted Child Quarterly,* Winter 1979, *23*(4), 757–767.

Related Research: Torrance, E. P., et al. (1977). Your Style of Learning and Thinking: Preliminary norms, abbreviated technical notes, scoring keys, and selected references. *Gifted Child Quarterly, 21,* 563–573.

CHAPTER 18
Problem Solving and Reasoning

2200

Test Name: ABSTRACT ORIENTATION SCALE

Purpose: To measure concreteness-abstractness.

Number of Items: 30

Format: Subjects indicate degree of agreement or disagreement on a 6-point scale. Only 18 items are used in the scoring.

Reliability: Test–retest reliability was .83 ($N = 192$).

Author: Hendrick, H. W.

Article: Differences in group problem-solving behavior and effectiveness as a function of abstractness.

Journal: *Journal of Applied Psychology*, October 1979, *64*(5), 518–525.

Related Research: O'Connor, J. (1972). Developmental changes in abstractness and moral reasoning (Doctoral dissertation, George Peabody College for Teachers, 1971). *Dissertation Abstracts International, 32*, 4109A. (University Microfilms No. 72–03831)

2201

Test Name: ABSTRACT REASONING TEST

Purpose: To measure abstract reasoning.

Number of Items: 15

Format: Includes the subject's ability to determine inductively the logical relationships among patterns of diagrams.

Reliability: Kuder-Richardson formula 20 reliability estimates .634 (senior boys) and .635 (senior girls).

Author: Alexander, K. L., et al.

Article: School SES influences—Composition or context?

Journal: *Sociology of Education*, October 1979, *52*(4), 222–237.

Related Research: Dailey, J. T., & Shaycoft, M. F. (1961). *Types of tests in project talent.* U.S. Department of Health, Education, and Welfare, Office of Education. Washington, DC: U.S. Government Printing Office.

2202

Test Name: ABSTRACT REASONING TEST

Purpose: To measure students' ability to identify and utilize concepts and principles, to recognize patterns and relationships, and to use simple inductive and deductive logic.

Number of Items: 10

Format: Requires the subject to differentiate between various number systems, to identify and utilize principles in the construction of mathematical series and Magic Squares, and to recognize the preservation of shape after rotation. Includes forms A, B, C, L, M, N, and X. Examples are given.

Validity: Correlations with CTMM for inner-city school students ranged from .18 to .28 for verbal total and .20 to .31 for nonverbal total. Correlations with end-of-year grade in mathematics ranged from .38 to .62.

Author: Gabor, G. M.

Article: Effect of differential teaching, and teacher's praise and reproof.

Journal: *California Journal of Educational Research*, May 1975, *26*(3), 155–166.

Related Research: See *DUEMM, 2,* 1978, 884.

2203

Test Name: ADAPTED MODIFIED ROLE REPERTORY TEST

Purpose: To measure cognitive complexity appropriate for use with children.

Number of Items: 10 role titles.

Format: Likert scale.

Reliability: Test–retest reliability for a group of elementary school children over a 4-week period was .81 (Vacc and Vacc, 1973).

Validity: Correlations of the test with Modified Role Repertory Test scores for two groups of college students were .51 and .55 (Vacc & Vacc, 1973).

Author: Vacc, N. A., and Vacc, N.

Article: Further development of the Adapted Modified Role Repertory Test.

Journal: *Measurement and Evaluation in Guidance*, January 1980, *12*(4), 216–222.

Related Research: Vacc, N. A., & Greenleaf, W. (1975). Sequential

Development of Cognitive Complexity. *Perceptual and Motor Skills*, August, *31*(1), 319–322.

Vacc, N., & Vacc, N. (1973). An adaptation of the Modified Role Repertory Test—A measure of cognitive complexity. *Psychological Reports, 33,* 771–776.

■ ■ ■

2204

Test Name: ARITHMETIC REASONING TEST

Purpose: To assess general reasoning.

Number of Items: 17

Time Required: 9 minutes.

Format: An arithmetic reasoning test in which the computations are "absurdly" simple.

Reliability: .86 (Kuder-Richardson coefficient).

Author: Undheim, J.

Article: Broad Ability factors in 12 to 13 year old children, the theory of fluid and crystallized intelligence, and the differentiation hypothesis.

Journal: *Journal of Educational Psychology,* June 1978, *70*(3), 433–443.

Related Research: Guilford, J., & Hoepfner, R. (1971). *The analysis of intelligence.* New York: McGraw-Hill.

■ ■ ■

2205

Test Name: ASSESSMENT OF CAREER DECISION MAKING

Purpose: To measure decision making styles, including rational, intuitive, and dependent.

Number of Items: 21

Format: Three 7-item scales.

Reliability: Test–retest reliabilities of 26 undergraduates over a

2-week interval: rational, .85; intuitive, .76; and dependent, .85.

Validity: Intercorrelations: rational with intuitive, $r = -.06$; rational with dependent, $r = -.03$; and intuitive with dependent, $r = .17$.

Author: Harren, V. A., and Biscardi, D. L.

Article: Sex roles and cognitive styles as predictors of Holland typologies.

Journal: *Journal of Vocational Behavior,* October 1980, *17*(2), 231–241.

Related Research: Harren, V. A. (1979). A model of career decision making for college students. *Journal of Vocational Behavior, 14,* 119–133.

■ ■ ■

2206

Test Name: ASSESSMENT OF CAREER DECISION MAKING

Purpose: To determine which of three decision-making styles (rational, intuitive, dependent) one primarily relies on in making important life decisions.

Number of Items: 140

Format: *Agree–disagree* response format.

Reliability: Internal consistency estimates of reliability are .72 (rational), .60 (intuitive), and .69 (dependent). Harren et al. (1978) reported the test–retest reliabilities to be .85 (rational), .76 (intuitive), and .85 (dependent).

Author: Rubinton, N.

Article: Instruction in career decision making and decision-making styles.

Journal: *Journal of Counseling Psychology,* November 1980, *27*(6), 581–588.

Related Research: Harren, V. A., et al. (1978). Influence of sex role

attitudes and cognitive styles on career decision-making. *Journal of Counseling Psychology, 25,* 390–398.

■ ■ ■

2207

Test Name: CAREER DECISION SCALE

Purpose: To measure career indecision in graduate students.

Number of Items: 19

Format: Items are given.

Reliability: Internal consistency coefficient (Cronbach's alpha) of $r = .92$. Test–retest reliability (Pearson correlation coefficient) was $r = .61$.

Validity: Pearson correlations between two raters and test scores (concurrent validity) were $r = .43$ ($p < .01$) and $r = .44$ ($p < .01$).

Author: Hartman, B. W., et al.

Article: Examining the reliability and validity of an adapted scale of educational-vocational undecidedness in a sample of graduate students.

Journal: *Journal of Vocational Behavior,* October 1979, *15*(2), 224–230.

Related Research: Osipow, S. H., et al. (1976). A scale of educational–vocational undecidedness: A typological approach. *Journal of Vocational Behavior, 9,* 223–243.

■ ■ ■

2208

Test Name: CAREER INDECISION SCALE

Purpose: To measure one's career decisiveness in terms of need for structure, perceived external barriers, positive choice conflict, and personal conflict.

Number of Items: 18

Format: Values of 1, 2, 3, or 4 are assigned to each response.

Reliability: Test–retest correlations on overall scores were .902 and .819 for groups of college students.

Author: Neice, D. E., and Bradley, R. W.

Article: Relationship of age, sex and educational groups to career decisiveness.

Journal: *Journal of Vocational Behavior*, June 1979, *14*(3), 271–278.

Related Research: Osipow, S., et al. (1976). A scale of educational–vocational undecidedness: A typological approach. *Journal of Vocational Behavior, 9*, 233–243.

■ ■ ■

2209

Test Name: CIRCLE REASONING TEST

Purpose: To measure inductive reasoning ability.

Number of Items: 17

Time Required: 6 minutes.

Format: Subjects are asked to discover the principle by which one small circle is blackened on each of four views of circles and dashes, then apply the rule to the fifth row.

Reliability: .89 (Kuder-Richardson coefficient).

Author: Undheim, J.

Article: Broad ability factors in 12 to 13 year-old-children, the theory of fluid and crystallized intelligence, and the differentiation hypothesis.

Journal: *Journal of Educational Psychology*, June 1978, *70*(3), 433–443.

Related Research: Guilford, J., & Hoepfner, R. (1971). *The analysis of intelligence.* New York: McGraw-Hill.

2210

Test Name: DEFINING ISSUES TEST

Purpose: To measure one's level of moral judgment.

Number of Items: 72

Format: Six moral dilemmas with 12 questions for each. Subject chooses the four most important questions for each dilemma and ranks them in order of importance.

Reliability: Median estimated reliability over 15 splits of the test into thirds by combining partial P-scores from pairs of dilemmas was .70.

Validity: The direction of significant differences between age groups was consistent with stage theory ($p < .05$).

Author: Martin, R. M., et al.

Article: The reliability, validity and design of the Defining Issues Test.

Journal: *Developmental Psychology*, September 1977, *13*(5), 460–468.

Related Research: Rest, J. R. (1975). Longitudinal study of the Defining Issues Test of moral judgment: A strategy for analyzing developmental change. *Developmental Psychology, 11*, 738–748.

■ ■ ■

2211

Test Name: DESIGN RECALL TEST

Purpose: To measure conceptual tempo.

Number of Items: 10

Format: Each item involves a standard Gibson figure with a set of seven transformations of the figure. Scoring is in terms of total

number of errors and mean latency in seconds.

Validity: Correlation of errors score with corrected level of aspiration was .14 ($n = 33$ boys) and .35 ($n = 30$ girls). Correlation of latency score with corrected level of aspiration was –.12 ($n = 33$ boys) and .12 ($n = 30$ girls).

Author: Gilpin, A. R., and Boyden, J. G.

Article: Children's conceptual tempo and level of aspiration.

Journal: *Perceptual and Motor Skills*, April 1978, *46*(2), 587–593.

Related Research: Kagan, J., et al. (1964). Information processing in the child: Significance of analytic and reflective attitudes. *Psychological Monographs, 78*(1, Whole No. 578).

■ ■ ■

2212

Test Name: ETHICAL REASONING INVENTORY

Purpose: To assess moral reasoning.

Number of Items: 26

Format: Includes six stories, each one followed by questions and possible reasons for an answer to each question. Examples are provided.

Reliability: Test–retest reliability was .69 (10 days, 51 college students).

Validity: Correlation with Moral Judgment Interview was .54; Defining Issues Test was .57; Moral Judgment Scale was .43.

Author: Page, R., and Bode, J.

Article: Comparison of measures of moral reasoning and development of a new objective measure.

Journal: *Educational and Psychological Measurement,* Summer 1980, *40*(2), 317–329.

2213

Test Name: GERIATRIC INTERPERSONAL EVALUATION SCALE

Purpose: To assess the cognitive functioning of psychogeriatric patients.

Number of Items: 16

Format: Includes measurement of such areas of functioning as orientation, immediate and remote memory, verbal and quantitative ability, concept formation, and perceptual motor ability.

Validity: Correlations with WAIS Verbal subtests ranged from .58 to .76; correlation with WAIS Verbal Total was .80.

Author: Smith, J. M., et al.

Article: Relationship between the Geriatric Interpersonal Evaluation Scale and the WAIS Verbal Scale.

Journal: *Perceptual and Motor Skills*, April 1977, *44*(2), 571–574.

Related Research: Plutchik, R., et al. (1971). Development of a scale (GIES) for assessment of cognitive and perceptual functioning in geriatric patients. *Journal of the American Geriatrics Society, 19*, 614–623.

■ ■ ■

2214

Test Name: INTEGRATIVE COMPLEXITY

Purpose: To measure the degree of integrative complexity.

Number of Items: 5

Format: Requires responses to incomplete sentence stems. Scores for the completions are added for all items with high scores indicating integrative complexity and low scores, integrative simplicity.

Reliability: Reliabilities ranged from .80 to .95 for two expert judges.

Validity: With Crockett's measure of cognitive differentiation, $r = .10$; with Bieri's role construct repertory test, $r = -.31$; with Harvey Conceptual Systems Test, $r = -.03$.

Author: Epting, F., and Wilkins, G.

Article: Comparison of cognitive structural measures for predicting person perception.

Journal: *Perceptual and Motor Skills*, June 1974, *38*(3, Part 1), 727–730.

Related Research: Schroder, H. M., et al. (1967). *Human information processing.* New York: Holt, Rinehart & Winston.

■ ■ ■

2215

Test Name: IT'S FUN TO THINK

Purpose: To test thinking skills.

Number of Items: 66

Format: Includes 11 subtests: memorizing, observing and inferring, collecting data, comparing, classifying, hypothesizing, coding, summarizing, looking for assumptions, evaluating, and problem solving. Includes two forms.

Reliability: Split-half reliabilities were .894 (Form A) and .946 (Form B) with $N = 21$.

Validity: Correlated with measures of Information hunt (.73), Interpreting data (.72), Fluency (.18), Flexibility (.23), Originality (.21), and Elaboration (.34).

Author: Jensen, L. R.

Article: Diagnosis and evaluation of creativity, research and thinking skills of academically talented elementary students.

Journal: *The Gifted Child Quarterly*, Spring 1978, *22*(1), 98–110.

2216

Test Name: LEARNING STYLE INVENTORY

Purpose: To measure an individual's emphasis on each of four learning modes: Concrete Experience (CE), Reflective Observation (RO), Abstract Conceptualization (AC), and Active Experimentation (AE).

Number of Items: Nine rows of four words.

Format: Individual assigns a 4 to the word that best describes her or his learning style, a 3 to the word that next best describes it, and so on down to a 1 for a word that is least characteristic of it.

Reliability: Test–retest reliabilities (31–day interval) were: Concrete Experience, .56; Reflective Observation, .52; Abstract Conceptualization, .59; Active Experimentation, .61; Abstract Conceptualization-Concrete Experience, .70; and Active Experimentation-Reflective Observation, .55.

Author: Geiler, L. M.

Article: Reliability of the Learning Style Inventory.

Journal: *Psychological Reports*, April 1979, *44*(2), 555–561.

Related Research: Kolb, D. A. (1976). *Learning Style Inventory technical manual.* Boston: McBer.

■ ■ ■

2217

Test Name: LISTENING TEST

Purpose: To measure immediate recall and ability to draw conclusions.

Time Required: 75 minutes.

Format: Includes two parts: The first part measures immediate recall of facts and the second part measures the ability to draw conclusions, make inferences, and identify speaker attitudes. The subject responds to multiple-choice questions following each part.

Reliability: Reliability coefficients were .76 for Part 1, .75 for Part 2, and .81 for the total.

Author: Devine, T. G.

Article: Listening: What do we know after fifty years of research and theorizing?

Journal: *Journal of Reading,* January 1978, *21*(4), 296–304.

Related Research: Blewett, T. (1951). An experiment in the measurement of listening at the college level. *Journal of Educational Research, 44,* 575–585.

■ ■ ■

2218

Test Name: MATURITY OF MORAL JUDGMENT SCALE

Purpose: To measure moral reasoning.

Number of Items: 15

Format: Includes conversational statements that require a projective, conversational response. Two points are assigned to any response that is clearly one of four pre-defined moral concerns and one point for each response that implies one of the four pre-defined moral concerns.

Reliability: Hoyt computation of test reliability is .82. Alpha reliabilities ranged from .68 to .72.

Validity: Correlation with the Objective Moral Judgment Scale was .17.

Author: Wilmoth, G. H., and McFarland, S. G.

Article: A comparison of four measures of moral reasoning.

Journal: *Journal of Personality*

Assessment, August 1977, *41*(4), 396–401.

Related Research: Hogan, R., & Dickstein, E. (1972). A measure of moral values. *Journal of Consulting and Clinical Psychology, 39,* 210–214.

■ ■ ■

2219

Test Name: MORAL JUDGMENT SCALE

Purpose: To assess the development of moral reasoning in Kohlberg's (1958) proposed invariant sequence of six stages.

Number of Items: 15 dilemmas.

Format: Objectively scored.

Reliability: Alpha coefficient was .49. Item-total correlations ranged from .06 to .32 with a median of .19.

Author: Bode, J., and Page, R.

Article: Comparison of measures of moral judgment.

Journal: *Psychological Reports,* August 1978, *43*(1), 307–312.

Related Research: Kohlberg, L. (1958). *The development of modes of moral thinking and choice in years ten to sixteen.* Unpublished doctoral dissertation, University of Chicago.

Maitland, K., & Goldman, J. R. (1974). Moral judgment as a function of peer group interaction. *Journal of Personality and Social Psychology, 30,* 699–704.

■ ■ ■

2220

Test Name: NECESSARY FACTS TEST

Purpose: To measure general reasoning ability.

Number of Items: 16

Time Required: 9 minutes.

Format: Subjects are asked to supply the needed fact that is missing in a statement of an arithmetic problem.

Reliability: .79 (Kuder-Richardson coefficient).

Author: Undheim, J.

Article: Broad ability factors in 12 to 13 year-old children, the theory of fluid and crystallized intelligence, and the differentiation hypothesis.

Journal: *Journal of Educational Psychology,* June 1978, *70*(3), 433–443.

Related Research: Guilford, J., & Hoepfner, R. (1971). *The analysis of intelligence.* New York: McGraw-Hill.

■ ■ ■

2221

Test Name: NUMBER SERIES

Purpose: To measure inductive reasoning ability.

Number of Items: 21

Time Required: 6 minutes.

Format: Subjects are asked to discover the rule for a series of numbers and indicate the next number in the series.

Reliability: .88 (Kuder-Richardson coefficient).

Author: Undheim, J.

Article: Broad ability factors in 12 to 13 year old children, the theory of fluid and crystallized intelligence, and the differentiation hypothesis.

Journal: *Journal of Educational Psychology,* June 1978, *70*(3), 433–443.

Related Research: Guilford, J., & Hoepfner, R. (1971). *The analysis of intelligence.* New York: McGraw-Hill.

2222

Test Name: OBJECTIVE MORAL JUDGMENT SCALE

Purpose: To measure moral reasoning.

Number of Items: 15

Format: Each item consists of a moral dilemma followed by a question answered by choosing one of six responses.

Reliability: Test–retest reliability was .83 (12–19 year olds), or .60 (11th and 12th graders). Split-half reliability coefficient was .71. Kuder-Richardson formula 20 yielded .67.

Author: Wilmoth, G. H., and McFarland, S. G.

Article: A comparison of four measures of moral reasoning.

Journal: *Journal of Personality Assessment,* August 1977, *41*(4), 396–401.

Related Research: Maitland, K., & Goldman, J. (1974). Moral judgment as a function of peer group interaction. *Journal of Personality and Social Psychology, 30,* 699–704.

■ ■ ■

2223

Test Name: PERSONNEL DECISION SIMULATION

Purpose: To measure information-seeking and decision-making strategies.

Number of Items: 2 decision problems.

Format: Includes the following decision processes: Information amount, decision time, processing role, decision accuracy, decision confidence, and decision flexibility.

Reliability: Reliabilities corrected by Spearman-Brown formula ranged from .68 to .98 ($N = 79$).

Validity: Correlations with Dogmatism ranged from –.34 to .23; Risk-taking propensity ranged from –.37 to .11; Intelligence ranged from –.45 to .39.

Author: Taylor, R. N., and Dunnette, M. D.

Article: Influence of dogmatism, risk-taking propensity, and intelligence on decision-making strategies for a sample of industrial managers.

Journal: *Journal of Applied Psychology,* August 1974, *59*(4), 420–423.

■ ■ ■

2224

Test Name: PICTORIAL PIAGETIAN TASKS

Purpose: To assess the cognitive level of children.

Number of Items: 40

Format: Includes the following concepts: number, substance, length, distance, perspective, horizontality, volume, and probability. An example is given.

Reliability: Cronbach's alpha ranged from .62 to .88 (ages 6 to 11).

Validity: Correlations with individually administered Piagetian tasks ranged from .42 to .99 (n ranged from 30 to 90).

Author: DeAvila, E., and Pulos, S.

Article: Group assessment of cognitive level by pictorial Piagetian tasks.

Journal: *Journal of Educational Measurement,* Fall 1979, *16*(3), 167–175.

Related Research: DeAvila, E. A., & Harassy, B. E. (1975). Piagetian alternative to I.Q.: Mexican-American Study. In N. Hobbs (Ed.), *Issues in the classification of exceptional children.* San Francisco: Jossey-Bass.

■ ■ ■

2225

Test Name: PROBLEM-SOLVING SKILLS INVENTORY

Purpose: To assess one's knowledge of problem-solving skills.

Number of Items: 25

Format: Likert items.

Reliability: A Cronbach alpha of .88 for the total inventory.

Validity: A significant multivariate F ratio ($p < .013$) was reported between subjects who participated in a problem-solving workshop and subjects without such experience.

Author: Heppner, P. P., and Dixon, D. N.

Article: Effects of client perceived need and counselor role on clients' behavior.

Journal: *Journal of Counseling Psychology,* November 1978, *25*(6), 514–519.

Related Research: Heppner, P. P., & Petersen, C. H. (1978, March). *Development, factor analysis, and initial validation of a problem-solving instrument.* Paper presented at the Meeting of the American Educational Research Association, Toronto, Ontario, Canada.

■ ■ ■

2226

Test Name: PURDUE ELEMENTARY PROBLEM SOLVING INVENTORY

Purpose: To measure problem solving ability.

Number of Items: 50

Format: Includes slides projected on a 3 x 5 foot screen portraying children in cartoon form in real life situations, tape recorded directions, and test booklet for recording responses. Measures sensing that a problem exists, defining the problem, asking questions, guessing causes, clarifying the goal of the problem situation, judging if more information is needed, analyzing details, redefining familiar objects for unusual uses, seeing implications, solving single- and multiple-solution problems, and verifying solutions.

Reliability: Kuder-Richardson formula 20 reliability is .79.

Author: Feldhusen, J., and Houtz, J.

Article: Problem solving and the concrete abstract dimension.

Journal: *The Gifted Child Quarterly*, Summer 1975, *19*(2), 122–129.

Related Research: Feldhusen, J. F., et al. (1972). The Purdue Elementary Problem Solving Inventory. *Psychological Reports, 31*, 891–901.

See *DUEMM, 2,* 1978, 894.

■ ■ ■

2227

Test Name: REASONING TEST

Purpose: To assess concrete and formal reasoning capabilities.

Number of Items: 19

Time Required: 45 minutes.

Reliability: Kuder-Richardson formula 20 estimated reliability was .85.

Validity: Correlation with Otis IQ was .50; concrete chemistry achievement was .39; formal chemistry achievement was .43.

Author: Carlson, J. S., et al.

Article: A comparison of the predictive validity of a measure of general intelligence and a Piaget-derived test relative to an

achievement examination in high school chemistry.

Journal: *Educational and Psychological Measurement,* Winter 1977, *37*(4), 999–1003.

Related Research: Lawson, A., & Blake, A. (1976). Concrete and formal thinking abilities in high school biology students as measured by three separate instruments. *Journal of Research in Science Teaching, 13*, 227–235.

■ ■ ■

2228

Test Name: RELATIONSHIPS INFLUENCING CAREER PLANNING SCALE

Purpose: To measure success avoidance, home–career conflict, and the importance of attitudes of significant members of the opposite sex as influences on college students' career planning.

Number of Items: 68

Format: 5-point Likert format ranging from *strongly agree* to *strongly disagree.*

Reliability: Reliability coefficients for all three subscales ranged from .84 to .91.

Author: Karpicke, S.

Article: Perceived and real sex differences in college students' career planning.

Journal: *Journal of Counseling Psychology,* May 1980, *27*(3), 240–245.

■ ■ ■

2229

Test Name: ROLE CONSTRUCT REPERTORY TEST-GRID FORM

Purpose: To measure cognitive complexity.

Format: Includes a 10 x 10 grid with 10 roles along one axis and 10 bipolar adjectives along another

with a 6-point semantic differential scale.

Reliability: Test–retest reliability ranged from .54 to .86.

Validity: Convergent validity was –.19.

Author: Schneier, C. E.

Article: Measuring cognitive complexity: Developing reliability, validity, and norm tables for a personality instrument.

Journal: *Educational and Psychological Measurement,* Autumn 1979, *39*(3), 599–612.

Related Research: Bieri, J., et al. (1966). *Clinical and social judgment.* New York: Wiley.

Wright, R. J., & Richardson, L. (1977). The effect of response style on cognitive complexity and course evaluation. *Educational and Psychological Measurement, 37*(1), 177–183.

■ ■ ■

2230

Test Name: ROLE CONSTRUCT REPERTORY TEST-MODIFIED

Purpose: To measure cognitive differentiation.

Number of Items: 64

Format: Subject nominates eight different role figures such as self, person you dislike, and so forth, and then rates these figures along eight provided construct dimensions from +3 to –3.

Validity: With Crockett's measure of cognitive differentiation, $r = -.06$; with Harvey conceptual systems test, $r = .31$; with Schroder's measure of integrative complexity, $r = -.31$.

Author: Epting, F., and Wilkins, G.

Article: Comparison of cognitive structural measures for predicting person perception.

Journal: *Perceptual and Motor Skills*, June 1974, *38*(3 Part 1), 727–730.

Related Research: Kelly, G. A. (1955). The psychology of personal constructs. New York: Norton.

■ ■ ■

2231

Test Name: SENTENCE SELECTION TEST

Purpose: To assess formal reasoning ability.

Number of Items: 14

Time Required: 6 minutes.

Format: Subjects select a sentence that is most probably true, using the information in a given statement.

Reliability: .77 (Kuder-Richardson coefficient).

Author: Undheim, J.

Article: Broad ability factors in 12 to 13 year old children, the theory of fluid and crystallized intelligence, and the differentiation hypothesis.

Journal: *Journal of Educational Psychology*, June 1978, *70*(3), 433–443.

Related Research: Guilford, J., & Hoepfner, R. (1971). *The analysis of intelligence.* New York: McGraw-Hill.

■ ■ ■

2232

Test Name: SPRINGS TASK

Purpose: To measure the ability to criticize and control experiments.

Format: Includes eight different springs suspended from hooks on a wooden frame and six flat fishing weights two, four, and eight

ounces. Two types of questions are asked.

Reliability: Split-half corrected reliabilities were .83 and .85 (13–year-olds, $n = 65$); .84 and .86 (12–year-olds, $n = 100$); .82 (high school seniors, $n = 60$).

Validity: Correlation with Bending Rods was .57; Spinning Wheels was .59; Ramp was .40; Pendulum was .68.

Author: Linn, M. C., and Rice, M.

Article: A measure of scientific reasoning: The Springs Task.

Journal: *Journal of Educational Measurement*, Spring 1979, *16*(1), 55–58.

Related Research: Levine, D., & Linn, M. C. (1977). Scientific reasoning ability in adolescence: Theoretical viewpoints and educational implications. *Journal of Research in Science Teaching, 14,* 371–384.

■ ■ ■

2233

Test Name: VOCATIONAL DECISION MAKING DIFFICULTY SCALE

Purpose: To assess the number of reasons given by subjects for vocational indecision.

Number of Items: 13

Format: True or false. Total score is the sum of true responses and higher scores indicate greater difficulty in vocational decision making.

Reliability: Kuder-Richardson formula 20 values for this scale for four samples of high school and college males and females was .86, .78, and .63.

Author: Slaney, R. B.

Article: Expressed vocational

choice and vocational indecision.

Journal: *Journal of Counseling Psychology*, March 1980, *27*(2), 122–129.

Related Research: Holland, J. L., & Holland, J. E. (1977). Vocational indecision: More evidence and speculation. *Journal of Counseling Psychology, 24,* 404–414.

■ ■ ■

2234

Test Name: VOCATIONAL DECISION SCALE

Purpose: To assess vocational decidedness; comfort with level of decidedness and reasons for being undecided.

Number of Items: 38

Format: Items are rated on a 6-point Likert scale in terms of the extent to which the respondent agreed that the reasons were true of him or her, 1 (*completely disagree*) to 6 (*completely agree*).

Reliability: Test–retest Pearson product–moment correlations for each item ranged between .36 and .64, with 74% having correlations of .50 or better.

Validity: Correlations of the scale with the *Assessment of Career Decision Making* scale, the *State-Trait Anxiety Inventory,* the *Identity Scale,* the *Career Salience Questionnaire,* and the *Anomy Scale* are given.

Author: Jones, L. K., and Chenery, M. F.

Article: Multiple subtypes among vocationally undecided college students; a model and assessment instrument.

Journal: *Journal of Counseling Psychology*, September 1980, *27*(5), 469–477.

CHAPTER 19
Status

2235

Test Name: CAREER SALIENCE QUESTIONNAIRE

Purpose: To measure work-role salience.

Number of Items: 28

Format: Twenty-seven of the items are rated on a 5-point Likert scale; 17 are positively worded and 10 negatively worded. The final item contains six areas of life that the individual ranks in terms of their importance.

Reliability: Coefficient alpha has been reported as .81 for both men and women by Greenhaus (1971) and as .85 for this population.

Author: Fannin, P. M.

Article: The relation between ego–identity status and sex-role attitude, work-role salience, a typicality of major and self-esteem in college women.

Journal: *Journal of Vocational Behavior,* February 1979, *14*(1), 12–22.

Related Research: Greenhaus, J. H. (1971). Self-esteem as an influence on occupational choice and occupational satisfaction. *Journal of Vocational Behavior, 1,* 75–83.

Illfelder, J. K. (1980). Fear of success, sex role attitudes and career salience and anxiety levels of college women. *Journal of Vocational Behavior, 16*(1), 7–17.

...

2236

Test Name: HIERARCHICAL INFLUENCE INDEX

Article: To measure hierarchical influence.

Number of Items: 15

Format: Likert items. Examples are presented.

Reliability: With teacher loyalty, r = .74.

Validity: Average correlation between item scores and total index score was .67; coefficient alpha was .83.

Author: Hoy, W. K., and Rees, R.

Article: Subordinate loyalty to immediate superior: A neglected concept in the study of educational administration.

Journal: *Sociology of Education,* Spring 1974, *47*(2), 268–286.

Related Research: Hills, R. J. (1963). The representative function: A neglected dimension of leadership behavior. *Administrative Science Quarterly, 8,* 83–101.

...

2237

Test Name: IDENTITY STATUS INCOMPLETE SENTENCES BLANK FOR WOMEN

Purpose: To classify one's identity status through the domains of occupation, religion, politics and attitudes toward premarital intercourse.

Number of Items: 40 stems

Format: Statements are scored on a scale ranging from –2 (*strong evidence of absence of the criterion*) to 0 (*no evidence of presence or absence of the criterion*) to +2 (*strong evidence of the presence of the criterion*).

Reliability: Interjudge reliability for status assignment ranged from .82 to .96; item-scale reliabilities ranged from .61 to .89.

Validity: Concurrent validity coefficients with the Marcia and Friedman (1970) identity status interview in the domain of attitudes toward premarital intercourse ranged from .40 to .86.

Author: Fannin, P. M.

Article: The relation between ego–identity status and sex-role attitude, work-role salience, atypicality of major, and self-esteem in college women.

Journal: *Journal of Vocational Behavior,* February 1979, *14*(1), 12–22.

Related Research: Marcia, J. E., & Friedman, M. L. (1970). Ego identity status in college women. *Journal of Personality, 38,* 249–263.

...

2238

Test Name: IDENTITY STATUS QUESTIONNAIRE

Purpose: To assess identity status.

Time Required: 10 minutes.

Format: Includes six subscales. Sample items are presented.

Reliability: Six test–retest correlations ranged from .45 to .81.

Author: Fry, P. S.

Article: Developmental changes in

identity status of university students from rural and urban backgrounds.

Journal: *Journal of College Student Personnel*, May 1974, *15*(3), 183–190.

Related Research: Constantinople, A. (1969). An Eriksonian measure of personality development in college students. *Developmental Psychology, 1*, 357–372.

■ ■ ■

2239

Test Name: SELF AND PRESTIGE SCALE

Purpose: To measure self-concept and one's sense of occupational prestige.

Number of Items: 38

Format: Four self-concept items in a Guttman scale format and 34 occupations rated by their "general standing or prestige." The rating categories are *excellent, good, average, below average* and *poor.*

Reliability: Self-concept statements have a coefficient of reproducibility of .96 and a coefficient of scalability of .73.

Author: Faulkner, G. L., et al.

Article: Self-concepts and occupational prestige among vocational-technical students.

Journal: *Journal of Vocational Behavior,* August 1977, *11*(1), 75–82.

Related Research: Rosenberg, M. (1965). *Society and the adolescent self-image.* Princeton, NJ: Princeton University Press.

CHAPTER 20
Trait Measurement

2240

Test Name: ACHIEVEMENT ANXIETY TEST

Purpose: To measure both facilitating anxiety and debilitating anxiety.

Number of Items: 26

Format: Subject responds to each item on a 5-point scale indicating degree of agreement with the statement.

Validity: Correlations with Opinion Leadership in fashion were −.37 (facilitating anxiety) and .28 (debilitating anxiety). Correlations with Field Dependence were .04 (facilitating anxiety) and .14 (debilitating anxiety). Correlations with external control were −.17 (facilitating anxiety) and .38 (debilitating anxiety).

Author: Brett, J. E., and Kernaleguen, A.

Article: Perceptual and personality variables related to opinion leadership in fashion.

Journal: *Perceptual and Motor Skills*, June 1975, *40*(3), 775–779.

Related Research: Alpert, R., & Haber, R. H. (1960). Anxiety in academic achievement situations. *Journal of Abnormal and Social Psychology, 61*, 207–215.

Towle, N. J., & Merrill, P. F. (1975). Effects of anxiety type and item-difficulty sequencing on mathematics test performance. *Journal of Educational Measurement, 12*, 241–249.

See *DUEMM, 2*, 1978, 908.

2241

Test Name: ADOLESCENT EGO IDENTITY SCALE

Purpose: To measure one's ego identity during Erickson's fifth developmental stage.

Number of Items: 24

Format: Responses are on a 5-point scale; one-half of the items are positive, the other half are negative.

Reliability: Cronbach's alpha coefficient of reliability for the total scale is .77.

Validity: Ego identity scores in the high grades were significantly higher ($p < .001$) than identity scores in the low grades.

Author: Tzuriel, D., and Klein, M. M.

Article: Ego identity: Effects of ethnocentrism, ethnic identification, and cognitive complexity in Israeli, Oriental, and Western ethnic groups.

Journal: *Psychological Reports*, June 1977, *40*(3), 1099–1110.

Related Research: Rasmussen, J. E. (1964). The relationship of ego identity to psycho-social effectiveness. *Psychological Reports, 15*, 815–825.

Wessman, A. E., & Ricks, D. F. (1966). *Mood and personality.* New York: Holt, Rinehart & Winston.

2242

Test Name: ADULT SELF-EXPRESSION SCALE

Purpose: Measure of assertiveness.

Number of Items: 48

Format: Self-report.

Reliability: .88 for 2-week and .91 for 5-week test–retest data.

Validity: Concurrent validity was reported, *t* test comparing subjects seeking personal-adjustment counseling with those not doing so was significant at the .01 level.

Author: Gay, M. L., et al.

Article: An assertiveness inventory for adults.

Journal: *Journal of Counseling Psychology*, July 1975, *22*, 340–344.

Related Research: Tanck, R. H., & Robbins, P. R. (1979). Assertiveness, locus of control and coping behaviors used to diminish tension. *Journal of Personality Assessment, 43*, 396–400.

2243

Test Name: AFFECTIVE SENSITIVITY SCALE

Purpose: To measure levels of empathy.

Format: Multiple-choice. After a videotaped sequence the subject is instructed to choose the statement that most nearly defines what the client in the videotape has been experiencing.

Reliability: Internal consistency coefficient ranged between .70 and .80, and a test–retest coefficient of correlation was .75 over a 6-month period.

Validity: Correlations between the Scale and ratings of counselors by peers, staff, and clients have ranged between .40 and .70.

Author: Breisinger, G. D.

Article: Sex and empathy, reexamined.

Journal: *Journal of Counseling Psychology*, May 1976, *23*(3), 289–290.

Related Research: Campbell, R., et al. (1971). The development and validation of a scale to measure effective sensitivity (empathy). *Journal of Counseling Psychology, 18*, 407–412.

■ ■ ■

2244

Test Name: AGREEMENT RESPONSE SCALE

Purpose: To measure acquiescence.

Number of Items: 15

Format: True–false version.

Reliability: Split-half reliability was .86.

Author: Millimet, C. R., and Votta, R. P.

Article: Acquiescence and the Bem Sex-Role Inventory.

Journal: *Journal of Personality Assessment*, April 1979, *43*(2), 164–165.

Related Research: Couch, A., & Keniston, K. (1960). Yeasayers and naysayers: Agreeing response set as a personality variable. *Journal of Abnormal and Social Psychology, 60*, 151–174.

■ ■ ■

2245

Test Name: AMBIGUITY TOLERANCE SCALE

Purpose: To measure one's tolerance for ambiguous situations.

Number of Items: 20

Format: Consists of the 16-item Rydell-Rosen test (1966) plus two items selected from the California Personality Inventory (1957) and two from Barron's (1953) conformity scale.

Reliability: Retest reliability was .63 ($p < .01$) over 6 months.

Author: Chabassol, D. J., and Thomas, D.

Article: Needs for structure, tolerance of ambiguity, and dogmatism in adolescents.

Journal: *Psychological Reports,* October 1975, *37*(2), 507–510.

Related Research: MacDonald, A. P., Jr. (1970). Revised scale for ambiguity tolerance: Reliability and validity. *Psychological Reports, 26*, 791–798.

■ ■ ■

2246

Test Name: ANGER INVENTORY

Purpose: To provide an index of anger reactions to a wide range of provocations.

Number of Items: 80

Format: Employs a 5-point Likert scale ranging from *not at all* to *very much.*

Reliability: Cronbach's alpha was .96.

Validity: Correlations with measures of anger and social desirability ranged from –.26 to .82.

Author: Biaggio, M. K.

Article: Assessment of anger arousal.

Journal: *Journal of Personality Assessment,* June 1980, *44*(3), 289–298.

Related Research: Novaco, R. W. (1977). Stress inoculation: A cognitive therapy for anger and its application to case of depression.

Journal of Consulting and Clinical Psychology, 45, 600–608.

■ ■ ■

2247

Test Name: ANGER SELF-REPORT

Purpose: To differentiate between the awareness and expression of aggression.

Number of Items: 64

Format: Provides separate scores for awareness of anger, expression of anger, guilt, condemnation of anger, and mistrust.

Validity: Correlations with measures of anger and social desirability ranged from –.49 to .78.

Author: Biaggio, M. K.

Article: Assessment of anger arousal.

Journal: *Journal of Personality Assessment,* June 1980, *44*(3), 289–298.

Related Research: Zelin, M. L., et al. (1972). Anger self-report: An objective questionnaire for the measurement of aggression. *Journal of Consulting and Clinical Psychology, 39*, 340.

■ ■ ■

2248

Test Name: ANXIETY SCALE

Purpose: To use verbal behavior to measure anxiety.

Time Required: 5 minutes.

Format: Uses Gottschalk and Gleser (1969) procedures.

Reliability: Interjudge reliability ranged from .51 to .92 with mean of –.73.

Validity: A curvilinear relationship with verbal communication level in psychotherapy patients was reported.

Author: Moxnes, P.

Article: Verbal communication level and anxiety in psychotherapeutic groups.

Journal: *Journal of Counseling Psychology*, September 1974, *21*(5), 399–403.

Related Research: Gottschalk, L., & Gleser, G. (1969). *The measurement of psychological states through the content analysis of verbal behavior.* Berkeley: University of California Press.

• • •

2249

Test Name: ASSERTIVENESS RATING INSTRUMENT

Purpose: To assess willingness of subjects to assert selves.

Number of Items: 8

Format: Anger producing situations presented to subjects who were asked to indicate how they would respond: responses were rated on a 7-point scale; examples of items are given.

Reliability: Interrater reliability was .947.

Validity: Significant differences between a treatment (assertive training) group and control were reported ($p < .05$); 23% of variance was accounted for.

Author: Rimm, D., et al.

Article: Group assertive training in treatment of expression of inappropriate anger.

Journal: *Psychological Reports,* June 1974, *34*(3), 791–798.

• • •

2250

Test Name: AUTHORITARIANISM SCALE

Purpose: To measure authoritarianism.

Number of Items: 4

Format: A Guttman scale.

Reliability: Coefficient of reproducibility was .90.

Validity: Correlations with the Rational Behavior Inventory ranged from .05 to –.34.

Author: Whiteman, V. L., and Shorkey, C. T.

Article: Validation testing of the Rational Behavior Inventory.

Journal: *Educational and Psychological Measurement,* Winter 1978, *38*(4), 1143–1149.

Related Research: Robinson, J. P., & Shaver, P. R. (1969). *Measures of social psychological attitudes.* Ann Arbor: University of Michigan, Institute for Social Research.

• • •

2251

Test Name: BECKER SEMANTIC DIFFERENTIAL

Purpose: To provide teachers a trait rating form with which to rate five child-behavior problem factors.

Number of Items: 47

Format: Consists of bipolar items including the following problem factors: relaxed disposition, withdrawn-hostile, lack of aggression, intellectual efficiency, and conduct problems.

Reliability: Test–retest reliability (4 weeks) ranged from .63 to .84.

Author: Bolstad, O. D., and Johnson, S. M.

Article: The relationship between teachers' assessment of students and the students' actual behavior in the classroom.

Journal: *Child Development,* June 1977, *48*(2), 570–578.

Related Research: Becker, W. C. (1960). The relationship of factors in parental ratings of self and each other to the behavior of kindergarten children as rated by

mothers, fathers, and teachers. *Journal of Consulting Psychology, 24,* 507–527.

• • •

2252

Test Name: BUSS DURKEE HOSTILITY INVENTORY

Purpose: To measure anger arousal.

Number of Items: 75

Format: True–false items including 8 types of hostility: assault, indirect hostility, irritability, negativism, resentment, suspicion, verbal hostility, and guilt.

Validity: Correlations with the Marlowe-Crowne Social Desirability Scale ranged from –.44 to –.68; authoritarianism was .25; role playing aggression was .36.

Author: Biaggio, M. K.

Article: Assessment of anger arousal.

Journal: *Journal of Personality Assessment,* June 1980, *44*(3), 289–298.

Related Research: Buss, A. H., & Durkee, A. (1957). An inventory for assessing different kinds of hostility. *Journal of Consulting Psychology, 21,* 343–349.

Holland, R. T., & Levi, M. (1980). Canonical versus factor analytic perspectives on the structure of associations between the MMPI and the Buss-Durkee Hostility Inventory. *Journal of Personality Assessment, 44,* 479–483.

• • •

2253

Test Name: CALIFORNIA F-SCALE

Purpose: To measure antidemocratic tendencies at a deep personality level without appearing to have that aim.

Number of Items: 37

Format: Includes nine subscales: conventionalism, authoritarian submission, authoritarian aggression, anti-intraception, superstition and stereotyping, power and toughness, destructiveness and cynicism, projectivity, sex-exaggerated concern with sexual goings-on. Each statement reflects an authoritarian point of view and is scored on the basis of a 5-point discrete scale ranging from 5 (*completely agree*) to 1 (*agree not at all*).

Reliability: Estimates by the Hoyt procedure for each subscale ranged from .21 to .68 with .78 for the total scale.

Author: Badgett, J. L., et al.

Article: The authoritarianism exhibited by intelligent men and women.

Journal: *Journal of College Student Personnel*, November 1974, *15*(6), 509–512.

Related Research: Adorno, T. W., et al. (1950). *The authoritarian personality*. New York: Harper.

■ ■ ■

2254

Test Name: CAREY SURVEY OF TEMPERAMENTAL CHARACTERISTICS

Purpose: To identify infant temperament characteristics.

Number of Items: 70

Format: Includes nine scales.

Validity: Correlations with the Infant Characteristics Questionnaire ranged from −.25 to .39.

Author: Bates, J. E., et al.

Article: Measurement of infant difficultness.

Journal: *Child Development*, September 1979, *50*(3), 794–803.

Related Research: Carey, W. B. (1973). Measurement of infant temperament in pediatric practice. In J. C. Westman (Ed.), *Individual differences in children*. New York: Wiley.

■ ■ ■

2255

Test Name: CHOICE DILEMMA QUESTIONNAIRE

Purpose: To categorize persons as high, moderate, or low risk takers.

Number of Items: 5

Time Required: 15 minutes.

Format: For each item the subject is faced with a choice between two alternative courses of action where one is more desirable and attractive than the other, but the probability of attaining or achieving it is less. The subject indicated the minimum odds of success he or she could demand before recommending that the more attractive and desirable alternative be chosen.

Author: Fischer, D. G., and Burdeny, T. C.

Article: Individual shifts and the group-shift phenomenon.

Journal: *Perceptual and Motor Skills*, October 1974, *39*(2), 939–954.

Related Research: Wallach, M. A., & Kogan, N. (1965). The roles of information, discussion and consensus in group risk taking. *Journal of Experimental Social Psychology, 1*, 1–19.

■ ■ ■

2256

Test Name: COLLEGE SELF-EXPRESSION SCALE

Purpose: To assess assertiveness.

Number of Items: 50

Format: Assesses expression of feelings related to family, strangers, business relations, authority figures, and same and opposite sex peers.

Reliability: Test–retest (2 weeks) reliability was .89, .90 (Galassi et al., 1974).

Validity: Correlation with ratings of assertiveness in college students by dorm counselors was .33 (*p* < .005). Significant differences were found between male college student legislators and three other groups (Math, Engineering, Dormitory Students).

Author: Galassi, J., and Galassi, M.

Article: Validity of a measure of assertiveness.

Journal: *Journal of Counseling Psychology*, May 1974, *21*(3), 248–250.

Related Research: Galassi, J., et al. (1974). The College Self Expression Scale: A measure of assertiveness. *Behavior Therapy, 5*, 165–171.

■ ■ ■

2257

Test Name: CONSERVATISM MEASURE

Purpose: To measure conservatism.

Number of Items: 10

Reliability: Coefficient alpha ranged from .67 to .81.

Validity: Correlation with dogmatism was .18 and with religiosity was .60.

Author: Rohrbaugh, J., et al.

Article: Measuring the relative importance of utilitarian and equalitarian values: A study of individual differences about fair distribution.

Journal: *Journal of Applied Psychology*, February, 1980, *65*(1), 34–49.

Related Research: Scott, W. A., & Rohrbaugh, J. (1975). Conceptions of harmful groups: Some correlates of group descriptions in three cultures. *Journal of Personality and Social Psychology, 31*, 992–1003.

• • •

2258

Test Name: DEGREE OF TOLERANCE SCALES

Purpose: To measure degree of tolerance.

Number of Items: 34

Format: Includes 4 scales: liberalism, conservatism, authoritarianism, and dogmatism.

Reliability: Test–retest reliability (1 week) was .96 (*N* = 100).

Validity: Correlation with level of education, Yule's *Q* = .16.

Author: Ogle, N. J., et al.

Article: Increased tolerance and reference group shifts: A test in the college environment.

Journal: *Educational Research Quarterly,* Fall 1978, *4*(3), 48–57.

• • •

2259

Test Name: DOGMATISM SCALE

Purpose: To measure inflexibility of beliefs in children.

Number of Items: 18

Format: True–not-true statements regarding beliefs about open-mindedness.

Reliability: .20

Author: Katz, P. A., et al.

Article: Perceptual concomitants of racial attitudes in urban grade-school children.

Journal: *Developmental Psychology,* March 1975, *11*(2), 135–144.

Related Research: Rokeach, M., et

al. (1960). Two kinds of prejudice or one? In M. Rokeach (Ed.), *The open and closed mind.* New York: Basic Books.

• • •

2260

Test Name: DOGMATISM SCALE

Purpose: To measure dogmatism.

Number of Items: 10

Reliability: Split-half reliability was .66.

Validity: Correlation with religiosity was .21 and with conservatism was .18.

Author: Rohrbaugh, J., et al.

Article: Measuring the relative importance of utilitarian and egalitarian values: A study of individual differences about fair distribution.

Journal: *Journal of Applied Psychology,* February 1980, *65*(1), 34–49.

Related Research: Troldahl, V., & Powell, F. A. (1965). A short form dogmatism scale for use in field studies. *Social Forces, 44,* 211–215.

• • •

2261

Test Name: DOGMATISM SCALE

Purpose: To measure dogmatism.

Number of Items: 10

Format: A Guttman scale.

Reliability: Coefficient of reproducibility was .83.

Validity: Correlations with the Rational Behavior Inventory ranged from .00 to –.36.

Author: Whiteman, V. L., and Shorkey, C. T.

Article: Validation testing of the Rational Behavior Inventory.

Journal: *Educational and*

Psychological Measurement, Winter 1978, *38*(4), 1143–1149.

Related Research: Robinson, J. P., & Shaver, P. R. (1969). *Measures of social psychological attitudes.* Ann Arbor: University of Michigan, Institute for Social Research.

• • •

2262

Test Name: EARLY CHILDHOOD MATCHING FAMILIAR FIGURES TEST

Purpose: To evaluate the child's ability to control impulsive responding when the task demands reflectivity.

Number of Items: 15

Format: The child is shown a picture that looks exactly like the object on another page. Half of the pictures are social in character (e.g., faces) and half involve geometric designs. One point is awarded for each correct matching. A high score indicates reflectivity.

Validity: Correlation with CATB Dog and Bone Test, .34; Color Recognition, .38; Weight Graduation, .19; WPPSI-Arithmetic, .45; WPPSI-Comprehension, .44; WPPSI-Sentences, .41; Wide Range Achievement, .32.

Author: Wexley, K., et al.

Article: An evaluation of Montessori and day care programs for disadvantaged children.

Journal: *Journal of Educational Research,* November 1974, *68*(3), 95–99.

Related Research: Banta, T. (1970). Tests for the evaluation of early childhood education: The Cincinnati Autonomy Test Battery. In J. Hellmuth (Ed.), *Cognitive studies* (pp. 424–490). New York: Brunner/Mazel.

2263

Test Name: F-SCALE

Purpose: To measure authoritarianism.

Number of Items: 28

Format: Subjects respond on a 5-point scale from *strongly agree* to *strongly disagree*.

Reliability: Corrected odd–even reliabilities of .82 for 110 students and .85 for 101 managers.

Validity: Correlations with the Miner Sentence Completion Scale ranged from .18 for 110 students and from –.20 to .17 for 101 managers. Correlations with the Ghiselli Self-Description Inventory ranged from –.35 to .21 for 110 students and from –.23 to .24 for 101 managers.

Author: Miner, J. B.

Article: Relationships among measures of managerial personality traits.

Journal: *Journal of Personality Assessment*, August 1976, *40*(4), 383–397.

Related Research: Adorno, T., et al. (1950). *The authoritarian personality*. New York: Harper.

■ ■ ■

2264

Test Name: F SCALE

Purpose: To measure authoritarianism.

Number of Items: 30

Format: Fifteen positive and 15 negative items.

Reliability: Reliabilities (Correlations between odd and even items, and test–retest) are in the .80s.

Author: Weller, L.

Article: Authoritarian personalities in the natural and social sciences.

Journal: *Journal of Vocational Behavior*, December 1979, *15*(3), 259–264.

Related Research: Lee, R., & Warr, P. (1969). The development and standardization of a balanced F scale. *Journal of General Psychology, 81*, 109–129.

■ ■ ■

2265

Test Name: GHISELLI SELF-DESCRIPTION INVENTORY

Purpose: To measure managerial traits.

Number of Items: 64

Format: Measures 13 traits: supervisory ability, need achievement, need self-actualization, self-assurance, decisiveness, need security, working class affinity, initiative, need financial reward, need power, maturity, masculinity–femininity, and intelligence.

Reliability: Corrected split-half reliabilities ranged from .06 to .50.

Validity: Correlations with the Miner Sentence Completion Scale ranged from –.19 to .31 for 110 students and from –.29 to .35 for 101 managers. Correlations with the F-Scale ranged from –.35 to .21 for 110 students and from –.23 to .24 for 101 managers.

Author: Miner, J. B.

Article: Relationships among measures of managerial personality traits.

Journal: *Journal of Personality Assessment*, August 1976, *40*(4), 383–397.

Related Research: Ghiselli, E. E. (1971). *Explorations in managerial talent*. Pacific Palisades, CA: Goodyear.

■ ■ ■

2266

Test Name: HAPTIC MATCHING TASK

Purpose: To measure reflection–impulsivity.

Number of Items: 8

Format: Consists of unfamiliar three-dimensional wooden forms. An example is presented.

Validity: Correlations with Matching Familiar Figures Test ranged from –.39 to .61.

Author: Kagan, J., et al.

Article: Infant antecedents of cognitive functioning: A longitudinal study.

Journal: *Child Development,* 1978, *49,* 1005–1023.

Related Research: Kagan, J., et al. (1964). Information processing in the child: Significance of analytic and reflective attitudes. *Psychological Monographs, 78*(Whole No. 578).

■ ■ ■

2267

Test Name: HELPING DISPOSITIONS SCALES

Purpose: To assess helping dispositions.

Number of Items: 55

Format: Includes 20 components scales and 14 composite indicators of predispositions to help. All items are presented.

Reliability: Median homogeneity ratio of the scales was .28 and their median estimated reliability was .84. Total score alpha was .94.

Validity: Correlation of the HDS total score with Harvey's need to help people was .70.

Author: Severy, L. J.

Article: Individual differences in helping dispositions.

Journal: *Journal of Personality Assessment*, June 1975, *39*(3), 382–392.

2268

Test Name: HOGAN EMPATHY SCALE

Purpose: To measure empathy.

Number of Items: 64

Format: Items were selected from the Minnesota Multiphasic Personality Inventory, California Psychological Inventory, and Institute of Personality Assessment and Research.

Reliability: .84.

Validity: Correlations ranged from .62 to .39.

Author: Gladding, S. T.

Article: Empathy, gender, and training as factors in the identification of normal infant cry-signals.

Journal: *Perceptual and Motor Skills,* August 1978, *47*(1), 267–270.

Related Research: Hogan, R. (1969). Development of an empathy scale. *Journal of Consulting and Clinical Psychology, 33,* 307–316.

■ ■ ■

2269

Test Name: INTERPERSONAL TRUST SCALE

Purpose: To measure interpersonal trust.

Number of Items: 40

Format: A Likert scale that includes 25 trust items and the rest filler items. An example is provided.

Validity: Correlations with behaviors, .06; negative intentions, –.25; positive intentions, .03; evaluation, .33; expertness-activity, .23 ($n = 307$).

Author: Wright, T. L., et al.

Article: Interpersonal trust and

attributions of source credibility: Evaluations of a political figure in a crisis.

Journal: *Perceptual and Motor Skills,* June 1977, *44*(3, Part 1), 943–950.

Related Research: Rotter, J. B. (1967). A new scale for the measurement of interpersonal trust. *Journal of Personality, 35,* 651–665.

■ ■ ■

2270

Test Name: INVENTORY OF ANXIETY IN DECISION MAKING

Purpose: To assess one's anxiety when faced with decision making.

Format: Subject is first required to indicate as clearly as possible the career decisions that troubled him or her, and in the second part to rate the extent to which he or she might experience 16 overt and covert anxiety symptoms while in the process of wrestling with these decisions.

Reliability: Internal consistency reliability was .85.

Validity: Correlates .44 and .58 with the School and Career subscales of the Decision-Difficulty Checklist.

Author: Mendonca, J. D., and Siess, T. F.

Article: Counseling for indecisiveness: Problem-solving and anxiety-management training.

Journal: *Journal of Counseling Psychology,* July 1976, *23*(4), 339–347.

Related Research: Mendonca, J. D. (1974). *Effectiveness of problem-solving and anxiety-management training in modifying vocational indecision.* Unpublished doctoral dissertation, University of Western Ontario.

2271

Test Name: LAWRENCE ASSERTIVE INVENTORY

Purpose: To assess assertiveness.

Number of Items: 112

Format: Multiple choice items.

Validity: A nonsignificant difference between an experimental (assertive training) group and control groups was reported.

Author: Rimm, D.

Article: Group-assertive training in treatment of expression of inappropriate anger.

Journal: *Psychological Reports,* June 1974, *34*(3), 791–798.

Related Research: Lawrence, P. S. (1970). *The assessment and modification of assertive behavior.* Unpublished doctoral dissertation, Arizona State University.

■ ■ ■

2272

Test Name: MATCHING FAMILIAR FIGURES TEST

Purpose: To measure reflection-impulsivity.

Format: Each item consists of a standard and six alternative stimuli exposed simultaneously. Latency to the first response and total number of errors were summed across all test items.

Reliability: Of mean latency measure, test–retest (3 months) reliability was .28 (*ns*); of mean number errors, test–retest (3 months) was .18 (*ns*).

Validity: Correlation with conceptual strategy assessment was .45 (Denny, 1973).

Author: Finch, A., et al.

Article: Reflection-impulsivity: Reliability of The Matching Familiar Figures Test with emotionally disturbed children.

Journal: *Psychological Reports,* December 1974, *35*(3), 1133–1134.

Related Research: Denny, D. (1973). Reflection and impulsivity as determinants of conceptual strategy. *Child Development, 44,* 614–623.

Denny, D. (1974). Relationship of three cognitive style dimensions to elementary reading abilities. *Journal of Educational Psychology, 66*(5), 702–709.

Kagan, J. (1964). Information processing in the child: Significance of analytic and reflective attitudes. *Psychological Monographs, 78*(1, Whole No. 578).

Kagan, J. (1966). Developmental studies in reflection and analysis. In A. H. Kidd & J. H. Rivoire (Eds.), *Perceptual Development in children* (pp. 487–522). New York: International Universities Press.

Kopfstein, D. (1973). Risk taking and cognitive style. *Child Development, 44,* 190–192.

See *DUEMM, 2,* 1978, 942; *DUEMM, 1,* 1974, 290.

• • •

2273

Test Name: MATERNAL VARIABLES

Purpose: To measure maternal responsiveness.

Number of Items: 15

Format: Employs a 0–10 scoring format whereby mothers are rated from *not in the least alike* to *almost exactly alike.*

Reliability: Test–retest reliability (2 weeks) was .84 (*N* = 12 families). Interrater reliability was .87.

Validity: Correlation with the Revised Carey Scale was –.54.

Author: Milliones, J.

Article: Relationship between perceived child temperament and maternal behaviors.

Journal: *Child Development,* 1978, *49,* 1255–1257.

Related Research: Allen, W. M. (1974). *Possible maternal and child variables influencing internalization.* Unpublished master's thesis, University of Pittsburgh.

• • •

2274

Test Name: MEASURE OF ACHIEVING TENDENCY

Purpose: To measure individual differences in achieving tendency.

Number of Items: 38

Format: Half the items are positively worded and half are negatively worded. Response to each item is made on a 9-point scale from +4 (*strong agreement*) through 0 to –4 (*strong disagreement*). Sample items are presented.

Reliability: Kuder-Richardson formula 20 reliability coefficient was .91.

Validity: Correlation with Crowne and Marlowe Scale was .02; Jackson's Achievement Scale was .74; Mehrabian's Measure of Achieving Tendency for males was .59; Mehrabian's Measure of Achieving Tendency for females was .68.

Author: Mehrabian, A., and Bank, L.

Article: A questionnaire measure of individual differences in achieving tendency.

Journal: *Educational and Psychological Measurement,* Summer 1978, *38*(2), 475–478.

Related Research: Mehrabian, A. (1969). Measures of achieving tendency. *Educational and Psychological Measurement, 29,* 445–451.

2275

Test Name: MOOD SURVEY

Purpose: To provide a trait measure of mood.

Number of Items: 18

Format: Includes two primary subscales: level and reactivity. All items are presented.

Reliability: Test–retest reliability was .80 for level and .85 for reactivity (3 weeks); .63 for level and .83 for reactivity (7 weeks).

Validity: Correlations of subscales with other personality measures ranged from –.39 to .63.

Author: Underwood, B., and Froming, W. J.

Article: The Mood Survey: A personality measure of happy and sad moods.

Journal: *Journal of Personality Assessment,* August 1980, *44*(4), 404–414.

• • •

2276

Test name: MOSHER RECORD CHOICE GUILT SCALE

Purpose: To measure dispositional guilt.

Number of items: 28

Format: Forced choice format.

Validity: Correlation with the Perceived Guilt Index was .03.

Author: Janda, L. H., et al.

Article: Affective guilt states in women and the Perceived Guilt Index.

Journal: *Journal of Personality Assessment,* February 1977, *41*(1), 79–84.

Related research: Mosher, D. L. (1966). The development and multitrait multimethod matrix analysis of three measures of three aspects of guilt. *Journal of Consulting Psychology, 30,* 25–29.

2277

Test name: MULTI-DIMEN-SIONAL AGGRESSION SCALE

Purpose: To assess aggression in a doll play interview for children.

Format: Doll play responses were scored along three dimensions: intensity, agent, and directionality.

Reliability: Mean interscorer reliability was .92.

Validity: Correlation with scoring system of Santrock (1970) was .92.

Author: Abramson, P., et al.

Article: The multidimensional aggression scale for the structured doll play interview.

Journal: *Journal of Personality Assessment*, October 1974, *38*(5), 436–440.

Related research: Santrock, J. (1970). Parental absence, sex typing, and identification. *Developmental Psychology, 2*, 264–272.

See *DUEMM, 2*, 1978, 927.

■ ■ ■

2278

Test name: O'CONNELL STORY TEST

Purpose: To measure humor, hostile wit, and resignation.

Number of items: 18

Format: Each anecdote has alternate endings for humor, hostile wit, and resignation. Rated on a 5-point scale.

Reliability: Interrater agreement was 87%; .85 (hostile wit); .79 (humor) (O'Connell, 1964).

Validity: Correlation was .336 between humor score and a measure of appreciation of absurd wit. Other correlations were nonsignificant and low.

Author: Groch, A.

Article: Generality of response to

humor and wit in cartoons, jokes, stories and photographs.

Journal: *Psychological Reports*, October 1974, *35*(2), 835–838.

Related research: O'Connell, W. (1964). Resignation, humor and wit. *Psychoanalytic Review, 51*, 49–56.

■ ■ ■

2279

Test name: PERCEIVED GUILT INDEX

Purpose: To provide an affective measure of guilt.

Number of items: 11

Format: Items are scaled to the degree to which they connote an affective guilt reaction. Items range from *innocent* with a scale value of 1.1 to *unforgivable* with a scale value of 10.4.

Validity: Correlation with the Mosher Forced Choice Guilt Scale was .03.

Author: Janda, L. H., et al.

Article: Affective guilt states in women and the perceived guilt index.

Journal: *Journal of Personality Assessment*, February 1977, *41*(1), 79–84.

Related research: Otterbacher, J. R., & Muntz, D. C. (1973). State-trait measure of experimental guilt. *Journal of Consulting and Clinical Psychology, 40*, 115–121.

■ ■ ■

2280

Test name: PERSONALITY TRAIT INFERENCES TEST

Purpose: To measure perceptions of student and teachers by students.

Number of items: 38

Time required: 6 minutes.

Format: There are 22 adjectives to

describe a child and 16 adjectives to describe a teacher. Ratings are done on 3- and 5-point Likert scales.

Reliability: Split-half reliability for trait ratings of the child was .98, test–retest after 5 days was .97. Split-half for trait ratings of the teacher was .98, test–retest, .95.

Validity: .96 for words used in describing a child and .97 for words used in describing a teacher (product-moment correlations between mean word values in this study and those presented by Anderson, 1960).

Author: Rice, W. K., Jr.

Article: Effects of discipline techniques on children's personality trait inferences.

Journal: *Journal of Educational Psychology*, August 1975, *67*(4), 570–575.

Related Research: Anderson, N. H. (1968). Likableness ratings of 555 personality-trait adjectives. *Journal of Personality and Social Psychology, 9*, 272–279.

■ ■ ■

2281

Test Name: PRINCIPAL'S AUTHORITARIANISM INDEX

Purpose: To determine the authoritarianism of the principal.

Number of Items: 7

Format: Teachers respond on a 4-point Likert scale from *rarely occurs* to *very frequently occurs*. Some examples are presented.

Validity: Coefficient alpha was .70.

Author: Hoy, W. K., and Rees, R.

Article: Subordinate loyalty to immediate superior: A neglected concept in the study of educational administration.

Journal: *Sociology of Education*, Spring 1974, *47*(2), 268–286.

Related Research: Blau, P. M., &

Scott, W. R. (1962). *Formal organizations*. San Francisco: Chandler.

■ ■ ■

2282

Test Name: RATHUS ASSERTION SCHEDULE

Purpose: To measure assertiveness.

Number of Items: 30

Format: Respondent rates items describing assertive or nonassertive behaviors as self-descriptive on a 7-point scale.

Reliability: Pearson product–moment correlation comparing odd and even scores yielded a value of .595 ($p < .001$).

Validity: Pearson product–moment correlation of .71 ($p < .001$) was obtained between self and external ratings on 71 scores.

Author: Mann, R. J., and Flowers, J. V.

Article: An investigation of the validity and reliability of the Rathus Assertion Schedule.

Journal: *Psychological Reports*, April 1978, *42*(2), 632–634.

Related Research: Chandler, T. A., et al. (1978). Sex differences in self-reported assertiveness. *Psychological Reports*, *43*(2), 395–402.

Rathus, S. A. (1973). A 30–item schedule for assessing assertive behavior. *Behavior Therapy*, *4*, 398–402.

■ ■ ■

2283

Test Name: REACTION INVENTORY

Purpose: To identify an individual's specific stimulus situations which result in anger.

Number of Items: 76

Format: Employs a Likert scale of

5 points ranging from *not at all* to *very much*.

Reliability: Mean item–test correlation coefficient was .46.

Validity: Correlations with the Buss Durkee Hostility Inventory were .52 and .57.

Author: Biaggio, M. K.

Article: Assessment of anger arousal.

Journal: *Journal of Personality Assessment*, June 1980, *44*(3), 289–298.

Related Research: Evans, D. R., & Strangeland, M. (1971). Development of the reaction inventory to measure anger. *Psychological Reports*, *29*, 412–414.

■ ■ ■

2284

Test Name: REACTION INVENTORY–GUILT

Purpose: To measure guilt.

Number of Items: 50

Format: Subjects enter the number of each item under one of five headings that indicate the extent of guilt they feel in each situation. Headings include: *not at all, a little, a fair amount, much, very much*. Includes four factors: intentional behavior disrupting interpersonal relations, self-destructive behavior, behavior contrary to moral or ethical principles, unintentional behavior disrupting interpersonal relationships.

Reliability: Estimate of internal consistency coefficient was .94.

Author: Evans, D. R., et al.

Article: Development of a reaction inventory to measure guilt.

Journal: *Journal of Personality Assessment*, August 1975, *39*(4), 421–423.

Related Research: Evans, D. R., et

al. (1974, April). *Development of a reaction inventory to measure guilt* (Research Bulletin #287). University of Western Ontario, Department of Psychology.

■ ■ ■

2285

Test Name: REVISED CAREY SCALE

Purpose: To measure child temperament.

Number of Items: 46

Format: Includes the following response categories: rhythmicity, adaptability, approach-withdrawal, intensity, and mood.

Validity: Correlation with Maternal Variables was –.54.

Author: Milliones, J.

Article: Relationship between perceived child temperament and maternal behaviors.

Journal: *Child Development*, 1978, *49*, 1255–1257.

Related Research: Carey, W. (1970). A simplified method for measuring infant temperament. *Journal of Pediatrics*, *77*, 188–194.

■ ■ ■

2286

Test Name: RIGIDITY TEST

Purpose: To measure rigidity.

Number of Items: 15

Format: A nonverbal test consisting of pairs of figures and numbers.

Validity: Between nonverbal rigidity and dispositional rigidity: a correlation of –.46.

Author: Joshi, R. T.

Article: Non-verbal rigidity and dispositional rigidity: A British sample.

Journal: *Perceptual and Motor*

Skills, February 1974, *33*(1), 102.

Related Research: Breskin, S. Measurement of rigidity, a non-verbal test. *Perceptual and Motor Skills,* 1968, *27*, 1203–1206.

See *D. U. E. M. M., 2,* 1978, 917.

■ ■ ■

2287

Test Name: ROKEACH DOGMATISM SCALE—SHORT FORM

Purpose: To measure the degree of dogmatism.

Number of Items: 20

Format: Subject indicates agreement or disagreement with each item.

Validity: Correlations with the 40-item scale was .94 and .95. Correlations with other variables (males) ranged from –.14 to .24 (men), –.06 to .31 (women).

Author: Muldrow, T. W., and Bayton, J. A.

Article: Men and women executives and processes related to decision accuracy.

Journal: *Journal of Applied Psychology,* April 1979, *64*(2), 99–106.

Related Research: Trodahl, V. C., & Powell, F. A. (1965). A short-form dogmatism scale for use in field studies. *Social Forces, 44,* 211–214.

■ ■ ■

2288

Test Name: ROTTER TRUST SCALE

Purpose: To measure interpersonal trust.

Number of Items: 25 plus 15 filler items.

Format: Likert format.

Reliability: Three factors identified

by cluster analysis: integrity of social agents, trustworthiness of human motives, dependability of people.

Validity: Principal components factor analysis with varimax rotation indicated three factors: institutional trust, sincerity, caution (Kaplan, 1973). No difference between peer and professionally counseled Black students (Williams, 1974).

Author: Stein, K., et al.

Article: Dimensions of the Rotter Trust Scale.

Journal: *Psychological Reports,* October 1974, *35*(2), 999–1004.

Related Research: Chun, K., & Campbell, J. (1974). Dimensionality of the Rotter Interpersonal Trust Scale. *Psychological Trust Scale,* December, *35*(3), 1059–1070.

Kaplan, R. (1973). Components of trust: Note on use of Rotter's Scale. *Psychological Reports, 33,* 13–14.

Rotter, J. (1967). A new scale for the measurement of interpersonal trust. *Journal of Personality, 35,* 651–665.

Rotter, J. (1971). Generalized expectancies for interpersonal trust. *American Psychologist, 26,* 443–452.

Williams, B. (1974). Trust and self disclosure among Black college students. *Journal of Counseling Psychology, 21,* 522–525.

See *D. U. E. M. M., 2,* 1978, 818, 954.

■ ■ ■

2289

Test Name: SCHEMATIZING TEST

Purpose: To assess a cognitive control style (leveling and sharpening).

Number of Items: 75 modified items.

Format: Performance test in which subjects asked to judge size of cardboard squares.

Reliability: Comparability of Long Form and Short Form: .97 and .77 (men), .93 and .66 (women) for two of the scores produced.

Author: Warren, W., and Staines, J.

Article: Leveling-Sharpening in aged persons.

Journal: *Psychological Reports,* August 1974, *35*(1), 181–182.

Related Research: Gardner, R., et al. (1959). Cognitive control: A study of individual consistencies in cognitive behavior. *Psychological Issues, 1*(4, Monog. 8).

■ ■ ■

2290

Test Name: SELF-REPORT MEASURE OF CONFORMITY

Purpose: To measure conformity.

Number of Items: 15

Format: Forced-choice format.

Validity: Correlation with Willis Anti-Conformity Measure, .02; with Peer Nominations for Conformity, –.12.

Author: Hoppe, C. F., and Loevinger, J.

Article: Ego development and conformity: A construct validity study of the Washington University Sentence Completion Test.

Journal: *Journal of Personality Assessment,* October 1977, *41*(5), 497–504.

Related Research: Hoppe, C. F. (1972). *Ego development and conformity behaviors.* Unpublished doctoral dissertation, Washington University.

2291

Test Name: SEMANTIC DIFFERENTIAL TEMPERAMENT SCALES

Purpose: To measure temperament.

Number of Items: 112

Format: Each item consists of a pair of adjectives separated by a 9-point scale. Includes three measures of pleasure–displeasure, level of arousal, and dominance–submissiveness.

Reliability: Kuder-Richardson formula 20 reliability coefficients for the three scales were .91 (pleasure), .60 (arousal), .84 (dominance).

Validity: Correlations of each of the three measures with several personality scales ranged from −.47 to .57.

Author: Mehrabian, A.

Article: Measures of individual differences in temperament.

Journal: *Educational and Psychological Measurement,* Winter 1978, *38*(4), 1105–1117.

Related Research: Mehrabian, A., & Russell, J. A. (1974). *An approach to environmental psychology.* Cambridge, MA: MIT Press.

■ ■ ■

2292

Test Name: SHORT-FORM DOGMATISM SCALE

Purpose: To measure open- and closed-mindedness.

Number of Items: 20

Format: Agree–disagree continuum.

Reliability: Split-half reliability coefficient was .79.

Validity: Correlation was .94 with

Rokeach's 40-item dogmatism scale.

Author: O'Reilly, R. R., and Fish, J. C.

Article: Dogmatism and tenure status as determinants of resistance toward educational innovation.

Journal: *Journal of Experimental Education,* Fall 1976, *45*(1), 68–70.

Related Research: Troldahl, V., & Powell, F. A. (1965). A short-form dogmatism scale for use in field studies. *Social Forces, 44,* 211–215.

■ ■ ■

2293

Test Name: SF TEST

Purpose: To measure authoritarianism symbolically.

Number of Items: 15

Format: Pairs of line drawings and number arrangements, for example, four lines that if connected would form a square and four connected lines forming a square; the digits 1 through 5 in ascending numerical order and the same digits in mixed order.

Reliability: Split-half reliability coefficients range from .84 to .93.

Validity: Convergent validity of .64 with verbal measures of authoritarianism.

Author: Hogan, H. W.

Article: Validity of a symbolic measure of authoritarianism.

Journal: *Psychological Reports,* October 1975, *37*(2), 539–543.

Related Research: Hogan, H. N. (1970). Reliability and convergent validity of a symbolic test for authoritarianism. *Journal of Psychology, 76,* 39–43.

2294

Test Name: TRODAHL AND POWELL DOGMATISM SCALE

Purpose: To measure dogmatism.

Number of Items: 10

Format: Scale is a shortened form of the Rokeach Scale: 5-point scale (*strongly agree* to *strongly disagree*).

Validity: Significant ($p < .001$) differences were found in attitude toward law and order between high and low dogmatics.

Author: Steffensmeier, D.

Article: Levels of dogmatism and attitudes toward law and order.

Journal: *Psychological Reports,* February 1974, *34*(1), 151–153.

Related Research: Trodahl, V., & Powell, F. (1965). A short form dogmatism scale for use in field studies. *Social Forces, 44,* 211–215.

■ ■ ■

2295

Test Name: ZAKS-WALTERS SCALE OF AGGRESSION

Purpose: To assess behavioral aggression.

Number of Items: 12

Format: MMPI type instrument.

Validity: Biserial correlation with Yuker Attitude Toward the Disabled Scale was .34 ($p < .05$).

Author: Evans, J.

Article: Attitude toward the disabled and aggression.

Journal: *Perceptual and Motor Skills,* December 1973, *37*(3), 834.

Related Research: Zaks, M., & Walters, R. (1959). First steps in the construction of a scale for the measurement of aggression. *Journal of Psychology, 47,* 199–208.

...
CHAPTER 21
Values

2296

Test Name: AMES PHILOSOPHICAL BELIEF INVENTORY

Purpose: To assess philosophical positions of counselors and counselor trainees.

Format: Scales: idealism, realism, pragmatism, phenomenology, and existentialism.

Reliability: .41 to .90 (Ames, 1965, 1968; Sawyer, 1971; Wise, 1966).

Validity: Five scales differentiated between religious Sisters and former Sisters group.

Author: Hart, G., et al.

Article: Philosophical positions of new and former nuns: A discriminant analysis.

Journal: *Psychological Reports,* August 1974, *35*(1), 675–678.

Related Research: Ames, K. (1965). *The development of an instrument for philosophical position of school counselors.* Unpublished doctoral dissertation, University of Wyoming.

Ames, K. (1968). The development of an instrument for philosophical position of school counselors. *Counselor Education and Supervision, 7,* 335–339.

Sawyer, R. (1971). The Ames Philosophical Belief Inventory: Reliability and validity. *Measurement and Evaluation in Guidance, 3,* 203–208.

Wise, D. (1966). *An initial study of the Ames Philosophical Belief Inventory with students in education.* Unpublished doctoral dissertation, University of Wyoming.

See *DUEMM, 2,* 1978, 968.

...

2297

Test Name: ANTI-BLACK PREJUDICE SCALE

Purpose: To measure anti-Black prejudice.

Number of Items: 17

Format: Part I contains 50 Likert scales; Part II contains 62 paired comparison items.

Reliability: Coefficient alpha reliability was .83.

Validity: Correlation with the FEM Scale was −.462.

Author: Singleton, Jr., R., and Christiansen, J. B.

Article: The construct validation of a shortform attitudes toward feminism scale.

Journal: *Sociology and Social Research,* April 1977, *61*(3), 294–303.

Related Research: Kramer, B. M. (1949). Dimensions of prejudice. *Journal of Psychology, 27,* 389–451.

...

2298

Test Name: AUTONOMOUS AND SOCIAL ACHIEVEMENT VALUES TEST

Purpose: To measure autonomous and social achievement standards.

Number of Items: 48

Format: Two scales: The Autonomous Achievement Values Scale and the Social Achievement Values Scale.

Reliability: Stability coefficients after 11 weeks were .85 for the Autonomous Achievement Values Scale and .77 for the Social Achievement Values Scale.

Validity: Autonomous Achievement Value Scale correlations were from .29 to .36 with the Crown-Marlowe (1964) Social Desirability Scale and from −.17 to −.38 for the Social Achievement Value Scale and the Social Desirability Scale.

Author: Strumpfer, D. J. W.

Article: Scales to measure autonomous and social achievement values.

Journal: *Psychological Reports,* February 1975, *36*(1), 191–208.

...

2299

Test Name: BELIEFS ABOUT EQUAL RIGHTS SCALE

Purpose: To measure beliefs about equal rights for men and women.

Number of Items: 28

Format: True or false responses are given to each item. All items are presented.

Reliability: Kuder-Richardson formula 20 reliability was .86 ($n = 63$).

Validity: Correlation with Attitudes Towards Women Scale was .14.

Author: Jacobson, L. I., et al.

Article: Construction and initial

validation of a scale measuring beliefs about equal rights for men and women.

Journal: *Educational and Psychological Measurement,* Winter 1976, *36*(4), 913–918.

■ ■ ■

2300

Test Name: COMPREHENSION OF SOCIAL-MORAL CONCEPTS TEST

Purpose: To test comprehension of social-moral concepts.

Number of Items: 10

Format: Subject picks from four statements the one that best interprets the main idea of a paragraph.

Reliability: Test–retest reliability (24 ninth graders) was .51; Kuder-Richardson consistency coefficient was .56 (*N* = 160).

Validity: Correlation with Defining Issues Test (a measure of moral judgment) was .58; Correlation with Differential Ability Tests (*n* = 73) was .41.

Author: Rest, J., et al.

Article: Judging the important issues in moral dilemmas–an objective measure of development.

Journal: *Developmental Psychology,* July 1974, *10*(4), 491– 501.

■ ■ ■

2301

Test Name: DEFINING ISSUES TEST

Purpose: To measure moral judgment.

Number of Items: 72

Format: Subject evaluates a set of 12 issues for each of 6 stories. Each issue is rated on a Likert scale of importance including

most, much, some, little, no. Some examples of items are given.

Reliability: Test–retest Pearson correlation was .81.

Validity: Correlations with age, .62 and .67; with Differential Ability Tests (*n* = 73), .35; with comprehension of social-moral concepts, .58.

Author: Rest, J., et al.

Article: Judging the important issues in moral dilemma—An objective measure of development.

Journal: *Developmental Psychology,* July 1974, *10*(4), 491– 501.

■ ■ ■

2302

Test Name: DEVELOPMENTAL INVENTORY OF FEMININE VALUES

Purpose: To ascertain one's degree of other or family orientation.

Number of Items: 34

Format: Value judgment statements related to a person's activities, satisfactions, and fulfillments to which one responds in accordance with a 5-point Likert scale that ranges from *completely agree, I have no opinion,* to *completely disagree.*

Reliability: Split-half reliability was .81 when corrected through the Spearman-Brown procedure.

Author: Konstam, V., and Gilbert, H. B.

Article: Fear of success, sex-role orientation, and performance in differing experimental conditions.

Journal: *Psychological Reports,* April 1978, *42*(2), 519–528.

Related Research: Steinmann, A., & Fox, D. J. (1966). Male–female perceptions of the female role in the U.S. *Journal of Psychology, 64,* 265–276.

2303

Test Name: INVENTORY OF FEMALE VALUES

Purpose: To measure perceptions of the female sex-role.

Number of Items: 34

Format: Items are rated on 5-point Likert scales ranging from *completely agree* to *completely disagree.*

Reliability: Spearman-Brown split-half reliability coefficient was .81.

Author: Voss, J. H., and Skinner, D. A.

Article: Concepts of self and ideal women held by college women: A replication.

Journal: *Journal of College Student Personnel,* May 1975, *16*(3), 210–213.

Related Research: Steinmann, A., & Fox, D. (1966). Male–female role in the United States. *Journal of Psychology, 64,* 265–276.

■ ■ ■

2304

Test Name: KILMANN INSIGHT TEST

Purpose: To measure the individual's interpersonal value constructs.

Number of Items: 18

Time Required: 10–15 minutes.

Format: The subject differentiate on a 7-point scale each interpersonal value construct according to how relevant it is to a series of six ambiguous pictures of interpersonal situations. Includes two factors: good fellowship versus functional task activity and interpersonal restraint versus boldness.

Author: Kilmann, R. H.

Article: A scaled-projective measure of interpersonal values.

Journal: *Journal of Personality Assessment,* February 1975, *39*(1), 34–40.

Related Research: Kilmann, R. H. (1972). *The development and validation of a projective measure of interpersonal values.* Unpublished doctoral dissertation, University of California, Los Angeles.

■ ■ ■

2305

Test Name: LIBERALISM–CONSERVATISM SCALE

Purpose: To measure the strength of general conservatism.

Number of Items: 5

Format: Subjects indicate their agreement or disagreement with each statement on a 4-point scale. All items are presented.

Validity: Correlation with income, .14; education, .26; self-reported status, .10; and age, –.16. Correlation with years of residence, –.03; home ownership, .14; political party registration, .14; and frequency of church attendance, –.12.

Author: Wilson, J., and Manton, K.

Article: Localism and temperance.

Journal: *Sociology and Social Research,* January 1975, *59*(2), 121–135.

Related Research: Matthews, D., & Prothro, J. (1966). *Negroes and the New Southern Politics.* New York: Harcourt, Brace & World.

McClosky, H. (1958). Conservatism and personality. *American Political Science Review, 52,* 27–45.

■ ■ ■

2306

Test Name: LOCALISM–COSMOPOLITANISM SCALE

Purpose: To measure the extent to which an individual has internalized the characteristic cosmopolitanism orientation of urban society.

Number of Items: 10

Format: Subjects respond indicating the extent of their agreement with each statement on a 4-point scale (*strongly agree, agree, disagree,* and *strongly disagree*). All items are presented.

Validity: Correlation with income, .06; education, .23; self-reported status, .01; and age, –.15. Correlation with: years of residence, –.18; home ownership, .05; political party registration, .09; and frequency of church attendance, –.01.

Author: Wilson, J., and Manton, K.

Article: Localism and temperance.

Journal: *Sociology and Social Research,* January 1975, *59*(2), 121–135.

Related Research: Dobriner, W. (1958). Local and cosmopolitan as contemporary suburban character types. In W. M. Dobriner (Ed.), *The suburban community* (pp. 132–143). New York: Putnam.

■ ■ ■

2307

Test Name: MEANING AND VALUE OF WORK SCALE

Purpose: To measure one's breadth of perception of the term *work* and one's work value orientation.

Number of Items: 112

Reliability: Part I has a Kuder-Richardson formula 20 reliability of .89; Part II has a Kuder-Richardson formula 20 reliability of .90.

Author: Kazanas, H. C.

Article: Relationship of job

satisfaction and productivity to work values of vocational education graduates.

Journal: *Journal of Vocational Behavior,* April 1978, *12*(2), 155–164.

Related Research: Kazanas, H. C., et al. (1975). An instrument to measure the meaning and value associated with work. *Journal of Industrial Teacher Education, 12,* 68–73.

■ ■ ■

2308

Test Name: MEASURE OF VALUES

Purpose: To identify personal values espoused by college students.

Number of Items: 134

Format: Items are phrases in the infinitive form expressing a value and are rated on a 5-point scale from *not at all important to me* to *overwhelmingly important to me.* There are 11 scales for men and 12 for women.

Reliability: Test–retest correlations (3 months) ranged from .70 to .80.

Author: Pierce, R. A., and Schwartz, A. J.

Article: Value similarity and satisfaction in suite-type living arrangements.

Journal: *Journal of College Student Personnel,* May 1974, *15*(3), 213–219.

Related Research: Pierce, R. A. (1972). *Measure of values.* Unpublished manuscript.

■ ■ ■

2309

Test Name: MODERNITY SCALE

Purpose: To measure modernity.

Number of Items: 8

Format: Subject responds on a 5-point scale from *agree strongly* to *disagree strongly*. All items are presented.

Reliability: Coefficient alpha was .55 ($n = 479$) and .77 ($n = 98$).

Validity: Correlation with Doob Modernity Scale was .34; Kahl Modernity Scale was .25; Stephenson Modernity Scale was .38.

Author: Gough, H. G.

Article: A measure of individual modernity.

Journal: *Journal of Personality Assessment,* February 1976, *40*(1), 3–9.

• • •

2310

Test Name: MORAL JUDGMENT INTERVIEW

Purpose: To gain a picture of a person's moral-judgment behavior.

Number of Items: 9

Format: Includes nine moral-dilemma situations. Yields a moral maturity score.

Reliability: Product–moment correlation between two sets of scores was .817.

Validity: With intelligence, $r = .432$.

Author: Moir, D. J.

Article: Egocentrism and the emergence of conventional morality in preadolescent girls.

Journal: *Child Development,* June 1974, *45*(2), 299–304.

Related Research: Kohlberg, L. (1958). *The development of modes of moral thinking and choice in the years ten to sixteen.* Unpublished doctoral dissertation, University of Chicago.

2311

Test Name: MORAL JUDGMENT TEST

Purpose: To measure the moral judgment of children.

Number of Items: 7

Format: Includes three situations measuring moral realism, two situations measuring expiatory punishment, and two situations assessing imminent justice.

Reliability: Reliability coefficients ranged from .77 to .90.

Author: LaVoie, J. C.

Article: Cognitive determinants of resistance to deviation in seven-, nine-, and eleven-year-old children of low and high maturity of moral judgment.

Journal: *Developmental Psychology,* May 1974, *10*(3), 393–403.

Related Research: Piaget, J. (1965). *The moral judgment of the child.* New York: The Free Press.

• • •

2312

Test Name: MOTHER'S RELIGIOSITY

Purpose: To assess a conventional orientation to religion.

Number of Items: 5

Format: Includes items dealing with the importance of participation in religious activities, regular attendance at religious services, turning to prayer when facing a personal problem, reliance on religious teachings, and belief in God. Scores range from 5 to 20.

Reliability: Scott's homogeneity ratio was .68. Cronbach's alpha was .91.

Validity: With the Problem Behavior Index, $rs = -.32$ (women) and $-.20$ (men).

Author: Jessor, S. L., and Jessor, R.

Article: Maternal ideology and adolescent problem behavior.

Journal: *Developmental Psychology,* March 1974, *10*(2), 246–254.

• • •

2313

Test Name: MOTHER'S TRADITIONAL BELIEFS SCALE

Purpose: To assess the mother's generalized orientation toward the norms and institutions of society along a conservative–liberal dimension.

Number of Items: 10

Format: Likert scale with items referring to family, the law, and social norms. Scores range from 10 to 40. Some examples are provided.

Reliability: Scott's homogeneity ratio was .23; Cronbach's alpha was .75.

Validity: With the Problem Behavior Index, $rs = -.29$ (women) and $-.34$ (men).

Author: Jessor, S. L., and Jessor, R.

Article: Maternal ideology and adolescent problem behavior.

Journal: *Developmental Psychology,* March 1974, *10*(2), 246–254.

• • •

2314

Test Name: OCCUPATION AUCTION

Purpose: To show what an individual does with respect to his or her personal values in a decision-making situation.

Number of Items: 8 job descriptions.

Format: Individuals choose between paired jobs coordinated with eight values.

Reliability: Test–retest reliability was .78 over a 5-week interval.

Validity: Median correlation was .79 (ranged from .42 to .94) between the Occupation Auction and the Work Values Inventory on seven similarly defined work values.

Author: Ohlde, C. D., and Vinitsky, M. H.

Article: Effect of values-clarification workshop on value awareness.

Journal: *Journal of Counseling Psychology,* September 1976, *23*(5), 489–491.

Related Research: Chapman, W., et al. (1973). *Report of a pilot study under field conditions.* Princeton, NJ: Educational Testing Service.

■ ■ ■

2315

Test Name: OCCUPATIONAL VALUE SURVEY

Purpose: To determine what one says his or her values are (helping others, high income, independence, leadership, leisure, prestige, security, and variety).

Number of Items: 10 occupational values.

Format: Individuals rank order from most important to least important 8 of the 10 occupational values.

Reliability: Test–retest reliability was .78 or higher over a 5-week interval.

Author: Ohlde, C. D., and Vinitsky, M. H.

Article: Effect of values-clarification workshop on value awareness.

Journal: *Journal of Counseling Psychology,* September 1976, *23*(5), 489–491.

Related Research: Chapman, W., et al. (1973). *Report of a pilot study under field conditions.* Princeton, NJ: Educational Testing Service.

■ ■ ■

2316

Test Name: OCCUPATIONAL VALUES SCALES

Purpose: To measure the importance of intrinsic and extrinsic values associated with work.

Number of Items: 30

Format: Each response is made on a 7-point Likert scale.

Reliability: Extrinsic: test–retest (3-week interval) Spearman rho was .84 ($n = 25$). Intrinsic: test–retest (3-week interval) Spearman rho was .79 ($n = 25$).

Author: Morrison, R. F.

Article: Career adaptivity: The effective adaptation of managers to changing role demands.

Journal: *Journal of Applied Psychology,* October 1977, *62*(5), 549–558.

Related Research: Kilpatrick, F. P., et al. (1964). *The image of the federal service.* Washington, DC: Brookings Institution.

■ ■ ■

2317

Test Name: OHIO WORK VALUES INVENTORY

Purpose: To measure the work values of elementary and secondary school-age children.

Number of Items: 77

Format: Values are altruism, object orientation, security, control, self-realization, independence, money, task satisfaction, solitude, ideas/data, prestige.

Reliability: Test–retest reliabilities were above .85.

Author: Hales, L. W., and Hartman, T. P.

Article: Measuring the work values of technical college students: The Ohio Work Values Inventory.

Journal: *Measurement and Evaluation in Guidance,* October 1978, *11*(3), 169–174.

Related Research: Hales, L. W., & Fenner, B. J. (1975). Measuring the work values of children: The Ohio Work Values Inventory. *Measurement and Evaluation in Guidance, 8,* 20–25.

■ ■ ■

2318

Test Name: POLITICO-ECONOMIC CONSERVATISM SCALE

Purpose: To identify a subject's political beliefs.

Number of Items: 12

Format: The items are counterbalanced.

Reliability: Alpha was .91.

Author: Nassi, A. J., and Abramowitz, S. I.

Article: Discriminant validity of Mirel's personal and political factors on Rotter's I-E Scale: Does a decade make a difference?

Journal: *Journal of Personality Assessment,* August 1980, *44*(4), 363–367.

Related Research: Kerpelman, L. C. (1972). *Activists and nonactivists: A psychological study of American college students.* New York: Behavioral Publications.

2319

Test Name: PROTESTANT WORK ETHIC SCALE

Purpose: To measure belief in the Protestant Work Ethic.

Number of Items: 8

Format: Four items measure the "pro-Protestant Ethic" and four items measure the "non-Protestant Ethic."

Reliability: Internal consistency with Spearman-Brown formula applied to the average item intercorrelation for "pro Protestant Ethic" items was .70.

Author: Wanous, J. P.

Article: Individual differences and reactions to job characteristics.

Journal: *Journal of Applied Psychology,* October 1974, *59*(5), 616–622.

Related Research: Blood, M. R. (1969). Work values and job satisfaction. *Journal of Applied Psychology, 53,* 456–459.

■ ■ ■

2320

Test Name: PROTESTANT ETHIC SCALE

Purpose: To measure work values and job satisfaction.

Number of Items: 4

Format: Responses to each item are made on a 7-point agree–disagree scale.

Reliability: .71

Validity: Correlation with Protestant Ethic Scale-Mirels and Garrett was .70; Survey of Work Values ranged from .27 to .49; Rotter's Internal–External Control of Reinforcement Scale was –.35; SAT was .03; cumulative grade point average was –.09.

Author: Waters, L. K., et al.

Article: Protestant ethic attitudes

among college students.

Journal: *Educational and Psychological Measurement,* Summer 1975, *35*(2), 447–450.

Related Research: Blood, M. R. (1969). Work values and job satisfaction. *Journal of Applied Psychology, 53,* 456–459.

■ ■ ■

2321

Test Name: PROTESTANT ETHIC SCALE

Purpose: To measure work values.

Number of Items: 19

Format: Yields a single overall score.

Reliability: .80

Validity: Correlation with Protestant Ethic Scale—Blood was .70; Survey of Work Values ranged from .26 to .49; Rotter's Internal–External Control of Reinforcement Scale was –.34; SAT was .08; cumulative grade point average was –.12.

Author: Waters, L. K., et al.

Article: Protestant ethic attitudes among college students.

Journal: *Educational and Psychological Measurement,* Summer 1975, *35*(2), 447–450.

Related Research: Merrens, M. R., & Garrett, J. B. (1975). The Protestant Ethic Scale as a predictor of repetitive work performance. *Journal of Applied Psychology,* February, *60,* 125–127.

Mirels, H. L., & Garrett, J. B. (1971). The Protestant ethic as a personality variable. *Journal of Consulting and Clinical Psychology, 36,* 40–44.

■ ■ ■

2322

Test Name: RELIGIOSITY SCALE

Purpose: To measure religiosity.

Number of Items: 8

Reliability: Cronbach's coefficient alpha was .90.

Validity: With dogmatism, $r = .21$, with conservatism, $r = .60$.

Author: Rohrbaugh, J., et al.

Article: Measuring the relative importance of utilitarian and egalitarian values: A study of individual differences about fair distribution.

Journal: *Journal of Applied Psychology,* February 1980, *65*(1), 34–49.

Related Research: Rohrbaugh, J., & Jessor, R. (1975). Religiosity in youth: A personal control against deviant behavior. *Journal of Personality, 43,* 136–155.

■ ■ ■

2323

Test Name: RELIGIOUS BELIEF QUESTIONNAIRE

Purpose: To assess religious beliefs.

Number of Items: 64 each form.

Format: Two forms: A and B, Subscales are God (20 items), Bible (4 items), Good and Evil (11 items), Organized Religion (7 items), Religious Practices (6 items), Duties of Daily Living (7 items).

Validity: Relationship with Study of Values (Religious) for eighth graders was .72 (boys), .53 (girls).

Author: Apfeldorf, M., and Smith, W.

Article: Religious beliefs and other values of high school students.

Journal: *Psychological Reports,* October 1974, *35*(2), 811–816.

Related Research: Smith, W., & Apfeldorf, M. (1969, October). *Multidenominational instruments* *for the assessment of religious beliefs and behavior.* Paper presented at the 20th Annual Meeting of the Society for the Scientific Study of Religion, Boston.

■ ■ ■

2324

Test Name: RELIGIOUS EXPERIENCE EPISODES MEASURE

Purpose: To measure mystical dimensions of intense religious experience.

Number of Items: 5

Format: Subjects indicate the extent to which they have had an experience similar to each item described by use of a 5-point scale (5 = *most similar*).

Reliability: Cronbach's alpha coefficient of internal reliability for 15 Caucasians and 15 Mexican Americans was .60.

Author: Hood, R. W., Jr., and Hall, J. R.

Article: Comparison of reported religious experience in Caucasian, American Indian, and two Mexican American samples.

Journal: *Psychological Reports,* October 1977, *41*(2), 657–658.

Related Research: Hood, R. W., Jr. (1970). Religious orientation and the report of religious experience. *Journal for the Scientific Study of Religion, 9,* 285–291.

■ ■ ■

2325

Test Name: ROKEACH VALUE SURVEY

Purpose: To provide a measure of an adolescent's value system.

Number of Items: 18

Format: Subject places a list of values in order of importance. Includes two value systems: terminal and instrumental.

Reliability: For terminal value system (intervals from 3 weeks to 17 months) .74 to .84; for instrumental value system in low .70s.

Author: Beech, R. P., and Schoeppe, A.

Article: Development of value systems in adolescents.

Journal: *Developmental Psychology,* September 1974, *10*(5), 644–656.

Related Research: Rokeach, M. (1969). Religious values and social compassion. *Review of Religious Research, 11,* 24–38.

■ ■ ■

2326

Test Name: ROKEACH VALUE SURVEY

Purpose: To discriminate more successful students from less successful.

Number of Items: 36

Format: Includes two categories of values: instrumental and terminal. A 7-point Likert scale was used.

Reliability: Cronbach's alpha was .76.

Validity: Correlation with grade point average was .56.

Author: Munson, V. M.

Article: Concurrent validity of a modified Rokeach value survey in discriminating more successful from less successful students.

Journal: *Educational and Psychological Measurement,* Summer 1980, *40*(II), 479–485.

Related Research: Rokeach, M. (1973). *The nature of human values.* New York: Free Press.

2327

Test Name: SELF- VERSUS OTHER-CENTERED VALUES SCALE

Purpose: To assess the relative importance of other-centered and self-centered values and goals.

Number of Items: 12

Format: Children rank the personal importance of 12 statements. Some items are presented.

Reliability: Test–retest reliability over a 10-day interval, determined on a sample of 27 fifth-grade children, was .83.

Author: Dlugokinski, E. L., and Firestone, I. J.

Article: Other centeredness and susceptibility to charitable appeals: Effects of perceived discipline.

Journal: *Developmental Psychology,* January 1974, *10*(1), 21–28.

Related Research: Rokeach, M. (1968). A theory of organization and change within value systems. *Journal of Social Issues, 24,* 13–33.

■ ■ ■

2328

Test Name: SURVEY OF WORK VALUES

Purpose: To measure work values, including Social Status of Job, Activity Preference, Job Involvement, Upward Striving, Attitude toward Earnings, and Pride in Work.

Number of Items: 54 statements

Format: Subjects endorse the statements on a 6-point scale of agreement.

Reliability: Internal consistency reliabilities of the subscales ranged from .55 to .66 and the test–retest reliabilities with a 1-month interval ranged from .65 to .76.

Author: Wijting, J. P., et al.

Article: Relationships between work values, socio-educational and work experiences, and vocational aspirations of 6th, 9th, 10th, and 12th graders.

Journal: *Journal of Vocational Behavior,* August 1977, *11*(1), 51–65.

Related Research: Waters, L. K., et al. (1975). Protestant ethic attitudes among college students. *Educational and Psychological Measurement,* Summer, *35*(2), 447–450.

Wollack, S., et al. (1971). The development of the Survey of Work Values. *Journal of Applied Psychology, 55,* 331–338.

CHAPTER 22
Vocational Evaluation

2329

Test Name: ADVISOR EFFECTIVENESS EVALUATION

Purpose: To evaluate college advisor effectiveness.

Number of Items: 19

Format: Eleven items on Interpersonal Advisor Behaviors, and 8 items on Academic Advisor Behavior all rated in 5-point scales from *never* to *very frequently*.

Reliability: Odd–even reliability coefficient of .82.

Validity: Factor loadings on the interpersonal behavior section ranged from .97 to .56 and for the academic behavior, from .54 to .84.

Author: Aiken, J., et al.

Article: Orientation advisor effectiveness: A continuing search.

Journal: *Journal of College Student Personnel*, January 1976, *17*(1), 16–21.

Related Research: Upcraft, M. L. (1971). Undergraduate students as academic advisors. *Personnel and Guidance Journal, 49*, 827–881.

■ ■ ■

2330

Test Name: ARIZONA CLINICAL INTERVIEW RATING SCALE

Purpose: To evaluate the interviewing techniques of medical students.

Number of Items: 16

Format: Includes six subsections: Organization, timeline,

transitional statements, questioning skills, documentation of data, and rapport. Subject responds to each item on a 5-point scale describing poor, average, and excellent performance. A sample item is presented.

Reliability: Reliability among three raters was .87 (Ebel method). Pearson product–moment coefficients were .85 and .90. Coefficients of internal consistency were .79 and .80 ($ns = 36, 60$).

Author: Stillman, P. L., et al.

Article: Construct validation of the Arizona Clinical Interview Rating Scale.

Journal: *Educational and Psychological Measurement,* Winter 1977, *37*(4), 1031–1038.

Related Research: Stillman, P. L., et al. (1976). Use of paraprofessionals to teach and evaluate interviewing skills in medical students. *Pediatrics, 55,* 769–774.

■ ■ ■

2331

Test Name: BEHAVIORAL EXPECTATION SCALES

Purpose: To evaluate faculty teaching.

Number of Items: 79

Format: Includes nine dimensions: ability to motivate, assignment and work load, delivery, depth of knowledge, grading, interpersonal relations, organization, relevance, and testing.

Reliability: Coefficients of

reproducibility ranged from .63 to .92.

Author: Kafry, D., et al.

Article: The scalability of behavioral expectation scales as a function of developmental criteria.

Journal: *Journal of Applied Psychology*, August 1976, *61*(4), 519–522.

Related Research: Smith, P. C., & Kendall, L. M. (1963). Retranslation of expectations: An approach to the construction of unambiguous anchors for rating scales. *Journal of Applied Psychology, 73*, 149–155.

■ ■ ■

2332

Test Name: BEHAVIORAL OBSERVATION SCALES

Purpose: To enable superintendents to evaluate supervisors.

Number of Items: 35

Format: The superintendent responds to each item on a 5-point scale indicating the extent to which the supervisor demonstrates each behavior.

Reliability: Cronbach's alpha was .95.

Validity: Correlation with the company's traditional performance appraisal instrument was .72.

Author: Latham, G. P., and Saari, L. M.

Article: Application of social-learning theory to training supervisors through behavioral modeling.

Journal: *Journal of Applied Psychology,* June 1979, *64*(3), 247–254.

Related Research: Latham, G. P., & Wexley, K. N. (1977). Behavioral observation scales for performance appraisal purposes. *Personnel Psychology, 30,* 239–246.

▪ ▪ ▪

2333

Test Name: COLLEGE TEACHING EFFECTIVENESS QUESTIONNAIRE

Purpose: To assess some of the characteristics ascribed to colleagues regarded as effective teachers.

Number of Items: 113 items.

Format: Subjects respond with *yes* or *no* to a series of statements when applied to the best teacher known by the respondent.

Reliability: Alpha reliabilities were .71 to .86, mode was .76.

Validity: Factor analysis resulted in five dimensions. Each scale correlated relatively low with each other. Research Activity and Recognition Scale was related to academic rank and discipline of teachers nominated as effective.

Author: Wilson, R., et al.

Article: Characteristics of effective college teachers as perceived by their colleagues.

Journal: *Journal of Educational Measurement,* 1973, *10*(1), 31–37.

▪ ▪ ▪

2334

Test Name: COLLEGE TEACHER–DESCRIPTION SCALES

Purpose: To provide colleagues with an instrument for judging the teaching effectiveness of others.

Number of Items: 113

Format: The items are grouped under the following 5 scales: each item is answered *yes* or *no:* Research Activity and Recognition, Participation in the Academic Community, Intellectual Breadth, Relation with Students, Concern for Teaching.

Reliability: .71 to .86.

Author: Wilson, R. C., et al.

Article: Characteristics of effective college teachers as perceived by their colleagues.

Journal: *Journal of Educational Measurement,* Spring 1973, *10*(1), 31–37.

Related Research: National Auxiliary Publications Service Document 01963 ASIS, National Auxiliary Publications Services, 909 Third Avenue, New York, NY 10022.

▪ ▪ ▪

2335

Test Name: COUNSELING EVALUATION INVENTORY

Purpose: To measure counselor effectiveness based upon client ratings of the counselor upon termination of the counseling relationship.

Number of Items: 21

Format: Three subscales: Counseling climate, Counselor comfort, and Client satisfaction.

Reliability: Average reliability coefficient was .72.

Author: Zarski, J., et al.

Article: Counseling effectiveness as a function of counselor social interest.

Journal: *Journal of Counseling Psychology,* January 1977, *24*(1), 1–5.

Related Research: Linden, J. D.,

et al. (1965). Development and evaluation of an inventory for rating counseling. *Personnel and Guidance Journal, 44,* 267–276.

▪ ▪ ▪

2336

Test Name: COUNSELING RATING FORM

Purpose: To assess client perceptions of counselor expertness, attractiveness, and trustworthiness.

Number of Items: 36

Format: Pairs of bipolar adjectives.

Reliability: Split-half reliabilities were .87, .84, and .90 for the three scales, respectively.

Author: Kerr, B. A., and Dell, D. M.

Article: Perceived interviewer expertness and attractiveness: Effects of interviewer behavior and attire and interview setting.

Journal: *Journal of Counseling Psychology,* November 1976, *23*(6), 553–556.

Related Research: Barak, A., & LaCrosse, M. (1975). Multidimensional perception of counselor behavior. *Journal of Counseling Psychology, 22,* 471–476.

La Crosse, M. B., & Barak, A. (1976). Differential perception of counselor behavior. *Journal of Counseling Psychology, 23,* 170–172.

▪ ▪ ▪

2337

Test Name: COUNSELOR EFFECTIVENESS SCALE

Purpose: To obtain an overall rating of the trainee's effectiveness.

Number of Items: 24

Format: A semantic differential scale.

Reliability: Interrater reliability coefficient was .79.

Author: DiMattia, D. J., and Arndt, G. M.

Article: A comparison of microcounseling and reflective listening techniques.

Journal: *Counselor Education and Supervision*, September 1974, *14*(1), 61–64.

Related Research: Ivan, A. E. (1971). *Microcounseling: Innovation in interview training*. Springfield, IL: Charles C Thomas.

■ ■ ■

2338

Test Name: COURSE EVALUATION INSTRUMENT

Purpose: To assess college instructor and course effectiveness.

Number of Items: 70

Format: Assesses instructor in class, instructor in general, subject matter, graded assignments and examinations, and text and/or other required reading.

Reliability: Test–retest reliabilities ranged from .87 to .92 for the five dimensions.

Validity: All scales differentiated ($p < .01$) between high and low learning.

Author: Schwab, D. P.

Article: Course and student characteristic correlates of the Course Evaluation Instrument.

Journal: *Journal of Applied Psychology*, December 1975, *60*(6), 742–747.

■ ■ ■

2339

Test Name: COUNSELOR EVALUATION RATING SCALE

Purpose: To rate counselor performance in counseling and supervision.

Number of Items: 27

Format: Likert scale.

Reliability: Split-half reliability was .95 and test–retest reliability was .94.

Author: Kingdon, M. A.

Article: A cost/benefit analysis of the interpersonal process recall technique.

Journal: *Journal of Counseling Psychology*, July 1975, *22*, 353–357.

Related Research: Jones, L. K. (1974, December). The counselor evaluation rating scale: A valid criterion of counselor effectiveness. *Counselor Education and Supervision, 14*(2), 112–116.

Myrick, R. D., & Kelly, F., Jr. (1971). A scale for evaluating practicum students in counseling and supervision. *Counselor Education and Supervision, 10*, 330–336.

■ ■ ■

2340

Test Name: COUNSELOR ORIENTATION QUESTIONNAIRE

Purpose: To assess counselor orientation.

Number of Items: 56

Time Required: 15 minutes.

Format: Responders indicate the degree to which they agreed or disagreed with the items on a 5-point Likert scale.

Validity: At least 83% (five out of six judges holding a PhD or EdD in counselor education or psychology) could correctly identify the item's theoretical base.

Author: Peterson, G., and Bradley, R. W.

Article: Counselor orientation and theoretical attitudes toward counseling: Historical perspective and new data.

Journal: *Journal of Counseling Psychology*, November 1980, *27*(6), 554–560.

■ ■ ■

2341

Test Name: COUNSELOR RATING FORM

Purpose: To measure counselor expertness, attractiveness, and trustworthiness.

Number of Items: 36

Format: Bipolar adjective pairs each separated by a 7-point bipolar scale.

Reliability: Split-half reliability coefficients were .87 (expertness), .84 (attractiveness), and .90 (trustworthiness; LaCrosse & Barak, 1976).

Author: Fitzgerald, L. F.

Article: Nontraditional occupations: Not for women only.

Journal: *Journal of Counseling Psychology*, May 1980, *27*(3), 252–259.

Related Research: Claiborne, C. D. (1979). Counselor verbal intervention, nonverbal behavior and social power. *Journal of Counseling Psychology, 26*, 378–383.

Freeman, H. R. (1980). Differential perceptions both between and within transcribed counselors as a function of level of facilitative conditions. *Journal of Counseling Psychology, 27*, 391–394.

LaCrosse, M. B. (1980). Perceived counselor social influence and counseling outcomes: Validity of the counselor rating form. *Journal of Counseling Psychology, 27*, 320–327.

LaCrosse, M. B., & Barak, A. (1976). Differential perception of counselor behavior. *Journal of Counseling Psychology, 23,* 170–172.

Lewis, K. N., & Walsh, W. B. (1980). Effects of value-communication style and similarity of values on counselor evaluation. *Journal of Counseling Psychology, 27,* 305–314.

■ ■ ■

2342

Test Name: COUNSELOR RATING FORM

Purpose: Assesses the client's perception of counselor expertness, attractiveness, and trustworthiness.

Number of Items: 36

Format: Bipolar adjectives scored on a 7-point scale.

Reliability: Interitem reliability coefficients were .874, .850, and .908 for expertness, attractiveness, and trustworthiness, respectively.

Author: Merluzzi, T. V., et al.

Article: Perceptions of counselor characteristics: Contributions of counselor sex, experience, and disclosure level.

Journal: *Journal of Counseling Psychology,* September 1978, *25*(5), 479–482.

Related Research: Corrigan, J. D. (1978). Salient attributes of two types of helpers: Friends and mental health professionals. *Journal of Counseling Psychology, 25,* 588–590.

Heppner, P. P., & Dixon, D. N. (1978). Effects of perceived need and counselor role on clients' behaviors. *Journal of Counseling Psychology, 25,* 514–519.

LaCrosse, M. B., & Barak, A. (1976). Differential perceptions of counselor behavior. *Journal of*

Counseling Psychology, 23, 170–172.

■ ■ ■

2343

Test Name: COUNSELOR RESPONSE QUESTIONNAIRE

Purpose: To measure beginning counseling skills.

Number of Items: 15

Format: Subject chooses which of three counselor responses of varying quality he or she thinks is most appropriate for a given client statement.

Reliability: Internal consistency alpha reliability coefficient was .77; test–retest reliability over 2 weeks was .85.

Validity: A significant difference, $t(189) = 12.40$, $p < .001$, was found between the scores of trained and untrained subjects; Wilks's lambda was .505 ($p < .001$) and there was a correlation of .704 ($p < .001$) for discriminant function scores and group membership.

Author: Stokes, J., and Lautenschlager, G.

Article: Development and validation of the counselor response questionnaire.

Journal: *Journal of Counseling Psychology,* March 1978, *25*(2), 157–163.

■ ■ ■

2344

Test Name: COUNSELOR'S FACILITATIVE CONDITIONS SCALES

Purpose: To assess the levels of three facilitative conditions offered by counselors.

Format: Includes 5 levels of each of the following: empathic understanding, communication of respect, and facilitative genuineness.

Reliability: Pearson product–moment interjudge reliabilities: .92 and .74 (empathic understanding); .82 and .75 (genuineness); .65 and .71 (respect).

Validity: Correlations with personality measures ranged from –.58 to .49.

Author: Jones, L. K.

Article: Toward more adequate selection criteria: Correlates of empathy, genuineness, and respect.

Journal: *Counselor Education and Supervision,* September 1974, *14*(1), 13–21.

Related Research: Carkhuff, R. R. (1969). *Helping and human relations.* New York: Holt, Rinehart & Winston.

■ ■ ■

2345

Test Name: DIAGNOSTIC SURVEY FOR LEADERSHIP IMPROVEMENT

Purpose: To measure satisfaction of subordinates for school leadership personnel.

Number of Items: 52

Format: Teachers respond to each item in the form of "is" or "should be" concerning their principal' s leadership.

Reliability: Reliability based upon two items from each of five scale factors was .99.

Author: Bledsoe, J. C., et al.

Article: Validity of the Mullen Diagnostic Survey for Leadership Improvement.

Journal: *Perceptual and Motor Skills,* June 1980, *50*(3, Part 1), 839–849.

Related Research: Mullen, D. J. (1976). *A diagnostic study of the human organization in schools* (Project No. 3–0476, Final

Report). Athens, GA: National Institute of Education, Department of Health, Education, and Welfare. (ERIC Document Reproduction Service No. ED 128 932, February 1977)

■ ■ ■

2346

Test Name: EXECUTIVE PARTICIPATION SCALE

Purpose: To measure the amount of influence the executive has on the decisions made in the organization.

Number of Items: 4

Reliability: Test–retest reliability was .63.

Validity: Correlation with propensity to leave the organization was –.23.

Author: Hamner, W. C., and Tosi, H. L.

Article: Relationship of role conflict and role ambiguity to job involvement measures.

Journal: *Journal of Applied Psychology*, August 1974, *59*(4), 497–499.

Related Research: Vroom, V. (1963). *Some personality determinants of the effects of participation*. Englewood Cliffs, NJ: Prentice-Hall.

■ ■ ■

2347

Test Name: HOYT-GRIM PUPIL REACTION INVENTORY

Purpose: To measure teaching effectiveness of secondary school student teachers.

Number of Items: 200

Format: Pupils make *agree, disagree,* or *no opinion* responses to each item. A few examples are provided.

Validity: With sixteen PF scores:

correlations ranged from –.66 to .60.

Author: Mattsson, K. D.

Article: Personality traits associated with effective teaching in rural and urban secondary schools.

Journal: *Journal of Educational Psychology*, February 1974, *66*(1), 123–128.

Related Research: Grim, P. R., et al. (1954). A study of instruments to appraise teaching competency. *Educational Research Bulletin, 33,* 69–72.

■ ■ ■

2348

Test Name: INSTRUCTOR EVALUATION FORM

Purpose: To provide for student evaluation of instructors.

Number of Items: 10

Format: Subject rates each item on a 5-point Likert scale ranging from *strongly agree* to *strongly disagree.*

Reliability: Coefficient alpha was .89.

Validity: Correlation with Rotter's I-E Scale was –.28.

Author: Reynolds, W. M.

Article: Relationship of affective characteristics of students to their evaluations of instructors.

Journal: *Educational and Psychological Measurement,* Winter 1979, *39*(4), 965–970.

Related Research: Battle, J. (1974). Reliability of college students evaluation of instructor's competence. *Psychological Reports,* June, *34,* 1086.

■ ■ ■

2349

Test Name: INSTRUCTOR RATING SCALE

Purpose: To evaluate the

instructor's perception of students' effort, maturity, leadership, extraversion, competence, and physical ability.

Number of Items: 40

Format: Opposing adjective pairs and 5-point scales with 1 representing the least favorable and 5 the most favorable evaluation.

Reliability: Odd–even reliability of .88.

Author: Baer, D. J., et al.

Article: Instructors' ratings of delinquents after outward bound survival training and their subsequent recidivism.

Journal: *Psychological Reports,* April 1975, *36*(2), 547–553.

Related Research: Keily, F. J., & Baer, D. J. (1968). *Outward Bound Schools as an alternative to institutionalization for adolescent delinquent boys.* Denver: Colorado Outward Bound School.

■ ■ ■

2350

Test Name: JOB INTERVIEW PERFORMANCE SELF-RATING SCALE

Purpose: To permit subjects to rate their job interview performance.

Number of Items: 17

Format: Subjects rate their performance in the job interview on 17 bipolar items.

Reliability: Internal consistency was .87.

Validity: Correlation with Body Satisfaction, .14; Self-Cathexis Scale, .31; Janis-Field-Eagly Scale, .47; Job interview expectations, .34; Judges' ratings, .22; Self-rating discrepancy scores, .59. (*N* = 87).

Author: King, M. R., and Manaster, G. J.

Article: Body image, self-esteem, expectations, self-assessments, and actual success in a simulated job interview.

Journal: *Journal of Applied Psychology,* October 1977, *62*(5), 589–594.

■ ■ ■

2351

Test Name:
MICROCOUNSELING SKILL DISCRIMINATION SCALE

Purpose: To measure the counselor-trainee's ability to discriminate between effective and ineffective counselor verbal and/or nonverbal behaviors.

Number of Items: 44 counselor–client interactions

Format: Raters rate the quality of the counselor response on a 7-point scale ranging from 1 (*most negative*) to 7 (*most positive*).

Reliability: Test–retest reliability on typescript segments based on 35 undergraduate students with 3-week time interval was .93.

Validity: Concurrent validity was established by Pearson product–moment correlations between the Scale and Carkhuff's Discrimination Rating Scale and Saltmarsh's Affective Recognition Scale. The correlations ranged between .50 and .70.

Author: Lee, D. Y., et al.

Article: Development and validation of a microcounseling skill discrimination scale.

Journal: *Journal of Counseling Psychology,* September 1976, *23*(5), 468–472.

■ ■ ■

2352

Test Name: PSYCHOTHERAPY PROCESS INVENTORY

Purpose: To rate the process of psychotherapy.

Number of Items: 74

Format: Each item was rated on a 5-point ordinal scale of either frequency or intensity and some items were rated for both.

Reliability: Aggregate ratings yielded an over-all intraclass correlation coefficient of .43 ($p <$ .05).

Author: Baer, P. E., et al.

Article: Therapists' perceptions of the psychotherapeutic process: Development of a Psychotherapy Process Inventory.

Journal: *Psychological Reports,* April 1980, *46*(2), 563–570.

Related Research: Strupp, H. H., et al. (1966). Longitudinal study of psychotherapy. In L. A. Gottschalk & A. H. Auerbach (Eds.), *Methods of research in psychotherapy* (pp. 424–476). New York: Appleton-Century-Crofts.

■ ■ ■

2353

Test Name: RELATIONSHIP INVENTORY

Purpose: Measures Empathic Understanding, Level of Regard, Unconditionality of Regard, and Congruence.

Number of Items: 64

Format: Items are scored on a 6-point agreement–disagreement scale ranging from +3 to –3.

Reliability: Test–retest reliabilities were Empathic Understanding, .89; Level of Regard, .84; Unconditionality, .90; and Congruence, .86.

Author: Bledsoe, J. C., and Layser, G. R.

Article: Effects of human relations training with houseparents on attainment of group facilitation skills.

Journal: *Psychological Reports,* June 1977, *40*(3), 787–791.

Related Research:
Barrett-Lennard, G. T. (1962). Dimension of therapist response as causal factors in therapeutic change. *Psychological Monographs, 76*(43, Whole No. 562).

■ ■ ■

2354

Test Name: RESIDENCE-HALL COUNSELOR EVALUATION SCALE

Purpose: To evaluate paraprofessional residence hall counselors.

Number of Items: 24

Format: Likert scale with five responses ranging from *strongly disagree* to *strongly agree.*

Reliability: Corrected split-half reliability was .9394.

Validity: Comparison of validating group with the original group was significant at the .05 level (validating group scores were higher than the original group).

Author: Rodgers, R. F., and Goodman, J.

Article: The development of a residence-hall counselor evaluation scale.

Journal: *Journal of College Student Personnel,* September 1975, *16*(5), 400–404.

Related Research: VanPelt, N. (1968, December). A study of the Edwards Personal Preference Record as related to residence hall counseling success. *Student Housing Research,* 1–2.

■ ■ ■

2355

Test Name: RESIDENT COUNSELOR EVALUATION SCALE

Purpose: To evaluate undergraduate residence hall counselors.

Number of Items: 24

Format: Includes six subscales: student contact, information, service, rule enforcement, interpersonal relationships, and personal qualities. Responses are made on a 5-point Likert scale from *strongly agree* to *strongly disagree.*

Reliability: Fall-Spring, $r = .489$.

Validity: With staff ranking, $r = .613$; with director's ranking, $r = .739$.

Author: Harshman, C. L., and Harshman, E. F.

Article: The evaluation of undergraduate residence hall staff: A model and instrumentation.

Journal: *Journal of College Student Personnel,* March 1974, *15*(2), 125–132.

CHAPTER 22 Vocational Evaluation
188■ ■ ■

2356

Test Name: RESIDENT EVALUATION FORM

Purpose: To assess the clinical performance of medical residents.

Number of Items: 33

Format: Includes nine categories of performance.

Reliability: Coefficients alpha ranged from .92 to .98.

Validity: Correlations with other measures ranged from .21 to .52.

Author: Keck, J. W., and Arnold, L.

Article: Development and validation of an instrument to assess the clinical performance of medical residents.

Journal: *Educational and Psychological Measurement,* Winter 1979, *39*(4), 903–908.

■ ■ ■

2357

Test Name: ROLE CONFLICT AND ROLE AMBIGUITY MEASURE

Purpose: To measure role conflict and role ambiguity.

Number of Items: 30

Reliability: Internal consistency reliabilities for conflict were .71 and for ambiguity .70.

Validity: Correlations with task perceptions and employee responses ranged from −.31 to .48.

Author: Brief, A. P., and Aldag, R. J.

Article: Correlates of role indices.

Journal: *Journal of Applied Psychology,* August 1976, *61*(4), 468–472.

Related Research: Rizzo, J., et al. (1970). Role conflict and ambiguity in complex organizations. *Administrative Science Quarterly, 15,* 150–163.

■ ■ ■

2358

Test Name: STUDENT EVALUATION OF INSTRUCTION QUESTIONNAIRE

Purpose: To measure college students' perceptions of instructor effectiveness.

Number of Items: 20

Format: Items pertain to lecturer knowledge, presentation manner, humor, enthusiasm, and student self-ratings of interest and learning gain.

Validity: Internal consistency of

.96 using the Kuder-Richardson formula 20.

Author: Williams, R. G., and Ware, J. E., Jr.

Article: Validity of student ratings of instruction under different incentive conditions: A further study of the Dr. Fox effect.

Journal: *Journal of Educational Psychology,* February 1976, *68*(1), 48–56.

Related Research: Pohlmann, J. T. (1975). A multivariate analysis of selected class characteristics and student ratings of instruction. *Multivariate Behavioral Research, 10,* 81–92.

■ ■ ■

2359

Test Name: TRUST IN SUPERVISOR SCALE

Purpose: To measure one's trust in the immediate superior, desire for promotion, and perceived supervisory influence.

Number of Items: 7

Format: Seven-point Likert scale. Items are given.

Reliability: Scale reliabilities: Trust, from .62 to .86 with a median of .68; Mobility, from .74 to .92 with a median of .82; Influence, from .53 to .77 with a median of .69.

Author: Yeager, S. J.

Article: Measurement of independent variables which affect communication: A replication of Roberts and O'Reilly.

Journal: *Psychological Reports,* December 1978, *43*(3), 1319–1324.

Related Research: Roberts, K., & O'Reilly, C. (1974). Measuring organizational communication. *Journal of Applied Psychology, 59,* 321–326.

CHAPTER 23
Vocational Interest

2360

Test Name: CAREER FACTOR CHECKLIST

Purpose: Measures the degree that career and sex role socialization factors affect people's career decisions and their awareness of these effects.

Number of Items: 28

Format: Respondents indicate on a 5-point Likert scale (*very much* to *not at all*) the degree to which the following factors affect their career decision making: (a) familial (4 items), (b) societal (4 items), (c) individual (6 items), (d) socioeconomic (5 items), (e) situational (3 items), (f) psychosocial emotional (6 items).

Reliability: Hoyt reliability coefficients for these six factors ranged from .65 to .81 and their test–retest reliabilities over a 4-week period have ranged from .49 to .83. The test–retest reliabilities for the total score over the same time interval was .83.

Author: O'Neill, J. M., et al.

Article: Research on a workshop to reduce the effects of sexism and sex role socialization on women's career planning.

Journal: *Journal of Counseling Psychology,* July 1980, *27*(4), 355–363.

Related Research: O'Neil, J. M., et al. (1980). Factors, correlates and problem areas affecting career decision making of a cross-sectional sample of students. *Journal of Counseling Psychology, 27,* 571–580.

2361

Test Name: CENTRAL LIFE INTEREST SCALE

Purpose: To assess the degree of the employee's work involvement compared with non-work activities.

Number of Items: 7

Format: Respondents rate each item on a 5-point scale from *strongly disagree* to *strongly agree.*

Reliability: Average item-total correlation was .69 and the average interitem correlation was .34. The alpha reliability was 76.

Author: Ben-Porat, A.

Article: Job involvement, central life interest and job satisfaction.

Journal: *Psychological Reports,* April 1980, *46*(2), 507–512.

Related Research: Dubin, R. (1956). Industrial workers' world: A study of the central life interests of industrial workers. *Social Problems, 3,* 131–142.

●●●

2362

Test Name: EMPLOYEES' EXPECTANCY SCALE

Purpose: To measure employees' satisfaction with their jobs.

Number of Items: 16

Format: Likert scales with responses ranging from 1 (*definitely not true of my job*) to 5 (*extremely true of my job*).

Reliability: Internal reliabilities ranged from .62 to .91.

Author: Schuler, R. S., and Kim, J. S.

Article: Employees' expectancy perceptions as explanatory variables for effectiveness of participation in decision making.

Journal: *Psychological Reports,* October 1978, *43*(2), 651–656.

Related Research: House, R. J., & Dessler, G. (1974). The path goal theory of leadership: Some post hoc and a priori tests. In J. Hunt & L. Larson (Eds.), *Contingency approaches to leadership* (pp. 29–55). Carbondale: Southern Illinois University Press.

Smith, P., et al. (1969). *The measurement of satisfaction with work and retirement: A strategy for the study of attitudes.* Chicago: Rand McNally.

Vroom, V. (1959). Some personality determinants of the effects of participation. *Journal of Abnormal and Social Psychology, 59,* 322–327.

●●●

2363

Test Name: FEMALE FACES SCALE

Purpose: To measure job satisfaction of women.

Number of Items: 11

Format: Employees "circle the face which best describes how you feel about your job in general."

Validity: Five of the 11 faces correlated at .05 or better with Kunin's (1955) male faces.

Author: Dunham, R. B., and Herman, J. B.

Article: Development of a Female Faces Scale for measuring job satisfaction.

Journal: *Journal of Applied Psychology,* October 1975, *60*(5), 629–631.

Related Research: Kunin, T. (1955). The construction of a new type of attitude measure. *Personnel Psychology, 8,* 65–78.

■ ■ ■

2364

Test Name: JOB INVOLVEMENT QUESTIONNAIRE

Purpose: To measure the extent to which one feels involved with one's job.

Number of Items: 6

Format: Items are rated on a 5-point Likert scale, reverse scored so that a high total score reflects high job involvement.

Author: Reliability was .73 and correlation was .87 with a larger 20-item composite (Lodahl & Kejner, 1965).

Author: Jones, A. P., et al.

Article: Perceived leadership behavior and employee confidence in the leader as moderated by job involvement.

Journal: *Journal of Applied Psychology,* February 1975, *60*(1), 146–149.

Related Research: Lodahl, T. M., & Kejner, M. (1965). The definition and measurement of job involvement. *Journal of Applied Psychology, 49,* 24–33.

■ ■ ■

2365

Test Name: JOB SATISFACTION MEASURE

Purpose: To determine one's satisfaction with his or her job.

Number of Items: 7

Format: Response alternatives are arranged on a 3-point scale ranging from *agree* to *disagree.*

Validity: A .70 correlation with Job Satisfaction Instrument (Brayfield & Rothe, 1951).

Author: Johnson, T. W., and Stinson, J. E.

Article: Role ambiguity, role conflict, and satisfaction: Moderating effects of individual differences.

Journal: *Journal of Applied Psychology,* June 1975, *60*(3), 329–333.

Related Research: Brayfield, A., & Rothe, H. (1951). An index of job satisfaction. *Journal of Applied Psychology, 35,* 307–311.

Johnson, T., & Graen, G. (1973). Organizational assimilation and role rejection. *Organizational Behavior and Human Performance, 10,* 72–87.

■ ■ ■

2366

Test Name: JOB SATISFACTION MEASURE

Purpose: To measure job satisfaction.

Number of Items: 12

Format: Items are rated on a 5-point scale ranging from *very dissatisfied* to *very satisfied.*

Reliability: Alpha was .92.

Validity: Correlation with conflict and ambiguity was –.28; leader facilitation and support, .29; work-group cooperation, .22; Navy satisfaction, .70; intent to reenlist, .45; self-esteem, .20; illness, –.12 (*N* = 3,725).

Author: La Rocco, J. M., and Jones, A. P.

Article: Co-worker and leader support as moderators of stress-strain relationships in work situations.

Journal: *Journal of Applied Psychology,* October 1978, *63*(5), 629–634.

Related Research: Porter, L. W., & Lawler, E. E., III. (1968). *Managerial attitudes and performance.* Havewood, IL: Irwin.

■ ■ ■

2367

Test Name: JOB SATISFACTION QUESTIONNAIRE

Purpose: To measure job satisfaction.

Number of Items: 19

Format: Includes six job facets: self-actualization, autonomy, personal worth, social affiliation, job security, and pay. Each item is answered on a 1–6 point Likert scale (*strongly agree* to *strongly disagree*). Examples are presented.

Reliability: Coefficient alpha reliability levels ranged from .70 to .85.

Author: Ivancevich, J. M.

Article: Effects of the shorter workweek on selected satisfaction and performance measures.

Journal: *Journal of Applied Psychology,* December 1974, *59*(6), 717–721.

Related Research: Porter, L. W., & Lawler, E. E., III. (1968). *Managerial attitudes and performance.* Homewood, IL: Irwin.

■ ■ ■

2368

Test Name: JOB SATISFACTION SCALE

Purpose: To measure job satisfaction.

Number of Items: 3

Format: Subjects respond to a 5-point scale with degrees ranging from *very much* to *very little.*

Reliability: Test–retest reliability was .75.

Validity: With role conflict, $r = .13$, with role ambiguity, $r = -.25$, with perceived threat and anxiety, $r = -.19$, with perceived upward influence, $r = .32$, with propensity to leave the organization, $r = -.12$.

Author: Hamner, W. C., and Tosi, H. L.

Article: Relationship of role conflict and role ambiguity to job involvement measures.

Journal: *Journal of Applied Psychology*, August 1974, *59*(4), 497–499.

Related Research: Vroom, V. (1963). *Some personality determinants of the effects of participation.* Englewood Cliffs, NJ: Prentice-Hall.

■ ■ ■

2369

Test Name: RAMAKE QUESTIONNAIRE

Purpose: To assess vocational preference in Israel.

Number of Items: 17 scores.

Format: Scored on a 3-point scale ranging from 1 (*low*) to 3 (*high*) and includes degree of attraction towards each of eight occupational fields, a prestige score of occupations selected in each field, and an average prestige score of occupations selected in all fields.

Reliability: Reliability was reported as .76.

Author: Grimm, V. E., and Nachmias, C.

Article: The effect of cognitive style and manifest anxiety on intellectual and vocational interest in adolescents.

Journal: *Journal of Vocational Behavior*, April 1977, *10*(2), 146–155.

Related Research: Meir, E. I., & Bark, A. (1974). A simple instrument for measuring vocational interests based on Roe's classification of occupations. *Journal of Vocational Behavior, 4,* 33–42.

Author Index

All numbers refer to test numbers for the current volume.

Blyth, D. A., 2134
Bochner, A., 1720
Bodden, J. L., 1707
Bode, J., 2212, 2219
Bödy, B., 2057
Boersma, F. J., 2147
Bohart, A. C., 1859
Bolstad, O. D., 2251
Bonjean, C. M., 1701
Boone, S. E., 2020
Borman, W. C., 1971
Bornstein, P. E., 1693
Boss, J. M., 1653
Boss, M., 1652
Boswell, D. A., 1774, 1812
Bower, P. M., 1695
Bowman, W. E., 1867
Boyden, J. G., 2211
Boyer, J., 1651
Boyle, D., 2139
Bradley, D. W., 2196
Bradley, R., 1705, 1948, 2086, 2208, 2340
Brannigan, G., 1708
Brant, W. D., 1754
Brantley, H. T., 1958, 2156
Braunstein, D. N., 2005, 2009, 2010
Brayfield, A., 2365
Brazelton, T. B., 1849
Breisinger, G. D., 2243
Brenneman, O. N., 1819, 1880
Breskin, S., 2286
Brett, J. E., 2104, 2240
Brief, A. P., 2357
Brigham, J. C., 1804
Brion-Meisels, L., 1852
Brodzinsky, D. M., 2170
Bronzaft, A., 1625
Brookhart, J., 1957
Brookover, W., 1850, 2128
Brooks, G. C., 1817
Brown, N. W., 1873
Brownfain, J. J., 2035
Bryant, B. K., 2076
Budner, S., 1796, 2077
Budoff, M., 1743
Bullock, D., 1840, 2190
Burbach, W. J., 1730
Burdney, T. C., 2255
Burke, R. J., 1638, 1886
Burlingame, M., 2117
Burns, D. S., 1833, 2033, 2188
Burns, K. A., 1597
Burns, M., 1800
Burns, W. J., 1597
Burr, R. G., 2067

Burstiner, I., 1925
Bush, E. S., 1635
Buss, A. H., 2252
Butler, M. C., 1866, 2067
Butterfield, D. A., 1970
Buttram, J., 1735
Byalick, R., 2189
Byrne, D., 1717, 1748, 1875

▪ ▪ ▪

Cabush, D. W., 1716
Cage, B. N., 2069
Caldwell, B., 1948
Cameron, A. E., 1987
Campbell, J., 2151, 2288
Campbell, R., 2243
Cantril, H., 2020, 2047
Caplan, R. D., 1686
Carey, R., 1656, 1693
Carey, W., 1845, 2285, 2254
Carifio, J., 1988
Carkhuff, R. R., 1714, 1716, 1889, 1890, 2344
Carlson, J. S., 2227
Carter, D. E., 2128
Cash, T. F., 1764, 1833, 2033, 2188
Cashman, J., 1968
Castenda, A., 1647
Castles, M. R., 1807
Caughren, H. J., Jr., 1994
Cautela, J., 1852, 2018
Cavin, R. S., 1707
Chabassol, D. J., 1991, 2175, 2245
Chandler, T. A., 2017, 2100, 2282
Chapman, J. W., 2147
Chapman, W., 2314, 2315
Chartier, G. M., 2146
Chelune, G. J., 1875
Chenery, M. F., 2234
Chess, S., 1884
Chester, R. D., 1787
Chiappone, D. I., 2125
Chissom, B. S., 2143
Cho, J. H., 1782
Christensen, D. L., 1990
Christiansen, J. B., 1789, 2297
Christie, R., 1721, 1775, 1821
Chun, K., 2151, 2288
Ciaoquinta, J. B., 2138
Claiborne, C. D., 2341
Clarkson, V., 1721
Clasen, R. E., 1867
Clayton, P. J., 1693
Cleland, J. F., 1703
Clifford, E., 1958, 2156

Clopton, J., 1739
Cloutier, R., 1614
Coan, R. W., 2162
Cockriel, I. W., 1605, 1609
Cohen, D., 2176
Cohen, L., 1759
Cole, C. W., 1648
Cole, J. L., 1993
Coleman, J., 2112
Coletta, A. J., 2038
Collins, B. E., 2091
Conley, J. J., 2176
Connor, J. M., 2060
Conrad, Sister C., 2043, 2124
Constantini, A., 1942, 2238
Constantinople, A., 1941
Cook, P. E., 1875, 2131
Cook, R., 1979
Cook, S. W., 1804
Cooke, R. A., 1827
Coopersmith, S., 1845, 1972, 2039, 2045, 2053, 2054, 2133
Corenblum, A. F., 1883
Corenblum, B., 1913
Corrigan, J. D., 2342
Couch, A., 2244
Coughlan, R. J., 1827
Counte, M. A., 1945
Coursey, R. D., 1914, 2024, 2187
Cowan, R., 1647, 1708, 2039, 2137
Cox, N., 1845, 1944
Crandall, C. V., 2086
Crandall, V., 1708, 2071, 2072, 2148
Crawford, J. E., 1761
Crawford, J. L., 1698
Crawford, T. J., 1761
Csoka, L. S., 2184
Cumming, E., 2173
Cunningham, D. J., 2181

▪ ▪ ▪

Dahl, H. G., 1756
Dailey, J. T., 2201
Dailey, R. C., 1712, 2088
Dansereau, F., 1896
Danzger, B., 1849
Dave, R. H., 1946
Davis, G., 1927, 1928, 2023, 2025, 2168
Davis, R. L., 1637
Dawley, H., 1629
Dean, D., 1698, 1727
DeAvila, E. A., 2224
DeCoster, D. A., 1863

Golden, C. J., 1934
Goldfried, M. R., 1672, 1673
Goldman, J., 2222
Goldman, J. A., 1941
Goldman, J. R., 2219
Goldschmid, M. L., 1614
Goldstein, I., 1759
Good, G., 1916
Good, K., 1657, 1658, 1676,
Good, L., 1657, 1658, 1676
Good, T. L., 1891
Goodkin, R., 1887
Goodman, J., 2354
Gordon, D. A., 1949, 2092
Gordon, M. E., 1836
Gosenpud, J., 1868
Gottlieb, J., 1759
Gottschalk, L., 2248
Gotz, K. O., 2034
Gough, H., 1792, 1809, 1933, 2007, 2309
Gould, S., 2083
Gouldner, A. W., 1996
Graen, G., 1896, 2365
Graybill, D., 2089
Greco, V. T., 1783
Green, R. A., 1862
Greene, C. N., 1711, 1998
Greene, R. J., 1945
Greenfeld, S., 1666
Greenhaus, J. H., 2011, 2105, 2139, 2235
Greenleaf, W., 2203
Greiler, M. M., 2036
Greiger, R. M., 1844
Griffore, R. J., 1626, 1659, 1660, 1850
Grim, P. R., 2347
Grimm, V. E., 1641, 2369
Grites, T. J., 1959
Groat, H. T., 1727
Groch, A., 2278
Grouws, D. A., 1891
Guevara, C., 1833
Guglielmino, L. M., 1742, 2193
Guiford, J., 1604, 1608, 1610, 1612, 1617, 1618, 1903, 1904, 1907, 1911, 1912, 1915, 1917, 1918, 1920, 2042, 2048, 2059, 2106, 2116, 2144, 2204, 2209, 2220, 2221, 2231
Gutkin, T. B., 2191
Guttentag, M., 2041
Guy, M. E., 2063

∎ ∎ ∎

Haber, R., 1625
Haber, R. H., 2240
Haber, R. M., 1633
Haber, R. N., 1626
Hackman, J. D., 1856
Hackman, J,R., 1981, 1999, 2000, 2001, 2036, 2182
Hales, L. W., 2317
Halinski, R. S., 1823
Hall, J., 1848, 1865, 2324
Hall, R. H., 1815
Hall, V. C., 1919
Halpern, A., 1603
Halpin, G., 1600
Halverson, C. F., 1844
Hamm, R. J., 2035
Hamner, W. C., 2121, 2346, 2368
Hane, M., 1828, 1829, 1879
Hansen, J. C., 1826
Hanson, R. A., 1947
Harassy, B. E., 2224
Hare, B. R., 2064
Harleston, B. W., 1633
Harper, F., 1625, 1629
Harren, V. A., 1757, 2205, 2206
Harris, C. L., 2141
Harris, J. E., 1707
Harris, M. B., 1864
Harris, R. E., 1664
Harris, T. L., 1873
Harshman, C. L., 2355
Harshman, E. F., 2355
Hart, G., 2296
Hartman, B. W., 2207
Hartman, T. P., 2317
Harvey, O. J., 1910
Hayes, M., 1735
Hays, C., 1691
Hawkins, J. G., 1648
Heath, R. W., 2179
Heck, E. J., 1908, 1910, 2077, 2078
Heilbrun, A. B., 1955
Heller, L. E., 1786
Helmreich, R., 1767, 1768, 2149
Hendel, D. D., 1768
Hendrick, H. W., 2200
Henry, W., 2173
Hensley, D. R., 1709
Hensley, W. E., 2138
Hepburn, M. A., 1806
Heppner, P. P., 2225, 2342
Herbert, T. T., 1838
Herbert, S., 1629
Herman, C. P., 1876
Herman, J. B., 2363
Hermans, H. J. M., 1986, 1989,

2017
Herron, W. G., 2158
Herschenson, D. B., 2172
Hertel, P., 2158
Hieronymous, A., 2028
Highlen, P. S., 1753
Hill, D. J., 1801, 2096
Hill, M. A., 1972
Hill, W. F., 1722
Hiller, J. H., 2073
Hills, R. J., 1892, 2236
Hinrichsen, J. J., 2176
Hirschfeld, R. M. A., 1715
Hocevar, D., 1921
Hock, E., 1957
Hoepfner, R., 1604, 1608, 1610, 1612, 1617, 1618, 1903, 1904, 1907, 1911, 1912, 1915, 1917, 1918, 2042, 2048, 2059, 2106, 2116, 2144, 2204, 2209, 2220, 2221, 2231
Hoffman, A. M., 1781
Hoftman, A. M., 1698
Hogan, H. W., 1777, 2293
Hogan, R., 2218, 2268
Holahan, C., 1965
Holland, J., 1921, 2233
Holland, T. R., 2252
Holland, W. E., 2008, 2124
Hollembeake, N., 1642
Holmes, G., 2183
Hood, R. W., Jr., 2324
Hoppe, C. F., 2290
Hopple, G. W., 1817
Horan, J., 1781, 1785
Horne, A. M., 2074
Horne, M. D., 1723
Horner, M. S., 1658
Hoskins, C. N., 1950
Hough, R. S., 1962
House, J., 1902
House, R. J., 1666, 1972, 2362
Houtz, J., 2226
Howat, G., 1996
Hoy, W. K., 1883, 1892, 2281, 2236
Hoyt, C. J., 1731, 1834
Huck, S., 1625
Hudgins, A. L., 2158
Hunt, J. G., 1793
Hunt, L. L., 1793
Hunt, S., 2142
Hurst, J. C., 1632
Husak, W. S., 2114
Husen, T., 1758
Hutchins, D. E., 1863
Huth, H., 2074
Hyde, E. M., 1596

Lichtenberg, J. W., 1908, 2077, 2078

Lieberman, M. A., 2107

Liebert, R. M., 1634, 1694

Lifshitz, M., 2071, 2072

Lifschitz, S., 2060

Lightsey, R., 1982

Lillesand, D. B., 1857

Linden, J. D., 2335

Lindgren, H., 1830, 2007

Lingoes, J. C., 1664

Linkowski, D. C., 1636

Linn, M. C., 2232

Lodahl, T. M., 1737, 2002, 2003, 2364

Loesch, L. C., 1936

Loevinger, J., 1944, 2290

Lollar, D., 2013

London, M., 1996

Long, B. H., 1728

Long, S., 1976, 1977, 2055, 2111

Lopez, E. M., 2011, 2139

Lorge, I., 1760

Lorr, M., 1720, 2169

Lorsch, J. W., 1865

Loucks, S., 1705

Lowman, J., 1951

Lubin, B., 1654

Lumenburg, F., 2117

Lundgren, D. C., 2140

Lutzker, D. R., 1795

Lyerly, S. B., 1871

Lynch, M., 1932

Lyon, H. L., 1643

■ ■ ■

MacDonald, A. P., 2081, 2094, 2245

Mack, D., 1876

MacKinnon, D., 1671

MacKinnon, N. J., 1667

MacMillan, A. M., 2067

Magill, R. A., 2114

Maitland, K., 2219, 2222

Mann, R. J., 2282

Manaster, G. J., 1736, 2044, 2082, 2126, 2350

Mandler, G., 1629

Mangelsdorff, D., 2149

Mann, B., 2037

Mansfield, A. F., 2032

Manson, M. P., 1639

Manton, K., 2305, 2306

Marantz, S. A., 2032

Marcia, J. E., 2237

Marcus, M., 2157

Marecek, J., 2033

Marion, P. B., 1795, 1821

Marks, D. F., 2154

Marshall, J., 1990

Marshall, S. J., 2022

Martin, C. J., 1615

Martin, H. J., 1775

Martin, J. D., 2164

Martin, R. M., 2210

Martin, W., 1654

Martinez, J. L., Jr., 1696

Mastie, M., 1938

Matranga, J. T., 1843

Matteson, D. R., 1830

Matthews, C. O., 1845

Matthews, D., 2305

Matthews, K. A., 1869

Mattocks, A., 1678

Martsson, K. D., 2347

Maxwell, B. A., 1961

Maw, E. W., 1778, 1818, 2021

Maw, W. H., 1778, 1818, 2021

McBain, G. D. M., 1796

McCarrey, M. W., 1805

McCarter, R. E., 2063

McClain, E., 1834

McClosky, H., 2305

McCutcheon, L., 1811

McDaniel, E. D., 2098

McDevitt, S. C., 1845, 1884

McDonald, T. F., 1611

McFall, R. M., 1857

McFarland, S. G., 2218, 2222

McGee, M. G., 2097

McIntire, W. G., 2054

McKechnie, G. E., 1997

McKelvie, S. J., 2154

McKinney, J. D., 1878

McPhillamy, D. J., 2188

McReynolds, P., 1833

Mahrabian, A., 1352, 1697, 1726, 1987, 1988, 2006, 2019, 2274, 2291

Meir, E. I., 2369

Melnick, J., 1899

Meltzer, G., 2158

Mendonca, J. D., 2180, 2270

Meredith, G. M., 1983

Mcrluzzi, T. V., 2342

Merrens, M. R., 2321

Merrill, L., 1840, 2190

Merrill, P. F., 2240

Messer, S. B., 2170

Metzler, J., 2097

Mezydle, L. S., 1768

Michael, J. J., 2115

Michael, W. B., 1613, 2056

Michener, A., 1882

Mijahira, S., 1995

Milgram, N. A., 2148

Milgram, R. M., 1924, 2148, 2176

Miller, J. C., 2049

Millimet, C. R., 2176, 2244

Milliones, J., 2273, 2285

Miner, J. B., 2263, 2265

Mirante, T. J., 1854

Mirels, H. L., 2321

Mischel, EW., 2146

Miskel, C., 1786

Moffett, L., 1776

Moir, D. J., 2310

Montague, J. C., Jr., 2069

Moorman, G. B., 1611

Moore, G., 1807

Moos, R. H., 1722

Morgan, B., 1636, 1873

Morgan, C. P., 1972

Morris, G. B., 1637

Morris, J. H., 2002, 2009, 2010, 2016, 2017, 2122

Morris, L. W., 1634, 1694

Morrison, J,K., 1771

Morrison, R. F., 2012, 2077, 2123, 2316,

Morse, J. J., 2070

Morstain, B. R., 1788

Mosher, D. L., 2276

Moss, H. A., 1940

Motowidlo, S. J., 1971

Mourad, S., 1742, 2193

Mouton, J. S., 1848

Mowday, R. L., 2014

Mowday, R. T., 2014

Moxnes, P., 2248

Moyer, D., 2189

Muchinsky, P. M., 1901

Muldrow, T. W., 2110, 2161, 2287

Mullen, D. J., 2345

Muller, D. G., 2115

Munson, V. M., 2326

Muntey, P. H., 1941

Muntz, D. C., 2279

Murphy, K. C., 2037

Murphy, T. J., 1668

Murray, P. 1649

Murray, V. V., 1883

Murrey, H., 1960, 2071

Musolino, R. F., 2172

Mussen, P. H., 1843

Mutran, E., 2139

Myrick, R. D., 2339

Myrow, D. L., 1616

Rosenberg, M., 2027, 2061, 2124, 2136, 2138, 2139, 2145
Rosenberg, M., 2239
Rosenkrantz, P., 2196
Rosenman, M. F., 1877
Rosenwald, G. C., 1875
Rosenzweig, S., 1675
Ross, A. C., 2044
Ross, S. M., 1616
Rothe, H., 2365
Rotter, J. B., 1718, 2068, 2074, 2075, 2091, 2112, 2269, 2288
Rowley, G., 1620, 1625, 1990
Rozswefszky, J., 1768
Rubin, Z., 1877
Rubinton, N., 2206
Runner, K., 2166
Russell, D., 1729
Russell, I., 1990
Russell, J. A., 2291
Russell, W. J. C., 1919
Ruter, M., 1872
Rychlak, J. F., 2177
Ryckman, D. B., 1854
Ryden, M. B., 2054
Ryman, D., 1669

■ ■ ■

Saal, F. E., 2003, 2017
Saari, L. M., 2332
Sales, S. M., 1886
Sallery, R., 1830
Sampson, D. L., 1795
Samuels, D. D., 1850
Sanders, M. G., 2074
Santrock. J., 2277
Sappenfield, B. R., 2141
Sarason, D., 1629
Sarason, S. B., 1635
Sassenrath, J., 1629
Sawyer, R., 2296
Schaefer, E., 2028
Scherer, S. E., 1674, 1702
Schiemann, W., 1896
Schmidt, J. P., 2176
Schneier, C. E., 2229
Schoeppe, A., 2325
Schriesheim, C. A., 1711, 1837, 1998
Schroder, H. M., 2214
Schuler, R. S., 2362
Schultz, C. B., 2017, 2019
Schuman, M. C., 1858
Schuster, D. H., 1622
Schutz, W. C., 1710

Schwab, D. P., 2338
Schwab, M. R., 2140
Schwartz, A. J., 2308
Schweisheimer, W., 1972
Schwertfeger, M., 1881
Scott, D. P., 2074
Scott, W. A., 2257
Scott, W. E., 1711, 1998
Scott, W. R., 2281, 1883
Seagren, A. T., 1894, 1897
Sease, W., 1724
Seay, T. A., 2163
Secord, P. F., 2126, 2141
Secord, P. J., 2043
Sedlacek, W. E., 1817
Segal, W., 1955, 2101, 2102
Sepie, A., 1630
Severance, L. J., 2074
Severy, L. J., 2267
Shannon, A. J., 1823
Shapiro, D. L., 1875
Shapiro, S. B., 1706
Shaver, P. R., 1685, 1706, 2142, 2261
Shavit, H., 2049
Shaw, W., 1847
Shaycoft, M. F., 2201
Sheehan, D. S., 1825, 2027, 2031, 2061, 2071, 2157
Sheehan, M. A., 1668
Sheehan, P. W., 2040, 2153
Sheffield, J. P., 1713
Shepard, R. N., 2097
Sheppard, D. I., 1936
Sherman, J. L., 1881
Sherwood, J. J., 2127
Shiflett, J. M., 1706
Shimota, H. E., 1992
Shoemaker, A. L., 2064
Shorkey, C. T., 1679, 1685, 1874, 2124, 2250, 2261
Siess, T. F., 2180, 2270
Silbergeld, S., 2050
Siler, J., 1780
Simmons, M., 1937, 2069
Simmons, R., 2027, 2061, 2134
Simpson, C. K., 2139
Sims, H. P., 2120
Sines, J. O., 1870
Singh, J. M., 1813
Singh, S., 2026
Singleton, R., Jr., 1789, 2297
Sisenwein, R. J., 1729
Skinner, D. A., 2303
Skoczylas, R. V., 1946
Slade, P., 1755

Slakter, M. J., 1620, 1826
Slaney, R. B., 2233
Slaughter, H., 1808
Slobin, M. S., 2158
Small, A. C., 2176
Smart, J. C., 1788
Smith, A., 1766
Smith, D. L., 1799
Smith, E. R., 1789
Smith, H. P., 1795
Smith, J. B., 1980
Smith, J. K., 1794
Smith, J. M., 2213
Smith, P., 2362
Smith, P. C., 2331
Smith, R. A., 2056
Smith, R. L., 2196
Smith, W., 2323
Smith, W. J., 1861
Snaith, R. P., 1692
Snyder, R. A., 2002, 2009, 2010, 2016, 2122
Solano, C. H., 1704, 1729
Soliday, S. M., 2065
Spaulding, R. I., 1878
Speas, C. M., 1864
Spence, J. T., 1766, 1767, 1768, 2110
Spencer, D. G., 2005, 2015
Spinelli, P., 1632
Spokane, A. R., 2090
Sprinthall, R. C., 1731
Srole, L., 1684
Staebler, B., 2071
Staines, J., 2289
Stapp, J., 2149
Starr, P., 1870
Steer, R. A., 1645
Steers, R. M., 2005, 2009, 2010, 2015
Steffensmeier, D., 2294
Stefic, E., 2169
Stein, K., 2288
Stein, M. I., 2022
Stein, S., 1768, 2165
Steinmann, A., 2302, 2303
Stewart, C. G., 2118
Stillman, P. L., 2330
Stinson, J. E., 2365
Stogdill, R. M., 2084
Stokes, J., 1860, 2343
Stone, E. F., 1999
Stone, L., 2176
Stott, D. H., 2191
Strahan. R., 1683, 2074
Strageland, M., 2283

Winett, B. A., 1741
Winston, R. B., Jr., 2062
Wise, D., 2296
Wittmer, J., 1745, 1890
Wolf, R. M., 1947
Wolpe, J., 1966
Wong, P. T. P., 2150
Woodbury, R., 1938
Woodley, K., 1621
Worden, J., 1649
Wright, R. J., 2229
Wright, G. Z., 2051
Wright, T. L., 1718, 2269
Wrightsman, L. S., 2151
Wurster, C. A., 2051

Wyatt, R. J., 1862

■ ■ ■

Yancey, A. V., 1813
Yeager, S. J., 2359
Yeatts, P., 2069
Yonge, G. D., 2080
Yost, E. B., 1838
Youngblood, R. L., 2138
Younis, R., 2169
Yuker, H., 1751

■ ■ ■

Zaks, M., 2295
Za'Rour, G. I., 1732
Zarski, J., 2335
Zax, M., 2174
Zedeck, S., 2183
Zelin, M. L., 2247
Zelniker, T., 1906
Zerega, W. D., Jr., 2074, 2094
Zimmerman, R. L., 1871
Zirtkel, P., 2039, 2133
Ziv, A., 2129
Zuckerman, M., 1660, 2023, 2024, 2025, 2172
Zung, W. W. K., 1682

Directory of Unpublished

Experimental Mental Measures

VOLUME 5

BERT ARTHUR GOLDMAN, EDD

Professor of Education

University of North Carolina at Greensboro

DAVID F. MITCHELL, PHD

Assistant Professor of Sociology

University of North Carolina at Greensboro

Contents

A cumulative subject index to Volumes 1 through 5 appears at the end of this book.

. . .

Preface

From the Original Printing of Volume 5, 1990

Purpose: This *Directory of Unpublished Experimental Mental Measures* Vol. 5, marks the fifth in a series of publications designed to fill a need for reference tools in behavioral and social science research. The authors recognized the need for the publication of a directory to experimental test instruments, i.e., tests that are not currently marketed commercially. It is intended that this reference provide researchers with ready access to sources of information about recently developed experimental measurement devices. The instruments are not evaluated, however it is anticipated that the directory stimulate further research of these experimental instruments. In essence, this directory provides references to nonstandardized, experimental mental measures currently undergoing development. The directory is not intended to provide evaluation of the instruments, nor is it intended to provide all necessary information for the researcher contemplating the use of a particular instrument; rather it should serve as a reference to enable the reader to identify potentially useful measures and to identify sources from which technical information concerning the instruments can be obtained.

Development: Thirty-seven relevant professional journals available to the authors were examined. The following list includes those journals which, in the judgment of the authors, contained research involving instruments of value to researchers in education, psychology, and sociology. Foreign journals were not surveyed for use in this directory. Measures identified in dissertations were excluded as a matter of expediency and because the microfilm abstracts generally contain minimal information.

American Journal of Sociology
Career Development Quarterly
Child Development
Child Study Journal
College Teaching
Comparative Social Research
Educational and Psychological Measurement
Educational Research Quarterly
Gifted Child Quarterly
Journal of Applied Psychology
Journal of College Student Personnel
Journal of Consulting and Clinical Psychology
Journal of Counseling Psychology
Journal of Creative Behavior
Journal of Educational Measurement
Journal of Educational Psychology
Journal of Educational Research
Journal of Experimental Education
Journal of General Education
Journal of Marriage and the Family
Journal of Occupational Psychology
Journal of Personality Assessment
Journal of Psychopathology and Behavioral Assessment

Journal of Reading
Journal of School Psychology
Journal of Social Psychology
Journal of Vocational Behavior
Measurement and Evaluation in Counseling and Development
Perceptual and Motor Skills
Personnel Psychology
Psychological Reports
Reading Research Quarterly
Social Psychology Quarterly
Sociological Methods and Research
Sociology and Social Research
Sociology of Education
The School Counselor

This directory lists tests described in the 1981–85 issues of the previously cited journals. An attempt was made to omit commercially published standardized tests, task-type activities such as memory word lists used in serial learning research and achievement tests developed for a single, isolated course of study. The reader should not assume that the instruments described herein form a representative sample of the universe of unpublished experimental mental measures.

Organization: This volume incorporates an additional category not found in the previous volumes, i.e., Adjustment—Vocational. Following is a brief description of each of the twenty-four categories under which the authors grouped the measures of Volume 5:

Achievement: Measure learning and/or comprehension in specific areas. Also include tests of memory and tests of drug knowledge.

Adjustment—Educational: Measure academic satisfaction. Also include tests of school anxiety.

Adjustment—Psychological: Evaluate conditions and levels of adjustment along the psychological dimension including, for example, tests of mood, fear of death, anxiety, depression, etc.

Adjustment—Social: Evaluate aspects of interactions with others. Also include tests of alienation, conformity, need for social approval, social desirability, instruments for assessing interpersonal attraction and sensitivity.

Adjustment—Vocational: Identify burnout, vocational maturity, job-related stress, job frustration, job satisfaction, etc.

Aptitude: Predict success in given activities.

Attitude: Measure reaction to a variety of experiences and objects.

Behavior: Measure general and specific types of activities such as classroom behavior and drug-use behavior.

Communication: Evaluate information exchange. Also include tests of self-disclosure and counselor/client interaction.

Concept Meaning: Test one's understanding of words and other concepts. Also include tests of conceptual structure, style, and information processing.

Creativity: Measure ability to reorganize data or information into unique configurations. Also include tests of divergent thinking.

Development: Measure emerging characteristics, primarily for preschool ages. Also include tests of cognitive and moral development.

Family: Measure intrafamily relations. Also include tests of marital satisfaction, nurturance, parental interest, and warmth.

Institutional Information: Evaluate institutions and their functioning.

Motivation: Measure goal strength. Also include measures of curiosity.

Perception: Determine how one sees self and other objects. Also include tests dealing with empathy, imagery, locus of control, self-concept, and time.

Personality: Measure general personal attributes. Also include biographical information and defense mechanisms.

Preference: Identify choices. Also include tests of preference for objects, taste preference, and sex-role preference.

Problem-Solving and Reasoning: Measure general ability to reason through a number of alternative solutions, to generate such solutions to problems, etc.

Status: Identify a hierarchy of acceptability.

Trait Measurement: Identify and evaluate unitary traits. Also include tests of anger, anxiety, authoritarianism, blame, and cheating.

Values: Measure worth one ascribes to an object or activity. Include tests of moral, philosophical, political, and religious values.

Vocational Evaluation: Evaluate a person for a specific position.

Vocational Interest: Measure interest in specific occupations and vocations as well as interest in general categories of activity.

The choice of the category under which each test was grouped was determined by the purpose of the test and/or its apparent content. The authors attempted to include the following facts regarding each test, however, in many cases not all of these facts were provided in the journal article:

Test Name
Purpose
Description
  Number of items
  Time required
  Format
Statistics
  Reliability (In most cases the particular design used to assess consistency is specified)
  Validity (Includes correlation with other tests and group difference information which help to define the characteristic being measured by the test)
Source
  Author
  Title
  Journal (Includes date of publication, volume, and page number)
Related Research
  Information identifying publications related to the source.

Volume 5 contains only those tests for which the journal article presented as a minimum: Test Name, Purpose, Source, and at least four facts from either Description, Statistics, and Related Research.

The reader is alerted to the fact that the numbers within the Index refer to test numbers rather than to page numbers as was the case with Volume 1. As a convenience to the reader, the authors have incorporated the indices from the four previous volumes in this Index and in so doing they converted all page numbers to test numbers. Thus, numbers 1 through 339 refer to tests of Volume 1, numbers 340 through 1034 refer to tests of Volume 2, numbers 1035 through 1595 refer to tests of Volume 3, numbers 1596 through 2369 refer to tests of Volume 4, and numbers 2370 through 3665 refer to tests of Volume 5. As was the case with Volume 4, a noncumulative author index is included.

The authors express their appreciation to Elizabeth House for typing the manuscript with assistance from Anita Hawkins. Additional thanks is extended to Ms. Katherine Poole and Deetra Thompson for their help in preparing the indices. Finally, the authors wish to thank the William C. Brown Publishers for taking over the publication of the directories.

Bert Arthur Goldman
David F. Mitchell

CHAPTER 1
Achievement

2370

Test Name: ANAPHORA TEST

Purpose: To measure understanding of anaphoric relations.

Number of Items: 50

Format: Sample item is presented.

Reliability: .87

Author: Johnson, B., and Johnson, D.

Article: Elementary students' comprehension of anaphora in well-formed stories.

Journal: *Journal of Educational Research*, March/April 1985, *78*(4), 221–223.

Related Research: Halliday, M. A., & Hasan, R. (1976). *Cohesion in English*. London: Longman.

...

2371

Test Name: BASIC MATHEMATICS TEST

Purpose: To measure basic mathematics skills.

Number of Items: 36

Format: Multiple-choice.

Reliability: Alpha was .89.

Validity: Correlations with Statistical Attitude Survey were .27 and .37.

Author: Roberts, D. M., and Saxe, J. E.

Article: Validity of a statistics attitude survey: A follow-up study.

Journal: *Educational and*

Psychological Measurement, Autumn 1982, *42*(3), 907–912.

...

2372

Test Name: BASIC STATISTICS TEST

Purpose: To measure basic statistics.

Number of Items: 20

Format: Covers descriptive statistics from frequency distributions to correlation.

Reliability: Alphas were .63 (pretest) and .55 (posttest).

Validity: Correlations with Statistical Attitude Survey ranged from .25 to .42.

Author: Roberts, D. M., and Saxe, J. E.

Article: Validity of a statistics attitude survey: A follow-up study.

Journal: *Educational and Psychological Measurement,* Autumn 1982, *42*(3), 907–912.

...

2373

Test Name: CHILDREN'S HANDWRITING SCALE

Purpose: To measure rate and quality of penmanship (grades 3–8).

Number of Items: 1 paragraph of 197 letters (except *x* and *z*) is evaluated on 5 characteristics.

Format: Children read paragraph, then copy it as well as they can. Progress in the first two minutes is marked. Characteristics rated are

form, slant, rhythm, space, and general appearance.

Reliability: For single rater, .64 to .82.

Validity: Significant relationship found between boys and girls on letter per minute rate.

Author: Phelps, J., et al.

Article: The Children's Handwriting Scale.

Journal: *Journal of Educational Research,* September/October 1985, *79*(1), 46–50.

...

2374

Test Name: COUNSELING INFORMATION SCALE

Purpose: To measure knowledge about counseling.

Number of Items: 8

Format: Multiple-choice.

Reliability: Split-half reliability was .67.

Validity: Counselors scored higher than students ($p < .001$).

Author: Davidshofer, C. O., and Richardson, G. G.

Article: Effects of precounseling training.

Journal: *Journal of College Student Personnel,* November 1981, *22*(6), 522–527.

...

2375

Test Name: DIAGNOSTIC INVENTORY

Purpose: To measure and evaluate

manuscript and cursive writing.

Number of Items: 7

Format: Trained raters rate writing on a 3-point scale.

Reliability: Interrater reliability was .43 or above on global score and .18 or above on separate facets of writing.

Author: Armitage, D., and Ratzlaff, H.

Article: The non-correlation of writing and print skills.

Journal: *Journal of Educational Research,* January/February 1985, *78*(3), 174–177.

Related Research: Herrick, V. E., & Erlenbacher, A. (1963). The Evolution of Legibility in Handwriting. In V. E. Herrick (Ed.), *New horizons for research in handwriting.* Madison: University of Wisconsin Press.

■ ■ ■

2376

Test Name: HANDWRITING LEGIBILITY

Purpose: To measure legibility of handwriting.

Number of Items: 6 letters.

Format: Letters are presented two at a time on worksheets and evaluated by a plastic overlay.

Reliability: Interscorer agreement was 96%.

Author: Sims, E. V., Jr., and Weisberg, P.

Article: Effects of page prompts on beginning handwriting legibility.

Journal: *Journal of Educational Research,* July/August 1984, *77*(6), 360–365.

Related Research: Helwig, J., et al. (1976). The measurement of manuscript letter strokes. *Journal of Applied Behavior Analysis, 9,* 231–236.

2377

Test Name: HEBREW VISUAL DISCRIMINATION TEST

Purpose: To measure nonverbal visual discrimination.

Number of Items: 50

Format: Match-to-model task employing Hebrew letter script with sets of items for letters, syllables, words, phrases, and a total score.

Reliability: Kuder-Richardson formula 20 internal-consistency reliability estimate for the total was .91.

Validity: Correlations with other variables ranged from –.13 to .57.

Author: Morrison, J. A., and Michael, W. B.

Article: Validity of measures reflecting visual discrimination and linguistic constructs for a sample of second-grade Hispanic children receiving reading instruction in Spanish.

Journal: *Educational and Psychological Measurement,* Summer 1984, *44*(2), 333–351.

Related Research: Velluntino, F. R., et al. (1973). Visual recall in poor and normal readers as a function of orthographic-linguistic familiarity. *Cortex, 9,* 368–384.

■ ■ ■

2378

Test Name: HUMOR PERCEPTIVENESS TEST— REVISED

Purpose: To measure humor comprehension.

Number of Items: 32

Format: Items are in the form of joke completions. All items are presented.

Reliability: Reliability coefficients (split-half, Kuder-Richardson,

alternate form) ranged from .84 to .93.

Validity: Correlation with WAIS IQ was .58.

Author: Feingold, A.

Article: Measuring humor ability: Revision and construct validation of the Humor Perceptiveness Test.

Journal: *Perceptual and Motor Skills,* February 1983, *56*(1), 159–166.

Related Research: Feingold, A. (1982). Measuring humor: A pilot study. *Perceptual and Motor Skills, 54,* 986.

■ ■ ■

2379

Test Name: JOBS-CAREER KEY

Purpose: To measure general occupational knowledge.

Number of Items: 147

Format: Multiple-choice items measuring three areas: education-training requirements, job conditions and characteristics, and worker relationships.

Reliability: Coefficient alphas were .79 and .83. Test–retest reliability was $r = .62$ (2 weeks).

Author: Taylor, M. S.

Article: The roles of occupational knowledge and vocational self-concept crystallization in students' school-to-work transition.

Journal: *Journal of Counseling Psychology,* October 1985, *32*(4), 539–550.

Related Research: Blank, J. R. (1979). Jobs-Career Key: A test of occupational information. *Vocational Guidance Quarterly, 26,* 9–17.

■ ■ ■

2380

Test Name: JOB KNOWLEDGE SURVEY

Purpose: To assess knowledge.

Number of Items: 48

Format: Each item is evaluated as having a high, medium, or low involvement with data, people, and things.

Reliability: Test–retest reliabilities ranged from .44 to .80.

Validity: Correlations with Work Values Inventory ranged from −.39 to .37.

Author: Sampson, J. P., and Loesch, L. C.

Article: Relationships among work values and job knowledge.

Journal: *Vocational Guidance Quarterly*, March 1981, *29*(3), 229–235.

Related Research: Loesch, L. C., et al. (1978). A field test of an instrument for assessing job knowledge. *Measurement and Evaluation in Guidance*, *11*, 26–33.

■ ■ ■

2381

Test Name: KINDERGARTEN PERFORMANCE PROFILE

Purpose: To measure and rate kindergarten children's performance.

Number of Items: 8 (4 classroom work skills and 4 classroom social skills).

Reliability: Test–retest reliability was .70–.84 for work skills, .69–.77 for social skills. Interrater reliability was .67–.77 for work skills, .45–.65 for social skills. Cronbach's alpha was .80–.82 for composite scores.

Author: Swartz, J. P., and Walker, D. K.

Article: The relationship between teacher ratings of kindergarten classroom skills and second grade

achievement scores: An analysis of gender differences.

Journal: *Journal of School Psychology*, 1984, *22*(2), 209–217.

Related Research: DiNola, A. J., et al. (1970). *Preschool and primary performance profile*. Ridgefield, NJ: Educational Performance Associates.

■ ■ ■

2382

Test Name: KNOWLEDGE OF BEHAVIORAL PRINCIPLES AS APPLIED TO CHILDREN SCALE

Purpose: To measure knowledge parents have of behavioral principles for child management.

Number of Items: 50

Format: Multiple-choice. Sample item is presented.

Reliability: Split-half ranged from .76 to .88. Kuder-Richardson formula 20 ranged from .59 to .88.

Author: McLoughlin, C. S.

Article: Utility and efficacy of knowledge of behavioral principles as applied to children.

Journal: *Psychological Reports*, April 1985, *56*(2), 463–467.

Related Research: O'Dell, S. L., et al. (1979). An instrument to measure knowledge of behavioral principles as applied to children. *Journal of Behavior Therapy and Experimental Psychiatry*, *10*, 29–34.

■ ■ ■

2383

Test Name: MATHEMATICS ACHIEVEMENT TEST

Purpose: To measure achievement in mathematics.

Number of Items: 70

Format: Test-type questions

covering concepts in skills. Sample items are presented in English, Japanese, and Chinese.

Reliability: Cronbach's alpha ranged from .93 to .95 across grades and countries.

Validity: United States students scored significantly lower than Japanese and Taiwanese students ($p < .05$).

Author: Stigler, J. W., et al.

Article: Curriculum and achievement in mathematics: A study of elementary school children in Japan, Taiwan, and the United States.

Journal: *Journal of Educational Psychology*, April 1982, *74*(2), 315–322.

■ ■ ■

2384

Test Name: MEMORY ASSESSMENT QUESTIONNAIRE

Purpose: To assess six aspects of a memory.

Number of Items: 7

Format: All but two items were in Likert scale form. All items are presented.

Reliability: Interjudge reliability for each item ranged from .23 to .93.

Author: Ireland, M. S., and Kernan-Schloss, L.

Article: Pattern analysis of recorded daydreams, memories, and personality type.

Journal: *Perceptual and Motor Skills*, February 1983, *56*(1), 119–125.

Related Research: Starker, S. (1973). Aspects of inner experience, autokinesis, daydreaming, dream recall and cognitive style. *Perceptual and Motor Skills*, *36*, 663–673.

2385

Test Name: MEMORY CHECK

Purpose: To measure mental status.

Number of Items: 15

Format: Instrument is administered directly to the person being evaluated. All items are presented.

Validity: Correlation with Competence Index was −.67; with Impairment Index was −.69; with Functional Behavior Survey was .71.

Author: Tobacyk, J., et al.

Article: Two brief measures for assessing mental competence in the elderly.

Journal: *Journal of Personality Assessment,* December 1983, *47*(6), 648–655.

Related Research: Dixon, J. C. (1965). Cognitive structure in senile conditions with some suggestions for developing a brief screening test of mental status. *Journal of Gerontology, 20,* 41–49.

■ ■ ■

2386

Test Name: MEMORY IMPAIRMENT SCALE

Purpose: To measure memory impairment.

Number of Items: 10

Format: Observation rating scale. All items are presented. Observers use a 6-point frequency scale (*always* to *not at all*).

Reliability: Item-remainder correlations ranged from .60 to .93. Interrater reliability (two raters) was .86. Generalizability coefficients ranged from .69 to .96.

Validity: Correlation with assorted memory tasks ranged from .48 to .86 (*p* < .05) and with Wechsler

Memory Scale was .68 (*p* < .01).

Author: Knight, R. G., and Godfrey, H. P. D.

Article: Reliability and validity of a scale for rating memory impairment in hospitalized amnesiacs.

Journal: *Journal of Consulting and Clinical Psychology,* October 1984, *52*(5), 769–773.

■ ■ ■

2387

Test Name: MORPHOGRAPHIC TRANSFER TEST

Purpose: To measure the ability to apply morphographic knowledge.

Number of Items: 15 (Test A).

Format: Multiple-choice. Sample item is presented.

Reliability: Cronbach's alpha was .81.

Author: Jacka, B.

Article: The teaching of defined concepts: A test of Gragne and Briggs' model of instructional design.

Journal: *Journal of Educational Research,* March/April 1985, *78*(4), 224–227.

Related Research: Gragne, R. M., & Briggs, L. J. (1974). *Principles of instructional design.* New York: Holt, Rinehart & Winston.

■ ■ ■

2388

Test Name: ORAL READING AND RECALL EVALUATION SCALE

Purpose: To measure reading comprehension ability.

Number of Items: 20

Format: 6-step scale from *highly ineffective* to *highly effective.*

Reliability: Alpha was .89.

Validity: Correlations with Reading Miscue Inventory ("moderately effective" RMI subjects yielded moderate scores on this scale).

Author: Taylor, J. B.

Article: Influence of speech variety on teachers' evaluation of reading comprehension.

Journal: *Journal of Educational Psychology,* October 1983, *73*(5), 662–667.

■ ■ ■

2389

Test Name: PERCEPTIVE LISTENING TEST

Purpose: To measure musical knowledge.

Number of Items: 20

Format: Test consists of 9 multiple-choice definition questions and 11 musical excerpts on audiotape. Sample items are presented.

Reliability: Cronbach's alpha was .83.

Validity: Correlated .45 with IQ.

Author: Bledsoe, J. C.

Article: Efficacy of popular music in learning music concepts in seventh grade general music classes.

Journal: *Psychological Reports,* April 1984, *51*(2), 381–382.

■ ■ ■

2390

Test Name: PRINT AWARENESS TEST

Purpose: To measure prereaders' understanding of the function of print.

Number of Items: 15

Format: Questions asked of child with pictures illustrating possible answers.

Reliability: Internal consistency was .85.

Validity: Correlations between print awareness scale and other measures of general ability and prereading skills ranged from –.05 to .77.

Author: Huba, M. E., and Kontos, S.

Article: Measuring print awareness in young children.

Journal: *Journal of Educational Research,* May/June 1985, *78*(5), 272–279.

■ ■ ■

2391

Test Name: READING MISCUE INVENTORY

Purpose: To measure comprehension effectiveness of oral reading by assessing how reader processes information being read.

Number of Items: Varies.

Format: Takes into account deviations made by readers while reading and how the deviations affect intended meaning and ability to recall information. Sample items given.

Reliability: Ranged from .89 to .95.

Author: Taylor, J. B.

Article: Influence of speech variety on teachers' evaluations of reading comprehension.

Journal: *Journal of Educational Psychology,* October 1983, *75*(5), 662–667.

Related Research: Goodman, Y., & Burke, C. (1972). *Reading miscue inventory manual: Procedures for diagnosis and evaluation.* New York: Macmillan.

■ ■ ■

2392

Test Name: READING SPAN TEST

Purpose: To measure ability to store and process information in working memory.

Number of Items: 6 (sets of unrelated sentences with 2–5 sentences preset).

Format: Sample item is presented. Sentences are presented on screens for 8 seconds, and then respondent is asked to write down the last word in each. Scores are percentage of final words recalled.

Validity: Correlates .53 ($p < .01$) with Nelson-Denny Reading Test.

Author: Masson, M. E. J., and Miller, J. A.

Article: Working memory and individual differences in comprehension and memory of text.

Journal: *Journal of Educational Psychology,* April 1983, *75*(2), 314–318.

Related Research: Daneman, M., & Carpenter, P. A. (1980). Individual differences in working memory and reading. *Journal of Verbal Learning and Verbal Behavior, 19,* 450–466.

■ ■ ■

2393

Test Name: SEX INFORMATION QUESTIONNAIRE

Purpose: To measure knowledge about human sexual functioning.

Number of Items: 30

Format: Multiple-choice format. Examples are presented.

Reliability: Test–retest reliability was .67.

Author: Alyn, J. H., and Becker, L. A.

Article: Feminist therapy with chronically and profoundly disturbed women.

Journal: *Journal of Counseling*

Psychology, April 1984, *31*(2), 202–208.

Related Research: McDermott, L. (1980). *Sex Information Questionnaire.* Unpublished manuscript, University of Colorado, Colorado Springs.

■ ■ ■

2394

Test Name: SPANISH VISUAL DISCRIMINATION TEST

Purpose: To measure second graders' verbally based Spanish visual discrimination.

Number of Items: 59

Format: Match-to-model task including sets of items for letters, syllables, words, phrases, and a total score.

Reliability: Kuder-Richardson formula 20 internal-consistency reliability coefficients were .82 and .85.

Validity: Correlations with other variables ranged from –.11 to .57.

Author: Morrison, J. A., and Michael, W. B.

Article: Validity of measures reflecting visual discrimination and linguistic constructs for a sample of second-grade Hispanic children receiving reading instruction in Spanish.

Journal: *Educational and Psychological Measurement,* Summer 1984, *44*(3), 333–351.

Related Research: Ransom, G. A. (1978). *Preparing to teach reading.* Boston: Little, Brown.

■ ■ ■

2395

Test Name: TEACHER RATING SCALE

Purpose: To obtain ratings of students by teachers on students' reading level.

Number of Items: 7

Format: Teachers choose the one item that best describes a student. All items are presented.

Reliability: Correlation between two raters was .58 ($p < .001$).

Validity: Correlates from .64 to .66 with California Achievement Test Reading Scores.

Author: Powers, S., and De La Garza, J.

Article: Stability and predictive validity of the Teacher Rating Scale.

Journal: *Psychological Reports,* October 1985, *52*(2), 543–546.

Related Research: Slaughter, H. B. (1980). *Teacher Rating Scale.* Unpublished manuscript, Tucson Unified School District, ECIA Chapter 1 project, Tucson, AZ.

■ ■ ■

2396

Test Name: TEST ON ECONOMIC DECISION-MAKING (TED)

Purpose: To assess the ability to apply and use economic principles.

Number of Items: 30

Format: Multiple-choice (4-choices per question).

Reliability: Guttman split-half reliability was .84.

Author: Kourilsky, M.

Article: Economic socialization of children: Attitude toward the distribution of rewards.

Journal: *Journal of Social Psychology,* October 1981, *115*(first half), 45–57.

■ ■ ■

2397

Test Name: VISUAL MEMORY TEST

Purpose: To measure the ability to remember pictures.

Number of Items: 14

Format: Multiple-choice.

Reliability: Kuder-Richardson formula reliability was .49.

Author: Shaw, G. A.

Article: The use of imagery by intelligent and by creative school children.

Journal: *Journal of General Psychology,* April 1985, *112*(2), 153–171.

Related Research: Marks, D. F. (1973). Visual imagery differences in the recall of pictures. *British Journal of Psychology, 61,* 17–24.

■ ■ ■

2398

Test Name: WORD READING TASK MEASURE

Purpose: To measure phonics achievement of learning disabled children.

Number of Items: 64 words.

Time Required: 6 seconds per word.

Format: Children presented words on index cards and responses recorded on tape and evaluated by trained examiners. Sample items are presented.

Reliability: Posttest split-half reliabilities ranged from .74 to .92.

Validity: Pretest scores were very low. IQ, age, and sex were not strongly related to posttest scores (.13 was maximum correlation).

Author: Fayne, H. R., and Bryant, N. D.

Article: Relative effects of various words synthesis strategies on the phonics achievement of learning disabled youngsters.

Journal: *Journal of Educational Psychology,* October 1981, *73*(5), 616–623.

CHAPTER 2
Adjustment—Educational

2399

Test Name: ACADEMIC AND SOCIAL INTEGRATION INSTRUMENT

Purpose: To measure the academic and social integration of students in their colleges.

Number of Items: 32

Format: Multiple-choice and Likert-format agreement scales.

Reliability: Alphas ranged from .46 to .64 across the two subscales.

Author: Pascarella, E. T., and Terenzini, P. T.

Article: Predicting voluntary freshmen year persistence/withdrawal behavior in a residential university: A path analytic validation of Tinto's Model.

Journal: *Journal of Educational Psychology*, April 1983, *75*(2), 215–226.

Related Research: Tinto, V. (1975). Dropout from higher education: A theoretical synthesis of recent research. *Review of Educational Research, 45,* 89–125.

•••

2400

Test Name: ADJUSTMENT TO COLLEGE SCALE

Purpose: To measure adjustment to college.

Number of Items: 67

Format: Students respond to each item on a 9-point scale. Includes four subscales: academic adjustment, social adjustment, personal/emotional, goal commitment/institutional attachment and the full scale. Some examples are presented.

Reliability: Coefficient alphas ranged from .78 to .95.

Author: Baker, R. W., et al.

Article: Expectation and reality in freshmen adjustment to college.

Journal: *Journal of Counseling Psychology,* January 1985, *32*(1), 94–103.

Related Research: Baker, R. W., & Siryk, B. (1984). Measuring adjustment to college. *Journal of Counseling Psychology, 31,* 179–189.

•••

2401

Test Name: ADJUSTMENT TO COLLEGE SCALE

Purpose: To measure adjustment to college.

Number of Items: 52

Format: Includes four subscales: academic, social, personal-emotional, general. Examples are provided.

Reliability: Cronbach's alpha ranged from .82 to .88 for the subscales and from .92 to .94 for the full scale.

Validity: Point-biserial correlations with attrition after 1 year ranged from –.02 to –.43 (Ns = 172 to 233). Point-biserial correlations with freshman year grade point average ranged from –.14 to .32 (Ns = 171 to 229).

Author: Baker, R. W., and Siryk, B.

Article: Measuring adjustment to college.

Journal: *Journal of Counseling Psychology,* April 1984, *31*(2), 179–189.

•••

2402

Test Name: CHECKLIST OF POSITIVE AND NEGATIVE THOUGHTS

Purpose: To measure positive and negative thoughts affecting concentration and performance on tests.

Number of Items: 37

Format: Checklist. All items are presented.

Reliability: Alpha was .77 for positive thoughts and .79 for negative thoughts.

Author: Gralassi, J. P., et al.

Article: Behavior of high, moderate and low test-anxious students during an actual test situation.

Journal: *Journal of Consulting and Clinical Psychology,* February 1985, *49*(1), 51–62.

Related Research: Sarason, I. G., et al. (1978). The test anxiety scale: Concept and research. In C. D. Spielberger & I. G. Sarason (Eds.), *Stress and anxiety, 5.* Washington, DC: Hemisphere.

•••

2403

Test Name: CHECKLIST OF POSITIVE AND NEGATIVE THOUGHTS—MODIFIED

Purpose: To enable students to provide data on the frequency of positive and negative thoughts outside of an actual testing situation and to assess frequency of control over negative thoughts.

Number of Items: 56

Format: Part one: Subjects rate each of 37 positive and negative thoughts on a 5-point scale, indicating how often each thought occurred to them while taking exams (1 = *never*, 5 = *very often*). Part two: Subjects rate each of the 19 negative thoughts on a 6-point scale indicating how often they can control each type of thought (0 = *never had a thought like this*, 1 = *can never stop this type of thought*, 5 = *can stop this type of thought very often*).

Reliability: Cronbach's alphas ranged from .86 to .94.

Author: Brown, S. D., and Nelson, T. L.

Article: Beyond the uniformity myth: A comparison of academically successful and unsuccessful test-anxious college students.

Journal: *Journal of Consulting Psychology*, July 1983, *30*(3), 367–374.

Related Research: Galassi, J. P., et al. (1981). Behavior of high, moderate, and low test-anxious students during an actual test situation. *Journal of Consulting and Clinical Psychology, 49,* 51–62.

■ ■ ■

2404

Test Name: CHILDREN'S ACADEMIC ANXIETY INVENTORY

Purpose: To measure academic anxieties.

Number of Items: 12 (3 per 4 subject areas).

Format: Items rated on 5-point Likert categories. Sample items are presented.

Reliability: Test–retest reliability was .70 to .85 for seventh graders; .50 to .65 for fourth graders. Alphas ranged from .50 to .65 across areas (all children).

Validity: Correlations with Otis-Lennon Mental Ability test ranged from −.20 to −.43.

Author: Gottfried, A. E.

Article: Relationships between academic intrinsic motivation and anxiety in children and young adolescents.

Journal: *Journal of School Psychology*, 1982, *20*(3), 205–215.

■ ■ ■

2405

Test Name: CHILDREN'S COGNITIVE ASSESSMENT QUESTIONNAIRE

Purpose: To measure perceived negative evaluations, off-task thoughts, positive evaluations, and on-task thoughts.

Number of Items: 40

Format: Yes–no response format. All items are presented.

Reliability: Alphas ranged from .67 to .82 across subscales. Test–retest reliability ranged from .63 to .71.

Validity: Discriminated between low, moderate, and highly anxious children (canonical correlation was .60, $p < .01$).

Author: Zatz, S., and Chassin, L.

Article: Cognitions of test-anxious children.

Journal: *Journal of Consulting and Clinical Psychology*, August 1983, *51*(4), 526–534.

■ ■ ■

2406

Test Name: CLASSROOM ADJUSTMENT SCALE

Purpose: To measure children's classroom adjustment.

Number of Items: 41

Format: Includes three factors of acting-out, moodiness, and learning.

Reliability: Test–retest reliability was .92.

Author: Jason, L. A., et al.

Article: Establishing supervising behaviors in eighth graders and peer-tutoring behaviors in first graders.

Journal: *Child Study Journal*, 1981, *11*(4), 201–219.

Related Research: Lorion, R. P., et al. (1975). Normative and parametric analysis of school maladjustment. *American Journal of Community Psychology, 3,* 291–301.

■ ■ ■

2407

Test Name: COLLEGE DESCRIPTIVE INDEX

Purpose: To measure a student's satisfaction with college experience.

Number of Items: 129

Format: Includes the following scales: teachers, administrators, self, courses, parents, other students, noncourse activities, and finances. All adjectives constituting the items are included.

Reliability: Alphas ranged from .73 to .91.

Validity: Correlations with variables ranged from .10 to .53.

Author: Reed, J. G., et al.

Article: Development of the college descriptive index: A measure of student satisfaction.

Journal: *Measurement and Evaluation in Counseling and Development*, July 1984, *17*(2), 67–82.

Related Research: Downey, R. G., et al. (1980). Development and validation of a set of university involvement scales. *Measurement and Evaluation in Guidance, 13,* 158–168.

. . .

2408

Test Name: COLLEGE OPTIMISM SCALE

Purpose: To measure optimism about college life.

Number of Items: 15

Format: Items rated on a 4-point scale. All items are presented.

Reliability: Alpha was .85.

Validity: Correlates −.26 with Taylor Manifest Anxiety Scale, −.44 with Zung Depression Inventory, and −.22 with Neuroticism.

Author: Prola, M.

Article: A scale to measure optimism about college life.

Journal: *Psychological Reports,* April 1984, *54*(2), 555–557.

. . .

2409

Test Name: COMPETENCE INVENTORY FOR COLLEGE STUDENTS

Purpose: To assess degree of competence students express in dealing with interpersonal and academic life while at college.

Number of Items: 52

Format: Raters evaluate subjects' role-played response on a 5-point continuum of competence.

Reliability: Alphas were .90 (all items); .85 (interpersonal items); and .79 (academic items).

Validity: Correlates with GPA (.32, $p < .01$), but not with the Beck's Depression Inventory (−.09, $p > .05$).

Author: Fisher-Beckfield, D., and McFall, R. M.

Article: Development of a competence inventory for college men and evaluation of relationships between competence and depression.

Journal: *Journal of Consulting and Clinical Psychology,* October 1982, *50*(5), 697–705.

Related Research: Goldfried, M. R., & D'Zurilla, T. J. (1969). A behavioral analytic model for assessing competence. In C. D. Spielberger (Ed.), *Current topics in clinical and community psychology* (Vol. 1). New York: Academic Press.

. . .

2410

Test Name: FEAR OF CONSEQUENCE OF SUCCESS SCALE

Purpose: To measure degree of fear if one were successful in academic work.

Number of Items: 18

Format: 7-point agree–disagree response categories. All items are presented.

Reliability: Test–retest (8-week interval) ranged from .54 to .57 over subscales. Cronbach's alpha ranged from .83 to .88 over subscales.

Validity: Correlates significantly (.60 or higher) with Fear of Success (Good & Good, 1973) and with Adult Audience Sensitivity Inventory (.24 or higher; Pavio, 1957, 1958).

Author: Ishiyama, F. I., and Chabassol, D. J.

Article: Fear of success consequence scale: Measure of fear of social consequences of academic success.

Journal: *Psychological Reports,* April 1984, *54*(2), 499–504.

2411

Test Name: FEAR OF SUCCESS QUESTIONNAIRE

Purpose: To identify people who fear academic success.

Number of Items: 83

Format: Yes–no responses are made to questions that specifically describe situations. Examples are provided.

Reliability: Kuder-Richardson formula 20 reliability was .90.

Validity: Correlations with debilitating anxiety, .57; internal-external control, .24; self-esteem, .47; and need to fail scale, .77.

Author: Pappo, M.

Article: Fear of success: The construction and validation of a measuring instrument.

Journal: *Journal of Personality Assessment,* February 1983, *47*(1), 36–41.

. . .

2412

Test Name: FEAR OF SUCCESS SCALE

Purpose: To measure success avoidance of college students.

Number of Items: 27

Format: A paper-and-pencil objective test with scores ranging from 27 to 189. High scores indicate high success avoidance.

Reliability: Coefficient alphas were estimated to be .69 (men) and .73 (women).

Validity: Correlation with the Intellectual Achievement Responsibility Questionnaire ranged from −.67 to .81 (Ns = 12 to 404); with the BEM sex-role inventory ranged from −.37 to .33 (Ns = 12 to 404).

Author: Ireland-Galman, M. M., and Michael, W. B.

Article: The relationship of a measure of the fear of success construct to scales representing the locus of control and sex-role orientation constructs for a community college sample.

Journal: *Educational and Psychological Measurement,* Winter 1983, *43*(4), 1217–1225.

Related Research: Zuckerman, M., & Allison, S. (1976). An objective measure of fear of success: Construction and validation. *Journal of Personality Assessment, 82,* 932–946.

• • •

2413

Test Name: FIRST GRADE ADJUSTMENT SCALE

Purpose: To measure student adjustment to first grade as perceived by their teachers in two dimensions: Academic ability and social adjustment.

Number of Items: 21

Time Required: 1 to 3 minutes per child.

Format: Teacher responds to 21 multiple-choice questions (example given).

Reliability: Hoyt reliabilities: academic ability, .92; social adjustment, .89.

Author: McClinton, S. L., and Topping, C.

Article: Extended day kindergartens: Are the effects tangible?

Journal: *Journal of Educational Research,* September/October 1981, *75*(1), 39–40.

• • •

2414

Test Name: HEALTH RESOURCES INVENTORY

Purpose: Measures teachers'

profiles of children's school-related competences.

Number of Items: 54

Format: Items rated on 5-point scales.

Reliability: Test–retest ranged from .72 to .91 across subscales.

Author: Weissberg, R. P., et al.

Article: The primary mental health project: Seven consecutive years of program outcome research.

Journal: *Journal of Consulting and Clinical Psychology,* October 1983, *51*(1), 100–107.

Related Research: Gesten, E. L. (1976). A health resources inventory: The development of a measure of the personal and social competence of primary grade children. *Journal of Consulting and Clinical Psychology, 44,* 775–786.

• • •

2415

Test Name: HOUSTON STRESS SCALE

Purpose: To measure student stress at the college level. (In four domains: academic, financial, family, and personal.)

Number of Items: Revision of College Environmental Stress Index (see Munoz & Garcia-Bahne).

Format: 7-point Likert response categories.

Reliability: Cronbach's alphas ranged from .78 to .84 over domains.

Author: Pliner, J. E., and Brown, D.

Article: Projections of reactions to stress and preference for helpers among students from four ethnic groups.

Journal: *Journal of College*

Student Personnel, March 1985, *26*(2), 147–151.

Related Research: Munoz, D., & Garcia-Bahne, B. *A study of the Chicano experience in higher education* (Final report for the Center for Minority Group Mental Health Programs and the National Institute of Mental Health, Contract No. NN24597-01). San Diego: University of California.

• • •

2416

Test Name: INVENTORY OF TEACHER–STUDENT RELATIONSHIPS

Purpose: To measure teacher–student relationships.

Number of Items: 17

Format: Rating scale format.

Reliability: Alpha ranged from .54 to .79 across subscales.

Author: Howell, F. M., and McBroom, L. W.

Article: Social relations at home and at school: An analysis of the correspondence principle.

Journal: *Sociology of Education,* January 1982, *55*(1), 40–52.

Related Research: Bachman, J. G., et al. (1972). *Blueprint for a longitudinal study of adolescent boys. Youth in transition* (Vol. 1). Ann Arbor, MI: Institute for Social Research.

• • •

2417

Test Name: MATHEMATICS ANXIETY RATING SCALE— REVISED

Purpose: To provide an index of mathematics course anxiety.

Number of Items: 24

Reliability: Coefficient alpha reliability was .97.

Validity: Correlations with

mathematics achievement, −.44; with achievement anxiety test, −.29 (facilitating) and .54 (debilitating); with state anxiety, .52; with trait anxiety, .52.

Author: Plake, B. S., et al.

Article: A validity investigation of the achievement anxiety test.

Journal: *Educational and Psychological Measurement,* Winter 1981, *41*(4), 1215–1222.

Related Research: Suinn, R. M., et al. (1972). The MARS, a measure of mathematics anxiety: Psychosomatic data. *Journal of Clinical Psychology, 28,* 373–375.

■ ■ ■

2418

Test Name: MATHEMATICS ANXIETY SCALE (COLLEGE)

Purpose: To measure mathematics anxiety among college students.

Number of Items: 10

Format: Likert format.

Reliability: Split-half reliability was .88.

Author: Bander, R. S., et al.

Article: A comparison of cue-controlled relaxation and study skills counseling in the treatment of mathematics anxiety.

Journal: *Journal of Educational Psychology,* February 1982, *74*(1), 96–103.

Related Research: Betz, N. E. (1977). *Math anxiety: What is it?* Paper presented at the 85th annual convention of the American Psychological Association, San Francisco.

■ ■ ■

2419

Test Name: MEDICAL SCHOOL ENVIRONMENTAL STRESS INVENTORY

Purpose: To measure stress in

terms of students' perceptions of significant problems in their learning environment.

Number of Items: 75

Format: Each statement described a situation that students rated as problematic on a 7-point Likert scale from 1 (*not at all a problem*) to 4 (*a moderate problem*) through 7 (*extremely problematic*). The first 62 items pertained to all students and the remainder to either ethnic, minority, or female students.

Reliability: Internal consistency reliability of the first 62 items was .94.

Author: Arnold, L., and Jensen, T. B.

Article: Students' perception of stress in a baccalaureate-MD degree program.

Journal: *Perceptual and Motor Skills,* April 1984, *52*(2), 651–662.

Related Research: Huebner, L. A., et al. (1981). The assessment and remediation of dysfunctional stress in medical schools. *Journal of Medical Education, 56,* 547.

■ ■ ■

2420

Test Name: MEIER BURNOUT ASSESSMENT SCALE

Purpose: To measure student burnout.

Number of Items: 27

Format: All items are presented.

Reliability: Cronbach's alpha was .82.

Author: Meier, S. T., and Schmeck, R. R.

Article: The burned-out college student: A descriptive profile.

Journal: *Journal of College Student Personnel,* January 1985, *26*(1), 63–69.

Related Research: Meier, S.

(1983). Toward a theory of burnout. *Human Relations, 36,* 899–910.

■ ■ ■

2421

Test Name: NEED FOR ACADEMIC COMPETENCE SCALE

Purpose: To measure competency needs in the academic realm.

Number of Items: 40

Format: True–false.

Reliability: Kuder-Richardson formula 20 was .80 (men) and .83 (women).

Author: Jordan, T. J.

Article: Self-concepts, motivations and academic achievement of Black adolescents.

Journal: *Journal of Educational Psychology,* August 1981, *73*(4), 509–517.

Related Research: Jordan, T. J. (1978). *Cognitive and personality factors related to academic achievement of inner-city junior high school students.* Unpublished doctoral dissertation, New York University.

■ ■ ■

2422

Test Name: RATING SCALE FOR KINDERGARTEN ADJUSTMENT

Purpose: To measure adjustment to nursery school.

Number of Items: 18

Format: Includes three factors: adjustment to learning tasks, emotional adjustment, and social adjustment. For each item the teacher identifies which of five sentences best describes the child.

Reliability: Alphas ranged from .69 to .88.

Author: Levy-Shiff, R.

Article: Adaptation and competence in early childhood: Communally raised kibbutz children versus family-raised children in the city.

Journal: *Child Development,* December 1983, *54*(6), 1606–1614.

Related Research: Smilanski, S., & Shephatia, L. (1976). *Manual for kindergarten teachers* (Research Report No. 181, Publication No. 534). Jerusalem: Szolel Institute. [In Hebrew.]

■ ■ ■

2423

Test Name: SOCIAL READJUSTMENT RATING SCALE—STRESSFUL LIFE EVENTS

Purpose: To measure student stress.

Number of Items: 15

Format: Yes–no. Sample items are presented.

Reliability: Cronbach's alpha was .87.

Author: Carson, N. D., and Johnson, R. E.

Article: Suicidal thoughts and problem solving preparation among college students.

Journal: *Journal of College Student Personnel,* November 1985, *26*(6), 484–487.

Related Research: Holmes, T. H., & Rahe, R. H. (1967). The social readjustment rating scale. *Journal of Psychosomatic Research, 11,* 213–218.

■ ■ ■

2424

Test Name: STRESSFUL LIFE EVENT SCALE

Purpose: To measure the perceived stress of events as experienced by students.

Number of Items: 20 events.

Format: Each event rated for stress on a 7-point continuum.

Validity: Correlations between stress ratings by two different ethnic groups was .93; with social standing (popularity) .81 or higher.

Author: Yamamoto, K., and Byrnes, D. A.

Article: Classroom social status, ethnicity and ratings of stressful events.

Journal: *Journal of Educational Research,* May/June 1984, *77*(5), 283–286.

Related Research: Yamamoto, K. (1979). Children's ratings of the stressfulness of experience. *Developmental Psychology, 116,* 163–171.

■ ■ ■

2425

Test Name: STRESS IN MEDICAL SCHOOL SCALE (SIMS)

Purpose: To measure stress in medical students.

Number of Items: 31

Format: 0–9 scale ranging from no stress to extreme stress.

Reliability: Ranged from .77 to .98.

Validity: Of 7 stress factors, 2 decreased over 3 months (as students changed major clerkship rotations).

Author: Linn, B. S., and Zeppa, R.

Article: Dimensions of stress in junior medical students.

Journal: *Psychological Reports,* June 1984, *54*(3), 964–966.

■ ■ ■

2426

Test Name: STUDENT SUPPORT AND ROLE CONGRUENCE QUESTIONNAIRE

Purpose: To measure harmony of student roles and perceived faculty and peer support of female doctoral students.

Number of Items: 30

Format: Items rated in 4-point Likert format. Sample items are presented.

Reliability: Test–retest reliabilities were role congruence, .82; faculty support, .88; peer support, .60.

Validity: Content validity was established by a panel of judges.

Author: Hite, L. M.

Article: Female doctoral students: Their perceptions and concerns.

Journal: *Journal of College Student Personnel,* January 1985, *26*(1), 18–22.

■ ■ ■

2427

Test Name: SUINN TEST ANXIETY BEHAVIOR SCALE

Purpose: To measure test anxiety.

Number of Items: 50

Format: Respondents rate themselves on amount of anxiety they experience in a wide range of academic situations.

Reliability: Test–retest reliability was .73 for graduate students (6 weeks); .74 for undergraduates (6 weeks).

Validity: Women report greater anxiety than men (1 = 3.87; df = 151).

Author: Ginter, E. J., et al.

Article: Suinn Test Anxiety Behavior Scale: Normative data for graduate students in education.

Journal: *Psychological Reports,* 1983, *50*(3) Part II, 1116–1118.

Related Research: Suinn, R. M. (1971). *Suinn Test Anxiety Behavior Scale (STABS):*

Information for users. Fort Collins, CO: Rocky Mountain Behavioral Science Institute.

■ ■ ■

2428

Test Name: SURVEY OF FEELINGS ABOUT TESTS

Purpose: To measure test anxiety.

Number of Items: 15

Format: Subjects respond by either *yes* or *no* to each question. The higher the score, the greater the expressed anxiety about test-taking. Some examples are presented.

Reliability: Cronbach's alphas were .73 (4th grade) and .80 (8th grade).

Validity: Correlations with science achievement test scores ranged from −.42 to .39.

Author: Payne, B. D., et al.

Article: Sex and ethnic differences in relationships of test anxiety to performance in science examinations by fourth and eighth grade students: Implications for valid interpretations of achievement test scores.

Journal: *Educational and Psychological Measurement,* Spring 1983, *43*(1), 267–270.

Related Research: Harnisch, D. L., et al. (1980). *Development of a shorter, more reliable and more valid measure of test motivation.* Paper presented at the annual meeting of the National

Council on Measurement in Education, Boston.

■ ■ ■

2429

Test Name: TEST ANXIETY INVENTORY

Purpose: To assess test anxiety.

Number of Items: 16

Format: Included Likert-scaled items.

Reliability: Test–retest reliability was .79 (*N* = 34).

Author: Shaha, S. H.

Article: Matching-tests: Reduced anxiety and increased test effectiveness.

Journal: *Educational and Psychological Measurement,* Winter 1984, *44*(4), 869–881.

Related Research: Osterhouse, R. A. (1972). Desensitization and study-skills training as treatment for two types of test-anxious students. *Journal of Counseling Psychology, 19,* 301–307.

■ ■ ■

2430

Test Name: TEST ANXIETY SCALE

Purpose: To measure general debilitative test anxiety.

Number of Items: 21

Format: True–false.

Reliability: Split-half reliability was .91; test–retest reliability was .82 (6-week interval).

Author: Bander, R. S., et al.

Article: A comparison of cue-controlled relaxation and study skills counseling in the treatment of mathematics anxiety.

Journal: *Journal of Educational Psychology,* February 1982, *74*(1), 96–103.

Related Research: Sarason, S. B., & Mandler, G. (1952). Some correlates of test anxiety. *Journal of Abnormal and Social Psychology, 47,* 561–565.

■ ■ ■

2431

Test Name: WRITING APPREHENSION INSTRUMENT

Purpose: To measure writing apprehension.

Number of Items: 26

Reliability: Internal consistency estimate was .94.

Validity: High apprehensives score lower on tests of writing skills than low apprehensives.

Author: Faigley, L., et al.

Article: The role of writing apprehension in writing performance and competence.

Journal: *Journal of Educational Research,* September/October 1981, *75*(1), 16–21.

Related Research: Daly, J. A., & Miller, M. D. (1975). The empirical development of an instrument to measure writing apprehension. *Research in the Teaching of English, 13,* 242–249.

CHAPTER 3
Adjustment—Psychological

2432

Test Name: ACCEPTANCE OF ILLNESS SCALE

Purpose: To measure subject's success in feeling valuable in spite of disease.

Number of Items: 8

Format: Items rated on a 5-point agree–disagree format. Sample items are presented, drawn from Linkowski (1971).

Reliability: Alpha was .83.

Author: Felton, B. J., and Revenson, T. A.

Article: Coping with chronic illness: A study of illness controllability and the influence of coping strategies on psychological adjustment.

Journal: *Journal of Consulting and Clinical Psychology*, June 1984, *52*(3), 343–353.

Related Research: Linkowski, D. S. (1971). A scale to measure acceptance of disability. *Rehabilitation Counseling Bulletin, 14*, 236–244.

• • •

2433

Test Name: ACHIEVEMENT ANXIETY TEST SCALE— REVISED

Purpose: To determine the extent to which one's anxiety either facilitates or debilitates one's performance.

Number of Items: 19

Format: Includes two scales: facilitating and debilitating. Examples are presented.

Reliability: Test–retest reliability was .80 (facilitating) and .42 (debilitating).

Validity: Correlations with other variables ranged from –.64 to .24.

Author: Sweeney, G. A., and Horan, J. J.

Article: Separate and combined effects of cue-controlled relaxation and cognitive restructuring in the treatment of musical performance anxiety.

Journal: *Journal of Counseling Psychology*, September 1982, *29*(5), 486–497.

Related Research: Alpert, R., & Haber, R. N. (1960). Anxiety in academic achievement situations. *Journal of Abnormal and Social Psychology, 61*, 207–215.

• • •

2434

Test Name: ACTIVATION– DEACTIVATION ADJECTIVE CHECKLIST

Purpose: To provide a measure of subjective level of stress.

Number of Items: 34

Format: Includes two factors: positive and negative arousal.

Reliability: Test–retest reliability was .75.

Author: Robbins, E. S., and Haase, R. F.

Article: Power of nonverbal cues in counseling interactions: Availability, vividness, or salience?

Journal: *Journal of Counseling*

Psychology, October 1985, *32*(4), 502–513.

Related Research: Thayer, R. E. (1967). Measurement of activation through self-report. *Psychological Reports, 20*, 663–678.

• • •

2435

Test Name: ADOLESCENT PERCEIVED STRESS SCALE

Purpose: To measure perceived stress.

Number of Items: 12

Format: Items rated in 5-point Likert format.

Reliability: Split-half reliability was .70.

Validity: Nonsmokers score lower on the scale than smokers (boys, $p < .05$; girls, $p < .05$).

Author: Mitic, W. R., et al.

Article: Perceived stress and adolescents' cigarette use.

Journal: *Psychological Reports*, December 1985, *53*(3, Part 2), 1043–1048.

• • •

2436

Test Name: AFFECT BALANCE SCALE

Purpose: To measure balance of positive and negative feelings and their rate of occurrence.

Number of Items: 11

Format: Agree–disagree. Sample items are presented.

Reliability: Alpha ranged from .73 to .77.

Author: Hanson, S. L., and Spanier, G. B.

Article: Family development and adjustment to marital separation.

Journal: *Sociology and Social Research*, October 1983, *68*(1), 19–40.

Related Research: Bradburn, N., & Caplovitz, D. (1965). *Reports on Happiness*. Chicago: University of Chicago.

■ ■ ■

2437

Test Name: AGGRESSION-ANXIETY SCALE

Purpose: To provide a projective measure of aggression-anxiety for five-year-old boys.

Number of Items: 24

Format: Includes high to low hostility value picture cards and four categories of behavior.

Reliability: Interscorer reliability was .92.

Validity: Biserial correlation coefficient with teacher ratings of aggression-anxiety was .59.

Author: Henry, R. M.

Article: Validation of a projective measure of aggression-anxiety for five-year-old boys.

Journal: *Journal of Personality Assessment*, August 1981, *45*(4), 359–369.

Related Research: Lesser, G. S. (1958). Conflict analysis of fantasy aggression. *Journal of Personality, 26*, 29–41.

■ ■ ■

2438

Test Name: AGORAPHOBIC COGNITIONS QUESTIONNAIRE

Purpose: To assess panic attack and fear of its occurrence.

Number of Items: 14

Format: 5-point frequency of occurrence scale.

Reliability: Item-total correlations ranged from .27 to .61 among agoraphobic sample and from –.08 to .70 in a normal sample.

Validity: Correlates .67 with Body Sensations Questionnaire; .38 with Beck Depression Inventory; .35 with Trait Anxiety-STAT; .43 with Eysenck Neuroticism.

Author: Chambliss, D. L., et al.

Article: Assessment of fear in agoraphobics: The body sensations questionnaire and the agoraphobics cognitions questionnaire.

Journal: *Journal of Consulting and Clinical Psychology*, December 1984, *52*(6), 1090–1097.

■ ■ ■

2439

Test Name: ALPERT-HABER ACHIEVEMENT ANXIETY TEST

Purpose: To measure achievement anxiety.

Number of Items: 28

Format: Multiple-choice.

Reliability: Ranged from .59 to .88 across subscales, by method of responding to items that subject must use, whether or not buffer items are included.

Validity: Correlates with the self-rating scale vary by item format, but not by presence of buffer items. There was no item-format–buffer interaction.

Author: Tuck, J. P.

Article: Will the real achievement anxiety test please stand up: Effects of removing buffer items and altering item format of the Alpert-Haber Achievement Anxiety Test.

Journal: *Psychological Reports*, 1982, *51*(2), 471–478.

Related Research: Huck, S. W., & Jacko, E. J. (1974). Effects of varying the response format of the Alpert-Haber Achievement Anxiety Test. *Journal of Counseling Psychology, 21*, 159–163.

■ ■ ■

2440

Test Name: ANXIETY DIFFERENTIAL

Purpose: To measure state of anxiety related to the emotional-autonomic domain.

Number of Items: 18

Format: A semantic differential format.

Reliability: Test–retest reliability was .41.

Validity: Correlations with other variables ranged from –.18 to .62.

Author: Sweeney, G. A., and Horan, J.

Article: Separate and combined effects of cue-controlled relaxation and cognitive restructuring in the treatment of musical performance anxiety.

Journal: *Journal of Counseling Psychology*, September 1982, *29*(5), 486–497.

Related Research: Husek, T. R., & Alexander S. (1963). The effectiveness of the anxiety differential in examination stress situations. *Educational and Psychological Measurement, 23*, 309–318.

■ ■ ■

2441

Test Name: ANXIETY SYMPTOM CHECKLIST

Purpose: To measure symptoms of anxiety.

Number of Items: 40 common physiological symptoms.

Format: 5-point scales indicating

the frequency, intensity, and interference in life of each symptom.

Reliability: Test–retest reliability (in past research) was .85.

Validity: Correlates .58 to .73 with measures of general anxiety (in past research).

Author: Deffenbacher, J. L., and Craun, A. M.

Article: Anxiety management training with stressed student gynecology patients: A collaborative approach.

Journal: *Journal of College Student Personnel*, November 1985, *26*(6), 513–518.

Related Research: Edie, C. A. (1973). Uses of AMT in treating trait anxiety. *Dissertation Abstracts International, 33,* 393–413. (University Microfilms No. 73-2789, 256)

• • •

2442

Test Name: AUTOMATIC THOUGHTS QUESTIONNAIRE

Purpose: To measure occurrence of automatic negative thoughts associated with depression.

Number of Items: 30

Format: Items are rated on a 5-point frequency scale.

Reliability: Alpha was .98; split-half reliability was .96; item total ranged from .56 to .91.

Validity: Correlates .85 with MMPI-D; correlates .87 with Beck Depression Inventory.

Author: Harrell, T. H., and Ryan, N. B.

Article: Cognitive–behavioral assessment of depression: Clinical validation of the automatic thoughts questionnaire.

Journal: *Journal of Consulting and*

Clinical Psychology, October 1983, *51*(5), 721–725.

Related Research: Hollon, S. D., & Kendall, P. C. (1980). Cognitive self-statements in depression: Development of an automatic thoughts questionnaire. *Cognitive Therapy and Research, 4,* 383–395.

• • •

2443

Test Name: AVOIDANCE OF EXISTENTIAL CONFRONTATION SCALE

Purpose: To measure failure, meaninglessness, uncertainty, frustration, and suffering.

Number of Items: 36

Format: Items are rated on a 7-point semantic differential scale. All items are presented.

Reliability: Reliability ranged between .62 and .73 (odd–even). Test–retest reliability was .75 (2-weeks).

Author: Thauberger, C. P., et al.

Article: Avoidance of existential–ontological confrontation: A review of research.

Journal: *Psychological Reports,* 1981, *49*(3), 747–764.

Related Research: Thauberger, P. C. (1969). *The relationship between an avoidance of existential confrontation and neuroticism and changes resulting from the basic encounter group learning experience.* Unpublished master's thesis, University of Saskatchewan, Saskatoon.

• • •

2444

Test Name: AVOIDANCE OF THE ONTOLOGICAL CONFRONTATION OF DEATH SCALE

Purpose: To measure avoidance of the harsh reality of death.

Number of Items: 20

Format: True–false. All items presented for forms A, B, and C.

Reliability: Kuder-Richardson formula 20 ranged from .82 to .96 across forms A, B, and C. Odd–even reliability ranged from .82 to .89 across forms A, B, and C. Test–retest reliability ranged from .76 to .91 across forms A, B, and C.

Validity: Does not correlate with Jackson's Social Desirability Scale (correlations –.04, .04, .07 across forms). Does correlate significantly with blood pressure. Correlates .37 with Eysenck's Neuroticism Scale.

Author: Thauberger, P. C., et al.

Article: Avoidance of existential–ontological confrontation: A review of research.

Journal: *Psychological Reports,* 1981, *49*(3), 747–764.

Related Research: Thauberger, P. C. (1979). The avoidance of ontological confrontation of death: A psychometric research scale. *Essence, 3,* 9–12.

• • •

2445

Test Name: BECK DEPRESSION INVENTORY

Purpose: To measure subjects' negative emotions.

Number of Items: 21

Format: Each item inquires about a specific symptom cluster with four levels of severity ranging from 0 to 3.

Reliability: Split-half reliability was .93.

Validity: Correlation with clinical judgments of depression was .65.

Author: Kraft, R. G., et al.

Article: Effects of positive reframing and paradoxical

directives in counseling for negative emotions.

Journal: *Journal of Counseling Psychology,* October 1985, *32*(4), 617–621.

Related Research: Beck, A. T. (1967). *Depression: Causes and treatments.* Philadelphia: University of Pennsylvania Press.

■ ■ ■

2446

Test Name: BECK DEPRESSION INVENTORY—ABRIDGED

Purpose: To serve as a depression screening device.

Number of Items: 13

Format: A self-report inventory whereby for each item the examinee selects from among four statements arranged in order of increasing level of depression the one statement which best describes the examinee's current feelings.

Reliability: Cronbach's alpha was .90.

Validity: Correlations with MMPI ranged from −.39 to .63.

Author: Scott, N. A., et al.

Article: Assessment of depression among incarcerated females.

Journal: *Journal of Personality Assessment,* August 1982, *46*(4), 372–379.

Related Research: Beck, A. T., & Beamesderfer, A. (1974). Assessment of depression: The depression inventory. In P. Pichot (Ed.), *Psychological measurements in psychopharmacology* (Vol. 7). Paris: Karger-Basel.

■ ■ ■

2447

Test Name: BOYAR'S FEAR OF DEATH SCALE

Purpose: To measure death anxiety.

Number of Items: 18

Format: Items are rated on 6-point Likert scales. Sample items are presented.

Reliability: Split-half reliability was .83; test-retest (10-day interval) reliability was .79.

Author: Downey, A. M.

Article: Relationship of religiosity to death anxiety of middle-aged males.

Journal: *Psychological Reports,* June 1984, *54*(3), 811–822.

Related Research: Boyar, J. I. (1964). The construction and partial validation of a scale for the measurement of the fear of death. *Dissertation Abstracts International, 25,* 2041.

■ ■ ■

2448

Test Name: BRIEF SYMPTOM INVENTORY

Purpose: To measure psychopathology.

Number of Items: 53

Time Required: 10 minutes.

Validity: Correlates .92 to .99 with Symptom Checklist–90.

Author: Hale, W. D., et al.

Article: Norms for the elderly on the brief symptom inventory.

Journal: *Journal of Consulting and Clinical Psychology,* April 1984, *52*(2), 321–322.

Related Research: Derogatis, L. R. (1977). *The SCL-90 Manual I: Scoring administration and procedures for the SCL-90.* Baltimore, MD: Johns Hopkins University School of Medicine, Clinical Psychometrics Unit.

■ ■ ■

2449

Test Name: CENTER FOR EPIDEMIOLOGIC STUDIES DEPRESSION SCALE

Purpose: To assess depression.

Number of Items: 20

Format: Subjects respond to each item on a 4-point scale indicating how often they feel the way described by the item. The scale runs from 0 (*rarely*) to 3 (*most*). Examples are presented.

Reliability: Cronbach's alphas were .90 (college students) and .86 (elderly women).

Validity: Correlations with loneliness scores ranged from .12 to .51.

Author: Schmitt, J. P., and Kurdek, L. A.

Article: Age and gender differences in and personality correlates of loneliness in different relationships.

Journal: *Journal of Personality Assessment,* October 1985, *49*(5), 485–496.

Related Research: Radloff, L. S. (1977). The CES-D scale: A self-report depression scale for research in the general population. *Applied Psychological Measurement, 1,* 385–401.

■ ■ ■

2450

Test Name: CHILDREN'S DEPRESSION INVENTORY

Purpose: To measure depression in children.

Number of Items: 27

Time Required: 10–20 minutes.

Format: Items are rated on 3-point frequency scales that best describe behavior over the past 2 weeks (children's self-reports).

Reliability: Test–retest ranged from .38 to .59; split-half ranged from .57 to .74; Kuder-Richardson formula ranged from .80 to .94.

Validity: Normal group scored lower than hospitalized group ($t = 2.48$, $p < .02$); correlation with Piers-Harris was $-.64$ ($p < .001$); correlation with Kestan was $.46$ ($p < .05$). Other validity data reported.

Author: Saylor, C. F., et al.

Article: The children's depression inventory: A systematic evaluation of psychosometric properties.

Journal: *Journal of Consulting and Clinical Psychology*, December 1984, *52*(6), 955–967.

Related Research: Kovacs, M. (1982). *The children's depression inventory: A self-rated depression scale for school-aged youngsters.* Unpublished manuscript, University of Pittsburgh.

Saylor, C. F., et al. (1984). Construct validity for measures of childhood depression: Application of multitrait-multimethod methodology. *Journal of Consulting and Clinical Psychology, 52,* 977–985.

■ ■ ■

2451

Test Name: CLIENT FEARS QUESTIONNAIRE

Purpose: To measure fears clients have of psychotherapy.

Number of Items: 15

Format: Items are rated on a 5-point concern scale. All items are presented.

Reliability: Alpha ranged from .84 to .92 across two factors.

Validity: Individuals not seeking therapy had greater fears than clients ($p < .001$).

Author: Pipes, R. B., et al.

Article: Measuring client fears.

Journal: *Journal of Consulting and Clinical Psychology*, December 1985, *53*(6), 933–934.

2452

Test Name: CLINICAL ASSESSMENT INVENTORY

Purpose: To measure psychiatric patients' progress.

Number of Items: 50 subcategories of behavior.

Format: Patients are observed twice daily on regular nursing rounds. Major behavior categories are presented.

Reliability: Agreements between pairs of observers ranged from 88.4% to 88.6%. Reliability was .85. Correlation of observations over 1-day interval was .945 (100 patients).

Validity: Correlates .77 with the Short Clinical Rating Scale.

Author: Brown, R. A., and Moss, G. R.

Article: Reliability and validation of a psychiatric assessment instrument for the hospital treatment of adults.

Journal: *Psychological Reports*, 1982, *51*(1), 142.

■ ■ ■

2453

Test Name: COLLETT-LESTER FEAR OF DEATH SCALE

Purpose: To assess fear of death.

Number of Items: 36

Format: Likert format with four scales: fear of death of self, fear of death of others, fear of dying of self, fear of dying of others.

Reliability: Subscale internal consistency reliability coefficients (alphas) ranged from .59 to .76.

Validity: Correlations with: Marlowe-Crowne Social Desirability Scale were .14 or less; Death Anxiety Scale ranged from .31 to .78.

Author: Wass, H., and Forfar, C. S.

Article: Assessment of attitudes toward death: Techniques and instruments for use with older persons.

Journal: *Measurement and Evaluation in Guidance*, October 1982, *15*(3), 210–220.

Related Research: Collett, L. J., & Lester, D. (1969). The fear of death and dying. *Journal of Psychology, 72,* 179–181.

■ ■ ■

2454

Test Name: COMBAT-RELATED POSTTRAUMATIC STRESS DISORDER SUBSCALE

Purpose: To assess combat-related posttraumatic stress.

Number of Items: 9

Format: Items taken from MMPI, Form R. Item numbers presented.

Validity: Correctly classified 82% of validation and cross-validation samples, compared with 74% with standard clinical scale rules.

Author: Keane, T. M., et al.

Article: Empirical development of an MMPI subscale for the assessment of combat-related posttraumatic stress disorder.

Journal: *Journal of Consulting and Clinical Psychology*, October 1984, *52*(5), 888–891.

Related Research: Fairbank, J. A., et al. (1983). Some preliminary data of the psychological characteristics of Vietnam veterans with posttraumatic stress disorders. *Journal of Consulting and Clinical Psychology, 51,* 912–919.

■ ■ ■

2455

Test Name: CONCERN OVER THE NEGATIVE CONSEQUENCES OF SUCCESS SCALE

Purpose: To measure concern about negative consequences of success.

Number of Items: 27

Format: Items are rated on a 4-point agreement scale.

Reliability: Alpha ranged from .46 to .78 across subscales and by sex.

Author: Hong, S., and Caust, C. D.

Article: A factor analytic evaluation of the concern over negative consequences of success scale.

Journal: *Psychological Reports,* February 1985, *56*(1), 331–338.

Related Research: Ho, R., & Zemaitis, R. (1981). Concern over the negative consequences of success. *Australian Journal of Psychology, 33,* 19–28.

■ ■ ■

2456

Test Name: CUE COUNT

Purpose: To assess behavioral anxiety.

Number of Items: 7

Format: Includes verbal speech disruption and nonverbal voice characteristics items. Responses are rated by trained raters.

Reliability: Interrater reliability was .94.

Author: Strohmer, D. C., et al.

Article: Cognitive style and synchrony in measures of anxiety.

Journal: *Measurement and Evaluation in Guidance,* April 1983, *16*(1), 13–17.

Related Research: Dibner, A. S. (1956). Cue counting: A measure of anxiety in interviews. *Journal of Consulting Psychology, 20,* 475–478.

2457

Test Name: CURRENT MOOD STATE SCALE

Purpose: To assess current mood state.

Number of Items: 9

Format: Subjects rate on a 5-point scale emotions felt during past 3 months, as well as questions concerning their marriage and current life concerns.

Reliability: Cronbach's alpha was .926.

Author: Berman, W. H., and Turk, D. C.

Article: Adaptation to divorce: Problems and coping strategies.

Journal: *Journal of Marriage and the Family,* February 1981, *43*(1), 179–189.

Related Research: Pearlin, L. I., & Schooler, C. (1978). The structure of coping. *Journal of Health and Social Behavior, 19,* 2–21.

■ ■ ■

2458

Test Name: DEATH ACCEPTANCE SCALE

Purpose: To measure death acceptance.

Number of Items: 7

Format: Likert scale.

Reliability: Internal consistency reliabilities (alpha) were .58 and .70.

Validity: Correlation with death anxiety was −.26.

Author: Wass, H., and Forfar, C. S.

Article: Assessment of attitude toward death: Techniques and instruments for use with older persons.

Journal: *Measurement and*

Evaluation in Guidance, October 1982, *15*(3), 210–220.

Related Research: Ray, J. J., & Najman, J. (1974). Death anxiety and acceptance: A preliminary approach. *Omega, 5,* 311–315.

■ ■ ■

2459

Test Name: DEATH ANXIETY SCALE

Purpose: To measure death anxiety.

Number of Items: 15

Format: Personal death-related questions answered true or false.

Reliability: Test–retest reliability (3 weeks) was .83. Internal consistency reliability coefficient (alpha) was .73.

Validity: Correlations with Manifest Anxiety Scale, .39; with Marlowe-Crowne Social Desirability Scale, .03, .21.; with a projective word association task, .25.

Author: Wass, H., and Forfar, C. S.

Article: Assessment of attitudes toward death: Techniques and instruments for use with older persons.

Journal: *Measurement and Evaluation in Guidance,* October 1982, *15*(3), 210–220.

Related Research: Templar, D. I. (1970). The construction and validation of a death anxiety scale. *Journal of General Psychology, 82,* 165–177.

■ ■ ■

2460

Test Name: DEATH CONCERN SCALE

Purpose: To measure concern for death.

Number of Items: 30

Format: Likert scale assessing conscious contemplation of death and negative evaluation of death.

Reliability: Split-half reliabilities for four administrations were above .85. Test–retest reliability (8 weeks) was .87.

Validity: Correlations with State and Trait Anxiety Inventory were .01, .16 (men), .48, .75 (women); with Marlowe-Crowne Social Desirability Scale, .40; with Death Anxiety Scale, .56; with Collett-Lester Fear of Death Scale, .38.

Author: Wass, H., and Forfar, C. S.

Article: Assessment and attitudes toward death: Techniques and instruments for use with older persons.

Journal: *Measurement and Evaluation in Guidance*, October 1982, *15*(3), 210–220.

Related Research: Dickstein, L. S. (1972). Death concern: Measurement and correlates. *Psychological Reports, 30,* 563–571.

• • •

2461

Test Name: DEPRESSION EXPERIENCES QUESTIONNAIRE

Purpose: To measure the subjective experiences of depression.

Number of Items: 66

Format: Agree–disagree format. Sample items presented.

Reliability: Alpha ranged from .72 to .81 across subscales.

Author: Blatt, S. J., et al.

Article: Dependency and self-criticism: Psychological dimensions of depression.

Journal: *Journal of Consulting and*

Clinical Psychology, February 1982, *50*(1), 113–124.

Related Research: Blatt, S. J., et al. (1976). *Depressive experiences questionnaire.* New Haven, CT: Yale University.

• • •

2462

Test Name: DEPRESSION PRONENESS RATING SCALE

Purpose: To measure proneness to depression.

Number of Items: Scale 3-3 items; Scale 11-11 items.

Format: Scale 3: Descriptor items followed by a 9-point scale (all items presented); Scale 11: Symptom (items) followed by a 5-point rating scale (all items presented).

Reliability: Test–retest reliabilities were .76 (Scale 3) and .57 (Scale 11).

Validity: Both scales correlate significantly with Scale 11, with Beck's Depression Inventory (short form), and with other's reports of depression. Correlations ranged from .29 to .91.

Author: Zemore, R.

Article: Development of a self-report measure of depression-proneness.

Journal: *Psychological Reports,* 1983, *52*(1), 211–216.

Related Research: Zemore, R., & Bretell, D. (1983). Depression-proneness, low self-esteem, unhappy outlook, and narcissistic vulnerability. *Psychological Reports, 52,* 223–230.

• • •

2463

Test Name: DEPRESSION SCALE

Purpose: To measure depression.

Number of Items: 11

Format: Responses are made on a 5-point frequency scale from 1 (*never*) to 5 (*very often*).

Reliability: Coefficient alpha was .78.

Validity: Correlation with employment characteristics ranged from .26 to .14 (husbands' depression) and −.35 to .15 (wives' depression).

Author: Keith, P. M., and Schafer, R. B.

Article: Employment characteristics of both spouses and depression in two-job families.

Journal: *Journal of Marriage and the Family,* November 1983, *45*(4), 877–884.

Related Research: Pearlin, L., & Johnson, J. (1977). Marital status, life-strains, and depression. *American Sociological Review, 42,* 704–715.

• • •

2464

Test Name: DEPRESSION SCALE

Purpose: To measure how "blue," "lonely," and "fearful" individuals feel.

Number of Items: 6

Format: 7-point response categories.

Reliability: Alpha was .79.

Author: Ross, C., and Mirowsky, J.

Article: Men who cry.

Journal: *Social Psychological Quarterly,* June 1984, *47*(2), 138–146.

Related Research: Radloff, L. S. (1977). The CES-D scale: A self-report depression scale for research in the general population. *Applied Psychological Research, 1,* 385–401.

2465

Test Name: DEPRESSION: SELF-RATING SCALE (Children's version)

Purpose: To measure depression in children.

Number of Items: 21

Format: Items are rated on a 0–2 scale (*always, sometimes, never present*).

Reliability: Alpha was .76 ($p <$ .01); split-half reliability was .67.

Validity: Depressed children score higher than nondepressed children ($p < .002$). Sensitivity was 51%; homogeneity was 91%; specificity was 95%; overall percentage of correct classifications was 74%. Correlates .81 with Child Depression Inventory.

Author: Asarnow, J. R., and Carlson, G. A.

Article: Depression self-rating scale: Utility with child psychiatric inpatients.

Journal: *Journal of Consulting and Clinical Psychology*, August 1985, *53*(4), 491–499.

Related Research: Birleson, A. T. (1981). The validity of depressive disorders and the development of a self-rating scale: A research report. *Journal of Child Psychiatry and Psychology, 22,* 73–88.

■ ■ ■

2466

Test Name: DISTRESS SCALE

Purpose: To measure feelings of distress and negative affect.

Number of Items: 22

Format: Responses are made on a 7-point scale. Sample items are presented.

Reliability: Alpha was .89.

Validity: Correlations with other variables ranged from –.67 to .49 ($N = 120$).

Author: Bhagat, R. S., et al.

Article: Total life stress: A multimethod validation of the construct and its effects on organizationally valued outcomes and withdrawal behaviors.

Journal: *Journal of Applied Psychology*, February 1985, *70*(1), 202–204.

Related Research: Bradburn, N. M. (1969). *The structure of psychological well-being.* Chicago: Aldine.

■ ■ ■

2467

Test Name: DYING AND DEATH SCALE

Purpose: To measure fear and beliefs about dying.

Number of Items: 12

Format: Items were rated on 5-point Likert response categories ranging from *strongly agree* to *strongly disagree.* All items are presented.

Reliability: Test–retest (48 hours) reliability was .80.

Validity: Age groups differed significantly.

Author: Westman, A. S., et al.

Article: Denial of fear of dying or of death in young and elderly populations.

Journal: *Psychological Reports*, October 1984, *55*(2), 413–444.

■ ■ ■

2468

Test Name: FEAR OF DEATH SCALE

Purpose: To measure fear of death.

Number of Items: 36

Format: Items rated on 6-point Likert response categories.

Validity: Cluster and factor analysis suggest that 4 or 5 subscales exist.

Author: Liveh, H.

Article: Brief note on the structure of the Collett-Lester Fear of Death Scale.

Journal: *Psychological Reports*, February 1985, *56*(1), 136–138.

Related Research: Collett, L., & Lester, D. (1969). The fear of death and the fear of dying. *Journal of Psychology, 72,* 179–181.

■ ■ ■

2469

Test Name: FEAR OF DEATH SCALE

Purpose: To measure one's fear of death.

Number of Items: 21

Format: Thurstone scale.

Reliability: Parallel form correlation was .58; internal consistency reliability coefficient (alpha) was .34.

Validity: Correlation with Marlowe-Crowne Social Desirability Scale, .10; with Collett-Lester Death of Self Subscale, .78.

Author: Wass, H., and Forfar, C. S.

Article: Assessment of attitudes toward death: Techniques and instruments for use with older persons.

Journal: *Measurement and Evaluation in Guidance*, October 1982, *15*(3), 210–220.

Related Research: Durlak, J. A. (1972). Measurement of the fear of death: An examination of some existing scales. *Journal of Clinical Psychology, 28,* 545–547.

2470

Test Name: FEAR OF SUCCESS AND FEAR OF APPEARING INCOMPETENT SCALES

Purpose: To measure fear of success and appearing incompetent.

Number of Items: 36 (incompetent), 29 (success).

Format: True–false.

Reliability: Kuder-Richardson formula 20, .89 (incompetent) and .81 (success).

Author: Brenner, O. C., and Tomkiewicz, J.

Article: Sex differences among business graduates on fear of success and fear of appearing incompetent as measured by objective instruments.

Journal: *Psychological Reports,* 1982, *51*(1), 179–182.

Related Research: Good, L. R., & Good, K. C. (1973). An objective measure of the motive to avoid appearing incompetent. *Psychological Reports, 33,* 1075–1078.

Good, L. R., & Good, K. C. (1973). An objective measure of the motive to avoid success. *Psychological Reports, 33,* 1009–1010.

• • •

2471

Test Name: FEAR OF SUCCESS SCALE

Purpose: To assess individual difference in the motive to avoid success.

Number of Items: 27

Format: Items are rated on 7-point Likert response scales.

Reliability: Alpha was .68, reported for college juniors and seniors.

Author: Taylor, K. M.

Article: An investigation of vocational indecision in college students: Correlates and Moderators.

Journal: *Journal of Vocational Behavior,* December 1982, *21*(3), 318–329.

Related Research: Zuckerman, M., & Allison, S. N. (1976). An objective measure of fear of success: Construction and validation. *Journal of Personality Assessment, 40,* 422–430.

• • •

2472

Test Name: FRUSTRATION SCALES

Purpose: To measure frustration.

Number of Items: 3

Format: Responses were made on a 7-point Likert scale. High scores represented greater frustration.

Reliability: Coefficient alphas were .76 and .68.

Validity: Correlations with other variables ranged from –.42 to .36.

Author: O'Connor, E. J., et al.

Article: Situational constraint effects on performance, affective reactions and turnover: A field replication and extension.

Journal: *Journal of Applied Psychology,* November 1984, *69*(4), 663–672.

Related Research: Peters, L. H., & O'Connor, E. J. (1980). Situational constraints and work outcomes: The influence of a frequently overlooked construct. *Academy of Management Review, 5,* 391–397.

• • •

2473

Test Name: GENERAL ANXIETY SCALE

Purpose: To measure general anxiety.

Number of Items: 17

Format: True–false format.

Reliability: Internal consistency coefficient was .75.

Validity: Correlations with other variables ranged from –.43 to .50.

Author: Llabre, M. M., and Suarez, E.

Article: Predicting math anxiety and course performance in college women and men.

Journal: *Journal of Counseling Psychology,* April 1985, *32*(2), 283–287.

Related Research: Sarason, I. G. (1978). The test anxiety scale: Concept and research. In C. D. Spielberger & I. G. Sarason (Eds.), *Stress and anxiety* (Vol. 5, pp. 193–216). Washington, DC: Hemisphere.

• • •

2474

Test Name: GENERAL WELL-BEING SCALE

Purpose: To measure subjective well-being and distress.

Number of Items: 18

Format: Fourteen items have 6-point responses that vary by item content. Four items have an 11-point response format.

Reliability: Alpha was .92.

Author: Himmelfarb, S.

Article: Age and sex differences in the mental health of older persons.

Journal: *Journal of Consulting and Clinical Psychology,* October 1984, *52*(5), 844–856.

Related Research: Fazio, A. F. (1977). *A concurrent validation study of the NCHS general well being schedule.* (U.S. Public Health Service, Vital and Health Statistics, Series 2, No. 73.) Washington, DC: U.S. Government Printing Office.

2475

Test Name: GERIATRIC DEPRESSION SCALE

Purpose: To assess depression in the elderly.

Number of Items: 30

Format: Items refer to affective, cognitive, and behavioral symptoms of depression. Examples are presented.

Validity: Correlations with other variables ranged from –.39 to .49.

Author: Fry, P. S.

Article: Development of a geriatric scale of hopelessness: Implications for counseling and intervention with the depressed elderly.

Journal: *Journal of Counseling Psychology,* July 1984, *31*(3), 322–331.

Related Research: Brink, T. L., et al. (1982). Screening test for geriatric depression. *Clinical Gerontologist, 1,* 37–43.

■ ■ ■

2476

Test Name: GERIATRIC HOPELESSNESS SCALE

Purpose: To assess hopelessness in nonpsychiatric, nonpatient, and subclinically depressed elderly.

Number of Items: 30

Format: Items are answered either *true* or *false.* All items are presented.

Reliability: Cronbach's coefficient alpha was .69; Spearman-Brown split-half coefficient was .73.

Validity: Correlations with other variables ranged from –.55 to .49.

Author: Fry, P. S.

Article: Development of a geriatric scale of hopelessness: Implication for counseling and intervention with the depressed elderly.

Journal: *Journal of Counseling*

Psychology, July 1984, *31*(3), 322–331.

Related Research: Beck, A. T., et al. (1974). The measurement of pessimism: The hopelessness scale. *Journal of Consulting and Clinical Psychology, 42,* 861–865.

■ ■ ■

2477

Test Name: GOLDFARB FEAR OF FAT SCALE

Purpose: To identify individuals at high risk for developing eating disorders.

Number of Items: 10

Format: Responses to each item are made on a 4-point Likert scale from 1 (*very untrue*) to 4 (*very true*). All items presented.

Reliability: Test–retest (1 week) reliability was .88 ($N = 23$).

Validity: Correlations with other variables ranged from –.64 to .65.

Author: Goldfarb, L. A., et al.

Article: The Goldfarb fear of fat scale.

Journal: *Journal of Personality Assessment,* June 1985, *49*(3), 329–332.

■ ■ ■

2478

Test Name: GOOD AND GOOD FEAR OF SUCCESS SCALE

Purpose: To assess fear of success.

Number of Items: 29

Format: True–false.

Reliability: Kuder-Richardson formula 20 was .81.

Validity: Correlates positively with Zuckerman and Allison and Pappo scales, except that it correlates negatively for men on the Zuckerman and Allison scales.

Author: Chabassol, D. J., and Ishiyama, F. I.

Article: Correlations among three measures of fear of success.

Journal: *Psychological Reports,* 1983, *52*(1), 55–58.

Related Research: Good, L. R., & Good, K. C. (1973). An objective measure of the motive to avoid success. *Psychological Reports, 33,* 1009–1010.

■ ■ ■

2479

Test Name: HAMILTON PSYCHIATRIC RATING SCALE FOR DEPRESSION

Purpose: To measure depression.

Number of Items: 17

Format: Items are presented by interviewer in a semistructured interview. Items scored 0 to 2 or 0 to 4 to reflect increasing severity of symptom.

Reliability: Interrater reliability ranged from .80 to .90.

Author: Atkeson, B. M., et al.

Article: Victims of rape: Repeated assessment of depressive symptoms.

Journal: *Journal of Consulting and Clinical Psychology,* February 1982, *50*(1), 96–102.

Related Research: Hamilton, M. (1960). A rating scale for depression. *Journal of Neurology, Neurosurgery and Psychiatry, 23,* 56–62.

■ ■ ■

2480

Test Name: HEALTH OPINION SURVEY

Purpose: To provide a general index of neurotic symptomatology focusing on psychosomatic complaints.

Number of Items: 18

Format: Subject responds to each

symptom by indicating *always, sometimes,* or *never.*

Validity: Correlations with other variables ranged from –.22 to .25.

Author: Ronchi, D., and Sparacino, J.

Article: Density of dormitory living and stress: Mediating effects of sex, self-monitoring and environmental affective qualities.

Journal: *Perceptual and Motor Skills,* December 1982, *55*(3, Part 1), 759–770.

Related Research: Leighton, D. C., et al. (1963). *The character of danger.* New York: Basic Books.

■ ■ ■

2481

Test Name: HIGH SCHOOL SOCIAL READJUSTMENT SCALE

Purpose: To measure stress.

Number of Items: 52

Format: Yes–no.

Reliability: Test–retest ranged from .40 to .63 (6-month interval).

Validity: Correlation with Epidemiological Studies Stress Scale ranged from .25 to .27 ($p < .02$) for girls but not significant ($r = .04$) for boys.

Author: Tolor, A., and Murphy, V. M.

Article: Stress and depression in high school students.

Journal: *Psychological Reports,* October 1985, *57*(2), 535–541.

Related Research: Tolor, A., et al. (1983). The high school social readjustment scale: An attempt to quantify stressful events in young people. *Research Communications in Psychology, Psychiatry and Behavior, 8,* 85–111.

Holmes, T. H., & Rahe, R. H. (1967). The social readjustment scale. *Journal of Psychosomatic Research, 11,* 213–218.

■ ■ ■

2482

Test Name: HOPELESSNESS SCALE FOR CHILDREN

Purpose: To measure hopelessness in children. Patterned on Beck et al. Hopelessness Scale.

Number of Items: 17

Format: True–not true format. All items presented.

Reliability: Item-total correlation ranged from .19 to .71 (all significant at $p < .05$); alpha was .75; split-half reliability was .70.

Validity: Correlates .49 ($p < .001$) with Children's Depression Inventory; .22 ($p < .05$) with Depression Symptom Checklist.

Author: Kazdin, A. E., et al.

Article: Hopelessness, depression, and suicidal intent among psychiatrically disturbed inpatient children.

Journal: *Journal of Consulting and Clinical Psychology,* August 1983, *51*(4), 504–510.

Related Research: Beck, A. T., et al. (1974). The measurement of pessimism: The hopelessness scale. *Journal of Consulting and Clinical Psychology, 42,* 861–865.

■ ■ ■

2483

Test Name: HOPELESSNESS SCALE

Purpose: To measure pessimism.

Number of Items: 20

Format: True–false. Sample items presented.

Reliability: Alpha was .93.

Author: Wolf, F. M., and Savickas, M. L.

Article: Time perspective and causal attributions for achievement.

Journal: *Journal of Educational Psychology,* August 1985, *77*(4), 471–480.

Related Research: Beck, A. T., et al. (1974). The measurement of pessimism: The hopelessness scale. *Journal of Consulting and Clinical Psychology, 42,* 861–865.

■ ■ ■

2484

Test Name: IMPACT OF EVENT SCALE

Purpose: To measure subjective stress.

Number of Items: 15

Format: Items rated on 4-point frequency of occurrence response scale (*not at all* to *often*). All items are presented.

Reliability: Alphas were .79 to .92.

Validity: Discriminates patient and field subject samples in expected direction.

Author: Zilberg, N. J., et al.

Article: Impact of event scale: A cross-validation study and some empirical evidence supporting a conceptual model of stress response syndromes.

Journal: *Journal of Consulting and Clinical Psychology,* June 1982, *50*(3), 407–414.

Related Research: Horowitz, M. J. (1979). Impact of event scale: A measure of subjective stress. *Psychosomatic Medicine, 41,* 209–218.

■ ■ ■

2485

Test Name: INDEX OF POTENTIAL SUICIDE— CLINICAL SCALE

Purpose: To predict future suicidal behavior in hospitalized attempted suicides over a 6-month period.

Number of Items: 50

Format: Includes six subscales: depression, emotional status, anxiety, alcoholism, suicidal behavior, and general health.

Reliability: Cronbach's alphas ranged from .38 to .75 for the subscales and was .84 for the total scale.

Validity: Correlations with other variables ranged from −.01 to .42.

Author: Petrie, K., and Chamberlain, K.

Article: The predictive validity of the Zung index of potential suicide.

Journal: *Journal of Personality Assessment,* February 1985, *49*(1), 100–102.

Related Research: Zung, W. W. K. (1974). Index of potential suicide. In A. T. Beck et al. (Eds.), *The prediction of suicide.* Maryland: Charles Press.

• • •

2486

Test Name: INTENSE AMBIVALENCE SCALE

Purpose: To measure tendency to endow diverse psychisms with a positive and negative indicator at the same time.

Number of Items: 45

Format: True–false.

Reliability: Test–retest (10–12 weeks) reliability was .81. Alpha ranged from .86 to .88.

Validity: Correlates .18 (depressed subjects) and .52 (schizophrenic subjects) with Beck Depression Inventory. Correlates .04 with Phillips Premorbid Adjustment Scale. Other validity data are presented.

Author: Raulin, M. L.

Article: Development of a scale to measure intense ambivalence.

Journal: *Journal of Consulting and Clinical Psychology,* February 1984, *52*(1), 63–72.

• • •

2487

Test Name: LEVY OPTIMISM– PESSIMISM SCALE

Purpose: To measure optimism– pessimism.

Number of Items: 16

Format: Multiple-choice. Sample items presented.

Reliability: Cronbach's alpha was .94.

Validity: Differentiates "morning" and "evening" persons ($t = 2.30$, $p < .025$), and thus may be associated with circadian rhythms.

Author: Levy, D. A.

Article: Optimism and pessimism: Relationships to circadian rhythms.

Journal: *Psychological Reports,* December 1985, *57*(3-II), 1123– 1126.

• • •

2488

Test Name: LIFE EVENTS CHECKLIST

Purpose: To measure total life stress.

Number of Items: 83

Format: Subjects use a 7-point scale from −3 to +3 to rate the degree of positive or negative impact that each event had on their life. Examples are presented.

Reliability: Cronbach's alpha ranged from .53 to .77 ($N = 282$).

Author: Bhagat, R. S., et al.

Article: Total life stress: A multimethod validation of the construct and its effects on organizationally valued outcomes and withdrawal behaviors.

Journal: *Journal of Applied Psychology,* February 1985, *70*(1), 202–214.

Related Research: Dohrenwend, B. S., et al. (1978). Exemplification of a method for scaling life events: The PERI life events scale. *Journal of Health and Social Behavior, 19,* 205–229.

• • •

2489

Test Name: LIFE EXPERIENCES SURVEY

Purpose: To measure life stress.

Number of Items: 57

Format: Subjects indicate events experienced during the previous year. Negative and positive stress scores represent the sum of ratings (4-point scale) of negative and positive events.

Reliability: Test–retest (5 or 6 weeks) reliability was .56 to .88.

Author: Heilbrun, A. B., Jr.

Article: Cognitive defenses and life stress: An information-processing analysis.

Journal: *Psychological Reports,* February 1984, *54*(1), 3–17.

Related Research: Johnson, J. H., & Sarason, I. G. (1979). Recent developments in research on life stress. In V. Hamilton & D. M. Warburton (Eds.), *Human stress and cognition: An information processing approach* (pp. 205– 233). New York: McGraw-Hill.

• • •

2490

Test Name: LOUISVILLE FEAR SURVEY FOR CHILDREN

Purpose: To measure fear in children.

Number of Items: 104

Format: Mothers rate children on a 5-point fear severity scale.

Reliability: Alphas ranged from .51 to .89 on subscales. Mean alpha was .76.

Validity: Correlations between child and mothers' reports ranged from −.13 to .86. Of 48 correlations, 27 are significant ($p <$ .05, .01, or .001), and in the correct direction.

Author: Dollinger, S. J., et al.

Article: Lightening-strike disaster: Effects of children's fears and worries.

Journal: *Journal of Consulting and Clinical Psychology*, December 1984, *52*(6), 1028–1038.

Related Research: Staley, A. A., & O'Donnell, J. P. (1984). A developmental analysis of mothers' reports of normal children's fears. *Journal of Genetic Psychology, 144*, 165–178.

■ ■ ■

2491

Test Name: MAINE SCALE OF PARANOID AND NONPARANOID SCHIZOPHRENIA

Purpose: To measure schizophrenia.

Number of Items: 10

Format: Multiple-choice. All items presented.

Reliability: Test–retest reliability ranged from .73 to .89 (4-day interval).

Validity: Correlations with other measures of schizophrenia ranged from .43 to .76. Correlations with expanded similarities test ranged from .02 to .26.

Author: Magaro, P. A., et al.

Article: The Maine scale of paranoid and nonparanoid schizophrenia.

Journal: *Journal of Consulting and Clinical Psychology*, June 1981, *49*(3), 438–447.

Related Research: Vojtisek, J. E. (1976). Signal detection and size estimation in schizophrenia. Doctoral dissertation, University of Maine (1975). *Dissertation Abstracts International, 36*, 5290B–5291B. (University Microfilms No. 76-7445)

■ ■ ■

2492

Test Name: MALADJUSTMENT SCALE

Purpose: To measure maladjustment.

Number of Items: 9

Format: Includes interpersonal, intrapersonal, and somatic problems. A 5-point Likert scale ranging from 1 (*not at all*) to 5 (*extremely*) was used to rate each problem.

Reliability: Coefficient alphas were .88 (200 clients) and .91 (200 counselors).

Author: Turner, C. J., and Schwartzbach, H.

Article: A construct validation study of the counseling expectation inventory.

Journal: *Measurement and Evaluation in Guidance*, April 1983, *16*(1), 18–24.

Related Research: Robinson, A. (1972). *Development and evaluation of a brief problem checklist for use in college counseling centers*. Unpublished doctoral dissertation, University of Tennessee.

■ ■ ■

2493

Test Name: MENTAL HEALTH INVENTORY

Purpose: To measure psychological distress and well-being in general populations.

Number of Items: 38

Format: Summated rating format.

Reliability: Internal consistency ranged from .83 to .91 across subscales. Stability ranged from .56 to .64.

Author: Veit, C. T., and Ware, J. E., Jr.

Article: The structure of psychological distress and well-being in general populations.

Journal: *Journal of Consulting and Clinical Psychology*, October 1983, *51*(5), 730–742.

Related Research: Dupuy, H. J. (1979). *A brief description of the research edition of the general psychological well-being schedule*. Fairfax, VA: National Center for Health Statistics.

■ ■ ■

2494

Test Name: MOOD QUESTIONNAIRE

Purpose: To assess mood.

Number of Items: 71

Format: Includes 6 mood dimensions: pleasantness, activation, calmness, extraversion, social orientation, and confidence.

Validity: Correlations with goals ranged from .04 to .56.

Author: Sjöberg, L., et al.

Article: Cathectic orientation, goal setting and mood.

Journal: *Journal of Personality Assessment*, June 1983, *47*(3), 307–313.

Related Research: Sjöberg, I., et al. (1979). The measurement of mood. *Scandinavian Journal of Psychology, 20*, 1–18.

■ ■ ■

2495

Test Name: MORALE SCALE

Purpose: To measure morale.

Number of Items: 6

Format: Responses to each item are made on a 4-point scale from *strongly agree* to *strongly disagree*. All items are presented.

Reliability: Cronbach's alphas were .85 (men) and .866 (women).

Validity: Correlations with other variables ranged from −.166 to .368.

Author: Lee, G. R., and Ellithorpe, E.

Article: Intergenerational exchange and subjective well-being among the elderly.

Journal: *Journal of Marriage and the Family,* February 1982, *44*(1), 217–224.

Related Research: Lee, G. R., & Ihinger-Tallman, M. (1980). Sibling interaction and morale: The effects of family relations on older people. *Research on Aging, 2,* 367–391.

■ ■ ■

2496

Test Name: MORALE SCALE

Purpose: To measure morale.

Number of Items: 14

Format: Three-category response scale: *high, depends, low.* All items are presented.

Reliability: Alpha was .82.

Author: Dowd, J. J., and LaRossa, R.

Article: Primary group contact and elderly morale: An exchange/power analysis.

Journal: *Sociology and Social Research,* January 1982, *66*(2), 184–197.

Related Research: Lawton, M. P. (1975). The Philadelphia geriatric morale scale: A revision. *Journal of Gerontology, 30,* 85–89.

2497

Test Name: MULTIDIMENSIONAL FEAR OF DEATH SCALE

Purpose: To measure fear of death.

Number of Items: 42

Format: Includes 8 dimensions: fear of dying process, fear of the dead, fear of being destroyed, fear for significant others, fear of the unknown, fear of conscious death, fear for the body after death, and fear of premature death.

Validity: Correlation of fear of the unknown subscale with a measure of religious orthodoxy was −.64.

Author: Wass, H., and Forfar, C. S.

Article: Assessment of attitude toward death: Techniques and instruments for use with older persons.

Journal: *Measurement and Evaluation in Guidance,* October 1982, *15*(3), 210–220.

Related Research: Hoelter, J. (1979). Multidimensional treatment of the fear of death. *Journal of Consulting and Clinical Psychology, 47,* 996–999.

■ ■ ■

2498

Test Name: MULTISCORE DEPRESSION INVENTORY— SHORT FORM

Purpose: To measure severity of depression and depressive features.

Number of Items: 47

Format: Includes 9 subscales: sad mood, guilt, instrumental helplessness, low energy level, social introversion, irritability, pessimism, cognitive difficulty, and low self-esteem.

Reliability: Test–retest reliabilities:

immediate (N = 108) ranged from .83 to .95 and 3 week (N = 108) ranged from .41 to .90. Coefficient alphas ranged from .71 to .92 (N = 133) and from .67 to .88 (N = 108).

Author: Berndt, D. J., et al.

Article: Multidimensional assessment of depression.

Journal: *Journal of Personality Assessment,* October 1984, *48*(5), 489–494.

Related Research: Berndt, D. J., et al. (1983). Readability of self-report depression inventories. *Journal of Consulting and Clinical Psychology, 51,* 627–628.

■ ■ ■

2499

Test Name: NEGATIVE WELL-BEING SCALE

Purpose: To measure negative well-being.

Number of Items: 32

Format: Items are rated on a 5-point rating scale.

Reliability: Alpha was .88.

Author: Litt, M. D., and Turk, D. C.

Article: Sources of stress and dissatisfaction in experienced high school teachers.

Journal: *Journal of Educational Research,* January/February 1985, *78*(3), 178–185.

Related Research: Zalezik, A., et al. (1977). Stress reactions in organizations: Syndromes, causes and consequences. *Behavior Science, 22,* 151–162.

■ ■ ■

2500

Test Name: PAPPO FEAR OF SUCCESS SCALE

Purpose: To measure self-doubt, preoccupation with competition, preoccupation with evaluation, repudiation of competence, and self-sabotage behavior.

Number of Items: 83

Format: Yes–no.

Reliability: .90

Validity: Correlations with Good and Good, and Zuckerman and Allison scales are generally positive, except for a negative correlation for men on the Zuckerman and Allison scales.

Author: Chabassol, D. J., and Ishiyama, F. I.

Article: Correlations among three measures of fear of success.

Journal: *Psychological Reports*, 1983, *52*(1), 55–58.

Related Research: Pappo, M. (1972). *Fear of success: An empirical and theoretical analysis.* Unpublished doctoral dissertation, Teacher's College, Columbia University.

■ ■ ■

2501

Test Name: PERCEIVED STRESS SCALE

Purpose: To measure perceived stress.

Number of Items: 4

Format: Frequency rating scale. Sample items presented.

Reliability: Alpha was .72. Test–retest (over 2 months) was .55.

Author: Glasgow, R. E., et al.

Article: Quitting smoking: Strategies used and variables associated with success in a stop-smoking contest.

Journal: *Journal of Consulting and Clinical Psychology*, December 1985, *53*(6), 905–912.

Related Research: Cohen, S., et al. (1983). A global measure of perceived stress. *Journal of Health and Social Behavior, 24*, 385–396.

2502

Test Name: PEER NOMINATION INVENTORY OF DEPRESSION (PNID)

Purpose: To assess depression.

Number of Items: 13

Format: Nomination format. Sample items presented. Children nominate (choose) other children who they believe "looks sad," "smiles," and so on.

Reliability: Reliability was .95.

Author: Lefkowitz, M. M., and Tesiny, E. P.

Article: Depression in children: Prevalence and correlates.

Journal: *Journal of Consulting and Clinical Psychology*, October 1985, *53*(5), 647–656.

Related Research: Lefkowitz, M. M., & Tesiny, E. P. (1980). Assessment of childhood depression. *Journal of Consulting and Clinical Psychology, 48*, 43–50.

Cantwell, D. P. (1983). Assessment of childhood depression: An overview. In D. P. Cantwell & G. A. Carlson (Eds.), *Affective disorders in childhood and adolescents–An update.* New York: Spectrum.

■ ■ ■

2503

Test Name: PEER RATING DEPRESSION SCALE

Purpose: To measure depression.

Number of Items: 9

Format: 4-point frequency scale.

Reliability: Alpha was .76

Validity: Correlates .44 with Beck Depression Inventory; correlates .39 with POMS-D scores.

Author: Malouff, J.

Article: Development and

validation of a behavioral peer-rating measured depression.

Journal: *Journal of Consulting and Clinical Psychology*, November 1984, *52*(6), 1108–1109.

■ ■ ■

2504

Test Name: PERSONAL LIFE SATISFACTION SCALE

Purpose: To measure personal life satisfaction.

Number of Items: 10

Format: Responses are made on a 7-point scale. Sample items are presented.

Reliability: Alpha was .83.

Validity: Correlations with other variables ranged from –.67 to .66.

Author: Bhagat, R. S., et al.

Article: Total life stress: A multimethod validation of the construct and its effects on organizationally valued outcomes and withdrawal behaviors.

Journal: *Journal of Applied Psychology*, February 1985, *70*(1), 202–214.

Related Research: Kornhauser, A. (1965). *Mental health of the industrial worker.* New York: Wiley.

■ ■ ■

2505

Test Name: PERSONALITY DATA FORM

Purpose: To measure irrational ideas, beliefs, and attitudes of individuals requesting psychotherapy.

Number of Items: 50

Format: Subjects indicate the frequency with which they experience the reactions and thoughts described in the items.

Reliability: Cronbach's alpha was .91.

Validity: Correlates –.60 with Rational Behavior Inventory (Shorkey & Whiteman, 1977); .66 with Trait Anxiety Inventory (Spielberger et al., 1970); and .56 with symptom checklist (Sutton-Simon & Shorkey, unpublished).

Author: Shorkey, C. T., and Sutton-Simon, K.

Article: Personality data form: Internal reliability and validity.

Journal: *Psychological Reports,* June 1983, *52*(3), 879–883.

■ ■ ■

2506

Test Name: PHILADELPHIA GERIATRIC CENTER MORALE SCALE

Purpose: To measure morale of the elderly.

Number of Items: 17

Format: *Yes–no* and *satisfied–not satisfied* response categories. All items presented.

Reliability: Agitation factor is most robust.

Validity: Four factors extracted from a factor analysis confirm four dimensions identified in other studies.

Author: Mancini, J. A., et al.

Article: Measuring morale: Note on use of factor scores.

Journal: *Psychological Reports,* February 1985, *56*(1), 139–144.

Related Research: Lawton, M. P. (1975). The Philadelphia geriatric center morale scale: A revision. *Journal of Gerontology, 30,* 85–89.

■ ■ ■

2507

Test Name: PHYSICAL ANHEDONIA SCALE

Purpose: To measure the lowered ability to experience pleasure.

Number of Items: 61

Format: True–false. Sample items presented.

Reliability: Alpha was .83 (men) and .78 (women).

Author: Chapman, L. J., et al.

Article: Reliabilities and intercorrelations of eight measures of proneness to psychosis.

Journal: *Journal of Consulting and Clinical Psychology,* April 1982, *50*(2), 187–195.

Related Research: Chapman, L. J., & Chapman, L. P. (1978). *Revised Psychical anhedonia scale.* Unpublished text.

Chapman, L. J., et al. (1976). Scales for physical and social anhedonia. *Journal of Abnormal Psychology, 85,* 374–392.

■ ■ ■

2508

Test Name: PIANO PERFORMANCE ANXIETY SCALE

Purpose: To provide a self-report state-anxiety measure.

Number of Items: 24

Format: Includes two subscales: cognitive–attentional and emotional–autonomic. Employs a true–false format. Examples are presented.

Reliability: Test–retest reliabilities were .49 (cognitive–attentional) and .27 (emotional–autonomic).

Validity: Correlations with other variables ranged from –.19 to .70.

Author: Sweeney, G. A., and Horan, J. J.

Article: Separate and combined effects of cue-controlled relaxation and cognitive restructuring in the treatment of musical performance anxiety.

Journal: *Journal of Counseling Psychology,* September 1982, *29*(5), 486–497.

Related Research: Sarason, I. G. (1978). The test anxiety scale: Concept and research. In C. D. Spielberger & I. G. Sarason (Eds.), *Stress and Anxiety* (Vol. 5). Washington, DC: Hemisphere.

■ ■ ■

2509

Test Name: PRESCHOOL OBSERVATIONAL SCALE OF ANXIETY

Purpose: To assess anxiety of children too young to accurately report their internal states.

Number of Items: 30

Format: Frequency of each behavior observed was recorded by observers. Examples are given.

Reliability: Interrater reliability was .93.

Author: Robinson, S. L., et al.

Article: Eye classification, sex, and math anxiety in learning disabled children: Behavioral observations on conservation of volume.

Journal: *Perceptual and Motor Skills,* December 1985, *61*(3, Part 2), 1311–1321.

Related Research: Glennon, B., & Weisz, J. B. (1978). An observational approach to the assessment of anxiety in young children. *Journal of Consulting and Clinical Psychology, 46,* 1246–1257.

■ ■ ■

2510

Test Name: PRIVATE SELF-CONSCIOUSNESS SCALE

Purpose: To measure private preoccupation with one's own characteristics.

Number of Items: 5

Format: Items are 3-category multiple-choice. All items are presented.

Reliability: Alpha was .603.

Author: Elliott, G. C., et al.

Article: Transient depersonalization in youth.

Journal: *Social Psychology Quarterly*, June 1984, *47*(2), 115–129.

Related Research: Fenigstein, A. M., et al. (1975). Public and private self-consciousness: Assessment and theory. *Journal of Counseling and Clinical Psychology*, *43*, 522–527.

• • •

2511

Test Name: PROCESSES OF CHANGE TEST

Purpose: To measure 10 processes of change (examples are consciousness raising, self-liberation, and self-reevaluation).

Number of Items: 40

Format: Items rated on 5-point Likert format. Sample items are presented for each of the 10 processes.

Reliability: Alpha ranged from .75 to .91 across processes.

Author: Prochaska, J. O., and DiClemente, C. C.

Article: Stages of processes of self-change of smoking: Toward an integrative model of change.

Journal: *Journal of Consulting and Clinical Psychology*, June 1983, *51*(3), 390–395.

Related Research: Prochaska, J. O., et al. (1981). *Measuring processes of change.* Paper presented at the annual meeting of the International Council of Psychologists, Los Angeles, CA.

2512

Test Name: PROBLEM AND ROLE PROJECTION SCALES

Purpose: To measure to what extent subjects project their problems and themselves into movies, plays, books, or television shows.

Number of Items: 5

Format: Multiple-choice. Sample items are presented.

Reliability: Alphas were .76 (problem) and .78 (role).

Author: Hirschman, E. C.

Article: Predictors of self-projection, fantasy, fulfillment, and escapism.

Journal: *Journal of Social Psychology*, June 1983, *120*(first half), 63–76.

Related Research: Hirschman, E. C., & Holbrook, M. B. (1982). Hedonic consumption: Emerging concepts, methods, propositions. *J. Market, 46*, 92–101.

• • •

2513

Test Name: PRONENESS TO DISORGANIZATION UNDER STRESS RATING

Purpose: To measure proneness to disorganization.

Number of Items: 1

Format: Test uses a 9-point rating scale.

Reliability: Interrater reliability was .95.

Author: Morgan, K. C., and Hock, E.

Article: A longitudinal study of the psychosocial variables affecting the career patterns of women with young children.

Journal: *Journal of Marriage and the Family*, May 1984, *46*(2), 383–390.

• • •

Related Research: Moss, H. (1971). *Manual for global variables–post-partum interview for determinants of maternal contract.* Unpublished manuscript, National Institutes of Mental Health, Washington, DC.

• • •

2514

Test Name: PSYCHIATRIC EVALUATION FORM

Purpose: To quantify pathology described in diagnostic interviews and structured interviews.

Number of Items: 19

Format: Six-point clinical scales.

Reliability: Interrater reliability ranged from .50 to .91.

Validity: Correlation of clinical impairment and cluster scores ranged from .32 to .50.

Author: Green, B. L., et al.

Article: Use of the psychiatric evaluation form to quantify children's interview data.

Journal: *Journal of Consulting and Clinical Psychology*, June 1983, *51*(3), 353–359.

Related Research: Endicott, J., & Spitzer, R. L. (1972). What! Another rating scale? The psychiatric evaluation form. *Journal of Nervous and Mental Disease, 154*, 88–104.

• • •

2515

Test Name: PSYCHIATRIC STATUS SCHEDULE

Purpose: To assess psychiatric symptomatology.

Number of Items: 321 (symptoms).

Format: Rating form completed by trained interviewers during a structured interview.

Reliability: Interrater reliability ranged from .91 to 1.00. Internal consistency ranged from .19 to .72 (reflecting low average covariance of symptom syndromes in normal populations).

Author: Kavanaugh, M. J., et al.

Article: The relationship between job satisfaction and psychiatric health symptoms for air traffic controllers.

Journal: *Personnel Psychology,* Winter 1981, *34*(4), 691–707.

Related Research: Spitzer, R. I., et al. (1967). Instruments and recording forms for evaluating psychiatric status and history: Rationale, method of development and description. *Comprehensive Psychiatry, 8,* 321–943.

■ ■ ■

2516

Test Name: PSYCHOSOMATIC COMPLAINTS SCALE

Purpose: To identify psychosomatic complaints.

Number of Items: 9

Format: Employs a 5-point scale. A sample question is presented.

Reliability: Cronbach's alpha was .84.

Author: Frese, M., and Okonek, K.

Article: Reasons to leave shiftwork and psychological and psychosomatic complaints of former shiftworkers.

Journal: *Journal of Applied Psychology,* August 1984, *69*(3), 509–514.

Related Research: Mohr, G. (1984). *Measuring psychological well-being in blue collar workers.* Unpublished manuscript, Freie Universitaet, Department of Psychology, Berlin.

Caplan, R. D., et al. (1975). *Job demands and worker health.* Washington, DC: National

Institute for Occupational Safety and Health, U.S. Department of Health, Education and Welfare.

■ ■ ■

2517

Test Name: PSYCHOLOGICAL STRESS SCALE

Purpose: To measure psychological stress.

Number of Items: 6

Format: Employs a 5-point answer scale. A sample question is presented.

Reliability: Cronbach's alpha was .80.

Author: Frese, M., and Okonek, K.

Article: Reasons to leave shiftwork and psychological and psychosomatic complaints of former shiftworkers.

Journal: *Journal of Applied Psychology,* August 1984, *69*(3), 509–514.

Related Research: Semmer, N. (1982). Stress at work, stress in private life, and psychological well-being. In W. Bachmann et al. (Eds.), *Mental load and stress in activity: European approaches.* Berlin: Deutscher Verlag der Wissenschaften.

■ ■ ■

2518

Test Name: PSYCHOPATHY IN CRIMINAL POPULATIONS CHECKLIST

Purpose: To measure psychopathy in criminal populations.

Number of Items: 22

Format: Checklist format. 3-point scale (0 = *does not apply,* 1 = *uncertainty,* 2 = *certain it does apply*).

Reliability: Interrater reliability

ranged from .88 to .93. Generalizability coefficient ranged from .85 to .90. Alpha ranged from .82 to .90.

Validity: Multiple correlation between checklist items and ratings of psychopathy was .86; 75% to 96% of cases were correctly classified in discriminant analyses.

Author: Schroeder, M. L., et al.

Article: Generalizability of a checklist for assessment of psychopathy.

Journal: *Journal of Consulting and Clinical Psychology,* August 1983, *51*(4), 511–516.

Related Research: Hare, R. D. (1980). A research scale for the assessment of psychopathy in criminal populations. *Personality and Individual Differences, 1,* 111–119.

■ ■ ■

2519

Test Name: PSYCHOTHERAPY PROBLEM CHECKLIST

Purpose: To measure difficult-to-change problems by self-report.

Number of Items: 21

Format: 21 items include these problems: headaches, anxiety, suicide intent, disturbed sleep, and so forth.

Reliability: $r = .81$.

Author: Morrison, J. K., and Heeder, R.

Article: Follow-up study of the effectiveness of emotive–reconstructive therapy.

Journal: *Psychological Reports,* February 1984, *54*(1), 149–150.

Related Research: Morrison, J. K., & Teta, D. C. (1978). Simplified use of the semantic differential to measure psychotherapy outcome. *Journal of Clinical Psychology, 34,* 751–753.

2520

Test Name: RATINGS OF BEHAVIORAL DEPRESSION

Purpose: To assess behavioral symptoms of depression.

Number of Items: 30

Format: Involves a semistructured interview procedure.

Validity: Correlations with other variables ranged from −.33 to .31.

Author: Fry, P. S.

Article: Development of a geriatric scale of hopelessness: Implications for counseling and intervention with the depressed elderly.

Journal: *Journal of Counseling Psychology*, July 1984, *31*(3), 322–331.

Related Research: Weinberg, J. (1975). Geriatric psychiatry. In A. M. Freeman, H. I. Kaplan, & B. J. Sadock (Eds.), *Comprehensive textbook of psychiatry, 2*, 2405–2420. Baltimore, MD: Williams & Wilkins.

■ ■ ■

2521

Test Name: REASONS FOR LIVING INVENTORY

Purpose: To measure range of belief potentially important as reasons for not committing suicide.

Number of Items: 48

Format: 6-point Likert scale.

Reliability: Alpha ranged from .72 to .89 across subscales.

Validity: Correlations with suicidal behaviors questionnaire generally confirm the validity of the inventory. Numerous *F* tests and correlations are presented.

Author: Linehan, M. M., et al.

Article: Reasons for staying alive when you are thinking of killing yourself: A reasons for living inventory.

Journal: *Journal of Consulting and Clinical Psychology*, April 1983, *51*(2), 276–286.

■ ■ ■

2522

Test Name: RECENT LIFE CHANGES QUESTIONNAIRE

Purpose: To provide a method of measuring life change.

Number of Items: 76

Format: Includes 5 categories: health, work, home and family, personal–social, and financial.

Reliability: Reliability was .84 (1-month interval).

Validity: Correlation with the schedule of recent experiences was .67.

Author: Pearson, J. E., and Long, T. J.

Article: Life change measurement: Scoring, reliability and subjective estimate of adjustment.

Journal: *Measurement and Evaluation in Counseling and Development*, July 1985, *18*(2), 72–80.

Related Research: Rahe, R. H. (1975). Epidemiological studies of life change and illness. *International Journal of Psychiatry in Medicine, 6*, 133–146.

■ ■ ■

2523

Test Name: REVISED WORRY–EMOTIONALITY SCALE

Purpose: To measure cognitive and emotional components of anxiety.

Number of Items: 10

Format: Items are rated in a 5-category multiple-choice format from *does not describe my present condition* to *describes my present condition very well.* All items are presented.

Reliability: Internal consistency correlations were .81 (worry) and .86 (emotionality).

Author: Morris, L. W., et al.

Article: Cognitive and emotional components of anxiety: Literature review and a revised worry–emotionality scale.

Journal: *Journal of Educational Psychology*, August 1981, *73*(4), 541–555.

Related Research: Liebert, R. M., & Morris, L. W. (1967). Cognitive and emotional components of test anxiety: A distinction and some initial data. *Psychological Reports, 20*, 975–978.

■ ■ ■

2524

Test Name: REVISED CHILDREN'S MANIFEST ANXIETY SCALE

Purpose: To measure chronic anxiety.

Number of Items: 37

Format: A self-report questionnaire. Includes 9 items to measure social desirability or lie scale.

Reliability: Internal consistency reliabilities were in the mid .80s.

Author: Reynolds, C. R.

Article: Long-term stability of scores on the revised Children's Manifest Anxiety Scale.

Journal: *Perceptual and Motor Skills,* December 1981, *53*(3), 702.

Related Research: Reynolds, C. R., & Richmond, B. O. (1978). What I think and feel: A revised measure of children's manifest anxiety. *Journal of Abnormal Child Psychology, 6*, 271–280.

■ ■ ■

2525

Test Name: ROLE AMBIGUITY SCALE

Purpose: To indicate role stress.

Number of Items: 6

Reliability: Cronbach's alpha was .84.

Validity: Correlation with other variables ranged from −.56 to .47.

Author: Chacko, T. I.

Article: Women and equal employment opportunity: Some unintended effects.

Journal: *Journal of Applied Psychology,* February 1982, *67*(1), 119–123.

Related Research: Rizzo, J. R., et al. (1970). Role conflict and ambiguity in complex organizations. *Administrative Science Quarterly, 15,* 150–163.

■ ■ ■

2526

Test Name: ROLE CONFLICT SCALE

Purpose: To indicate role stress.

Number of Items: 8

Reliability: Cronbach's alpha was .73.

Validity: Correlation with other variables ranged from −.56 to −.07.

Author: Chacko, T. I.

Article: Women and equal employment opportunity: Some unintended effects.

Journal: *Journal of Applied Psychology,* February 1982, *67*(1), 119–123.

Related Research: Rizzo, J. R., et al. (1970). Role conflict and ambiguity in complex organizations. *Administrative Science Quarterly, 15,* 150–163.

■ ■ ■

2527

Test Name: ROLE STRESS SCALE

Purpose: To measure role stress.

Number of Items: 16

Format: Items are rated on a 5-point Likert scale.

Reliability: Alphas ranged from .70 to .88 across subscales.

Author: Keenan, A., and Newton, T. J.

Article: Frustration in organizations: Relationships to role stress, climate and psychological strain.

Journal: *Journal of Occupational Psychology,* March 1984, *57*(1), 57–65.

Related Research: Rizzo, J. R., et al. (1970). Role conflict and ambiguity in complex organizations. *Administrative Science Quarterly, 15,* 150–163.

■ ■ ■

2528

Test Name: ROSENZWEIG PICTURE-FRUSTRATION STUDY

Purpose: To assess typical modes of reaction to frustration.

Number of Items: 24

Format: Subjects write in what they think an anonymous person would say who is pictured to the right of each of 24 cartoon-like pictures depicting an everyday, interpersonally frustrating situation. Provides six scores: extraggression, intraggresion, imaggression, obstacle-dominance, ego-defense, and need-persistence.

Reliability: Correlations between raters ranged from .50 to .90.

Author: Graybill, D., et al.

Article: Effects of playing violent versus nonviolent video games on the aggressive ideation of aggressive and non-aggressive children.

Journal: *Child Study Journal,* 1985, *15*(3), 199–205.

Related Research: Rosenzweig, S. (1978). *Aggressive behavior and the Rosenzweig Picture Frustration Study.* New York: Praeger.

■ ■ ■

2529

Test Name: SATISFACTION WITH LIFE SCALE

Purpose: To measure global life satisfaction.

Number of Items: 5

Format: Responses to each item are made on a scale from 1 (*strongly disagree*) to 7 (*strongly agree*).

Reliability: Test–retest (2 months) correlation coefficient was .82. Coefficient alpha was .87.

Validity: Correlations with other variables ranged from −.37 to .68 ($N = 176$) and from −.32 to .66 ($N = 163$).

Author: Dicner, E., et al.

Article: The satisfaction with life scale.

Journal: *Journal of Personality Assessment,* February 1985, *49*(1), 71–75.

■ ■ ■

2530

Test Name: SCALE FOR SUICIDE IDEATORS

Purpose: To assess and quantify degree of suicide intent in suicide ideators.

Number of Items: 19

Format: Interviewer rated format.

Validity: Self-report form correlates .90 with interviewer form.

Author: Schotte, D. E., and Clum, G. A.

Article: Suicide ideation in a college population: A test of a model.

Journal: *Journal of Consulting and Clinical Psychology*, October 1982, *50*(5), 690–696.

Related Research: Beck, A., et al. (1979). Assessment of suicidal ideation: The scale for suicide ideators. *Journal of Consulting and Clinical Psychology, 47*, 343–352.

■ ■ ■

2531

Test Name: SCHEDULE OF RECENT EVENTS

Purpose: To measure the amount of stress experienced from readjustment to life events.

Number of Items: 43

Format: Life events included are: work, family, personal, and financial.

Reliability: Cronbach's alpha was .83 ($N = 120$).

Validity: With ego-permissiveness, $r = .57$ ($N = 120$); with field-dependent perception, $r = -.73$ ($N = 120$).

Author: Daly, E. B.

Article: Relationship of stress and ego energy to field-dependent perception in older adults.

Journal: *Perceptual and Motor Skills*, December 1984, *59*(3), 919–926.

Related Research: Holmes, T. H., & Masuda, M. (1973). Life change and illness susceptibility. In J. P. Scott & E. C. Senay (Eds.), *Separation and depression: Clinical and research aspects* (pp. 161–186) [Symposium presented at the Chicago meeting of the American Association of the Advancement of Science, December 27, 1970]. Washington, DC: American Association for the Advancement for Science.

2532

Test Name: SCHEDULE OF RECENT EXPERIENCES

Purpose: To provide a tool for recording and studying the impact of life changes on stress-related illness.

Number of Items: 42

Format: Items are weighted according to seriousness of impact and degree of adjustment required.

Reliability: Test–retest reliability ranged from .87 to .90 (1-week interval); and from .55 to .70 (6- to 9-month intervals).

Validity: Correlation with the Recent Life Changes Questionnaire was .67 ($N = 109$).

Author: Pearson, J. E., and Long, T. J.

Article: Life change measurement: Scoring, reliability, and subjective estimates of adjustment.

Journal: *Measurement and Evaluation in Counseling and Development*, July 1985, *18*(2), 72–80.

Related Research: Rahe, R. H. (1972). Epidemiological studies of life change and illness. *International Journal of Psychiatry in Medicine, 6*, 133–146.

■ ■ ■

2533

Test Name: SCHEDULE OF RECENT EXPERIENCES (SRE)

Purpose: To measure stressful life events.

Number of Items: 43

Format: Items (events) are checked if they have occurred in the last 12 months. A score is obtained by summing the weight of each checked item.

Validity: Correlated .40 with

Organizational Readjustment Rating Scale (Naismith, 1975).

Author: Weiss, H. M., et al.

Article: Effects of life and job stress on information search behaviors of organizational members.

Journal: *Journal of Applied Psychology*, February 1982, *67*(1), 60–66.

Related Research: Holmes, T. H., & Rahe, R. H. (1967). The social readjustment rating scale. *Journal of Psychosomatic Research, 11*, 213–218.

■ ■ ■

2534

Test Name: SHORT FORM MULTISCORE DEPRESSION INVENTORY

Purpose: To assess severity of depressive symptoms.

Number of Items: 47

Reliability: Kuder-Richardson formula was .92.

Validity: Correlated .63 with Beck Depression Inventory.

Author: Berndt, D. J.

Article: Evaluation of a short form of the multiscore depression inventory.

Journal: *Journal of Consulting and Clinical Psychology*, October 1983, *51*(5), 790–791.

Related Research: Berndt, D. J., et al. (1980). Development and initial evaluation of a multiscore depression inventory. *Journal of Personality Assessment, 44*, 396–404.

■ ■ ■

2535

Test Name: STRESS ASSESSMENT PACKAGE

Purpose: To measure stress-related variables.

Number of Items: 160

Format: Includes 20 factors and 12 single item variables.

Reliability: Coefficient alphas for the 20 factors ranged from .67 to .94.

Author: Hendrix, W. H., et al.

Article: Behavioral and physiological consequences of stress and its antecedent factors.

Journal: *Journal of Applied Psychology,* February 1985, *70*(1), 188–201.

Related Research: Fye, S. P & Staton, C. W. (1981). *Individual and organizational variables relationship to coronary heart disease* (Report No. LSSR 3-81). Wright-Patterson AFB, OH: Air Force Institute of Technology.

Martin, W. H., & Simard, L. C. (1982). *Stress and coronary heart disease in organizational, extraorganizational and individual environments* (Report No. LSSR8-82). Wright-Patterson AFB, OH: Air Force Institute of Technology.

■ ■ ■

2536

Test Name: STRESS RESPONSE SCALE

Purpose: To assess the behavioral pattern that the child is likely to adopt in response to stress.

Number of Items: 40

Format: The scale is completed by the person perceiving the child's problematic behavior. Included is a total score and subscale scores for each of five response patterns: impulsive (acting out), passive–aggressive, impulsive (overactive), repressed, and dependent. A 6-point rating scale is employed ranging from *never* (0) to *always* (5).

Reliability: Test–retest (1 month) reliability coefficient was .86 (*N*= 25). Coefficient alpha was .94.

Author: Chandler, L. A., and Shermis, M. D.

Article: Assessing behavioral responses to stress.

Journal: *Educational and Psychological Measurement,* Winter 1985, *45*(4), 825–844.

Related Research: Chandler, L. A. (1983). The Stress Response Scale: An instrument for use in assessing emotional adjustment reactions. *School Psychology Review, 12,* 260–265.

■ ■ ■

2537

Test Name: STRESS SCALE

Purpose: To measure affective states indicative of psychological strain and stress.

Number of Items: 19

Format: Includes three subscales: depression, anxiety, and irritation.

Reliability: Internal consistency, alpha was .89.

Author: Colarelli, S. M.

Article: Methods of communication and mediating processes in realistic job previews.

Journal: *Journal of Applied Psychology,* November 1984, *69*(4), 633–642.

Related Research: Caplan, R. D., et al. (1975). Job demands and worker health. Washington, DC: U.S. Government Printing Offices.

■ ■ ■

2538

Test Name: SUICIDAL TENDENCIES TESTING PROCEDURE

Purpose: To assess suicidal tendencies.

Number of Items: 4

Time Required: 15–25 minutes.

Format: Four stories are followed by a question to which a child responds by indicating a response on a color-coded ruler. All stories are presented.

Reliability: Test–retest ranged from .23 to .78 (7 of 8 statistically significant, $p < .05$).

Validity: Subscales correlate with themselves at two different times more strongly than with each other.

Author: Orbach, I., et al.

Article: Attraction and repulsion by life and death in suicidal and normal children.

Journal: *Journal of Consulting and Clinical Psychology,* October 1983, *51*(5), 661–670.

■ ■ ■

2539

Test Name: SYMPTOM CHECKLIST–90

Purpose: To measure psychiatric symptoms by self-report.

Number of Items: 90

Format: Items are rated on a 5-point scale of distress.

Reliability: Alpha ranged from .56 to .96 across nine subscales.

Validity: Most variance accounted for by first unrotated factor. Scale may measure mainly general discomfort, not specific dimensions of symptomatology.

Author: Holcomb, W. R., et al.

Article: Factor structure of the Symptom Checklist–90 with acute psychiatric inpatients.

Journal: *Journal of Consulting and Clinical Psychology,* August 1983, *51*(4), 535–538.

Related Research: Derogatis, L. R., & Cleary, P. A. (1977). Confirmation of the dimensional structure of the SCL-90: A study in construct validation. *Journal of Clinical Psychology, 33,* 981–989.

* * *

2540

Test Name: TEDIUM MEASURE

Purpose: To measure physical, mental, and emotional exhaustion.

Number of Items: 21

Format: Items are rated on a 7-point scale (*never* to *always*).

Reliability: Alpha ranged between .91 and .93. Test–retest (1 month) reliability was .89.

Validity: Significant correlation with job satisfaction and health problems was reported.

Author: Stout, J. K., and Posner, J. L.

Article: Stress, role ambiguity and role conflict.

Journal: *Psychological Reports,* December 1984, *55*(3), 747–753.

Related Research: Pines, A. M., et al. (1981). *Burnout: From tedium to personal growth.* New York: Free Press.

Stout, J. K., & Williams, J. M. (1983). A comparison of two measures of burnout. *Psychological Reports, 53,* 283–289.

* * *

2541

Test Name: TEMPLAR DEATH ANXIETY SCALE

Purpose: To measure the degree of acceptance of death.

Number of Items: 15

Format: True–false.

Reliability: Test–retest reliability was .83; split-half reliability ranged from .43 to .83; Spearman-Brown correlation coefficient was .60.

Author: Schell, B. H., and Zinger, J. T.

Article: Death anxiety scale means and standard deviations for Ontario undergraduates and funeral directors.

Journal: *Psychological Reports,* April 1984, *54*(2), 439–446.

Related Research: Templar, D. I. (1970). The construction and validation of a death anxiety scale. *Journal of General Psychology, 82,* 165–177.

* * *

2542

Test Name: TENSION INDEX

Purpose: To measure tension.

Number of Items: 9

Format: Responses were made on a 5-point scale from *never* to *nearly all the time.*

Reliability: Alpha was .86.

Validity: Zero-order correlations with role ambiguity was .41 and with role conflict was .69.

Author: Bedeian, A. G., et al.

Article: The relationship between role stress and job-related, interpersonal and organizational climate factors.

Journal: *Journal of Social Psychology,* April 1981, *113*(second half), 247–260.

Related Research: Lyons, T. F. (1971). Role clarity, need for clarity, satisfaction, tension and withdrawal. *Organizational Behavior and Human Performance, 6,* 99–110.

* * *

2543

Test Name: TOTAL LIFE STRESS SCALE

Purpose: To measure stress.

Number of Items: 83

Format: Checklist format for occurrence; 7-point Likert format (–3 to 3) to assess positive or negative impact.

Reliability: Alpha ranged from .53 to .77 across subscales.

Validity: All correlations between subscales and six validation scales were significant (*r*s ranged from .23 to .67 in absolute value) and were in predicted directions.

Author: Bhagat, R. S., et al.

Article: Total life stress: A multimethod validation of the construct and its effects on organizationally valued outcomes and withdrawal behaviors.

Journal: *Journal of Applied Psychology,* February 1985, *70*(1), 202–214.

Related Research: Dohrenwend, B. S., et al. (1978). Exemplification of a method for scaling life events: The PERI life events scale. *Journal of Health and Social Behavior, 19,* 205–229.

Johnson, J. H., & Sarason, I. G. (1979). Recent developments in research on life stress. In V. Hamilton & D. M. Warburton (Eds.), *Human stress and cognition: An information processing approach* (pp. 205–236). New York: Wiley.

* * *

2544

Test Name: WELL-BEING SCALE

Purpose: To measure psychological and physical well-being.

Number of Items: 18

Format: Forced choice format. All items presented.

Reliability: Item-scale correlations ranged from .30 to .63.

Validity: Correlated .44 ($p < .01$) with seeing a doctor in last 6 months, and .35 with number of days sick in last 6 months.

Author: Davidson, W. B., and Cotter, P.

Article: Adjustment to aging and relationship with offspring.

Journal: *Psychological Reports,* 1982, *50*(3, Part I), 731–738.

Related Research: Pfeiffer, E. (1976). *Multidimensional functional assessment: The OARS methodology—A manual.* Durham, NC: Center for the Study of Aging and Human Development.

■ ■ ■

2545

Test Name: ZUCKERMAN AND ALLISON FEAR OF SUCCESS SCALE

Purpose: To measure fear of success.

Number of Items: 27

Format: Items are rated on a 7-point Likert scale.

Validity: Correlated positively with Pappo and Good and Good scales, except among men, for whom the correlation was negative.

Author: Chabassol, D. J., and Ishiyama, F. I.

Article: Correlations among three measures of fear of success.

Journal: *Psychological Reports,* 1983, *52*(1), 55–58.

Related Research: Zuckerman, M., & Allison, S. N. (1976). An objective measure of fear of success: Construction and validation. *Journal of Personality Assessment, 40,* 422–430.

■ ■ ■

2546

Test Name: ZUNG SELF-RATING DEPRESSION SCALE

Purpose: To assess behavioral changes, cognitive processes, and affective concomitants of depression.

Number of Items: 20

Format: Items are rated on 4-point Likert type categories (*most of the time* to *none or little of the time*).

Reliability: Cronbach's alpha ranged from .88 to .93 across criterion groups.

Validity: Discriminated between depressed and nondepressed clients ($p < .001$).

Author: Gabrys, J. B., and Peters, K.

Article: Reliability, discriminant, and predictive validity of the Zung Self-Rating Depression Scale.

Journal: *Psychological Reports,* December 1985, *57*(3–11), 1091–1096.

Related Research: Zung, W. K. (1965). A self-rating depression scale. *Archives of General Psychiatry, 12,* 63–70.

CHAPTER 4
Adjustment—Social

2547

Test Name: ACCULTURATION RATING SCALE FOR MEXICAN-AMERICANS

Purpose: To measure degree of acculturation.

Number of Items: 20

Format: Likert format (1 = *Mexican/Spanish* to 5 = *Anglo/ English*).

Reliability: Alpha was .88; test–retest reliability was .72.

Author: Franco, J. N., et al.

Article: Ethnic and acculturation differences in self-disclosure.

Journal: *Journal of Social Psychology*, February 1984, *122*(first half), 21–32.

Related Research: Cuellar, I., et al. (1980). An acculturation scale for Mexican American normal and clinical populations. *Hispanic Journal of Behavioral Science*, *2*(3), 199–217.

• • •

2548

Test Name: ACQUAINTANCE DESCRIPTION FORM

Purpose: To measure different aspects of the strength and rewardingness of an interpersonal relationship.

Number of Items: 80

Format: Responses to each item are made on a 7-point scale from 0 to 6 indicating to what extent the item applies to the subject's relationship with a designated person. Includes seven scales.

Reliability: Test–retest correlations for the scales ranged from .70 to .93. Split-half reliabilities ranged from .79 to .94.

Author: Wright, P. H., and Keple, T. W.

Article: Friends and parents of a sample of high school juniors: An exploratory study of relationship intensity and interpersonal rewards.

Journal: *Journal of Marriage and the Family*, August 1981, *43*(3), 559–570.

Related Research: Wright, P. H. (1974). The delineation and measurement of some key variables in the study of friendship. *Representative Research in Social Psychology, 5,* 93–96.

• • •

2549

Test Name: ADOLESCENT ALIENATION SCALE

Purpose: To measure adolescent alienation.

Number of Items: 41

Format: Items are rated on 4-point *agree–disagree* response categories.

Reliability: Alpha ranged from .67 to .80 across subscales.

Author: James, N. L., and Johnson, D. W.

Article: The relationship between attitudes toward social interdependence and psychological health within three criminal populations.

Journal: *Journal of Social Psychology*, October 1983, *121*(first half), 131–143.

Related Research: Mackey, J., & Ahlgren, A. (1977). A dimension of adolescent alienation. *Applied Psychological Measurement, 1*(2), 219–232.

• • •

2550

Test Name: ADULT ORIENTATION TO CHILD AUTONOMY SCALE

Purpose: To assess adults' orientations to control or autonomy in interactions with children.

Number of Items: 32

Format: Four vignettes followed by 4 items that can be rated as appropriate or not on a 7-point scale. Sample items presented.

Reliability: Cronbach's alpha ranged from .63 to .80 across subscales.

Validity: Correlated positively and significantly with intrinsic motivation and self-esteem. Correlations ranged from .27 to .56. Did not correlate with perceived physical competence.

Author: Deci, E. L., et al.

Article: An instrument to access adults' orientations toward control versus autonomy with children: Reflections on intrinsic motivation and perceived competence.

Journal: *Journal of Educational Psychology*, October 1981, *73*(5), 642–650.

2551

Test Name: AUDIENCE ANXIOUSNESS SCALE

Purpose: To measure audience anxiousness independent of specific social behaviors.

Number of Items: 12

Format: Subjects respond to each item on a 5-point scale to identify the degree to which the item is true. The scale ranged from *not at all* to *extremely characteristic.* All items are presented.

Reliability: Cronbach's alphas were .88 and .91.

Validity: Correlations with other variables ranged from −.24 to .84.

Author: Leary, M. R.

Article: Social anxiousness: The construct and its measurement.

Journal: *Journal of Personality Assessment,* February 1983, *47*(1), 66–75.

■ ■ ■

2552

Test Name: AVOIDANCE OF THE ONTOLOGICAL CONFRONTATION OF LONELINESS SCALE

Purpose: To measure the avoidance of the harsh reality of loneliness.

Number of Items: 40

Format: True–false. All items are presented.

Reliability: Cronbach's alpha was .81; odd–even reliability was .78.

Validity: Correlated .37 with Jackson's Social Desirability Scale. Did not correlate with Eysenck's Neuroticism Scale.

Author: Thauberger, P. C.

Article: Avoidance of existential–ontological confrontations: A review of research.

Journal: *Psychological Reports,* 1981, *49*(3), 747–764.

Related Research: Thauberger, P., & Cleland, J. (1979). *Measuring the abyss: Avoidance of the ontological confrontations of loneliness.* Paper presented at the UCLA Research Conference on Loneliness.

■ ■ ■

2553

Test Name: BRADLEY LONELINESS SCALE— MODIFIED

Purpose: To measure loneliness.

Number of Items: 37

Format: Items are rated on a 6-point Likert scale (*rarely true* to *always true*).

Reliability: Internal consistency was .92.

Author: Ponzetti, J. J., and Cate, R. M.

Article: Sex differences in the relationship between loneliness and academic performance.

Journal: *Psychological Reports,* June 1981, *48*(3), 758.

Related Research: Bradley, R. (1969). Measuring loneliness (Doctoral dissertation, Washington State University). *Dissertation Abstracts International, 30,* 3382B. (University Microfilms No. 70-1048)

■ ■ ■

2554

Test Name: CHILDREN'S LONELINESS SCALE

Purpose: To measure loneliness.

Number of Items: 16

Format: Items are rated on a 5-point truth scale (*always true* to

not true at all). All items presented.

Reliability: Alpha was .90.

Validity: Correlated −.39 with play rating of same-sex peer; −.37 with positive nomination of same-sex peer; .37 to negative nomination of same-sex peer. All correlations, *p* < .001.

Author: Asher, S. R., and Wheeler, V. A.

Article: Children's loneliness: A comparison of rejected and neglected peer status.

Journal: *Journal of Consulting and Clinical Psychology,* August 1985, *53*(4), 500–505.

Related Research: Asher, S. R., et al. (1984). Loneliness in children. *Child Development, 55,* 1457–1464.

■ ■ ■

2555

Test Name: COGNITION OF BEHAVIORAL UNITS

Purpose: To measure social intelligence.

Number of Items: 34

Format: For the first 16 items, the subject selects one of four pictures that best illustrates the feelings described in a verbal statement read to the examinees. For the remaining 18 items, the subject selects one of four facial pictures that best corresponds to a picture of a face.

Reliability: Test–retest reliability was .40.

Validity: Correlations with CIRCUS ranged from .22 to .46 (*N*s = 69 to 74).

Author: Snyder, S. D., and Michael, W. B.

Article: The relationship of performance on standardized tests in mathematics and reading to two measures of social intelligence and one of academic self-esteem for two samples of primary school children.

Journal: *Educational and Psychological Measurement,* Winter 1983, *43*(4), 1141–1148.

Related Research: Favero, J. (1979). *Tests of SOI behavior skills and classroom activities for improving behavioral skills.* Unpublished manuscript. Glendora, CA: Glendora Unified School District.

■ ■ ■

2556

Test Name: COLLEGE PEER RATING SYSTEM

Purpose: To measure peer ratings on task orientation, classroom behavior, and social acceptance.

Number of Items: 3

Format: Each child rates all others on each sociometric item. Items presented along with 5-point response categories.

Reliability: Test–retest reliability over 4 months ranged from .64 to .78.

Validity: Correlations between ratings were significant and in expected direction.

Author: Bailey, D. B., Jr., et al.

Article: Generalized effects of a highly structured time-on-task intervention.

Journal: *Psychological Reports,* April 1984, *54*(2), 483–490.

■ ■ ■

2557

Test Name: COMPREHENSIVE SOCIAL DESIRABILITY SCALE FOR CHILDREN

Purpose: To assess social desirability.

Number of Items: 27

Format: True–false.

Reliability: Correlation between alternate forms was .92; alpha (internal consistency) was .57.

Validity: Correlation was .36 with Crandall, Crandall, and Katkovsky Social Desirability Scale (1965).

Author: Malizio, A. G., et al.

Article: Relationship of social desirability, age, and sex with task persistence and contingent self-reinforcement.

Journal: *Psychological Reports,* 1982, *50*(1), 39–47.

■ ■ ■

2558

Test Name: CONCERN FOR APPROPRIATENESS SCALE

Purpose: To measure the tendency to adopt protective self-presentation styles.

Number of Items: 20

Format: Includes two subscales: cross-situational variability and attention to social comparison.

Reliability: Coefficient alpha ranged from .82 to .89. Test–retest (3 weeks) reliability was .84.

Validity: Correlations with other variables ranged from –.08 to .41.

Author: Cutler, B. L., and Wolfe, R. N.

Article: Construct validity of the concern for appropriateness scale.

Journal: *Journal of Personality Assessment,* June 1985, *49*(3), 318–323.

Related Research: Lennox, R. D., & Wolfe, R. N. (1984). Revision of the self-monitoring scale. *Journal of Personality and Social Psychology, 46,* 1349–1364.

■ ■ ■

2559

Test Name: COUPLES THERAPY ALLIANCE SCALE

Purpose: To measure client's view of therapeutic relationship.

Number of Items: 28

Format: Items rated on 5-point Likert scales.

Reliability: Internal consistency was .96 (total test); consistency ranged from .85 to .92 across subscales.

Author: Johnson, S. M., and Greenberg, L. S.

Article: Differential effects of experiential and problem-solving interventions in resolving marital conflict.

Journal: *Journal of Consulting and Clinical Psychology,* April 1985, *53*(2), 175–184.

Related Research: Pinsof, W., & Catherall, D. (1983). *The couples' therapy alliance scale manual.* Chicago, IL: The Chicago Center for Family Studies, Northwestern University.

■ ■ ■

2560

Test Name: CULTURAL MISTRUST INVENTORY

Purpose: To measure cultural mistrust among Blacks.

Number of Items: 48

Format: Responses are made to each item on a 7-point Likert scale that ranged from *strongly agree* to *strongly disagree.*

Reliability: Test–retest (2 weeks) reliability estimate was .82.

Author: Terrell, F., and Terrell, S.

Article: Race of counselor, client sex, cultural mistrust level, and premature termination from counseling among Black clients.

Journal: *Journal of Counseling Psychology,* July 1984, *31*(3), 371–375.

Related Research: Terrell, F., & Terrell, S. L. (1981). An inventory to measure cultural mistrust among Blacks. *Western Journal of Black Studies, 5,* 180–184.

■ ■ ■

2561

Test Name: DIFFERENTIAL LONELINESS SCALE

Purpose: To assess dissatisfaction with four types of relationships.

Number of Items: 60

Format: Subjects respond by answering *true* or *false* to items regarding the quality and quantity of interaction in relationships. Includes four scales: family, larger groups, friendship, and romantic/sexual.

Reliability: Cronbach's alpha ranged from .46 to .89.

Validity: Correlations with other variables ranged from −.89 to .54.

Author: Schmitt, J. P., and Kurdek, L. A.

Article: Age and gender differences in and personality correlates of loneliness in different relationships.

Journal: *Journal of Personality Assessment,* October 1985, *49*(5), 485–496.

Related Research: Schmidt, N., & Sermat, V. (1983). Measuring loneliness in different relationships. *Journal of Personality and Social Psychology, 44,* 1038–1047.

■ ■ ■

2562

Test Name: DYADIC TRUST SCALE

Purpose: To measure trust between two people.

Number of Items: 8

Format: 7-point Likert format. Sample items presented.

Reliability: Alpha was .85.

Author: Hansen, G.

Article: Perceived threats and marital jealousy.

Journal: *Social Psychology Quarterly,* September 1985, *48*(3), 262–268.

Related Research: Larzelere, R. E., & Huston, T. L. (1980). The dyadic trust scale: Toward understanding interpersonal trust in close relationships. *Journal of Marriage and the Family, 42,* 595–604.

■ ■ ■

2563

Test Name: ENLARGED ANOMIA SCALE

Purpose: To measure anomia.

Number of Items: 9

Format: Agree–disagree response categories. All items are presented.

Reliability: Part–whole correlations were .91, .89, and .89 in each of 3 consecutive years. Test–retest reliability ranged from .41 to .56 from 1st to 2nd year, 2nd to 3rd year, and 1st to 3rd year.

Author: Poresky, R. H., et al.

Article: Anomia in rural women: A longitudinal comparison of two measures.

Journal: *Psychological Reports,* 1981, *49*(2), 480–482.

Related Research: Robinson, J. P., & Shover, P. R. (1973). *Measures of psychological attitudes.* Ann Arbor: University of Michigan, Survey Research Center.

■ ■ ■

2564

Test Name: EVALUATION OF BEHAVIORAL IMPLICATIONS

Purpose: To measure social intelligence.

Number of Items: 20

Format: Each item contains a verbal stem describing a social dilemma, followed by four alternative pictures from which the examinee selects the one that depicts the most appropriate resolution of the dilemma.

Reliability: Test–retest reliability was .55.

Validity: Correlations with CIRCUS ranged from .11 to .46 (*N*s = 69 to 74).

Author: Snyder, S. D., and Michael, W. B.

Article: The relationship of performance on standardized tests in mathematics and reading to two measures of social intelligence and one of academic self-esteem for two samples of primary school children.

Journal: *Educational and Psychological Measurement,* Winter 1983, *43*(4), 1141–1148.

Related Research: Favero, J. (1979). *Tests of SOI behavioral skills and classroom activities for improving behavioral skills.* Unpublished manual, Glendora, CA: Glendora Unified School District.

■ ■ ■

2565

Test Name: FRIENDLINESS QUESTIONNAIRE

Purpose: To assess the components of friendliness.

Number of Items: 40

Format: Includes four components: self-concept, accessibility, rewardingness, and alienation.

Reliability: Test–retest (3 to 4 weeks) correlations ranged from .73 to .81 (*N* = 66).

Author: Reisman, J. M.

Article: SACRAL: Toward the meaning and measuring of friendliness.

Journal: *Journal of Personality Assessment*, August 1983, *47*(4), 405–413.

Related Research: Dean, D. G. (1969). Alienation: Its meaning and measurements. In D. G. Dean (Ed.), *Dynamic social psychology*. New York: Random House.

Wright, P. H. (1969). A model and a technique for the studies of friendship. *Journal of Experimental Social Psychology, 5*, 295–309.

■ ■ ■

2566

Test Name: GERIATRIC EVALUATION BY RELATIVE'S RATING INSTRUMENT

Purpose: To measure cognitive and social functioning, mood, and somatic functioning of elderly outpatients.

Number of Items: 49

Format: A 5-point frequency scale follows each specific and behavioral item (*almost all of the time* to *almost never*).

Reliability: Interrater reliability was .96 for total score and ranged between .63 and .96 across subscales. Cronbach's alpha ranged from .66 to .96.

Validity: Differentiates between three groups of elderly outpatients who differ in severity of global deterioration (Reisberg, 1982).

Author: Schwartz, G. E.

Article: Development and validation of the geriatric evaluation by relatives rating instrument (GERRI).

Journal: *Psychological Reports*, October 1983, *53*(2), 479–488.

■ ■ ■

2567

Test Name: GREENWOOD'S POSITIVE SOCIAL BEHAVIOR SCALE

Purpose: To enable teachers to evaluate kindergarten children's social competence.

Number of Items: 9

Format: Includes only social behaviors of a positive nature. Teachers respond to each item on a 7-point Likert scale from *accurate* (7) to *false* (1) description of the child's behavior. Some examples are provided.

Validity: Correlations with other social competence scales ranged from –.67 to .57.

Author: Begin, G.

Article: Convergent validity of four instruments for teachers' assessing social competence of kindergarten children.

Journal: *Perceptual and Motor Skills*, December 1983, *57*(3-Part 1), 1007–1012.

Related Research: Greenwood, C. R., et al. (1978). *Social assessment manual for preschool level* (SAMPLE). Eugene: Center at Oregon for Research in the Behavioral Education of the Handicapped.

■ ■ ■

2568

Test Name: GROUP ATMOSPHERE SCALE

Purpose: To provide a description of group atmosphere.

Number of Items: 10

Format: Includes an 8-point semantic differential for each item. Examples are provided.

Reliability: Median alpha was .91.

Validity: Correlations with the Job Descriptive Index Co-Worker and Supervision subscales ranged from .38 to .68.

Author: Vecchio, R. P.

Article: A further test of leadership effects due to between-group

variation and within-group variation.

Journal: *Journal of Applied Psychology*, April 1982, *67*(2), 200–208.

Related Research: Fiedler, F. E. (1967). *A theory of leadership effectiveness*. New York: McGraw-Hill.

■ ■ ■

2569

Test Name: GROUP COHESIVENESS INDEX

Purpose: To measure group cohesiveness.

Number of Items: 4

Format: Items are rated on a 4-point scale. All items are presented.

Reliability: Alpha was .85.

Author: O'Reilly, C. A., III, and Caldwell, D. F.

Article: The impact of normative social influence and cohesiveness on task perceptions and attitudes: A social information processing approach.

Journal: *Journal of Occupational Psychology*, September 1985, *58*(3), 193–206.

Related Research: Seashore, S. (1954). *Group cohesiveness in the industrial work group*. Institute for Social Research, University of Michigan.

■ ■ ■

2570

Test Name: HETEROSOCIAL ASSESSMENT INVENTORY FOR WOMEN

Purpose: To evaluate five dimensions that may influence performance in 12 heterosocial situations.

Number of Items: 60

Format: Five questions are

presented for each of 12 heterosocial situations to provide a self-assessment. An example is presented.

Reliability: Split-half reliabilities ranged from .74 to .94. Cronbach's alphas ranged from .88 to .96. Test–retest (3 weeks) reliability coefficients ($N = 31$) ranged from .80 to .87.

Validity: Correlations with other variables ranged from −.43 to .78 (Study I) and from −.75 to .86 (Study II).

Author: Kolko, D. J.

Article: The heterosocial assessment inventory for women: A psychometric and behavioral evaluation.

Journal: *Journal of Psychopathy and Behavioral Assessment,* March 1985, *7*(1), 49–64.

Related Research: Klaus, D., et al. (1977). Survey of dating habits of male and female college students: A necessary precursor to measurement and modification. *Journal of Clinical Psychology, 33,* 369–375.

■ ■ ■

2571

Test Name: INDIVIDUALISM–SOCIAL DETERMINISM SCALE

Purpose: To measure individualist and social determinist beliefs.

Number of Items: 11

Format: Matched-pair format. All items presented.

Reliability: Alpha was .66. Item-total correlations ranged from .38 to .55.

Validity: Did not correlate with Rosenberg Self-Esteem Scale or Srole Anomie Scale or the F-Scale. Correlated .00 to .15 across three dimensions of locus of control. Additional discriminant and construct validation presented.

Author: Zeitz, G., and Lincoln, J. R.

Article: Individualism–social determinism: A belief component in the formation of sociopolitical attitudes.

Journal: *Sociology and Social Research,* April 1981, *65*(3), 283–298.

■ ■ ■

2572

Test Name: INTERACTION ANXIOUSNESS SCALE

Purpose: To measure interaction anxiousness independent of specific social behaviors.

Number of Items: 15

Format: Subjects respond to each item on a 5-point scale to identify the degree to which the item is true. The scale ranged from *not at all* to *extremely characteristic.* All items are presented.

Reliability: Cronbach's alphas were .88 and .89.

Validity: Correlations with other variables ranged from −.33 to .87.

Author: Leary, M. R.

Article: Social anxiousness: The construct and its measurement.

Journal: *Journal of Personality Assessment,* February 1983, *47*(1), 66–75.

■ ■ ■

2573

Test Name: INTERPERSONAL CONFLICT RESPONSE INVENTORY

Purpose: To measure how accurately individuals classify responses to conflict situations into assertive, nonassertive, and aggressive behavior.

Number of Items: 36

Time Required: 15 minutes.

Format: Situations are described,

response is described and respondent asked to choose the best description of the response. All items presented.

Author: Warehime, R. G., and Lowe, D. R.

Article: Assessing assertiveness in work settings: A discrimination measure.

Journal: *Psychological Reports,* December 1983, *53*(3-Part 1), 1007–1012.

Related Research: Lange, A. J., & Jakubowski, P. (1976). *Responsible assertive behavior: Cognitive/behavioral procedures for trainers.* Champaign, IL: Research Press.

■ ■ ■

2574

Test Name: INTERPERSONAL DEPENDENCY INVENTORY

Purpose: To assess three components of interpersonal dependency in adults.

Number of Items: 48

Format: Includes three components: emotional reliance on another, lack of social self-confidence, and assertion of autonomy.

Reliability: Internal consistency reliabilities for the three components ranged from .72 to .91.

Author: Brown, S. D., and Reimer, D. A.

Article: Assessing attachment following divorce: Development and psychometric evaluation of the divorce reaction inventory.

Journal: *Journal of Counseling Psychology,* October 1984, *31*(4), 520–531.

Related Research: Hirschfield, R. M. A., et al. (1977). A measure of interpersonal dependency.

Journal of Personality Assessment, 41, 610–618.

•••

2575

Test Name: INTERPERSONAL JEALOUSY SCALE

Purpose: To measure interpersonal jealousy.

Number of Items: 28

Format: Subjects respond to each item on a 9-point scale ranging from (1) *absolutely false, disagree completely* to (9) *absolutely true, agree completely.* Some examples are presented.

Reliability: Estimate of internal consistency reliability was .92.

Validity: Correlations with threat level were .44 (men) and .51 (women); with degree of affirmation in answer (reflecting possessiveness) were −.40 (men) and −.37 (women).

Author: Mathes, E. W., et al.

Article: Behavioral correlates of the Interpersonal Jealousy Scale.

Journal: *Educational and Psychological Measurement,* Winter 1982, *42*(4), 1227–1231.

Related Research: Mathes, E. W., & Severa, N. (1981). Jealousy, romantic love and liking: Theoretical considerations and preliminary scale development. *Psychological Reports, 49,* 23–31.

•••

2576

Test Name: INTERPERSONAL PROBLEM-SOLVING ASSESSMENT TECHNIQUE

Purpose: To provide a free response test of interpersonal effectiveness.

Number of Items: 46

Format: Each item is a problematic interpersonal situation in which

the respondent imagines being present at the moment. Respondents write alternative ways of handling each situation and which solution they would choose. Includes six classes of interpersonal situations.

Reliability: Average reliability among four scores ranged from .82 to .99

Validity: Correlations with College Self-Expression Scale ranged from −.42 to .29; Edwards Personal Preference Schedule ranged from −.42 to .36; Psychological Screening Inventory ranged from −.29 to .25.

Author: Getter, H., and Nowinski, J. K.

Article: A free response test of interpersonal effectiveness.

Journal: *Journal of Personality Assessment,* June 1981, *45*(3), 301–308.

•••

2577

Test Name: INTERPERSONAL RELATIONS SCALE

Purpose: To measure openness of interpersonal relations in schools.

Number of Items: 4

Format: Multiple-choice. All items are presented.

Reliability: Alpha was .87.

Validity: Correlates significantly (*p* < .05) with teacher leadership behavior and teachers' assessment of students (*r*s = .17 and .20, respectively).

Author: Peterson, M. F., and Cooke, R. A.

Article: Attitudinal and contextual variables explaining teachers' leadership behavior.

Journal: *Journal of Educational Psychology,* February 1983, *75*(1), 50–62.

2578

Test Name: INTERPERSONAL SUPPORT EVALUATION LIST

Purpose: To assess general social support.

Number of Items: 10

Format: Sample items presented. Response categories not presented.

Reliability: Alpha ranged from .70 to .92. Test–retest ranged from .87 (4 weeks) to .60 (6 months).

Author: Glasgow, R. E., et al.

Article: Quitting smoking: Strategies used and variables associated with success in a stop-smoking contest.

Journal: *Journal of Consulting and Clinical Psychology,* December 1985, *53*(6), 905–912.

Related Research: Cohen, S., et al. (1983). Measuring the functional components of social support. In I. G. Sarason & B. Sarason (Eds.), *Social support: Theory, research and applications.* The Hague, Holland: Martines Nijhoff.

•••

2579

Test Name: INTIMACY ATTITUDE SCALE—REVISED

Purpose: To measure intimacy attitudes.

Number of Items: 50

Format: Each item is rated on a 5-point scale (*strongly disagree, mildly disagree, agree/disagree equally,* and *strongly agree*).

Reliability: Cronbach's alphas ranged from .78 to .87 (*N*s ranged from 15 to 217). Test–retest reliability was .57 (*N* = 29) for an interval of 30 days.

Author: Amidon, E., et al.

Article: Measurement of intimacy attitudes: The Intimacy Attitude Scale—Revised.

Journal: *Journal of Personality Assessment*, December 1983, *47*(6), 635–639.

Related Research: Treadwell, T. W. (1981). *Intimacy Attitude Scale: Its structure, reliability, and validity.* Unpublished doctoral dissertation, Temple University.

■ ■ ■

2580

Test Name: INTIMACY SCALE

Purpose: To measure intimacy.

Number of Items: 42

Format: Includes 6 dimensions: ease of communication, confidence sharing, egocentrism, empathy, voluntary interdependence, and person as unique other. Responses to each item are made on a 6-point scale ranging from *strong disagreement* to *strong agreement.*

Reliability: Alphas ranged from .63 to .84.

Author: Devlin, P. K., and Cowan, G. A.

Article: Homophobia, perceived fathering and male intimate relationships.

Journal: *Journal of Personality Assessment*, October 1985, *49*(5), 467–473.

Related Research: Fischer, J. L. (1981). Transitions in relationship style from adolescence to young adulthood. *Journal of Youth and Adolescence, 10*, 11–23.

■ ■ ■

2581

Test Name: LIFE EVENTS QUESTIONNAIRE

Purpose: To measure the number of events that require a wide range of social readjustment (for college students).

Number of Items: 65

Format: Checklist format.

Reliability: Split-half reliability was .76.

Author: Miller, A., and Cooley, E.

Article: Moderator variables for the relationship between life cycle change and disorders.

Journal: *Journal of General Psychology*, April 1981, *104*(second half), 223–233.

Related Research: Cooley, E., et al. (1979). Self-report assessment of life change and disorders. *Psychological Reports, 44*, 1079–1086.

■ ■ ■

2582

Test Name: LIKING PEOPLE SCALE

Purpose: To measure interpersonal orientation.

Number of Items: 15

Format: A 5-point Likert scale was used from *strongly agree* to *strongly disagree.* All items are presented.

Reliability: Coefficients alpha were .85 ($N = 140$) and .75 ($N = 73$).

Validity: With Social Anxiety Scale, $r = -.18$; with Misanthropy Scale, $r = .38$; with Social Self-Esteem, $r = .49$; with Judgmental Ability, $r = .31$; with Social Desirability, $r = .10$.

Author: Filsinger, E. E.

Article: A measure of interpersonal orientation: The Liking People Scale.

Journal: *Journal of Personality Assessment*, June 1981, *45*(3), 295–300.

■ ■ ■

2583

Test Name: LONELINESS AND SOCIAL DISSATISFACTION MEASURE

Purpose: To assess children's feelings of loneliness and social dissatisfaction.

Number of Items: 16

Format: Items focus on children's feelings of loneliness. All items are presented.

Reliability: Cronbach's alpha was .90; split-half correlation between forms was .83; Spearman-Brown reliability coefficient was .91; Guttman split-half reliability coefficient was .91.

Validity: Correlations with sociometric status ranged from −.19 to −.37.

Author: Asher, S. R., et al.

Article: Loneliness in children.

Journal: *Child Development*, August 1984, *55*(4), 1456–1464.

■ ■ ■

2584

Test Name: LOVE ADDICTION SCALE

Purpose: To measure love "addiction," "mania," and "possessiveness."

Number of Items: 20

Time Required: 15 minutes.

Format: Items are rated on a 5-point Likert agreement scale. Sample items are presented.

Reliability: Test–retest was .99 (2-week interval).

Author: Hunter, M. S., et al.

Article: A scale to measure love addiction.

Journal: *Psychological Reports*, April 1981, *48*(2), 582.

■ ■ ■

2585

Test Name: MARLOWE-CROWNE SOCIAL DESIRABILITY SCALE

Purpose: To provide a measure of social desirability.

Number of Items: 33

Format: Measures social desirability in terms of the need of subjects to respond in culturally sanctioned ways.

Reliability: Internal consistency Kuder-Richardson formula 20 reliability was .88 ($N = 39$). Test–retest reliability was .89 (1-month interval).

Author: Caillet, K. C., and Michael, W. B.

Article: The construct validity of three self-report instruments hypothesized to measure the degree of resolution for each of the first six stage crises in Erikson's developmental theory of personality.

Journal: *Educational and Psychological Measurement,* Spring 1983, *43*(1), 197–209.

Related Research: Crowne, D. P., & Marlowe, D. (1960). A new scale of social desirability independent of psychotherapy. *Journal of Consulting Psychology, 24,* 349–354.

■ ■ ■

2586

Test Name: MARTIN-LARSEN APPROVAL MOTIVATION SCALE

Purpose: To measure need for social approval.

Number of Items: 20

Format: Subjects respond to each item on a 5-point scale from *disagree strongly* (1) to *agree strongly* (5). All items are presented.

Reliability: Cronbach's alpha ranged from .64 to .75 (Ns ranged from 129 to 185).

Validity: Correlations with other variables ranged from –.50 to .61.

Author: Martin, H. J.

Article: A revised measure of

approval motivation and its relationship to social desirability.

Journal: *Journal of Personality Assessment,* October 1984, *48*(5), 508–519.

Related Research: Larsen, K. S., et al. (1976). Approval seeking, social cost and aggression: A scale and some dynamics. *Journal of Psychology, 94,* 3–11.

■ ■ ■

2587

Test Name: MILLER SOCIAL INTIMACY SCALE

Purpose: To provide a measure of the maximum level of intimacy currently experienced.

Number of Items: 17

Format: Six items require an answer indicating frequency on a 10-point scale. Eleven items require an answer indicating intensity on a 10-point scale. All items are presented.

Reliability: Cronbach's alphas were .91 ($N = 45$) and .86 ($N = 39$). Test–retest reliabilities were .96 (2-month interval) and .84 (1-month interval).

Validity: With IRS, $r = .71$ ($N = 45$); with UCLA Loneliness Scale, $r = -.65$ ($N = 59$); with Tennessee Self-Concept Scale, $r = .48$ ($N = 45$).

Author: Miller, R. S., and Lefcourt, H. M.

Article: The assessment of social intimacy.

Journal: *Journal of Personality Assessment,* October 1982, *46*(5), 514–518.

■ ■ ■

2588

Test Name: MINES-JENSEN INTERPERSONAL RELATIONSHIP INVENTORY

Purpose: To measure tolerance

level and quality of relationships.

Number of Items: 42

Format: 4-point response scale. Sample items provided.

Reliability: Kuder-Richardson reliabilities were in the .65–.70 range.

Author: Riahinejad, A. R., and Hood, A. B.

Article: The development of interpersonal relationships in college.

Journal: *Journal of College Student Personnel,* November 1984, *25*(6), 498–502.

Related Research: Mines, R. A. *Change in college students along Chickering's vector of freeing of interpersonal relationships* (Iowa Student Development Project, Technical Report No. 26). Unpublished manuscript, The University of Iowa.

■ ■ ■

2589

Test Name: NETWORK ORIENTATION SCALE

Purpose: To measure degree to which personal network is useless in time of need.

Number of Items: 20

Format: 4-point agree–disagree scale. All items are presented.

Validity: Three factors are presented: Advisability/Independence, History, Mistrust.

Author: Vaux, A.

Article: Factor structure of the network orientation scale.

Journal: *Psychological Reports,* December 1985, *57*(3-II), 1181–1182.

Related Research: Tolsdorf, C. (1976). Social networks, support and coping: An exploratory study. *Family Process, 15,* 407–417.

2590

Test Name: PEER GROUP ROLE AND STUDENT ROLE SCALES (FROM ABIC)

Purpose: To measure behavior in peer group and student roles.

Number of Items: 70

Format: Items rated on 5-point SOMPA rating categories.

Reliability: Interrater reliability high. Comparison of rating categories revealed no difference between interviewers ($z = .69$, not significant).

Validity: Mothers give more and higher scoring ratings than teachers.

Author: Wall, S. M., and Paradise, L. V.

Article: A comparison of parent and teacher reports of selected adoptive behaviors of children.

Journal: *Journal of School Psychology*, 1981, *19*(1), 73–77.

Related Research: Goodman, J. F. (1979). Is tissue the issue? A critique of SOMPA's models and tests. *School Psychology Digest, 8*, 47–62.

■ ■ ■

2591

Test Name: PEER NETWORK FUNCTIONS SCALE

Purpose: To measure the functions of peer networks.

Number of Items: 24

Format: Yes–no format.

Reliability: Alpha ranged from .60 to .82 across subscales.

Validity: No differences reported by sex and ambition, but one was found between ethnic and nonethnic respondents.

Author: Burke, R. J.

Article: Relationships in and around organizations: It's both

who you know and what you know that counts.

Journal: *Psychological Reports,* August 1984, *55*(1), 299–307.

■ ■ ■

2592

Test Name: PERSONAL ASSESSMENT OF INTIMACY IN RELATIONSHIPS INVENTORY

Purpose: To measure intimacy in relationships.

Number of Items: 36

Format: Items rated on a 5-point disagree–agree Likert format.

Reliability: Total reliability was .70. Subscales ranged from .57 to .79.

Author: Johnson, S. M., and Greenberg, L. S.

Article: Differential effects of experiential and problem-solving interventions in resolving marital conflict.

Journal: *Journal of Consulting and Clinical Psychology,* April 1985, *53*(2), 175–188.

Related Research: Schaefer, M. T., & Olson, D. H. (1981). Assessing intimacy: The PAIR Inventory. *Journal of Marital and Family Therapy, 1,* 47–60.

■ ■ ■

2593

Test Name: PICTORIAL SCALE OF PERCEIVED COMPETENCE AND SOCIAL ACCEPTANCE FOR YOUNG CHILDREN

Purpose: To assess perceived competence and social acceptance in young children, ages 4–7.

Number of Items: 24

Format: Two versions: one for preschool-kindergarten; one for first–second grade. Includes two factors, each defined by two

subscales. General competence includes cognitive and physical competence subscales. Social acceptance includes peer and maternal acceptance subscales.

Reliability: Reliabilities ranged from .50 to .89.

Author: Harter, S., and Pike, R.

Article: The pictorial scale of perceived competence and social acceptance for young children.

Journal: *Child Development,* December 1984, *55*(6), 1969–1982.

Related Research: Harter, S. (1982). The perceived competence scale for children. *Child Development, 53,* 87–97.

■ ■ ■

2594

Test Name: PREMORBID SOCIAL COMPETENCE SCALE

Purpose: To measure social competence before schizophrenia.

Number of Items: 5

Format: Multiple-choice. All items and responses presented.

Reliability: Agreement in categorizing patients from records is 99%.

Validity: Factor structure of items differs by gender and by type of hospital.

Author: Zigler, E., and Levine, J.

Article: Premorbid competence in schizophrenia: What is being measured?

Journal: *Journal of Consulting and Clinical Psychology,* February 1981, *49*(1), 96–105.

Related Research: Zigler, E., & Levine, J. (1973). Premorbid adjustment and paranoid-nonparanoid status in schizophrenia: A further investigation. *Journal of Abnormal Psychology, 82,* 189–199.

2595

Test Name: PROBLEM INVENTORY FOR ADOLESCENT GIRLS (MULTIPLE-CHOICE VERSION)

Purpose: To assess social competence in adolescent girls.

Number of Items: 52

Format: Subjects select a response on a 5-point scale that expresses what they would do in a situation being described.

Validity: 51 of 52 items showed significant differences ($p < .05$) with delinquent and nondelinquent girls. Correlated .52 with IQ and .32 with socioeconomic status. Correlated −.83 with delinquent behavior checklist.

Author: Gaffney, L. R.

Article: A multiple-choice test to measure social skills in delinquent and nondelinquent adolescent girls.

Journal: *Journal of Consulting and Clinical Psychology,* October 1984, *52*(5), 911–912.

Related Research: Graffney, L. R., & McFall, R. M. (1981). A comparison of social skills in delinquent and nondelinquent adolescent girls using a behavioral role-playing inventory. *Journal of Consulting and Clinical Psychology, 49,* 959–967.

■ ■ ■

2596

Test Name: PURSUING-DISTANCING SCALE

Purpose: To measure interpersonal pursuing and distancing.

Number of Items: 92

Format: Half the items reflect distancing; the other half reflect tendencies to pursue. Includes 6 domains: cognitive style,

emotionality, social style, communication style, sensation seeking, and reflecting anality. All items are presented.

Reliability: Type reliability ranged from $r = .23$ to $r = .70$; item reliability ranged from $r = .07$ to $r = .50$.

Author: Bernstein, D. M., et al.

Article: Pursuing and distancing: The construct and its measurement.

Journal: *Journal of Personality Assessment,* June 1985, *49*(3), 273–281.

Related Research: Fogarty, R. (1976). Marital crisis. In P. Guerin, Jr. (Ed.), *Family therapy.* New York: Gardner Press.

■ ■ ■

2597

Test Name: RELATIONSHIP EVENTS SCALE

Purpose: To provide a self-report measure of courtship progress.

Number of Items: 13

Format: A Guttman scale. All items are presented.

Reliability: Correlation between scores of male and female members of couples was .81 ($N = 55$).

Validity: Correlations with other variables ranged from .16 to .59.

Author: King, C. E., and Christensen, A.

Article: The relationship events scale: A Guttman scaling of progress in courtship.

Journal: *Journal of Marriage and the Family,* August 1983, *45*(3), 671–678.

Related Research: Christensen, A., & King, C. E. *The Relationship Events Scale* (item pool and final scale). (Available from the authors, Department of Psychology, University of

California, Los Angeles, CA 90024.)

■ ■ ■

2598

Test Name: REWARD LEVEL SCALE

Purpose: To measure reward levels in six resource areas (love, status, services, goods, money, information, and sexuality).

Number of Items: 7

Format: 9-point Likert format.

Reliability: Alpha was .90.

Author: Lloyd, S. A., et al.

Article: Predicting premarital relationship stability: A methodological refinement.

Journal: *Journal of Marriage and the Family,* February 1984, *46*(1), 71–76.

Related Research: Foa, U. G., & Foa, E. G. (1974). *Societal structures of the mind.* Springfield, IL: Charles C Thomas.

■ ■ ■

2599

Test Name: ROMANTIC LOVE SYMPTOM CHECKLIST

Purpose: To measure feelings of romantic love.

Number of Items: 76

Format: Respondents check any of the 76 feelings that are elicited by the thought of their beloved.

Reliability: Internal consistency was .95.

Author: Mathes, E. W.

Article: Mystical experience, romantic love and hypnotic susceptibility.

Journal: *Psychological Reports,* 1982, *50*(3 Part 1), 701–702.

Related Research: Rubin, Z. (1974). Measurement of romantic love. *Journal of Personality and Social Psychology, 83,* 268–277.

■ ■ ■

2600

Test Name: ROMANTIC LOVE SYMPTOM CHECKLIST

Purpose: To measure feelings of romantic love.

Number of Items: 35

Format: Subjects check or do not check items. Sample items presented.

Reliability: Internal consistency was .92 for men and .91 for women.

Validity: Correlated .37 (men) and .48 (women) with Rubin's Romantic Love Scale.

Author: Mathes, E. W., and Wise, P. S.

Article: Romantic love and ravages of time.

Journal: *Psychological Reports,* December 1983, *53*(3 Part 1), 839–846.

Related Research: Mathes, E. W. (1982). Mystical experiences, romantic love and hypnotic susceptibility. *Psychological Reports, 50,* 701–702.

■ ■ ■

2601

Test Name: SELLS AND ROFF SCALE OF PEER RELATIONS

Purpose: To evaluate the degree to which a child is accepted or rejected by peers.

Format: A teacher rating form.

Reliability: Ranged from .58 to .75.

Validity: Correlations with the Battelle Developmental Inventory ranged from .16 to .56 (*N*= 50). Correlations with the Wide Range Achievement Test ranged from .00 to .22 (*N*= 50).

Author: Guidubaldi, J., and Perry, J. D.

Article: Concurrent and predictive validity of the Battelle Development Inventory at the first grade level.

Journal: *Educational and Psychological Measurement,* Winter 1984, *44*(4), 977–985.

Related Research: Sells, S., & Roff, M. (1967). *Peer acceptance–rejection and personality development in children.* Washington, DC: U.S. Government Printing Office.

■ ■ ■

2602

Test Name: SIMULATED SOCIAL INTERACTION TEST

Purpose: To assess social skills.

Number of Items: 8

Format: Consists of 8 social simulations in which subjects are asked to role play. All items are presented.

Reliability: Reliability coefficients ranged from .76 to .82.

Author: Steinberg, S. L., et al.

Article: The effects of confederate prompt delivery style in a standardized social simulation test.

Journal: *Journal of Behavioral Assessment,* September 1982, *4*(3), 263–272.

Related Research: Curran, J. P. (1982). A procedure for the assessment of social skills: *The Simulated Social Interaction Test.* In J. P. Curran & P. M. Monti (Eds.), *Social skills training: A practical handbook for assessment and treatment.* New York: Guilford Press.

■ ■ ■

2603

Test Name: SOCIAL ACTIVITY QUESTIONNAIRE

Purpose: To measure dating experience.

Number of Items: 7

Format: Evaluates dating frequency, comfort, and skill and satisfaction with present dating situation.

Validity: Correlations with Heterosocial Assessment Inventory for Women ranged from .06 to .32.

Author: Kolko, D. J.

Article: The Heterosocial Assessment Inventory for Women: A psychometric and behavioral evaluation.

Journal: *Journal of Psychopathology and Behavioral Assessment,* March 1985, *7*(1), 49–64.

Related Research: Christensen, A., and Arkowitz, H. (1974). Preliminary report on practice dating and feedback as treatment for college dating problems. *Journal of Counseling Psychology, 21,* 92–95.

■ ■ ■

2604

Test Name: SOCIAL ANXIETY SCALE

Purpose: To measure social anxiety.

Number of Items: 28

Format: True–false questions concerning how one feels in a variety of social contexts and what situations one tends to avoid.

Reliability: Test–retest (1-month) reliability coefficient was .68.

Author: Oppenheimer, B. T.

Article: Short-term small group intervention for college freshmen.

Journal: *Journal of Counseling Psychology,* January 1984, *31*(1), 45–53.

Related Research: Watson, D., & Friend, R. (1969). Measurement of social-evaluative anxiety. *Journal of Consulting and Clinical Psychology, 33,* 448–457.

• • •

2605

Test Name: SOCIAL ANXIETY SUBSCALE OF THE SELF-CONSCIOUSNESS SCALE

Purpose: To assess social anxiety.

Number of Items: 6

Format: Subjects respond to each item on a 5-point scale indicating how well the item describes them. The scale ranges from 0 (*extremely not like me*) to 4 (*extremely like me*). An example is presented.

Reliability: Test–retest (2 weeks) correlation was .73.

Validity: Correlations with other variables ranged from –.45 to .63.

Author: Schmidt, J. P., and Kurdek, L. A.

Article: Correlates of social anxiety in college students and homosexuals.

Journal: *Journal of Personality Assessment,* August 1984, *48*(4), 403–409.

Related Research: Fenigstein, A., et al. (1975). Public and private self-consciousness: Assessment and theory. *Journal of Consulting and Clinical Psychology, 43,* 522–527.

• • •

2606

Test Name: SOCIAL COMPETENCE OBSERVATION MEASURE

Purpose: To assess children's behavior with peers, with teacher, and when alone.

Number of Items: 28

Format: Time-sampling format in which observers record incidences of 28 behaviors at 5-s intervals. All items are presented.

Reliability: Interrater ranged from .92 to .98.

Validity: Factor 1 items correlated .64 (*p* < .01) with Factor 1 of KPI (men only) and .71 (*p* < .01) with Factor 2 of KPI (women only).

Author: Ali Khan, N., and Hoge, R. D.

Article: A teacher-judgement measure of social competence: Validity data.

Journal: *Journal of Consulting and Clinical Psychology,* December 1983, *51*(6), 809–814.

Related Research: Connolly, J., & Doyle, A. (1981). Assessment of social competence in preschoolers: Teachers vs. peers. *Developmental Psychology, 17,* 454–462.

• • •

2607

Test Name: SOCIAL FUNCTIONING INDEX

Purpose: To measure energy, self-control, hygiene practices, communication, and awareness of environment's structure.

Number of Items: 51

Format: Raters indicate on a 5-point adequacy scale the behavior of patients on each of the 51 items. All items are presented.

Reliability: Interrater reliability ranged from .19 to .94 across items. Total score reliability across raters was .85.

Validity: Three rehabilitation consultants verified content validity, following determination that related scales were not valid for the purpose of the present scale.

Author: Peterson, L.

Article: Social functioning assessment of aftercare psychiatric patients in socialization therapy.

Journal: *Psychological Reports,*

December 1983, *53*(3 Part 2), 1123–1130.

• • •

2608

Test Name: SOCIAL PERFORMANCE SURVEY SCHEDULE

Purpose: To measure range of behaviors that contribute to social skill.

Number of Items: 50 positive behaviors.

Format: A 5-point frequency response scale for each of the 50 behaviors indicates how often each respondent demonstrates it.

Reliability: Cronbach's alpha was .94.

Validity: Correlated –.40 with Beck Depression Inventory; –.59 with MMPI Depression; .59 with Social Activity; .64 with Social Skills; –.54 with MMPI Social Introversion; .55 with MMPI Social Desirability (*p* < .01 for all correlations).

Author: Lowe, M. R.

Article: Validity of the positive behavior subscale of the Social Performance Survey Schedule in a psychiatric population.

Journal: *Psychological Reports,* 1982, *50*(1), 83–87.

• • •

2609

Test Name: SOCIAL PERFORMANCE SURVEY SCHEDULE

Purpose: To measure social skill.

Number of Items: 100

Format: Includes positive and negative subscales and seven factors.

Reliability: Coefficient alpha was .94. Test–retest reliability was .87.

Author: Lowe, M. R., and D'Illio, V.

Article: Factor analysis of the Social Performance Survey Scale.

Journal: *Journal of Psychopathology and Behavioral Assessment*, March 1985, *7*(1), 13–22.

Related Research: Lowe, M. R., & Cautela, J. R. (1978). A self-report measure of social skill. *Behavior Therapy, 9,* 535–544.

■ ■ ■

2610

Test Name: SOCIAL PERFORMANCE SURVEY SCHEDULE–REVISED

Purpose: To measure social skills.

Number of Items: 31

Format: The items describe various behaviors and respondents indicate how frequently they emit such behaviors.

Reliability: Interrater reliability coefficients ranged from .47 to .76. Alpha coefficients ranged from .83 to .86.

Author: Wessberg, H. W., et al.

Article: Evidence for the external validity of a social simulation measure of social skills.

Journal: *Journal of Behavioral Assessment*, September 1981, *3*(3), 209–220.

Related Research: Lowe, M. R., & Cautela, J. R. (1978). A self-report measure of social skill. *Behavior Therapy, 9,* 535–544.

■ ■ ■

2611

Test Name: SOCIAL PROPENSITY SCALE

Purpose: To measure social propensity.

Number or items: 50

Format: Items are rated on a 19-asterisk continuum from *Applies very closely* at one end to *Doesn't apply to me at all* at other end.

Reliability: Cronbach's alphas were .94, .95, and .92 over 3 years of testing.

Validity: Correlations with social adjustment ranged from .29 to .45. Correlates .33 with campus activities. Correlates –.25 with attrition.

Author: Baker, R. W., and Siryk, B.

Article: Social propensity and college adjustment.

Journal: *Journal of College Student Personnel*, July 1983, *24*(4), 331–336.

■ ■ ■

2612

Test Name: SOCIAL ANOMIA SCALE

Purpose: To examine comparative feelings of anomia among married women.

Number of Items: 9

Format: Response to each item is either *disagree* (0) or *agree* (1). All items are presented.

Reliability: Coefficient alpha was .73.

Author: Lovell-Troy, L. A.

Article: Anomia among employed wives and housewives: An exploratory analysis.

Journal: *Journal of Marriage and the Family*, May 1983, *45*(2), 301–310.

Related Research: Srole, L., et al. (1962). *Mental health in the metropolis: The midtown Manhattan study.* New York: McGraw-Hill.

2613

Test Name: TAXONOMY OF PROBLEMATIC SOCIAL SITUATIONS FOR CHILDREN

Purpose: To identify and classify problematic social situations.

Number of Items: 44

Format: Consisted of a 1–5 scale on which teachers indicated how much of a problem the item (situation) was for the child.

Reliability: Alphas ranged from .89 to .97 ($p < .001$) across subscales. Total alpha was .96. Test–retest ranged from .57 to .72 (total = .79).

Validity: Teachers rated situations more problematic for rejected children than for adaptive children ($p < .001$).

Author: Dodge, K. A., et al.

Article: Situational approach to the assessment of social competence in children.

Journal: *Journal of Consulting and Clinical Psychology*, June 1985, *53*(3), 344–353.

■ ■ ■

2614

Test Name: TEXAS SOCIAL BEHAVIOR INDEX

Purpose: To measure personal worth and social interaction.

Number of Items: 32

Format: Likert format.

Reliability: Alternate forms was .89.

Validity: Correlated .50–.52 with self-esteem scale of California Personality Inventory.

Author: McIntire, S. A., and Levine, E. L.

Article: An empirical investigation of self-esteem as a composite construct.

Journal: *Journal of Vocational Behavior*, December 1984, *25*(3), 290–303.

Related Research: Helmreich, R., & Stapp, J. (1974). Short forms of the Texas Social Behavior Inventory (TSBI), an objective measure of self-esteem. *Bulletin of the Psychonomic Society*, *4*(5A), 473–475.

■ ■ ■

2615

Test Name: UCLA REVISED LONELINESS SCALE

Purpose: To measure loneliness.

Number of Items: 20

Format: Ten positively and ten negatively worded statements followed by 4-point (*never* to *often*) response categories. Sample items presented.

Validity: Correlated significantly (r

= .41, $p < .001$) with time spent alone, and with a self-labeling loneliness scale ($r = .71$).

Author: Booth, R.

Article: An examination of college GPA, composite ACT scores, IQs, and gender in relation to loneliness of college students.

Journal: *Psychological Reports*, October 1983, *53*(2), 347–352.

Related Research: Russell, D., et al. (1980). The revised UCLA Loneliness Scale, concurrent and discriminant validity evidence. *Journal of Personality and Social Psychology*, *39*, 472–480.

■ ■ ■

2616

Test Name: VANDERBILT PSYCHOTHERAPY PROCESS SCALE

Purpose: To measure patient

characteristics, therapist characteristics, and their interaction.

Number of Items: 80

Format: Consists of 5-point Likert scales. Judges rate patient, therapist, and their interaction. All items are presented.

Reliability: Interrater reliability was .90 (experienced raters). Alpha ranged from .82 to .96 across subscales.

Author: O'Malley, S. S., et al.

Article: The Vanderbilt Psychotherapy Process Scale: A report on the scale development and process-outcome study.

Journal: *Journal of Consulting and Clinical Psychology*, August 1983, *51*(4), 581–586.

Related Research: Strupp, H. H., et al. (1981). *Vanderbilt Psychotherapy Process Scale*. Vanderbilt University.

CHAPTER 5
Adjustment—Vocational

2617

Test Name: ADMINISTRATIVE STRESS INDEX

Purpose: To measure perceived job-related stress for administrators.

Number of Items: 25

Format: Items are rated on a 5-point Likert scale. All items are presented.

Reliability: Alphas exceeded .70.

Validity: Four subscales were identified by factor analysis. Role-Based Stress correlated −.02 with age, −.01 with years of administrative experience, and −.11 ($p < .01$) with position. A second factor correlated −.10, −.10 ($p < .01$), and −.02 with the three measures, respectively. Boundary-Spanning Stress correlated .11 ($p < .01$), .23 ($p < .001$), and .23 ($p < .001$) with the three measures, respectively. Conflict-Mediating Stress correlated −.05 ($p < .05$), −.10 ($p < .01$), and −.38 ($p < .001$) with the three measures, respectively.

Author: Koch, J. L., et al.

Article: Job stress among school administrators: Factorial dimensions and differential effects.

Journal: *Journal of Applied Psychology,* August 1982, *67*(4), 493–499.

Related Research: Indik, B., et al. (1964). Demographic correlates of psychological strain. *Journal of Abnormal and Social Psychology, 69,* 26–38.

2618

Test Name: ADULT VOCATIONAL MATURITY ASSESSMENT INTERVIEW

Purpose: To assess an individual's ability to cope with tasks associated with choosing, preparing for, and entering an occupation.

Number of Items: 120

Format: Includes eight scales: orientation to work, orientation to education, concern with choice, self-appraisal—interests and abilities, self-appraisal—personality characteristics, self-appraisal—values, exploring occupations, and using resources.

Reliability: Internal consistency reliability estimates ranged from .52 to .91.

Validity: Correlations with other variables ranged from −.25 to .75 ($N = 20$).

Author: Manuele, C. A.

Article: Modifying vocational maturity in adults with delayed career development: A life skills approach.

Journal: *Vocational Guidance Quarterly,* December 1984, *33*(2), 101–112.

Related Research: Manuele, C. (1983). The development of a measure of vocational maturity for adults with delayed career development. *Journal of Vocational Behavior, 23,* 45–63.

2619

Test Name: BURNOUT MEASURE

Purpose: To measure burnout.

Number of Items: 21

Format: Includes three components: physical exhaustion, emotional exhaustion, and mental exhaustion. Responses are recorded on a 7-point scale.

Reliability: Cronbach's alpha was .89.

Author: Etzion, D.

Article: Moderating effect of social support on the stress-burnout relationship.

Journal: *Journal of Applied Psychology,* November 1984, *69*(4), 615–622.

Related Research: Pines, A., et al. (1981). *Burnout: From tedium to personal growth.* New York: Free Press.

...

2620

Test Name: COUNSELOR OCCUPATIONAL STRESS INVENTORY (COSI)

Purpose: To measure occupational stress among school counselors.

Number of Items: 50

Format: Likert format.

Reliability: Alpha ranged from .81 to .95 across subscales.

Author: Moracco, J. C., et al.

Article: Measuring stress in school counselors: Some research findings and implications.

Journal: *The School Counselor,* November 1984, *32*(2), 110–118.

Related Research: Moracco, J. C., & Gray, P. (1983). *The COSI: Development of an instrument to assess stress in counselors.* Paper presented at the annual convention of the American Personnel and Guidance Association, Washington, DC.

■ ■ ■

2621

Test Name: DEPRESSION AND IRRITATION SCALES

Purpose: To measure job-related stress and irritation.

Number of Items: 9

Format: Items rated on 4-point response scales. Sample items are presented.

Reliability: Alpha (depression) was .81; alpha (irritation) was .80.

Author: Ganster, D. C., et al.

Article: Managing organizational stress: A field experiment.

Journal: *Journal of Applied Psychology,* October 1982, *67*(5), 533–542.

Related Research: Cobb, S. (1970). *A variable from the Card Sort Test: A study of people changing jobs* (Project Analysis Memo No. 12). Ann Arbor: University of Michigan, ISR.

■ ■ ■

2622

Test Name: EMPLOYEE ATTITUDE SURVEY

Purpose: To assess employee attitudes including satisfaction with pay, staffing, and performance appraisal.

Number of Items: 31

Format: Items rated on 5-point

Likert scales. All items are presented.

Reliability: Alphas ranged from .70 to .95 across subscales.

Author: Gomez-Mejia, L. R.

Article: Dimensions and correlates of the personnel audit as an organizational assessment tool.

Journal: *Personnel Psychology,* Summer 1985, *38*(2), 293–308.

Related Research: Gomez-Mejia, L. R. (1983). Sex differences during political socialization. *Academy of Management Journal, 26,* 492–499.

■ ■ ■

2623

Test Name: FRUSTRATION SCALE

Purpose: To measure job frustration.

Number of Items: 3

Format: Items rated on a 7-point Likert scale.

Reliability: Alpha ranged from .68 to .76.

Author: O'Connor, E. J., et al.

Article: Situational constraint effects on performance, affective reactions, and turnover: A field replication and extension.

Journal: *Journal of Applied Psychology,* November 1984, *69*(4), 663–672.

Related Research: Peters, L. H., & O'Connor, E. J. (1980). Situational constraints and work outcomes: The influence of a frequently overlooked construct. *Academy of Management Review, 5,* 391–397.

■ ■ ■

2624

Test Name: HOPPOCK JOB SATISFACTION BLANK— SHORT FORM

Purpose: To measure overall job satisfaction.

Number of Items: 4

Format: The items measure affect, duration, social comparison, and behavioral intention.

Reliability: Cronbach's alphas were .79 and .81; test–retest (6 months) reliability was .73.

Author: Scandura, T. A., and Graen, G. B.

Article: Moderating effects of initial leader-member exchange status on the effects of a leadership intervention.

Journal: *Journal of Applied Psychology,* August 1984, *69*(3), 428–436.

Related Research: Hoppock, R. (1935). *Job satisfaction.* New York: Harper.

■ ■ ■

2625

Test Name: INDEX OF JOB SATISFACTION

Purpose: To measure general job satisfaction.

Number of Items: 18

Format: Each item was rated on a 5-point Likert scale from minimum to maximum job satisfaction.

Reliability: Odd–even reliability corrected by Spearman-Brown formula was .87 ($N = 231$). Cronbach's alpha was .94.

Author: Rahim, A.

Article: Demographic variables in general job satisfaction in a hospital: A multivariate study.

Journal: *Perceptual and Motor Skills,* December 1982, *55*(3, Part 1), 711–719.

Related Research: Brayfield, A. H., & Rothe, H. F. (1951). An index of job satisfaction. *Journal* *of Applied Psychology, 35,* 307–311.

■ ■ ■

2626

Test Name: INFLUENCE SCALE

Purpose: To measure perceived influence at work.

Number of Items: 4

Format: 5-point scale (*never true* to *always true*). All items presented were taken from Vroom's influence scale.

Reliability: Alpha was .83.

Author: Jackson, S. E.

Article: Participation in decision making as a strategy for reducing job-related stress.

Journal: *Journal of Applied Psychology,* February 1983, *69*(1), 3–19.

Related Research: Vroom, V. H. (1959). Some personality determinants of the effects of participation. *Journal of Abnormal and Social Psychology, 59,* 322–327.

■ ■ ■

2627

Test Name: IRRITATION/ STRAIN SCALE

Purpose: To measure irritation/ strain from work.

Number of Items: 4

Format: Employs a 5-point scale. A sample question is presented.

Reliability: Cronbach's alpha was .88.

Author: Frese, M., and Okonek, K.

Article: Reasons to leave shiftwork and psychological and psychosomatic complaints of former shiftworkers.

Journal: *Journal of Applied*

Psychology, August 1984, *69*(3), 509–514.

Related Research: Mohr, G. (1984). *Measuring psychological well-being in blue collar workers.* Unpublished manuscript, Freie Universitaet, Department of Psychology, Berlin.

■ ■ ■

2628

Test Name: JOB BURNOUT INVENTORY

Purpose: To measure job burnout.

Number of Items: 15

Format: Items rated on 7-point Likert response categories. All items presented.

Reliability: Cronbach's alpha ranged from .67 to .82 across subscales.

Validity: Correlated nonsignificantly with health symptoms, episodic stress, and chronic job stress, but significantly ($p < .05$) with sick days taken.

Author: Ford, D. L., Jr., and Murphy, C. J.

Article: Exploratory development and validation of a perceptual job burnout inventory: Comparison of corporate sector and human services professionals.

Journal: *Psychological Reports,* June 1983, *52*(3), 995–1006.

■ ■ ■

2629

Test Name: JOB DESCRIPTIVE INDEX

Purpose: To measure job satisfaction.

Format: Includes the following: pay, promotions, work, co-workers, and supervision.

Reliability: Coefficient alpha ranged from .15 to .90.

Validity: Correlation with

absenteeism ranged from –.49 to .23.

Author: Teborg, J. R., et al.

Article: Extension of the Schmidt and Hunter validity generalization procedure to the prediction of absenteeism behavior from knowledge of job satisfaction and organizational commitment.

Journal: *Journal of Applied Psychology,* August 1982, *67*(4), 440–449.

Related Research: Smith, P. C., et al. (1969). *The measurement of satisfaction in work and retirement.* Chicago: Rand McNally.

Johnson, S. M., et al. (1982). Response format of the Job Descriptive Index: Assessment of reliability and validity by the multitrait–multimethod matrix. *Journal of Applied Psychology, 67*(4), 500–505.

■ ■ ■

2630

Test Name: JOB DESCRIPTIVE INDEX—MODIFIED

Purpose: To measure job satisfaction.

Number of Items: 70

Format: Includes separate scores to measure satisfaction with the work itself, promotion, supervision, co-workers, and pay. Utilizes a 5-point Likert scale.

Reliability: Coefficient alphas for separate scores ranged from .81 to .98.

Validity: Correlations with other measures ranged from –.82 to .74.

Author: Adler, S., and Golan, J.

Article: Lateness as a withdrawal behavior.

Journal: *Journal of Applied Psychology,* October 1981, *66*(5), 544–554.

Related Research: Smith, P. C., et al. (1969). *The measurement of satisfaction in work and retirement.* Chicago: Rand McNally.

■ ■ ■

2631

Test Name: JOB DIAGNOSTIC SURVEY

Purpose: To measure the apprentices' general job satisfaction.

Number of Items: 5

Format: A 7-point scale format is employed.

Reliability: Alpha coefficient was .89 (*N* = 166).

Validity: Correlations with other variables ranged from .09 to .52.

Author: Tharenou, P., and Harker, P.

Article: Moderating influence of self-esteem on relationships between job complexity, performance and satisfaction.

Journal: *Journal of Applied Psychology,* November 1984, *69*(4), 623–632.

Related Research: Hackman, J. R., & Oldham, G. R. (1974). *The Job Diagnostic Survey: An instrument for the diagnosis of jobs and the evaluation of redesign projects* (Technical Report No. 4). New Haven, CT: Yale University, Department of Administrative Sciences.

■ ■ ■

2632

Test Name: JOB INVOLVEMENT QUESTIONNAIRE

Purpose: To measure job satisfaction.

Number of Items: 6

Format: 7-point scale.

Reliability: Test–retest reliability was .65.

Author: Barling, J., and Van Bart, D.

Article: Mothers' subjective employment experiences and the behavior of their nursery school children.

Journal: *Journal of Occupational Psychology,* March 1983, *57*(1), 49–56.

Related Research: Warr, P., et al. (1979). Scales for the measurement of some attitudes as aspects of psychological well-being. *Journal of Occupational Psychology, 52,* 129–148.

■ ■ ■

2633

Test Name: JOB PERCEPTION SCALES

Purpose: To measure satisfaction with job.

Number of Items: 21

Format: Semantic differential scales modified to five anchor points.

Reliability: Test–retest (3-week interval) ranged from .64 to .80.

Validity: Principal components factor analysis revealed the five hypothesized dimensions initially expected: work, pay, promotions, supervision, and co-workers. Significant multitrait–multimethod procedures indicate convergent and discriminant validity.

Author: Hatfield, J. D., et al.

Article: An empirical evaluation of a test for assessing job satisfaction.

Journal: *Psychological Reports,* February 1985, *56*(1), 39–45.

■ ■ ■

2634

Test Name: JOB SATISFACTION SCALE

Purpose: To measure job satisfaction.

Number of Items: 18

Format: Likert format.

Reliability: Alpha was .83.

Author: Jamal, M.

Article: Shiftwork related to job attitudes, social participation and withdrawal behavior: A study of nurses and industrial workers.

Journal: *Personnel Psychology,* Autumn 1981, *34*(3), 535–547.

Related Research: Brayfield, A. H., & Rathe, F. H. (1951). An index of job satisfaction. *Journal of Applied Psychology, 35,* 307–311.

■ ■ ■

2635

Test Name: JOB SATISFACTION SCALE

Purpose: To measure job satisfaction.

Number of Items: 13

Format: Items rated on a 7-point scale.

Reliability: Alpha was .85.

Author: Litt, M. D., and Turk, D. C.

Article: Sources of stress and dissatisfaction in experienced high school teachers.

Journal: *Journal of Educational Research,* January/February 1985, *78*(3), 178–185.

Related Research: Hackman, J. R., & Oldham, G. R. (1974). *The Job Diagnostic Survey: An instrument for the diagnosis of jobs and the evaluation of job redesign projects* (Technical Report No. 4). New Haven, CT: Yale University, Department of Administrative Sciences.

2636

Test Name: JOB SATISFACTION SCALE

Purpose: To measure job satisfaction.

Number of Items: 2

Format: Items rated on 5- and 7-point response scales. Both items presented.

Reliability: Alpha was .86.

Author: Louis, M. R., et al.

Article: The availability and helpfulness of socialization practices.

Journal: *Personnel Psychology*, Winter 1983, *36*(4), 857–866.

Related Research: O'Reilly, C., & Caldwell, D. F. (1980). Job choice: The impact of intrinsic and extrinsic factors on subsequent satisfaction and commitment. *Journal of Applied Psychology, 65,* 559–565.

■ ■ ■

2637

Test Name: JOB SATISFACTION SCALE

Purpose: To measure job satisfaction as a chronic mood state.

Number of Items: 20

Format: Items are bipolar adjectives separated by a 7-point scale. A few examples are presented.

Reliability: Coefficient alpha was .84.

Validity: Correlations with other variables ranged from −.21 to .31.

Author: Smith, C. A., et al.

Article: Organizational citizenship behavior: Its nature and antecedents.

Journal: *Journal of Applied Psychology*, November 1983, *68*(4), 653–663.

Related Research: Scott, W. E., Jr. (1967). The development of semantic differential scales as measures of "morale." *Personnel Psychology, 20,* 179–198.

■ ■ ■

2638

Test Name: JOB-RELATED TENSION INDEX

Purpose: To provide an overall measure of perceived psychological tension or strain associated with stresses at work.

Number of Items: 15

Format: Likert scale.

Reliability: Reported internal consistency ranged from .73 to .87.

Author: Abush, R., and Burkhead, E. J.

Article: Job stress in midlife working women: Relationships among personality type, job characteristics, and job tension.

Journal: *Journal of Counseling Psychology*, January 1984, *31*(1), 36–44.

Related Research: Kahn, R. L., et al. (1964). *Organizational stress: Studies in role conflict and role ambiguity*. New York: Wiley.

■ ■ ■

2639

Test Name: JOB-RELATED TENSION INDEX

Purpose: To measure organizational stress.

Number of Items: 14

Format: Likert items.

Reliability: Test–retest reliability coefficient was .724.

Author: West, D. J., Jr., et al.

Article: Component analysis of occupational stress inoculation applied to registered nurses in an acute care hospital setting.

Journal: *Journal of Counseling Psychology*, April 1984, *31*(2), 209–218.

Related Research: Kahn, R. L., et al. (1964). *Organizational stress: Studies in role conflict and role ambiguity*. New York: Wiley.

■ ■ ■

2640

Test Name: JOB-RELATED TENSION INDEX

Purpose: To measure job-related tension.

Number of Items: 9

Format: Items rated on 5-point Likert response categories. Sample items are presented.

Reliability: Median item intercorrelation was .27. Split-half reliability was .69.

Author: Wright, D., and Thomas, J.

Article: Role strain among psychologists in the midwest.

Journal: *Journal of School Psychology*, 1982, *20*(2), 96–102.

Related Research: Lyons, T. F. (1971). Role clarity, need for clarity, satisfaction, tension and withdrawal. *Organizational Behavior and Human Performance, 6,* 99–110.

■ ■ ■

2641

Test Name: JOB STRESS QUESTIONNAIRE

Purpose: To measure role conflict, role ambiguity, organizational conflict, and workgroup cooperation.

Number of Items: 36

Format: Items rated on a 5-point Likert scale. Sample items are presented.

Reliability: Alpha ranged from .55 to .84 across subscales.

Author: Burr, R. G.

Article: Smoking among U.S. Navy enlisted men: Some contributing factors.

Journal: *Psychological Reports,* February 1984, *54*(1), 287–294.

Related Research: Butler, M. C., & Burr, R. G. (1980). Utility of a multidimensional locus of control scale in predicting health and job related outcomes in military environments. *Psychological Reports, 47,* 719–728.

■ ■ ■

2642

Test Name: JOB STRESS SCALES

Purpose: To measure environmental and psychological stress.

Number of Items: 16 (10 environmental, 6 psychological).

Format: Items rated on a 5-point answering scale. Sample items presented.

Reliability: Alphas were .84 (environmental); and .80 (psychological).

Author: Frese, M., and Okonek, K.

Article: Reasons to leave shiftwork and psychological and psychosomatic complaints of former shiftworkers.

Journal: *Journal of Applied Psychology,* August 1984, *69*(3), 509–514.

Related Research: Semmer, N. (1982). Stress at work, stress in private life, and psychological well-being. In W. Bachmann et al., (Eds.), *Mental load and stress in activity: European approaches.* Berlin: Deutscher Verlag der Wissenschaften.

■ ■ ■

2643

Test Name: JOB TEDIUM SCALE

Purpose: To measure physical, emotional, and mental exhaustion.

Number of Items: 21

Format: Items rated on 7-point scale (1 = *never*, 7 = *always*).

Reliability: Test–retest (1 month) reliability was .89; 2 month reliability was .76; 6 months reliability was .66. Alpha (internal consistency) ranged from .91 to .93.

Validity: Significant ($p < .05$) correlations in expected direction with job satisfaction, desire to leave job and negative attitude toward clients, and Maslach Burnout Scale.

Author: Stout, J. K., and Williams, J. M.

Article: Comparison of two measures of burnout.

Journal: *Psychological Reports,* August 1983, *53*(1), 283–289.

Related Research: Pines, A. M., et al. (1981). *Burnout: From tedium to personal growth.* New York: Free Press.

■ ■ ■

2644

Test Name: JOB TIME-DEMANDS SCALE

Purpose: To measure job time demands experienced by people who have family and employment responsibilities.

Number of Items: 15

Format: Items rated on 4-point Likert response categories (*almost never* to *almost always*). Each item describes time–demand situations. All items are presented.

Reliability: Cronbach's alpha on composite scale was .80. Alpha ranged from .66 to .82 on three subscales derived by factor analysis.

Validity: People who reported job-family difficulties scored higher on the Job Time-Demand Scale ($t = 9.61$, $p < .001$).

Author: Johnson, P.

Article: Development of a measure of job-time demands.

Journal: *Psychological Reports,* December 1982, *51*(3, Part 2), 1087–1094.

■ ■ ■

2645

Test Name: MARKET DISSATISFACTION SCALE

Purpose: To measure how secure and well-paid a respondent's job is.

Number of Items: 7

Format: Items rated on 5-point Likert format. All items are presented.

Reliability: Alpha ranged from .51 to .55.

Validity: Correlated with potential grievance ($r = .25$ and .30, $p < .01$).

Author: Blyton, P., et al.

Article: Job status and White-collar members' union activities.

Journal: *Journal of Occupational Psychology,* March 1981, *54*(1), 33–45.

■ ■ ■

2646

Test Name: MEIER BURNOUT ASSESSMENT

Purpose: To measure cognitions and expectations related to burnout.

Number of Items: 23

Format: True–false.

Reliability: Alpha was .79.

Validity: Correlated .58 with Maslach Burnout Inventory.

Author: Meier, S. T.

Article: The construct validity of burnout.

Journal: *Journal of Occupational Psychology*, September 1984, *57*(3), 211–219.

Related Research: Meier, S. (1983). Toward a theory of burnout. *Human Relations, 36,* 899–910.

■ ■ ■

2647

Test Name: NEED FOR CLARITY INDEX

Purpose: To measure respondent need for clear assessment of job performance.

Number of Items: 4

Format: Items rated on 5-point Likert response categories.

Reliability: Median item intercorrelation was .40. Split-half reliability was .65.

Author: Wright, D., and Thomas, J.

Article: Role strain among psychologists in the midwest.

Journal: *Journal of School Psychology*, 1982, *20*(2), 96–102.

Related Research: Lyons, T. F. (1971). Role clarity, need for clarity, satisfaction, tension and withdrawal. *Organizational Behavior and Human Performance, 6,* 99–110.

■ ■ ■

2648

Test Name: NURSING STRESS SCALE

Purpose: To measure the frequency with which certain nursing situations are perceived as stressful by nurses.

Number of Items: 34

Format: Subjects respond to each item on a scale from 0 (*never*) to 3 (*very frequently*). Includes 7

factors: death and dying, conflict with physicians, inadequate preparation, lack of support, conflict with other nurses, work load, and uncertainty concerning treatment. All items are presented.

Reliability: Test-retest reliability ranged from .42 to .86. Spearman-Brown coefficients ranged from .57 to .84. Guttman split-half coefficients ranged from .46 to .79. Coefficient alphas ranged from .64 to .89. Standardized item alphas ranged from .65 to .89.

Validity: Correlations with other variables ranged from –.15 to .39.

Author: Gray-Toft, P., and Anderson, J. G.

Article: The Nursing Stress Scale: Development of an instrument.

Journal: *Journal of Behavioral Assessment*, March 1981, *3*(1), 11–23.

■ ■ ■

2649

Test Name: OCCUPATIONAL STRESS SCALE

Purpose: To measure occupational stress.

Number of Items: 34

Format: True–false–undecided response categories. Sample items are presented.

Reliability: Split-half and test–retest reliabilities ranged from .60 to .87.

Author: Petrie, K., and Rotherham, M. J.

Article: Insulators against stress: Self-esteem and assertiveness.

Journal: *Psychological Reports,* 1982, *50*(3, Part 1), 963–966.

Related Research: Weyer, G., & Hodapp, V. (1974). Development of a questionnaire for measuring perceived stress. *Archiv für Psychologie, 127,* 161–188.

2650

Test Name: ORGANIZATIONAL READJUSTMENT RATING SCALE

Purpose: To measure stressful events on the job.

Number of Items: 31

Format: A total of 31 events are checked if they have occurred in the last 12 months. Sum of item weights yields a stress score.

Validity: Correlated .40 with Holmes and Rahe Schedule of Recent Experiences Scale.

Author: Weiss, H. M., et al.

Article: Effects of life and job stress on information search behaviors of organizational members.

Journal: *Journal of Applied Psychology,* February 1982, *67*(1), 60–66.

Related Research: Naismith, D. C. (1975). *Stress among managers as a function of organizational change.* Doctoral dissertation, George Washington University.

■ ■ ■

2651

Test Name: PAY INCREASE SCALE

Purpose: To measure meaningfulness of pay increases.

Number of Items: 16

Format: Paired comparison. Money-oriented responses paired with recognition-oriented responses.

Reliability: Internal consistency was .96.

Author: Frzystofiak, F., et al.

Article: Pay, meaning, satisfaction and size of a meaningful pay increase.

Journal: *Psychological Reports,* 1982, *51*(2), 660–662.

Related Research: Krefting, L. A., & Mahoney, T. A. (1977). Determining the size of meaningful pay increase. *Industrial Relations, 16,* 89–93.

■ ■ ■

2652

Test Name: PAY SATISFACTION SCALE

Purpose: To measure satisfaction with pay.

Number of Items: 7

Format: Four items were concerned with perceived fairness of pay and three items were concerned with satisfaction of pay.

Reliability: Cronbach's alpha was .89.

Validity: Correlations with other variables ranged from –.39 to .51.

Author: Motowidlo, S. J.

Article: Predicting sales turnover from pay satisfaction and expectation.

Journal: *Journal of Applied Psychology,* August 1983, *68*(3), 484–489.

Related Research: Motowidlo, S. J. (1982). Relationship between self-rated performance and pay satisfaction among sales representatives. *Journal of Applied Psychology, 67,* 209–213.

■ ■ ■

2653

Test Name: PERCEIVED INFLUENCE SCALE

Purpose: To measure how much influence respondent would like to have at work.

Number of Items: 4

Format: Items rated on 9-point Likert format.

Reliability: Alpha was .86.

Author: Rafaeli, A.

Article: Quality circles and employee attitudes.

Journal: *Personnel Psychology,* Autumn 1985, *38*(3), 603–615.

Related Research: Hackman, J. R., & Lawler, E. E. (1971). Employee reactions to job characteristics. *Journal of Applied Psychology, 55,* 259–286.

■ ■ ■

2654

Test Name: PHYSICAL AND PSYCHOLOGICAL STRESS SCALES

Purpose: To measure stress at work.

Number of Items: 15

Format: Varies. All items are presented.

Reliability: Reliability ranged from .64 to .90 across component subscales.

Author: Frese, M.

Article: Stress at work and psychosomatic complaints: A causal interpretation.

Journal: *Journal of Applied Psychology,* May 1985, *70*(2), 314–328.

Related Research: Zapf, D., et al. *Scale documentation of the research project–Psychological stress at work: Factors promoting and impeding humane working conditions.* Institut für Psychologie, Freie Universität Berlin, 1000 Berlin 33, Germany.

■ ■ ■

2655

Test Name: POTENTIAL AND ACTUAL STRESSORS SCALES

Purpose: To measure teacher stress.

Number of Items: 9 separate scales contain from 3 to 7 items each.

Format: Multiple-choice. Sample items presented.

Reliability: Alpha ranged from .58 to .94 across scales.

Author: Tellenback, S., et al.

Article: Teacher stress: Exploratory model building.

Journal: *Journal of Occupational Psychology,* March 1983, *56*(1), 19–33.

Related Research: Tellenback, S., et al. Teacher stress: A structural-comparative analysis. *Pedagogical Reports, 14.* Lund: Department of Education.

■ ■ ■

2656

Test Name: POTENTIAL GRIEVANCE SCALE

Purpose: To measure how much a respondent might want his or her union to help with job problems.

Number of Items: 5

Format: Items rated in 5-point Likert format. All items presented.

Reliability: Alpha ranged from .71 to .73.

Validity: Correlated with market dissatisfaction (rs = .25 and .30, p < .01).

Author: Blyton, P., et al.

Article: Job status and White-collar members' union activity.

Journal: *Journal of Occupational Psychology,* March 1981, *54*(1), 33–45.

■ ■ ■

2657

Test Name: PROPENSITY TO LEAVE SCALE

Purpose: To assess likelihood of leaving an organization.

Number of Items: 3

Format: A 5-point multiple-choice.

Reliability: Alpha was .83.

Author: Bedeian, A. G.

Article: The relationship between role stress and job-related interpersonal and organizational climate factors.

Journal: *Journal of Social Psychology*, April 1981, *113*(second half), 247–260.

Related Research: Lyons, T. F. (1971). Role clarity, need for clarity, satisfaction, tension and withdrawal. *Organizational Behavior and Human Performance*, *6*, 99–110.

■ ■ ■

2658

Test Name: PSYCHOLOGICAL STRESS AT WORK SCALE

Purpose: To measure psychological stress at work.

Number of Items: 14

Format: Includes items relating to: uncertainty in the job, organizational problems, environmental stress, danger of accidents, and intensity.

Reliability: Coefficient alphas ranged from .52 to .79.

Validity: Correlations with physical stress ranged from −.22 to .42.

Source: Frese, M.

Article: Stress at work and psychosomatic complaints: A causal interpretation.

Journal: *Journal of Applied Psychology*, May 1985, *70*(2), 314–328.

■ ■ ■

2659

Test Name: SATISFACTION SCALE

Purpose: To measure overall satisfaction with work, salary, research and teaching support,

colleagues, and the power and decision-making structure within the university.

Number of Items: 16

Format: Responses were made on a 5-point scale ranging from *very dissatisfied* to *very satisfied*.

Reliability: Internal consistency reliability was .91.

Validity: Correlations with other variables ranged from −.53 to .87.

Author: Zalesny, M. D.

Article: Comparison of economic and noneconomic factors in predicting faculty vote preference in a union representation election.

Journal: *Journal of Applied Psychology*, May 1985, *70*(2), 243–256.

Related Research: Terborg, J. R., et al. (1982, August). *University faculty dispositions toward unionization: A test of Triandis' model.* Paper presented at the meeting of the American Psychological Association, Washington, DC.

■ ■ ■

2660

Test Name: SATISFACTION WITH 3/38 WORK SCHEDULE SCALE

Purpose: To measure satisfaction with working 38 hours in 3 work days.

Number of Items: 7

Format: Items rated in 7-point Likert format. All items presented.

Reliability: Alpha was .93.

Validity: A group actually on a 3-day/38-hour schedule scored higher than a group on a 5-day/40-hour schedule.

Author: Latack, J. C., and Foster, L. W.

Article: Implementation of

compressed work schedules: Participation and job design as critical factors for employee acceptance.

Journal: *Personnel Psychology*, Spring 1985, *38*(1), 75–92.

■ ■ ■

2661

Test Name: SATISFACTION WITH THE NAVY SCALE

Purpose: To measure satisfaction with the Navy.

Number of Items: 6

Format: Likert format.

Reliability: Alpha was .80.

Author: James, L. R., et al.

Article: Perceptions of psychological influence: A cognitive information processing approach for explaining moderated relationships.

Journal: *Personnel Psychology*, Autumn 1981, *34*(3), 453–475.

Related Research: Jones, A. P., et al. (1977). Black-White differences in job satisfaction and its correlates. *Personnel Psychology*, *30*, 5–16.

■ ■ ■

2662

Test Name: SCHOOL PSYCHOLOGIST STRESS INVENTORY

Purpose: To identify and measure sources of stress among school psychologists.

Number of Items: 35 job-related events.

Format: Respondents indicate how stressful each event is on a scale of 1 to 9.

Validity: Factor analysis yielded 9 factors with eigenvalues greater than one. Statistically significant differences by gender reported on 6 factors, significant differences by age on 5 factors, significant differences by salary on 4 factors.

Author: Wise, P. S.

Article: School psychologists' rankings of stressful events.

Journal: *Journal of School Psychology*, 1985, *23*(1), 31–41.

• • •

2663

Test Name: TASK SATISFACTION SCALE

Purpose: To measure subjects' overall task satisfaction.

Number of Items: 7

Format: Responses are made on a 7-point Likert scale. Sample items are presented.

Reliability: Coefficient alpha was .85.

Validity: Correlation with performance was .21.

Author: Phillips, J. S., and Freedman, S. M.

Article: Contingent pay and intrinsic task interest: Moderating effects of work values.

Journal: *Journal of Applied Psychology*, May 1985, *70*(2), 306–313.

• • •

2664

Test Name: TEACHER BURNOUT SURVEY

Purpose: To measure and assess burnout.

Number of Items: 65

Format: Items rated on Likert scales.

Reliability: Spearman-Brown split-half reliability was .88.

Author: Farber, B. A.

Article: Stress and burnout in suburban teachers.

Journal: *Journal of Educational Research*, July/August 1984, *77*(6), 325–331.

Related Research: Maslach, C., & Jackson, S. (1981). The measure of experienced burnout. *Journal of Occupational Behavior*, *2*, 1–15.

• • •

2665

Test Name: TEACHER OCCUPATIONAL STRESS FACTOR QUESTIONNAIRE

Purpose: To identify the perceived occupational stress factors of teachers.

Number of Items: 30

Format: Responses are made on a scale from not stressful to extremely stressful. Includes four factors: Relationships with teachers, work and compensation, working with students, perceptions of respect from others. All items are presented.

Reliability: Cronbach's alpha coefficients ranged from .79 to .92. Overall reliability was .93.

Author: Foxworth, M. D., et al.

Article: The factorial validity of the Teacher Occupational Stress Factor Questionnaire for the teacher of the gifted.

Journal: *Educational and Psychological Measurement*, Summer 1984, *44*(2), 527–532.

Related Research: Clark, E. H. (1980). *An analysis of occupational stress factors as perceived by public school teachers.* Unpublished doctoral dissertation, Auburn University.

Halpin, G., et al. (1985). Teacher stress as related to locus of control, sex and age. *Journal of Experimental Education, 53*(3), 136–140.

Harris, K., et al. (1985). Teacher

characteristics and stress. *Journal of Educational Research, 78*(6), 346–350.

• • •

2666

Test Name: TEACHER STRESS INVENTORY

Purpose: To measure occupational stress in teachers.

Number of Items: 38

Format: Items rated on Likert scales (two responses per item: one for strength and one for frequency of stress.)

Reliability: Alpha ranged from .62 to .95 across subscales and across samples of respondents.

Validity: Items factored similarly in different samples (types) of teachers (regular and special education).

Author: Fimian, M. J.

Article: The development of an instrument to measure occupational stress in teachers: The Teacher Stress Inventory.

Journal: *Journal of Occupational Psychology*, December 1984, *57*(4), 277–293.

• • •

2667

Test Name: TENSION SCALE

Purpose: To measure feelings of being bothered by work-related factors.

Number of Items: 9

Format: A 5-category multiple-choice test.

Reliability: Alpha was .86.

Author: Bedeian, A. G., et al.

Article: The relationship between role stress and job-related interpersonal and organizational climate factors.

Journal: *Journal of Social*

Psychology, April 1981, *113*(second half), 247–260.

Related Research: Kahn, R. L., et al. (1964). *Organizational stress: Studies in role conflict and role ambiguity*. New York: Wiley.

■ ■ ■

2668

Test Name: TRIPLE AUDIT OPINION SURVEY (TAOS)

Purpose: To measure job satisfaction.

Number of Items: 104

Format: Items are rated on 5-point Likert format.

Reliability: Ranged from .74 to .95.

Author: Lee, R., et al.

Article: Sex, wage-earner status, occupational level and job satisfaction.

Journal: *Journal of Vocational Behavior*, June 1981, *18*(3), 362–373.

Related Research: The TAOS is a variation of the Minnesota Satisfaction Questionnaire.

■ ■ ■

2669

Test Name: UNION INSTRUMENTALITY SCALE

Purpose: To measure how much nurses perceive joining a union as leading to various outcomes.

Number of Items: 13

Format: Items are rated on a 5-point scale (*never* to *always*).

Reliability: Alphas ranged from .72 to .82 for extrinsic and intrinsic items.

Validity: Does not correlate significantly ($r = .11$) with locus of control (Rotter, 1966), or pro-Strike attitudes ($R = .19$). Does correlate significantly with

intention to join a union ($r = .34$).

Author: Beutell, N. J., and Biggs, D. L.

Article: Behavioral intentions to join a union: Instrumentality x valence, locus of control and strike attitudes.

Journal: *Psychological Reports*, August 1984, *55*(1), 215–222.

■ ■ ■

2670

Test Name: WARR JOB SATISFACTION QUESTIONNAIRE

Purpose: To measure satisfaction with intrinsic and extrinsic job factors.

Number of Items: 15

Format: Items rated in 7-point Likert format.

Reliability: Test–retest reliability was .63.

Author: Barling, J., and Van Bart, D.

Article: Mothers' subjective employment experience and the behavior of their nursery school children.

Journal: *Journal of Occupational Psychology*, March 1984, *57*(1), 49–56.

Related Research: Warr, P., et al. (1979). Scales for the measurement of some attitudes as aspects of psychological well-being. *Journal of Occupational Psychology, 52*, 129–148.

■ ■ ■

2671

Test Name: WORK ALIENATION–INVOLVEMENT SCALE

Purpose: To measure work alienation–involvement.

Number of Items: 15

Format: Items rated on 5-point

Likert agreement scales.

Reliability: Alpha was .89.

Author: Lefkowitz, J., et al.

Article: The role of need level and/or need salience as moderators of the relationship between need satisfaction and work alienation–involvement.

Journal: *Journal of Vocational Behavior*, April 1984, *24*(2), 142–158.

Related Research: Lefkowitz, J., & Somers, M. (1982). *Work alienation-involvement: Scale construction, validation, and a developmental model*. Poster Session I (Division 14) at the meeting of the American Psychological Association, Washington, DC.

■ ■ ■

2672

Test Name: WORK ROLE CENTRALITY SCALE

Purpose: To determine the degree to which the work role dominates the attention and interests of the employee relative to nonorganizational roles.

Number of Items: 5

Format: A 5-point format was employed.

Reliability: Coefficient alpha was .74.

Author: Drasgow, F., and Miller, H. E.

Article: Psychometric and substantive issues in scale construction and validation.

Journal: *Journal of Applied Psychology*, June 1982, *67*(3), 268–279.

Related Research: Dubin, R. (1956). Industrial workers' worlds: A study of the "central life interests" of industrial workers. *Social Problems*, 131–140.

2673

Test Name: WORK SATISFACTION SCALE

Purpose: To measure degree to which respondent obtained specific rewards from work.

Number of Items: 25

Format: Items rated on 5-point scales. Sample items are presented.

Reliability: Alpha was .94.

Author: Pistrang, N.

Article: Women's work involvement and experience of new motherhood.

Journal: *Journal of Marriage and the Family*, May 1984, *46*(2), 433–447.

Related Research: Robinson, J. P., et al. (1974). *Measures of occupational attitudes and occupational characteristics.* Ann Arbor, MI: Survey Research Center of the Institute for Social Research.

■ ■ ■

2674

Test Name: WORK TEDIUM QUESTIONNAIRE

Purpose: To measure work tedium.

Number of Items: 21

Format: Subjects indicate their frequency of experiencing mental, emotional, and physical exhaustion at work on a 7-point frequency scale.

Reliability: Coefficient alpha was .79.

Validity: Correlations with other variables ranged from −.10 to −.82.

Author: Adler, S., and Golan, J.

Article: Lateness as a withdrawal behavior.

Journal: *Journal of Applied Psychology*, October 1981, *66*(5), 544–554.

Related Research: Kafry, D., and Pines, A. (1980). The experience of tedium in life and work. *Human Relations, 33*, 477–503.

■ ■ ■

2675

Test Name: WORKER OPINION SURVEY

Purpose: To measure shop-floor job satisfaction.

Number of Items: 48

Time Required: 6–8 minutes.

Reliability: Kuder-Richardson formula values were .71 to .86.

Validity: Multitrait–multimethod validity with Job Descriptive Index met all Campbell and Fiske criteria.

Author: Soutar, G. N., and Weaver, J. R.

Article: The measurement of shop-floor job satisfaction: The convergent and discriminant validity of the worker opinion survey.

Journal: *Journal of Occupational Psychology*, March 1982, *55*(1), 27–33.

Related Research: Cross, D. (1973). The worker opinion survey: A measure of shop-floor satisfaction. *Occupational Psychology, 47*, 193–208.

■ ■ ■

2676

Test Name: WORK ORIENTATION SCALE

Purpose: To measure orientation to work.

Number of Items: 10

Format: *Yes–no* or frequency (i.e., *never* to *often*) format. Sample items are presented.

Reliability: Cronbach's alpha was .63.

Validity: Correlated significantly with burnout (−.16 to −.19).

Author: Nagy, S.

Article: Burnout and selected variables as components of occupational stress.

Journal: *Psychological Reports*, February 1985, *56*(1), 195–200.

CHAPTER 6
Aptitude

2677

Test Name: CHILD'S LEARNING ABILITY RATING SCALE

Purpose: To measure child's learning.

Number of Items: 16

Time Required: 4 seconds per item.

Format: Children are asked to match geometric design with eight concrete and eight abstract nouns.

Reliability: Split-half (Spearman-Brown) reliability was .85. Interrater reliability was .71.

Author: Dean, R. S., and Kundert, D. K.

Article: Intelligence and teachers' ratings as predictors of abstract and concrete learning.

Journal: *Journal of School Psychology*, 1981, *19*(1), 78–85.

...

2678

Test Name: COGNITIVE TASKS

Purpose: To measure cognitive ability of elementary school children in Japan, China, and the United States.

Number of Items: Ranged from 138 (1st graders) to 149 (5th graders).

Format: Includes 10 tasks: coding, spatial relations, perceptual speed, auditory memory, verbal-spatial, serial memory (words), serial memory (numbers), verbal memory, vocabulary, general information.

Reliability: Cronbach's alpha ranged from .47 to .98.

Author: Stevenson, H. W., et al.

Article: Cognitive performance and academic achievement of Japanese, Chinese, and American children.

Journal: *Child Development*, June 1985, *56*(3), 718–734.

Related Research: Stigler, J. W., et al. (1982). Curriculum and achievement in mathematics: A study of elementary school children in Japan, Taiwan, and the United States. *Journal of Educational Psychology, 74*, 315–322.

...

2679

Test Name: COMPUTER SCIENCE SUCCESS PREDICTOR TEST

Purpose: To measure level of success in beginning computer science courses.

Number of Items: 30

Time Required: 1 class period.

Format: Questions on logic, reading comprehension, alphabetic and numeric sequences, algorithmic execution, and alphanumeric translation.

Reliability: Kuder-Richardson formula 20 was .76.

Validity: Multiple correlation was .25 with final examination.

Author: Wileman, S., et al.

Article: Factors influencing success in beginning computer science courses.

Journal: *Journal of Educational Research,* March/April 1987, *74*(4), 223–226.

...

2680

Test Name: HUMOR PERCEPTIVENESS TEST

Purpose: To measure humor aptitude.

Number of Items: 18

Format: Each item is a sentence-completion item taken from a fairly common joke. A few examples are presented.

Reliability: Corrected split-half reliability was .75 ($n = 56$).

Validity: Correlation with the Humor Achievement Test was .66 ($N = 45$). Correlation with GPA was −.24 ($n = 35$).

Author: Feingold, A.

Article: Measuring humor: A pilot study.

Journal: *Perceptual and Motor Skills*, June 1982, *54*(3, Part 1), 986.

...

2681

Test Name: LATERALITY INDEX

Purpose: To assess cognitive impairment resulting from unilateral hemispheric damage to the brain using the WAIS-R.

Format: The Index is devised from Factor 2 of the WAIS-R (Worksheet provided).

Reliability: Split-half reliability was .78. Test–retest reliability was .79.

Validity: An LI that is more extreme than 10th or 90th percentile is indicative of probable damage.

Author: Lawson, J. S., et al.

Article: A laterality index of cognitive impairment devised from a principal-components analysis of the WAIS-R.

Journal: *Journal of Consulting and Clinical Psychology,* December 1983, *51*(6), 841–847.

Related Research: Lawson, J. S., & Inglis, J. (1983). A laterality index of cognitive impairment after hemispheric damage: A measure devised from a principal-components analysis of the Wechsler Adult Intelligence Scale. *Journal of Consulting and Clinical Psychology, 51,* 832–840.

■ ■ ■

2682

Test Name: LEADERSHIP OPINION QUESTIONNAIRE

Purpose: To measure leadership potential in college students.

Number of Items: 40

Format: Multiple-choice.

Validity: Significant expected differences between known leaders and non-leaders on the consideration and structure dimensions.

Author: DeJulio, S. S., et al.

Article: The measurement of leadership potential in college students.

Journal: *Journal of College Student Personnel,* May 1981, *22*(3), 202–213.

Related Research: Fleishman, E. A. (1957). A leader behavior description for industry. In R. M. Stogdill & A. E. Coons (Eds.), *Leader behavior: Its description and measurement.* Columbus, OH: Bureau of Business Research.

2683

Test Name: MULTIVARIATE ACHIEVEMENT PREDICTOR TEST

Purpose: To predict academic achievement.

Number of Items: 64

Time Required: Less than one class period.

Reliability: Alphas ranged from .56 to .86.

Author: Foshay, W. R., and Misanchuk, E. R.

Article: Toward the multivariate modeling of achievement, aptitude, and personality.

Journal: *Journal of Educational Research,* May/June 1981, *74*(5), 352–357.

Related Research: Misanchuk, E. R. (1977). A model-based prediction of scholastic achievement. *Journal of Educational Research, 71,* 30–35.

■ ■ ■

2684

Test Name: NON-COGNITIVE QUESTIONNAIRE

Purpose: To predict academic success by race.

Number of Items: 21

Format: Includes 18 Likert items and 3 open-ended questions dealing with present goals, past accomplishments, group memberships, and offices held.

Reliability: Test–retest reliability (2 weeks, *N* = 18) on the Likert items ranged from .70 to .94.

Author: Tracey, T. S., and Sedlacek, W. E.

Article: Non-cognitive variables in predicting academic success by race.

Journal: *Measurement and Evaluation in Guidance,* January 1984, *16*(4), 171–178.

Related Research: Sedlacek, W. E., & Brooks, G. C., Jr. (1976). *Racism in American education: A model for change.* Chicago: Nelson-Hall.

■ ■ ■

2685

Test Name: PERCEPTUAL ACUITY TEST

Purpose: To assess non-transformational intellectual functions.

Number of Items: 30

Time Required: 20 minutes.

Format: Five geometric figures are presented to subjects on a screen. Subjects are asked to choose one that meets specified criteria.

Validity: Correlates .21 to .33 with age. Correlates .38 with Gollschaldt Hidden Figures Test, .28 with Cane-Ruch Spatial Relations Test, and –.41 with Witkin's rod-and-frame test.

Author: Gough, H. G., and Weiss, D. S.

Article: A nontransformational test of intellectual competence.

Journal: *Journal of Applied Psychology,* February 1981, *66*(1), 102–110.

Related Research: Gough, H. G., & McGurk, E. A. (1967). A group test of perceptual acuity. *Perceptual and Motor Skills, 24,* 1107–1115.

■ ■ ■

2686

Test Name: REAL ESTATE CAREER SCALE

Purpose: To measure, with biographical data, a person's probable success in the career of real estate agent.

Number of Items: 85

Format: Multiple-choice. Scoring done by the England "weighted application blank" (WAB) method.

Reliability: Test–retest (1 week) reliability was .84 ($n = 13$).

Validity: Using obtaining a real estate license as a criterion, 60 to 62 % of "failures" were eliminated and 69 to 80% of "successes" were retained.

Author: Mitchell, T. W., and Klimoski, R. J.

Article: Is it rational to be empirical? A test of methods for scoring biographical data.

Journal: *Journal of Applied Psychology*, August 1982, *67*(4), 411–418.

Related Research: England, G. W. (1971). *Development and use of weighted application blanks* (Rev. ed.) Minneapolis: University of Minnesota, Industrial Relations Center.

■ ■ ■

2687

Test Name: RIGHT HEMISPHERE ORIENTATION SCALE

Purpose: To measure hemispheric orientation.

Number of Items: 7

Format: Seven pairs of metaphoric characteristics said to typify hemispheric (left–right) orientation are presented to subjects at the ends of a 7-point scale. All items presented.

Reliability: Internal consistency was .82.

Author: Hirschman, E. C.

Article: Psychological sexual identity and hemispheric orientation.

Journal: *Journal of General Psychology*, April 1983, *108*(second half), 153–168.

Related Research: Springer, S. P., & Deutsch, G. (1981). *Left brain/right brain*. San Francisco: Freeman.

■ ■ ■

2688

Test Name: SIMON-DOLE LISTENING COMPREHENSION TEST

Purpose: To measure listening comprehension as a predictor of reading comprehension.

Number of Items: 38

Format: For each item, the child places an X on one of three pictures that best answers a question. Also included are 19 short passages.

Reliability: Kuder-Richardson formula 20 estimated reliability was .84.

Validity: Correlations with the Boehm Test of Basic Concepts were .42, .62. Correlation with the Comprehensive Test of Basic Skills was .34.

Author: Dole, J. A., et al.

Article: The development and validation of a listening comprehension test as a predictor of reading comprehension: Preliminary results.

Journal: *Educational Research Quarterly*, 1984–1985, *9*(4), 40–46.

■ ■ ■

2689

Test Name: THUMIN TEST OF MENTAL DEXTERITY

Purpose: To measure intelligence.

Number of Items: 100

Time Required: 60 minutes.

Format: Multiple-choice.

Validity: Product–moment correlation with WAIS full scale was .84.

Author: Thumin, F. J., et al.

Article: Relationship between the Thumin Test of Mental Dexterity and the WAIS.

Journal: *Perceptual and Motor Skills*, October 1983, *57*(2), 599–603.

Related Research: Thumin, F. J., & Stern, A. (1977). Two construct validity studies of the Thumin Test of Mental Dexterity. *Psychological Reports, 40*, 884–886.

■ ■ ■

2690

Test Name: YOUR STYLE OF LEARNING AND THINKING— FORM C-A

Purpose: To determine hemispheric preferences.

Number of Items: 36

Format: Respondents select one of three choices that represent left, right, or the integrative capacity of right and left hemispheres. Examples are presented.

Reliability: Reliability coefficients ranged from .58 to .97.

Author: Shannon, M., and Rice, D. R.

Article: A comparison of hemispheric preference between high ability and low ability elementary children.

Journal: *Educational Research Quarterly*, Fall 1983, *7*(3), 7–15.

Related Research: Kalsounis, B. (1979). Evidence for the validity of the scale. Your style of learning and thinking. *Perceptual and Motor Skills, 48*, 177–178.

CHAPTER 7
Attitude

2691

Test Name: ATTITUDES OF ELEMENTARY TEACHERS QUESTIONNAIRE

Purpose: To measure teachers' attitudes about students and teaching.

Number of Items: 30

Format: Items rated on a 5-point agreement–disagreement scale. Sample item is presented.

Reliability: Alphas ranged from .54 to .84 over subscales. Alpha for total scale was .694.

Author: Mitman, A. L.

Article: Teachers' differential behavior toward higher and lower achieving students and its relation to selected teacher characteristics.

Journal: *Journal of Educational Psychology*, April 1985, *77*(2), 149–161.

Related Research: Mitman, A. L. Effects of teachers' naturally occurring expectations and a feedback treatment on teachers and students. *Dissertation Abstracts International, 42,* 618-A. (University Microfilms No. 8115812)

■ ■ ■

2692

Test Name: ATTITUDE TOWARD COLLEGE INVENTORY

Purpose: To measure attitudes toward college.

Number of Items: 12

Format: Items rated on a 5-point Likert scale. Sample item is presented.

Reliability: Cronbach's alphas were .68 (pretest), .68 (posttest). Test–retest (10 day interval) reliability was .63.

Validity: Significant correlation (*p* < .01) with interest in college, perceived affordability, perceived difficulty, and perceived intelligence.

Author: Johanson, R. P., and Vopava, J. R.

Article: Attitude assessment and prediction of college attendance among economically disadvantaged students.

Journal: *Journal of College Student Personnel*, July 1985, *26*(4), 339–342.

■ ■ ■

2693

Test Name: ATTITUDES TOWARD DISABLED PERSONS SCALE

Purpose: To measure attitudes toward disabled persons.

Number of Items: 20

Format: Likert format. (6-point scale.)

Reliability: Median stability coefficient was .73. Split-half reliability was .75 to .85.

Author: Antonak, R. F.

Article: Prediction of attitudes toward disabled persons: A multivariate analysis.

Journal: *Journal of General Psychology,* January 1981, *104*(first half), 119–123.

Related Research: Yuker, H. E., et al. (1966). *A scale to measure attitudes toward disabled persons* (Human Resources Study No. 5). Albertson, NY: Human Resources Center.

■ ■ ■

2694

Test Name: ATTITUDES TOWARD MAINSTREAMING SCALE

Purpose: To measure teacher attitudes toward mainstreaming individuals with different handicaps.

Number of Items: 18

Format: Includes three dimensions: learning capabilities, general mainstreaming, and traditional limiting disabilities.

Reliability: Internal consistency reliabilities for the three subscales ranged from .78 to .88 and .91 for the total scale.

Author: Green, K., and Harvey, D.

Article: Cross-cultural validation of the attitudes toward mainstreaming scale.

Journal: *Educational and Psychological Measurement,* Winter 1983, *43*(4), 1255–1261.

Related Research: Berryman, J. D., & Neal, W. R. (1980). The cross validation of the Attitudes Toward Mainstreaming Scale (ATMS). *Educational and Psychological Measurement, 40,* 469–474.

2695

Test Name: ATTITUDES TOWARD NUCLEAR DISARMAMENT SCALE (AND)

Purpose: To measure attitudes toward nuclear disarmament.

Number of Items: 21

Format: Likert format.

Reliability: Split-half reliability was .84 ($p < .01$).

Validity: ROTC respondents differed significantly from nuclear freeze proponents ($t = 10.59$, $p < .001$) in predicted direction. Correlated .51 with negative Soviet Union attitudes ($p < .01$).

Author: Larsen, K. S.

Article: Attitudes toward nuclear disarmament and their correlates.

Journal: *Journal of Social Psychology,* February 1985, *125*(1), 17–21.

■ ■ ■

2696

Test Name: ATTITUDES TOWARD NURSES SCALE

Purpose: To measure attitudes toward nurses.

Number of Items: 20

Format: Items rated on 4-point Likert format. All items presented.

Reliability: Alpha ranged from .80 to .84.

Validity: Participants in a Summer program with nurses scored higher than nonparticipants and those who did not apply, $F(2, 64) = 3.73$, $p < .05$.

Author: Hojat, M., and Herman, M. W.

Article: Developing an instrument to measure attitudes toward nurses: Preliminary psychometric findings.

Journal: *Psychological Reports,* April 1985, *56*(2), 571–579.

2697

Test Name: ATTITUDES TOWARD OLD PEOPLE

Purpose: To measure attitudes toward older persons.

Number of Items: 137

Format: Includes 13 categories: conservatism, activities and interests, financial, physical, family, personality traits, attitude toward the future, best time of life, insecurity, mental deterioration, sex, interference, and cleanliness.

Reliability: Test–retest ranged from .36 to .62.

Author: Finnerty-Fried, P.

Article: Instruments for the assessment of attitudes toward older persons.

Journal: *Measurement and Evaluation in Guidance,* October 1982, *15*(3), 201–209.

Related Research: Tuckman, J., & Lorge, I. (1953). Attitudes toward old people. *Journal of Social Psychology, 37,* 249–260.

■ ■ ■

2698

Test Name: ATTITUDES TOWARD SEEKING PROFESSIONAL PSYCHOLOGICAL HELP SCALE

Purpose: To identify attitudes toward using professional counseling services.

Number of Items: 29

Format: Includes four subscales: stigma, need, openness, and confidence.

Reliability: Test–retest reliability was .83.

Author: Sanchez, A. R., and Atkinson, D. R.

Article: Mexican-American cultural commitment, preference for counselor ethnicity, and

willingness to use counseling.

Journal: *Journal of Counseling Psychology,* April 1983, *30*(2), 215–220.

Related Research: Fischer, E. H., & Turner, J. L. (1970). Orientations to seeking help: Development and research utility of an attitude scale. *Journal of Consulting and Clinical Psychology, 35,* 79–90.

■ ■ ■

2699

Test Name: ATTITUDES TOWARD SEX ROLES SCALE

Purpose: To measure perceptions of sex-appropriate attitudes and behaviors, with emphasis on those that may influence career development directly or indirectly.

Number of Items: 35

Format: Low scores indicate responses toward an androgynous end of a scale (no differentiation made between the sexes) as opposed to high scores that indicate responses toward a dichotomous end of the scale (roles divided into male and female categories).

Reliability: Alpha coefficients ranged from .80 to .92.

Validity: Correlations with other variables ranged from .18 to .36.

Author: Hawley, P., and Even, B.

Article: Work and sex-role attitudes in relation to education and other characteristics.

Journal: *Vocational Guidance Quarterly,* December 1982, *31*(2), 101–108.

Related Research: Goldman, R. D., et al. (1973). Sex differences in the relationship of attitudes toward technology to choice of field of study. *Journal of Counseling Psychology, 20,* 412–418.

2700

Test Name: ATTITUDES TOWARD OCCUPATIONS SCALE

Purpose: To measure attitudes about traditional and nontraditional occupations.

Number of Items: 16

Format: Semi-projective. Students must complete each of 16 sentences. Sample items presented.

Reliability: Interrater reliability was .95.

Author: Haring, M. J., and Beyard-Tyler, K. C.

Article: Career development: Counseling with women: The challenge of nontraditional careers.

Journal: *The School Counselor*, March 1984, *31*(4), 301–309.

Related Research: Getzels, J. W., & Walsh, J. J. (1958). The method of paired direct and projective questionnaires in the study of attitude structure and socialization. *Psychological Monographs, 72* (1, Whole No. 454).

■ ■ ■

2701

Test Name: ATTITUDES TOWARD STATISTICS

Purpose: To measure attitude change in introductory statistics students.

Number of Items: 29

Format: Includes two subscales: attitude toward field of statistics and attitude toward course. Employs a Likert format with a 5-point response scale from *strongly disagree* to *strongly agree*.

Reliability: Coefficient alphas were .92 (for field) and .90 (for course). Test–retest reliabilities (2 weeks) were .82 (field) and .91 (course).

Validity: Correlation of grade with course subscale was .27; with field subscale was –.04.

Author: Wise, S. L.

Article: The development and validation of a scale measuring attitudes toward statistics.

Journal: *Educational and Psychological Measurement,* Summer 1985, *45*(2), 401–405.

■ ■ ■

2702

Test Name: ATTITUDES TOWARD THE HANDICAPPED SCALE

Purpose: To measure attitudes of third graders toward the handicapped.

Number of Items: 12

Format: Employed a Likert scale ranging from *very happy* to *very unhappy*. An example is presented. Five items involved the handicapped, five did not.

Reliability: Coefficient alpha for the questions that involved the handicapped was .77. Coefficient alpha for the questions that did not involve the handicapped was .79.

Author: Beardsley, D. A.

Article: Using books to change attitudes toward the handicapped among third graders.

Journal: *Journal of Experimental Education,* Winter 1981/1982, *50*(2), 52–55.

Related Research: Yuker, H. E., et al. (1966). *The measurement of attitudes toward disabled persons* (Human Resources Study No. 7). Albertson, NY: Human Resources Center. (Reprinted 1970, Albertson, NY: Insurance Company of North America.)

2703

Test Name: ATTITUDES TOWARD WOMEN SCALE

Purpose: To measure attitudes toward women's roles.

Number of Items: 25

Format: The items depict various roles women may enact. The higher the score, the greater the pro-feminist attitude.

Reliability: Alpha was .90 (women) and .89 (men).

Author: Beutell, N. J., and Greenhaus, J. H.

Article: Integration of home and nonhome roles: Women's conflict and coping behavior.

Journal: *Journal of Applied Psychology,* February 1973, *68*(1), 43–48.

Related Research: Spence, J. T., et al. (1973). A short version of the Attitudes Toward Women Scale. *Bulletin of the Psychometric Society, 2,* 219–220.

■ ■ ■

2704

Test Name: ATTITUDES TOWARD WOMEN SCALE— ADAPTED

Purpose: To measure attitudes toward the appropriate roles of women in society.

Number of Items: 15

Format: Subjects respond to each item on a 4-point scale ranging from *agree strongly* to *disagree strongly*.

Reliability: Internal consistency coefficients were .89 and .86.

Validity: Correlations with other variables ranged from –.27 to .35.

Author: Stafford, I. P.

Article: Relation of attitudes toward women's roles and

occupational behavior to women's self-esteem.

Journal: *Journal of Counseling Psychology*, July 1984, *31*(3), 332–338.

Related Research: Spence, J. T., & Helmreich, R. L. (1978). *Masculinity and femininity: Their psychological dimensions, correlates, and antecedents.* Austin: University of Texas Press.

McHale, S. M., & Huston, T. L. (1984). Men and women as parents: Sex role orientations, employment, and parental roles with infants. *Child Development, 55*(4), 1349–1361.

■ ■ ■

2705

Test Name: ATTITUDES TOWARD WORKING MOTHERS SCALE

Purpose: To measure educators' attitudes toward working mothers.

Number of Items: 32

Format: 7-point Likert format (*strongly agree* to *strongly disagree*).

Reliability: Cronbach's alpha ranged from .94 to .95 for men and women.

Author: Tetenbaum, T. J., et al.

Article: Educators' attitudes toward working mothers.

Journal: *Journal of Educational Psychology*, June 1981, *73*(3), 369–375.

Related Research: Tetenbaum, T. J., et al. (1983). The construct validation of an attitudes toward working mothers scale. *Psychology of Women Quarterly, 8*(1), 69–78.

■ ■ ■

2706

Test Name: ATTITUDE TOWARD AGGRESSION SCALE

Purpose: To measure attitudes toward aggression.

Number of Items: 4

Format: 5-point response categories (*almost always true* to *never true*). All items presented.

Reliability: Alpha was .70.

Author: Liska, A. E., et al.

Article: Estimating attitude-behavior reciprocal effects within a theoretical specification.

Journal: *Social Psychology Quarterly*, March 1984, *47*(1), 15–23.

Related Research: Backman, J., et al. (1967). *Youth in transition* (Vol. 1). Ann Arbor, MI: Survey Research Center.

■ ■ ■

2707

Test Name: ATTITUDE TOWARD CONTROVERSY SCALE

Purpose: To measure attitudes toward controversy.

Number of Items: 5

Format: 5-point Likert format. All items presented.

Reliability: Alpha was .94.

Author: Smith, K. A., et al.

Article: Effects of controversy on learning in cooperative groups.

Journal: *Journal of Social Psychology*, April 1984, *122*(second half), 199–209.

Related Research: Johnson, D. W., et al. (1978). The effects of cooperative and individualized instruction on student attitudes and achievement. *Journal of Social Psychology, 104*, 207–216.

■ ■ ■

2708

Test Name: ATTITUDE TOWARD COUNSELING SCALE

Purpose: To measure attitudes toward counseling.

Number of Items: 32

Format: Items rated on 5-point Likert scales.

Reliability: Split-half reliability was .76.

Validity: Counselors (and counseling graduate students) differed significantly from a group of former clients who gave negative evaluations of services.

Author: Davidshafter, C. O., and Richardson, G. G.

Article: Effects of precounseling training.

Journal: *Journal of College Student Personnel*, November 1981, *22*(6), 522–527.

■ ■ ■

2709

Test Name: ATTITUDE TOWARD DREAMS SCALE

Purpose: To measure attitudes toward dreams.

Number of Items: 17

Format: The first item was not scored. Three subscales were formed by the remaining 16 items: person's own attitude toward dreams; person's perceptions of attitudes of significant others toward dreams; and the person's perception of attitudes of other people in general toward dreams or toward individuals who publicly discuss dreams. All items are presented.

Reliability: Cronbach's alpha coefficients of internal consistency ranged from .66 to .76 for the subscales and .69 for the 16 items scored.

Validity: Correlation of the 16 items with dream recall frequency was .31.

Author: Cernovsky, Z. Z.

Article: Dream recall and attitude toward dreams.

Journal: *Perceptual and Motor Skills,* June 1984, *58*(3), 911–914.

. . .

2710

Test Name: ATTITUDE TOWARD EDUCATIONAL INQUIRY

Purpose: To measure attitude toward educational research.

Number of Items: 38

Format: Subject responds to each item on a 5-point scale from *very unfavorable* (1) to *very favorable* (5).

Reliability: Gulliksen estimate of reliability was .79.

Validity: Correlations with perceived confidence in competencies was .14, with perceived importance of competencies was .48.

Author: Stauffer, A. J.

Article: The validity of selected measures to predict success on a non-traditional criterion development for an educational research program.

Journal: *Educational and Psychological Measurement,* Spring 1983, *43*(1), 237–241.

Related Research: Stauffer, A. J. (1974). An investigation of the procedures for developing and validating the classroom attitude toward educational inquiry. *Educational and Psychological Measurement, 34,* 893–898.

. . .

2711

Test Name: ATTITUDE TOWARD EVANGELISM SCALE

Purpose: To measure attitudes

toward evangelism.

Number of Items: 21

Format: 5-point Likert format. Sample items presented.

Reliability: Split-half reliability was .83.

Validity: Correlates .76 with fanaticism. Evangelism scores higher for Protestants than non-Protestants ($t = 3.00, p < .001$). No difference by age or sex.

Author: Seyfarth, L. H., et al.

Article: Attitude toward evangelism: Scale development and validity.

Journal: *Journal of Social Psychology,* June 1984, *123*(first half), 55–61.

. . .

2712

Test Name: ATTITUDE TOWARD INSTRUCTION SCALE

Purpose: To measure positive or negative affect toward experimental instructional treatments.

Number of Items: 10

Format: 7-point bipolar adjective scales. All scales presented.

Reliability: Spearman-Brown coefficient was .92.

Author: Alesandrini, K. L.

Article: Pictorial-verbal and analytic-holistic learning strategies in science learning.

Journal: *Journal of Educational Psychology,* June 1981, *73*(3), 358–368.

Related Research: Snow, R. E. (1974). Representative and quasi-representative designs for research on teaching. *Review of Educational Research, 44,* 265–291.

2713

Test Name: ATTITUDE TOWARD MALE HOMOSEXUALITY SCALE

Purpose: To measure homophobia.

Number of Items: 28

Format: Responses to each item are made on a 9-point scale ranging from *strongly disagree* to *strongly agree.* Scores ranged from 28 to 252.

Reliability: Internal consistency was .934.

Validity: Correlations with other variables ranged from –.26 to .24.

Author: Devlin, P. K., and Cowan, G. A.

Article: Homophobia, perceived fathering, and male intimate relationships.

Journal: *Journal of Personality Assessment,* October 1985, *49*(5), 467–473.

Related Research: MacDonald, A. P., Jr., & Games, R. G. (1974). Some characteristics of those who hold positive and negative attitudes toward homosexuals. *Journal of Homosexuality, 1,* 9–27.

. . .

2714

Test Name: ATTITUDE TOWARD SELF-CONTROL SCALE

Purpose: To measure attitude toward self-control.

Number of Items: 6

Format: There were 6 response categories (*very good* to *very bad*). All items are presented.

Reliability: Alpha ranged between .74 and .78.

Author: Liska, A. E., et al.

Article: Estimating attitude-behavior reciprocal effects within a theoretical specification.

Journal: *Social Psychology Quarterly,* March 1984, *47*(1), 15–23.

Related Research: Backman, J., et al. (1967). *Youth in transition* (Vol. 1). Ann Arbor, MI: Survey Research Center.

● ● ●

2715

Test Name: ATTITUDES TOWARD MATHEMATICS SCALE

Purpose: To measure attitudes toward mathematics and its teaching.

Number of Items: 11

Format: Each of 11 concepts is measured with 10, 7-point bipolar scales.

Reliability: Alphas were .94 (mathematics) and .88 (the teacher when teaching mathematics).

Author: Schofield, H. L.

Article: Teacher effects on cognitive and affective pupil outcomes in elementary school mathematics.

Journal: *Journal of Educational Psychology,* August 1981, *73*(4), 462–471.

Related Research: Schofield, H. L., & Start, K. B. (1978). Mathematics attitude and achievement among student teachers. *Australian Journal of Education, 22*(1), 72–82.

● ● ●

2716

Test Name: ATTITUDE TOWARD TEACHING SCALE

Purpose: To measure general attitude toward career.

Number of Items: 11

Format: Items are rated on a 6-response Likert scale.

Reliability: Split–half reliability was .71. Test–retest coefficient was .79.

Validity: Correlations with other variables ranged from –.24 to .69.

Author: Thomas, R. G., and Bruning, C. R.

Article: Validities and reliabilities of minor modifications of the Central Life Interests and Career Salience Questionnaire.

Journal: *Measurement and Evaluation in Guidance,* October 1981, *14*(3), 128–135.

Related Research: Merwin, J. C., & DiVesta, F. J. (1959). A study of need and theory and career choice. *Journal of Counseling Psychology, 6,* 302–308.

● ● ●

2717

Test Name: ATTITUDE TOWARD TREATMENT OF DISABLED STUDENTS SCALE

Purpose: To measure attitude toward disabled students.

Number of Items: 32

Format: Likert items.

Reliability: Cronbach's alpha was .88.

Validity: Correlations of .32 with Attitude Toward Disabled Persons Scale.

Author: Fonosch, G. G., and Schwab, L. O.

Article: Attitudes of selected university faculty members towards disabled students.

Journal: *Journal of College Student Personnel,* May 1981, *22*(3), 229–235.

● ● ●

2718

Test Name: ATTITUDINAL TEST

Purpose: To measure students' attitudes toward achievement tests.

Number of Items: 12

Format: Responses to each item are made on a scale from 0 (*strongly disagree*) to 7 (*strongly agree*). All items are presented.

Reliability: Test–retest reliability was .87 (*N* = 45).

Validity: Correlations with achievement scores ranged from –.18 to .45.

Author: Karmos, A. H., and Karmos, J. S.

Article: Attitudes toward standardized achievement tests and their relation to achievement test performance.

Journal: *Measurement and Evaluation in Counseling and Development,* July 1984, *17*(2), 56–66.

● ● ●

2719

Test Name: BARGAINING OF JOB-RELATED ISSUES SCALE

Purpose: To measure approval of union-management cooperation.

Number of Items: 14

Format: Items rated on a 3-point rating scale. Sample items are presented.

Reliability: Alpha ranged from .65 to .71 across subscales.

Author: Holley, W. H., et al.

Article: Negotiating quality of worklife, productivity and traditional issues: Union members preferred roles of their union.

Journal: *Personnel Psychology,* Summer 1981, *34*(2), 309–328.

Related Research: Dyer, L., et al. (1977). Union attitudes toward management cooperation. *Industrial Relations, 16,* 163–172.

2720

Test Name: BIAS IN ATTITUDE SURVEY SCALE

Purpose: To assess attitudes and beliefs about sex roles.

Number of Items: 35

Format: The items are declarative statements dealing with the facts and beliefs about men and women and their personalities. A 5-point Likert scale from *strongly agree* to *strongly disagree* is used.

Reliability: Coefficient alphas ranged from .85 to .94.

Author: Phifer, S. J., and Plake, B. S.

Article: The factorial validity of the Bias in Attitude Survey Scale.

Journal: *Educational and Psychological Measurement,* Autumn 1983, *43*(3), 887–891.

Related Research: Jean, P. J., & Reynolds, C. R. (1980). Development of the Bias in Attitude Survey: A sex-role questionnaire. *The Journal of Psychology, 104,* 269–277.

■■■

2721

Test Name: CALCULATOR ATTITUDE SCALE

Purpose: To measure attitudes about calculators.

Number of Items: 20

Format: Likert scale.

Reliability: Alpha of .82 (pretest) and alpha of .85 (posttest).

Validity: Correlations with Statistical Attitude Survey ranged from −.04 to .17.

Author: Roberts, D. M., and Saxe, J. E.

Article: Validity of a statistics attitude survey: A follow-up study.

Journal: *Educational and*

Psychological Measurement, Autumn 1982, *42*(3), 907–912.

Related Research: Geisinger, K. F., & Roberts, D. M. (1978). *Individual differences in calculator attitudes and performance in a statistics course.* Paper presented at American Educational Research Association, Toronto.

■■■

2722

Test Name: CHILDREN'S ATTITUDES TOWARD TELEVISION COMMERCIALS

Purpose: To measure children's attitudes toward TV commercials.

Number of Items: 7

Format: Items rated on a 4-point agreement scale. All items are presented.

Reliability: Alpha was .57. Test–retest reliability was .34 to .80.

Validity: Items do not always form one factor.

Author: Macklin, M. C.

Article: Psychometric investigation of Rossiter's short test measuring children's attitudes toward T.V. commercials.

Journal: *Psychological Reports,* April 1984, *54*(2), 623–627.

Related Research: Rossiter, J. R. (1977). Reliability of a short test measuring children's attitudes toward T.V. commercials. *Journal of Consumer Research, 3,* 179–184.

■■■

2723

Test Name: CHILDREN'S ATTITUDE TOWARD AUTHORITY SCALE

Purpose: To measure attitude toward authority among children in grades 7 to 11.

Number of Items: 28

Format: Likert format. All items presented.

Reliability: Alpha was .86.

Validity: Correlates .65 with authoritarian personality.

Author: Ray, J. J., and Jones, J. M.

Article: Attitude to authority and authoritarianism among schoolchildren.

Journal: *Journal of Social Psychology,* April 1983, *119* (second half), 199–203.

■■■

2724

Test Name: COGNITIVE AND AFFECTIVE COMPUTER ATTITUDE SCALES

Purpose: To measure computer attitudes.

Number of Items: 14

Format: Includes two subscales: cognitive and affective. Responses are made on a 5-point Likert scale ranging from *strongly agree* (0) to *strongly disagree* (4). All items are presented.

Reliability: Alpha coefficients were .929 for cognitive items and .896 for affective items.

Author: Bannon, S. H., et al.

Article: Cognitive and affective computer attitude scales: A validity study.

Journal: *Educational and Psychological Measurement,* Autumn 1985, *45*(3), 679–681.

Related Research: Ahl, D. (1976). Survey of public attitudes toward computers in society. In D. H. Ahl (Ed.), *The best of creative computering* (Vol. 1). Morristown, NJ: Creative Computing Press.

2725

Test Name: COMMUNITY DENTAL HEALTH IDEOLOGY SCALE

Purpose: To measure a student's attitude and attitude change with respect to community dental health care and private practice.

Number of Items: 23

Format: Students indicate level of agreement with each item from 1 (*low*) to 4 (*high*). Includes two factors. Most items are presented.

Reliability: Coefficient alpha for Factor 1 was .70 and for Factor 2 was .55.

Author: Stein, M. I., et al.

Article: Factor analytic study of the Kurtzman Community Dental Health Ideology Scale.

Journal: *Perceptual and Motor Skills,* February 1983, *56*(1), 79–82.

Related Research: Kurtzman, C. (1977). A scale of community dental health ideology: Establishing a valid means of measurement for evaluation. *Journal of Public Health Dentistry, 37,* 275–280.

■ ■ ■

2726

Test Name: COMPUTER ATTITUDE SCALE

Purpose: To measure attitudes about computers.

Number of Items: 20

Format: Items rated in 5-point Likert format. All items presented.

Reliability: Alpha ranged from .79 to .84.

Validity: Correlates negatively with computer aptitude (−.22, $p < .001$).

Author: Dambrot, F. H., et al.

Article: Correlates of sex

differences in attitudes toward and involvement with computers.

Journal: *Journal of Vocational Behavior,* August 1985, *27*(1), 71–86.

■ ■ ■

2727

Test Name: COMPUTER ATTITUDE SCALE

Purpose: To measure teachers' attitudes toward computers.

Number of Items: 40

Format: Includes four subscales: computer anxiety, computer confidence, computer liking, and computer usefulness. Examples are presented.

Reliability: Coefficient alphas for the four subscales ranged from .82 to .90. Coefficient alpha for the total score was .95.

Author: Loyd, B. H., and Loyd, D. E.

Article: The reliability and validity of an instrument for the assessment of computer attitudes.

Journal: *Educational and Psychological Measurement,* Winter 1985, *45*(4), 903–908.

Related Research: Loyd, B. H., & Gressard, C. (1984). Reliability and factorial validity of computer attitude scales. *Educational and Psychological Measurement, 44,* 501–505.

■ ■ ■

2728

Test Name: COMPUTER-RELATED ATTITUDES SCALE

Purpose: To assess computer-related attitudes.

Number of Items: 10

Format: Test uses a 7-point Likert response format.

Reliability: Alpha was .85.

Validity: Correlated .83 with computer beliefs.

Author: Stone, D. L., et al.

Article: Relationship between rigidity, self-esteem, and attitudes about computer-based information systems.

Journal: *Psychological Reports,* December 1984, *55*(3), 991–998.

■ ■ ■

2729

Test Name: COMPUTER-RELATED BELIEFS SCALE

Purpose: To assess computer-related beliefs on 4 dimensions.

Number of Items: 21

Format: Test uses a 7-point Likert response format.

Reliability: Alpha was .86.

Validity: Correlated −.63 with rigidity ($p < .01$) and .02 with self-esteem ($p < .05$).

Author: Stone, D. L., et al.

Article: Relationship between rigidity, self-esteem and attitudes about computer-based information systems.

Journal: *Psychological Reports,* December 1984, *55*(3), 991–998.

■ ■ ■

2730

Test Name: CONSEQUENCES OF WORKING AND NOT WORKING SCALE

Purpose: To measure attitudes toward consequence of working and not working.

Number of Items: 29

Format: Each item is responded to on three 5-point Likert scales: (a) Desirability in general, (b) desirability if working, and (c) desirability if not working. Difference between 2 and 3 yielded a single score. All items presented.

Reliability: Alpha was .88.

Author: Granrose, C. S.

Article: A Fishbein-Ajzen model of intention to work following childbirth.

Journal: *Journal of Vocational Behavior*, December 1984, *25*(3), 359–372.

Related Research: Fishbein, M., & Ajzen, I. (1975). *Belief, attitude, intention and behavior*. Reading, MA: Addison-Wesley.

■ ■ ■

2731

Test Name: CONSERVATISM SCALE

Purpose: To measure conservatism of American public opinion.

Number of Items: 22

Format: Likert format. All items presented.

Reliability: Alpha was .85. Correlation between positively and negatively scored halves was .45.

Author: Ray, J. J.

Article: A scale to measure conservatism of American public opinion.

Journal: *Journal of Social Psychology*, April 1983, *119*(second half), 293–294.

Related Research: Ray, J. J. (1982). Authoritarianism/ libertarianism as the second dimension of social attitudes. *Journal of Social Psychology, 117*, 33–34.

■ ■ ■

2732

Test Name: CONSERVATISM SCALE FOR URBAN AFRIKANERS

Purpose: To measure conservatism.

Number of Items: 14

Format: Likert format. (Subset of items from Ray Conservatism Scale used in California.)

Reliability: Alpha was .73.

Author: Ray, J. J., and Heavan, P. C. L.

Article: Conservatism and Authoritarianism among urban Afrikaners.

Journal: *Journal of Social Psychology*, April 1984, *122*(second half), 163–170.

Related Research: Ray, J. J. (1983). A scale to measure conservatism of American public opinion. *Journal of Social Psychology, 119*, 293–294.

■ ■ ■

2733

Test Name: CONTROVERSY ATTITUDE SCALE

Purpose: To measure attitudes toward controversy.

Number of Items: 5

Format: Likert format.

Reliability: Cronbach's alpha was .94.

Author: Lowry, N., and Johnson, D. W.

Article: Effects of controversy on epistemic curiosity, achievement and attitudes.

Journal: *Journal of Social Psychology*, October 1981, *115*(first half), 31–43.

Related Research: Johnson, D. W., et al. (1978). The effects of cooperative and individualized instruction on student attitudes and achievement. *Journal of Social Psychology, 104*, 207–216.

■ ■ ■

2734

Test Name: CONVENTIONALITY SCALE

Purpose: To measure conventional attitudes.

Number of Items: 7

Format: Guttman format. Includes 5 items from Nettler.

Reliability: Reproducibility was .87 for 74 undergraduates.

Author: Raden, D.

Article: Dogmatism and conventionality.

Journal: *Psychological Reports*, 1982, *50*(3), 1020–1022.

Related Research: Nettler, G. (1957). A measure of alienation. *American Sociological Review, 22*, 670–677.

■ ■ ■

2735

Test Name: COURSE STRUCTURE INVENTORY

Purpose: To identify student attitudes toward course structure.

Number of Items: 66

Format: Includes two subscales: attitude toward course structure and attitude toward course difficulty.

Reliability: Coefficient alpha reliabilities for the two subscales were .74 and .76.

Validity: Correlation of the subscales with three personality measures of arousal, dogmatism, and achievement motivation, and with grade point average ranged from −.37 to .26.

Author: Strom, B., et al.

Article: The course structure inventory: Discriminant and construct validity.

Journal: *Educational and Psychological Measurement*, Winter 1982, *42*(4), 1125–1133.

2736

Test Name: CREECH MENTAL ILLNESS QUESTIONNAIRE

Purpose: To measure opinions and attitudes about mental illness.

Number of Items: 64

Format: Items rated in 6-point Likert format.

Reliability: Pretest reliability was .81 (Hoyt).

Author: Napoletano, M. A.

Article: Correlates of changes in attitudes towards mental illness among vocational nursing students.

Journal: *Psychological Reports,* 1981, *49*(1), 147–150.

Related Research: Creech, S. (1977). Changes in attitudes about mental illness among nursing students following a psychiatric practicum. *Journal of Psychiatric Nursing and Mental Health Services, 15,* 9–14.

■ ■ ■

2737

Test Name: DREAM QUESTIONNAIRE

Purpose: To measure attitudes to and experience of dreaming.

Number of Items: 17

Format: Subjects respond to each item on a 4-point scale from *never* to *always*. All items are presented.

Validity: Correlation with the Harvard Group Scale of Hypnotic Susceptibility was .50.

Author: Gibson, H. B.

Article: Dreaming and hypnotic susceptibility: A pilot study.

Journal: *Perceptual and Motor Skills,* April 1985, *60*(2), 387–394.

Related Research: Arkin, A. M., et al. (Ed.). (1978). *The mind in sleep: Psychology and Psychophysiology.* Hillside, NJ: Erlbaum.

Cohen, D. B. (1979). *Sleep and dreaming: Origins, nature and functions.* Oxford: Pergamon.

Wolman, B. B. (Ed.). (1979). *Handbook on dreams.* New York: Van Nostrand.

■ ■ ■

2738

Test Name: EDUCATIONAL ATTITUDES INVENTORY

Purpose: To identify the general content of teacher attitudes relative to the educational process.

Number of Items: 34

Format: Responses from *agree* to *disagree* to each item were made on a 5-point scale. Includes four factors: affective, cognitive, directive, and interpretive.

Reliability: Split-half reliability coefficients ranged from .73 to .89.

Author: Bunting, C. E.

Article: Dimensionality of teacher education beliefs: An exploratory study.

Journal: *Journal of Experimental Education,* Summer 1984, *52*(4), 195–198.

Related Research: Bunting, C. E. (1981). The development and validation of the educational attitudes inventory. *Educational and Psychological Measurement, 41,* 559–565.

■ ■ ■

2739

Test Name: EDUCATION SCALE VII

Purpose: To measure traditional and progressive educational attitudes.

Number of Items: 30

Format: Items rated on a 7-point agreement scale.

Reliability: Alpha ranged from .65 to .87.

Author: Borko, H., and Cadwell, J.

Article: Individual differences in teachers' decision strategies: An investigation of classroom organization and management decisions.

Journal: *Journal of Educational Psychology,* August 1982, *74*(4), 598–610.

Related Research: Kerlinger, F. N., & Pedhazur, E. J. (1968). Educational attitudes and perceptions of desirable traits of teachers. *American Educational Research Journal, 5,* 543–559.

■ ■ ■

2740

Test Name: ENJOYMENT OF MATHEMATICS SCALE

Purpose: To measure attitude toward mathematics.

Number of Items: 11

Format: Employs a 5-point Likert format from 0 (*strongly disagree*) to 4 (*strongly agree*). All items are presented.

Reliability: Coefficient alpha was .88.

Validity: Correlations with other variables ranged from −.246 to .566.

Author: Watson, J. M.

Article: The Aiken attitude to mathematics scales: Psychometric data on reliability and discriminant validity.

Journal: *Educational and Psychological Measurement,* Winter 1983, *43*(4), 1247–1253.

Related Research: Aiken, L. R. (1974). Two scales of attitude toward mathematics. *Journal for Research in Mathematics Education, 5,* 67–71.

2741

Test Name: ESTES READING ATTITUDE SCALE

Purpose: To measure attitudes toward reading.

Number of Items: 20

Format: Likert items whereby students respond on a 5-point scale ranging from *strongly disagree* to *strongly agree*.

Reliability: Coefficient alpha reliability indices ranged from .78 to .93.

Author: Plake, B. S., et al.

Article: The relationship of ethnic group membership to the measurement and meaning of attitudes towards reading: Implications for validity of test score interpretations.

Journal: *Educational and Psychological Measurement,* Winter 1982, *42*(4), 1259–1267.

Related Research: Estes, T. H. (1971). A scale to measure attitudes towards reading. *Journal of Reading, 15,* 135–138.

■ ■ ■

2742

Test Name: FEMALE ROLES QUESTIONNAIRE

Purpose: To measure attitudes toward female roles.

Number of Items: 25

Format: Items rated on 4-point Likert response categories. All items presented.

Reliability: For Great Britain version, split-half reliability was .92; test–retest reliability was .94. For the 20-item Dutch version: Test–retest reliability was .92 (10 days).

Validity: Women in traditional occupations score lower than women in nontraditional

occupations ($p < .04$). Discriminates between men and women with high school and elementary school educations (p ranged from .03 to .04).

Author: Hubbard, F. O. A., et al.

Article: Validation of a questionnaire measuring attitudes toward females' social roles for a Dutch population.

Journal: *Psychological Reports,* 1982, *51*(2), 491–498.

Related Research: Slade, P., & Jenner, F. A. (1978). Questionnaire measuring attitudes to female social roles. *Psychological Reports, 43,* 351–354.

■ ■ ■

2743

Test Name: FISCHER PRO–CON ATTITUDE SCALE

Purpose: To assess attitudes about seeking psychological help.

Format: Items rated in 5-point Likert format.

Reliability: Test–retest reliability ranged from .73 to .89 over 2-week to 2-month interval. Internal consistency was .86.

Validity: Seekers of help and nonseekers of help differed significantly ($p < .001$).

Author: Hall, L. E., and Tucker, C. M.

Article: Relationships between ethnicity, conceptions of mental illness, and attitudes associated with seeking psychological help.

Journal: *Psychological Reports,* December 1985, *57*(3, I), 907–916.

Related Research: Fischer, E. H., and Turner, J. L. (1972). Orientations to seeking professional psychological help. *Journal of Consulting and Clinical Psychology, 30,* 70–74.

2744

Test Name: FOREIGN LANGUAGE ATTITUDE SCALE

Purpose: To measure attitude toward foreign language.

Number of Items: 22

Format: Subjects respond to items on a 5-point Likert scale. Examples are provided.

Reliability: Internal consistency reliability was approximately .90.

Validity: Correlations with other variables ranged from –.07 to .47.

Author: Raymond, M. R., and Roberts, D. M.

Article: Development and validation of a foreign language attitude scale.

Journal: *Educational and Psychological Measurement,* Winter 1983, *43*(4), 1239–1246.

■ ■ ■

2745

Test Name: GABLE-ROBERTS ATTITUDES TOWARD SCHOOL SUBJECTS

Purpose: To measure attitudes toward specified school subjects.

Number of Items: 23

Format: Likert items responded to on a 5-point scale from *strongly agree* to *strongly disagree*. Eleven items were written in a negative direction. All items are presented.

Reliability: Alpha reliabilities ranged from .59 to .94.

Author: Gable, R. K., and Roberts, A. D.

Article: An instrument to measure attitude toward school subjects.

Journal: *Educational and Psychological Measurement,* Spring 1983, *43*(1), 289–293.

Related Research: Remmers, H. H.

(Ed.). (1960). *A scale to measure attitude toward any school subject.* Lafayette: Purdue Research Foundation.

■ ■ ■

2746

Test Name: GENDER ROLE ORIENTATION

Purpose: To measure traditional and nontraditional gender role attitudes.

Number of Items: 10

Format: 7-point Likert format. Sample items presented.

Reliability: Alpha was .89.

Author: Hansen, G.

Article: Perceived threats and marital jealousy.

Journal: *Social Psychology Quarterly,* September 1985, *48*(3), 262–268.

Related Research: Brogan, D., & Kutner, N. G. (1976). Measuring sex-role orientation. *Journal of Marriage and the Family, 38,* 31–40.

■ ■ ■

2747

Test Name: GENERAL ATTITUDE TO INSTITUTIONAL AUTHORITY SCALE (GAIAS)

Purpose: To measure attitude toward institutional authority.

Number of Items: 16 (short form).

Format: Same format as 32-item full scale.

Reliability: Alpha was .89. Subscale alphas ranged from .62 to .82.

Validity: Correlates negatively with age (−.54) and positively with The Authority Behavior Inventory (.76). Not correlated with Ray's Directiveness Scale (.03).

Author: Rigby, K.

Article: Acceptance of authority and directiveness as indicators of authoritarianism: A new framework.

Journal: *Journal of Social Psychology,* April 1984, *122*(second half), 171–180.

■ ■ ■

2748

Test Name: HETEROSEXUAL ATTITUDES TOWARD HOMOSEXUALITY SCALE

Purpose: To measure attitudes toward homosexuality.

Number of Items: 20

Format: Likert format. Sample items presented.

Reliability: Item-total correlations ranged between .57 and .74. Split-half reliability was .92.

Author: Nevid, J. S.

Article: Exposure to homoerotic stimuli: Effects on attitudes and affects of heterosexual viewers.

Journal: *Journal of Social Psychology,* April 1983, *119*(second half), 249–255.

Related Research: Larsen, K. S., et al. (1980). Attitudes of heterosexuals toward homosexuality: A Likert scale and construct validity. *Journal of Sex Research, 16,* 245–257.

■ ■ ■

2749

Test Name: HOMOSEXISM SCALE

Purpose: To measure prejudicial attitudes toward homosexuals.

Number of Items: 53 (long form); 15 (short form).

Format: Items rated in 5-point Likert format. Sample items are presented.

Reliability: Alphas were .98 (long) and .96 (short).

Validity: Males score higher than females (*t* = 1.85, *p* < .05). Subjects who knew homosexuals scored lower than those who did not (*t* = 5.44, *p* < .001).

Author: Hansen, G. L.

Article: Measuring prejudice against homosexuality (homosexism) among college students: A new scale.

Journal: *Journal of Social Psychology,* August 1982, *117*(second half), 233–236.

■ ■ ■

2750

Test Name: HOMOSEXISM SCALE—SHORT FORM

Purpose: To measure prejudicial attitudes towards homosexuals.

Number of Items: 15

Format: Subjects respond on a 5-point scale from *strongly agree* to *strongly disagree*.

Reliability: Alpha reliability coefficient was .96.

Author: Hansen, G. L.

Article: Measuring prejudice against homosexuality (homosexism) among college students: A new scale.

Journal: *Journal of Social Psychology,* August 1982, *117*(second half), 233–236.

Related Research: Lumby, M. E. (1976). Homophobia: The quest for a valid scale. *Journal of Homosexuality, 2,* 39–47.

■ ■ ■

2751

Test Name: INFORMATION-PRIVACY VALUES, BELIEFS, AND ATTITUDES INTERVIEW SCHEDULE

Purpose: To obtain data concerning information-privacy values, information-privacy beliefs, information-privacy attitudes, information experiences, future intentions concerning information control activities, and demographic characteristics.

Number of Items: 69 plus several demographic items.

Format: Generally responses were made on either a 7-point scale from 1 = *strongly disagree* to 7 = *strongly agree*, or on a *yes–no* basis. Sample items are presented.

Reliability: Coefficient alphas ranged from .68 to .93.

Author: Stone, E. F., et al.

Article: A field experiment comparing information-privacy values, beliefs, and attitudes across several types of organizations.

Journal: *Journal of Applied Psychology,* August 1983, *68*(3), 459–468.

Related Research: Stone, E. F., et al. (1980). *Development of a measure to assess individuals' values, beliefs, and attitudes concerning control over personal information.* Unpublished manuscript, Purdue University.

■ ■ ■

2752

Test Name: INVASION OF PRIVACY SCALE

Purpose: To measure attitudes toward invasion of privacy in employment situations.

Number of Items: 5

Format: Items rated in 5-point Likert format (*strongly agree* to *strongly disagree*).

Reliability: Alpha was .87.

Author: Tolchinsky, P. D., et al.

Article: Employee perceptions of invasion of privacy: A field simulation experiment.

Journal: *Journal of Applied*

Psychology, June 1981, *66*(3), 308–313.

Related Research: Ganster, D. C., et al. (1979). *Information privacy in organizations: An examination of employee perceptions and attitudes.* Proceedings of the 39th Annual Conference of the National Academy of Management, 262–266.

■ ■ ■

2753

Test Name: INVENTORY OF CAREER ATTITUDES

Purpose: To measure perceived realism of career-planning beliefs.

Number of Items: 28

Format: Items rated on a 5-point agreement scale.

Reliability: Alpha was .76.

Author: Pinkney, J. W., and Ramirez, M.

Article: Career-planning myths of Chicano students.

Journal: *Journal of College Student Personnel,* July 1985, *26*(4), 300–305.

Related Research: Woodrick, C. P. (1979). *The development and standardization of an attitude scale designed to measure myths held by college students.* Unpublished doctoral dissertation, Texas A&M University, Galveston.

■ ■ ■

2754

Test Name: JOB ATTITUDE SURVEY

Purpose: To measure attitude towards supervisor, general management, work group, working conditions, pay, and locus of control.

Number of Items: 47

Format: Likert format.

Reliability: Alpha was .84 (split-half).

Author: Kasperson, C. J.

Article: Locus of control and job satisfaction.

Journal: *Psychological Reports,* 1982, *50*(3, Part 1), 823–826.

Related Research: Smith, P., et al. (1969). *The measurement of satisfaction in work and retirement.* Chicago: Rand-McNally.

■ ■ ■

2755

Test Name: KOGAN'S ATTITUDES TOWARD OLD PEOPLE SCALE

Purpose: To identify sentiments toward older persons.

Number of Items: 17

Format: Items are matched positive–negative pairs of statements. Items include: residence, homogeneity, intergenerational relations, dependence, cognitive style, personal appearance, and power.

Reliability: Odd–even reliability coefficients ranged from .66 to .85.

Author: Finnerty-Fried, P.

Article: Instruments for the assessment of attitudes toward older persons.

Journal: *Measurement and Evaluation in Guidance,* October 1982, *15*(3), 201–209.

Related Research: Kogan, N. A. (1961). Attitudes toward old people: The development of a scale and an examination of correlates. *Journal of Abnormal and Social Psychology, 62,* 44–54.

■ ■ ■

2756

Test Name: LANGUAGE ATTITUDE SCALE

Purpose: To measure teachers' attitudes toward Black English.

Number of Items: 25

Format: Items rated in 5-point Likert format.

Reliability: Alpha was .95. Item-total correlations ranged from .42 to .82.

Author: Taylor, J. B.

Article: Influence of speech variety on teachers' evaluation of reading comprehension.

Journal: *Journal of Educational Psychology*, October 1983, *75*(5), 662–667.

Related Research: Taylor, O. (1962). Teachers' attitudes toward Black and nonstandard English as measured by the Language Attitude Scale. In R. Shuy & R. Fasold (Eds.), *Language attitudes: Current trends and prospects*. Washington, DC: Georgetown University Press.

■ ■ ■

2757

Test Name: LEARNING ORIENTATION / GRADE ORIENTATION SCALE

Purpose: To measure learning and grade orientation in college students.

Number of Items: 20

Format: Forced choice.

Reliability: Test–retest reliability was .71 ($p < .001$).

Author: Meredith, G. M.

Article: Course- and instructor-related correlates of student's orientation toward grades and learning.

Journal: *Psychological Reports*, 1981, *49*(3), 794.

Related Research: Eison, J. A. (1981). A new instrument for assessing student's orientations towards grades and learning.

Psychological Reports, 48, 919–924.

■ ■ ■

2758

Test Name: LIBRARY ATTITUDE SCALE

Purpose: To indicate student attitudes toward the school library/librarian.

Number of Items: 16

Format: Responses are made anonymously on a 3-option scale (*Yes, ?, No*).

Reliability: Hoyt reliability index was .92.

Author: Schon, I., et al.

Article: A special motivational intervention program and junior high school students' library use and attitudes.

Journal: *Journal of Experimental Education*, Winter 1984–1985, *53*(2), 97–101.

Related Research: Schon, I., et al. (1984). The effects of a special school library program on elementary students' library use and attitudes. *School Library Media Quarterly, 12*(3), 227–231.

Davies, R. A. (1979). *The school library media center: Instructional force for excellence* (3rd ed.). New York: R. R. Bowker.

■ ■ ■

2759

Test Name: MACHO SCALE

Purpose: To measure masculine attitudes.

Number of Items: 18

Format: Items rated in 5-point Likert format.

Reliability: Alpha was .89.

Author: Brinkerhoff, M. B., and Mackle, M.

Article: Religion and gender: A

comparison of Canadian and American student attitudes.

Journal: *Journal of Marriage and the Family*, May 1985, *47*(2), 415–429.

Related Research: Villemez, W. J., & Touhey, J. C. (1977). A measure of individual differences in sex stereotyping and sex discrimination: The "macho" scale. *Psychological Reports, 41*, 411–415.

■ ■ ■

2760

Test Name: MALE SEX-ROLE ATTITUDE SURVEY

Purpose: To assess male sex-role attitudes.

Number of Items: 29

Format: Includes two scales: one focuses on traditional attitudes, the other emphasizes liberated attitudes. Responses are made on a 7-point scale from very *strongly agree* to very *strongly disagree*.

Reliability: Test–retest (3 weeks) correlations were .85 and .92.

Author: Fiebert, M. S., and Vera, W.

Article: Test–retest reliability of a male sex-role attitude survey: The traditional liberated content scale.

Journal: *Perceptual and Motor Skills*, February 1985, *60*(1), 66.

Related Research: Biggs, P., & Fiebert, M. S. (1984). A factor analytic examination of American male attitudes. *Journal of Psychology, 116*, 113–116.

■ ■ ■

2761

Test Name: MATHEMATICS ATTITUDE SCALE

Purpose: To measure student attitudes toward mathematics.

Number of Items: 24

Reliability: Alpha ranged between .50 and .91 across subscales.

Validity: Correlates significantly with arts and sciences grades and education grades, but not business and technology grades ($p < .05$). Significant rs ranged between .28 and .49.

Author: Gadzella, B. M., et al.

Article: Mathematics course grades and attitudes in mathematics for students enrolled in three university colleges.

Journal: *Psychological Reports,* December 1985, *57*(3,I), 767–772.

Related Research: Aiken, L. R. Attitudes toward mathematics and science in Iranian middle schools. *School Science and Mathematics, 79,* 229–234.

■ ■ ■

2762

Test Name: MATHEMATICS ATTITUDE SCALE

Purpose: To measure student self-concept as a mathematician and opinion of mathematics.

Number of Items: 14

Format: Likert items. Sample items presented.

Reliability: Alpha was .25.

Validity: Significantly associated with achievement as determined by F test ($p < .05$).

Author: Tsai, S.-L., and Walberg, H. J.

Article: Mathematics achievement and attitude productivity in junior high students.

Journal: *Journal of Educational Research,* May/June 1983, *76*(5), 267–272.

■ ■ ■

2763

Test Name: MIKULECKY BEHAVIORAL READING ATTITUDE MEASURE

Purpose: To measure secondary and postsecondary respondents' attitudes toward reading.

Number of Items: 20

Format: Response to each item is made on a scale of 1 (*very unlike me*) to 5 (*very like me*).

Reliability: Coefficient alpha for the total instrument was .89 ($N=$ 411).

Author: Hawk, J. W., et al.

Article: The factor structure of the Mikulecky Behavioral Reading Attitude Measure.

Journal: *Educational and Psychological Measurement,* Winter 1984, *44*(4), 1059–1065.

Related Research: Mikulecky, L. J. (1976). *The developing, field testing, and initial norming of a secondary/adult level reading attitude measure that is behaviorally oriented and based on Krathwohl's taxonomy of the affective domain.* Unpublished doctoral dissertation, University of Wisconsin—Madison.

■ ■ ■

2764

Test Name: MONEY ATTITUDE SCALE

Purpose: To measure money attitudes.

Number of Items: 29

Format: Includes five factors: power-prestige, retention-time, distrust, quality, and anxiety. Subjects respond to each item on a 7-point Likert scale. All items are presented.

Reliability: Coefficient alphas for total score and factors ranged from .69 to .80. Test–retest reliability coefficients ranged from .87 to .95 (5 weeks).

Validity: Correlations with related measures ranged from −.33 to .48.

Author: Yamauchi, K. T., and Templer, D. I.

Article: The development of a money attitude scale.

Journal: *Journal of Personality Assessment,* October 1982, *46*(5), 522–528.

■ ■ ■

2765

Test Name: MOVIE ATTITUDE SCALE

Purpose: To measure attitudes about motion pictures.

Number of Items: 40

Format: Items rated on 5-point response categories. Sample items presented.

Validity: Factor analysis revealed several dimensions, not one overall favorable/unfavorable dimension.

Author: Austin, B. A.

Article: A factor analytic study of attitudes toward motion pictures.

Journal: *Journal of Social Psychology,* August 1982, *117*(second half), 211–217.

Related Research: Bannerman, J., & Lewis, J. M. (1977). College students' attitudes toward movies. *Journal of Popular Film, 6,* 126–139.

■ ■ ■

2766

Test Name: MULTIRACIAL ATTITUDE QUESTIONNAIRE (MAQ)

Purpose: To measure multiracial attitudes of teachers in five dimensions.

Format: Likert items.

Reliability: Alpha reliability ranged from .39 to .92 across dimensions.

Validity: Intercorrelation among the five dimensions ranged from .05 to .76. Correlations presented with several other instruments suggest considerable construct validity.

Author: Giles, M. B., and Sherman, T. M.

Article: Measurement of multiracial attitudes of teacher trainees.

Journal: *Journal of Educational Research*, March/April 1982, *75*(4), 204–209.

■ ■ ■

2767

Test Name: NURSES ATTITUDES TOWARDS ARTHRITIS SCALE

Purpose: To measure nurses' attitudes toward arthritis.

Number of Items: 25

Format: Items rated in 5-point Likert format.

Reliability: Alpha was .74.

Validity: Nurses who completed a clinical rotation in rheumatology scored more favorably than nurses who did not complete the rotation, $F(1,103) = 6.17$, $p < .02$.

Author: Nambayan, A., et al.

Article: Scale for assessing nurses attitudes towards arthritis.

Journal: *Psychological Reports*, August 1985, *57*(1), 57.

■ ■ ■

2768

Test Name: PERCEPTIONS OF MEXICAN-AMERICANS SCALE

Purpose: To measure sixth-graders' attitudes toward and perceptions of Mexican-Americans.

Number of Items: 24

Format: Responses were made on a 3-point scale of *yes*, *?*, and *no*. Some examples are presented.

Reliability: Hoyt reliability

estimates ranged from .86 to .92.

Validity: Correlation with teachers' ratings was .1.

Author: Schon, I., et al.

Article: The effects of special curricular study of Mexican culture on Anglo- and Mexican-American students' perceptions of Mexican-Americans.

Journal: *Journal of Experimental Education*, Summer 1982, *50*(4), 215–218.

■ ■ ■

2769

Test Name: PROCRASTINATION INVENTORY

Purpose: To assess subjects' attitudes about their procrastination.

Number of Items: 36

Format: Includes two subscales: controllability and expectation to change. Subjects rated all items on a 7-point scale ranging from *true* to *false*. Examples are presented.

Reliability: Cronbach's alphas were .76 and .89.

Author: Lopez, F. G., and Wambach, C. A.

Article: Effects of paradoxical and self-control directives in counseling.

Journal: *Journal of Counseling Psychology*, March 1982, *29*(2), 115–124.

Related Research: Strong, S., et al. (1979). Motivational and equipping functions of interpretation in counseling. *Journal of Counseling Psychology*, *26*, 98–107.

■ ■ ■

2770

Test Name: PUNITIVENESS SCALE

Purpose: To measure punitiveness towards criminals.

Number of Items: 12

Format: Likert-format. Sample items presented.

Reliability: Alpha ranged from .78 to .82.

Author: Ray, J. J.

Article: The punitive personality.

Journal: *Journal of Social Psychology*, June 1985, *125*(3), 329–333.

Related Research: Ray, J. J. (1982). Prison sentence and public opinion. *Australian Quarterly*, *54*, 435–443.

■ ■ ■

2771

Test Name: PUPIL CONTROL IDEOLOGY SCALE

Purpose: To measure beliefs and attitudes teachers have about pupil control.

Number of Items: 20

Format: Items rated on 5-point Likert scales.

Reliability: Alpha was .89.

Author: Harris, K. R., et al.

Article: Teacher characteristics and stress.

Journal: *Journal of Educational Research*, July/August 1985, *78*(6), 346–350.

Related Research: Willower, D. J. (1975). Some comments on inquiries on schools and student control. *Teachers' College Record*, *77*, 32–59.

■ ■ ■

2772

Test Name: RACIAL IDENTITY ATTITUDE SCALE

Purpose: To measure racial identity attitudes.

Number of Items: 24

Format: Includes 4 subscales: pre-encounter, encounter, immersion–emersion, and internalization.

Reliability: Coefficient alphas ranged from .66 to .72.

Author: Parham, T. A., and Helms, J. E.

Article: The influence of Black students' racial identity attitudes on preferences for counselor's race.

Journal: *Journal of Consulting Psychology*, May 1981, *28*(3), 250–257.

Related Research: Hall, W. S., et al. (1972). Stages in the development of Black awareness: An exploratory investigation. In R. L. Jones (Ed.), *Black psychology*. New York: Harper & Row.

■ ■ ■

2773

Test Name: RACIAL IDENTITY ATTITUDE SCALE

Purpose: To measure attitudes associated with various stages of Black identity development.

Number of Items: 30

Format: Includes four subscales: pre-encounter, encounter, immersion–emersion, and internalization.

Reliability: Internal consistency reliability coefficients ranged from .66 to .72.

Author: Parham, T. A., and Helms, J. E.

Article: Relation of racial identity attitudes to self-actualization and affective states of Black students.

Journal: *Journal of Counseling Psychology*, July 1985, *32*(3), 431–440.

Related Research: Parham, T. A., & Helms, J. E. (1981). The

influence of Black students' racial identity attitudes on preference for counselor's race. *Journal of Counseling Psychology, 28,* 250–256.

■ ■ ■

2774

Test Name: RATIONAL BEHAVIOR INVENTORY—LOW READING LEVEL

Purpose: To measure the average degree and nature of rational beliefs.

Number of Items: 37

Format: Designed for assessment of adolescents with mild to moderate reading difficulties who may require special education or counseling services.

Reliability: Cronbach's alpha was .82.

Validity: Correlation with Rosenberg Self-Esteem Scale was .30; with Buss-Durkee Hostility Inventory—Negativism Scale was –.24.

Author: Shorkey, C. T., and Saski, J.

Article: A low reading-level version of the Rational Behavior Inventory.

Journal: *Measurement and Evaluation in Guidance*, July 1983, *16*(2), 95–99.

■ ■ ■

2775

Test Name: READING ATTITUDE SCALE

Purpose: To indicate student attitude toward reading.

Number of Items: 17

Format: Responses are made anonymously on a 3-option scale (*Yes, ?, No*).

Reliability: Hoyt reliability was .91.

Author: Schon, I., et al.

Article: A special motivational intervention program and junior high school students' library use and attitudes.

Journal: *Journal of Experimental Education,* Winter 1984–1985, *53*(2), 97–101.

Related Research: Schon, I., et al. (1984). The effects of a special school library program on elementary students' library use and attitudes. *School Library Media Quarterly, 12*(3), 227–231.

■ ■ ■

2776

Test Name: RISK-TAKING INVENTORY

Purpose: To measure attitudes toward situations that involve tension, risk, and adventure.

Number of Items: 38

Format: *Yes, doubtful, no* response categories. Sample items presented.

Reliability: Alpha was .89. Split-half reliability was .87. Test–retest reliability was .90.

Validity: People with risky jobs scored higher than people with no-risk jobs ($p < .05$).

Author: Keinan, G., et al.

Article: Measurement of risk takers' personality.

Journal: *Psychological Reports,* August 1984, *55*(1), 163–167.

■ ■ ■

2777

Test Name: ROMANTIC ATTITUDES SCALES

Purpose: To measure romantic attitudes of university students.

Number of Items: 84

Format: Items rated on 5-point Likert response categories (*very*

romantic to *very unromantic*). Sample items presented.

Reliability: Exceeded .90 on each of three subscales identified by a factor analysis.

Validity: Three factors extracted: traditional romance, sexual behavior, and routine activities.

Author: Prentice, D. S., et al.

Article: Romantic attitudes of American university students.

Journal: *Psychological Reports,* December 1983, *53*(3, Part 1), 815–822.

■ ■ ■

2778

Test Name: SCHOOL ATTITUDE SCALE

Purpose: To measure attitudes towards school.

Number of Items: 8

Format: Agree–disagree format. Sample item presented.

Reliability: Cronbach's alpha was .74.

Author: Brader, P. K., et al.

Article: Further observations on the link between learning disabilities and juvenile delinquency.

Journal: *Journal of Educational Psychology,* December 1981, *73*(6), 838–850.

Related Research: Educational Testing Service (1971). *Michigan Assessment of Basic Skills, Form UMT, Book 2.* Unpublished manuscript. Princeton, NJ: Educational Testing Service.

■ ■ ■

2779

Test Name: SCHOOL SENTIMENT INVENTORY

Purpose: To measure school attitudes.

Number of Items: 37

Format: Includes five subscales: attitudes toward teachers, school subjects, school structure and climate, peers, and a general estimate of school attitudes. Responses are either *yes* or *no.*

Reliability: Test–retest reliability was .87.

Author: Sloan, V. J., et al.

Article: A comparison of orientation methods for elementary school transfer students.

Journal: *Child Study Journal,* 1984, *14*(1), 47–60.

Related Research: Frith, S., & Narikawa, D. (1972). *Measures of self-concept, grades K-12.* Los Angeles: Instructional Objectives Exchange.

■ ■ ■

2780

Test Name: SEAT BELT SCALES

Purpose: To measure reported use and beliefs about seat belt use.

Number of Items: 4 (reported use) and 14 (beliefs).

Format: Use items rated on a 7-point use scale (*not at all likely to use* to *very likely*). Belief items rated on a 7-point scale. Sample items presented.

Reliability: Alphas were .93 (use) and .80 (belief).

Validity: Use scale items all load on one factor. Belief items factor into three subscales (convenience, effectiveness, comfort).

Author: Jonah, B. A.

Article: Legislation and the prediction of reported seat belt use.

Journal: *Journal of Applied Psychology,* August 1984, *69*(3), 401–407.

2781

Test Name: SEX KNOWLEDGE AND ATTITUDE TEST

Purpose: To collect information about sexual attitudes, knowledge, degree of experience in a variety of sexual behaviors.

Number of Items: 106

Format: Knowledge portion contains 71 true–false items, the attitude portion has 35 five-alternative Likert items.

Reliability: Internal consistency reliability (coefficient alpha) estimates for attitude scales from .68 to .86 and .87 for the knowledge scale.

Author: Smith, P., et al.

Article: Training teachers in human sexuality: Effect on attitude and knowledge.

Journal: *Psychological Reports,* April 1981, *48*(2), 527–530.

Related Research: Lief, H. I., & Reed, D. M. (1970). *Sex knowledge and attitude test.* Philadelphia: Center for the Study of Sex Education in Medicine, Department of Psychiatry, University of Pennsylvania School of Medicine.

Miller, W. R., & Lief, H. I. (1979). The sex knowledge and attitude test. *Journal of Sex and Marital Counseling, 5,* 282–287.

■ ■ ■

2782

Test Name: SEX-ROLE EGALITARIANISM SCALE

Purpose: To measure attitudes toward the equality of males and females.

Number of Items: 95

Format: Includes five domains of adult living: marital roles, parental roles, employment roles, social-interpersonal-heterosexual roles, and educational roles. Responses are made on a 5-point Likert rating scale ranging from *strongly agree* to *strongly disagree*. There are two forms. Examples are presented.

Reliability: Internal consistency estimates were .97 for both forms and ranged from .84 to .89 for the domains. Equivalence coefficient for the total score was .93 and ranged from .84 to .88 for the domains. Stability coefficients ranged from .81 to .91.

Author: King, D. W., and King, L. A.

Article: Measurement precision of the Sex-Role Egalitarianism Scale: A generalizability analysis.

Journal: *Educational and Psychological Measurement,* Summer 1983, *43*(2) 435–447.

Related Research: King, L. A., et al. (1981). *A new measure of sex-role attitudes.* Paper presented at the meeting of the Midwestern Psychological Association.

■ ■ ■

2783

Test Name: SEX-ROLE ORIENTATION SCALE

Purpose: To identify sex-role orientation.

Number of Items: 36

Format: Responses were made on a 5-point scale from *strongly agree* (1) to *strongly disagree* (5). High scores indicate more nontraditional attitudes toward sex roles. An example is presented.

Reliability: Alpha reliability was .95.

Author: Keith, P. M.

Article: Sex-role attitudes, family plans, and career orientations: Implications for counseling.

Journal: *Vocational Guidance*

Quarterly, March 1981, *29*(3), 244–252.

Related Research: Brogan, D., & Kutner, N. (1976). Measuring sex-role orientation: A normative approach. *Journal of Marriage and the Family, 38,* 31–40.

■ ■ ■

2784

Test Name: SITUATIONAL ATTITUDE SCALE— HANDICAPPED

Purpose: To measure attitudes toward handicapped.

Number of Items: 100 (10 situations with 10 bipolar semantic differential scales).

Format: A 5-point semantic differential (situations presented).

Reliability: Split-half reliability ranged between .67 and .90 across situations.

Author: Stovall, C., and Sedlacek, W. E.

Article: Attitudes of male and female university students toward students with different physical disabilities.

Journal: *Journal of College Student Personnel,* July 1983, *24*(4), 325–330.

Related Research: Sedlacek, W. E., & Brooks, G. C. (1972). *Situational attitude scale (SAS Manual).* Chicago: Natresources.

■ ■ ■

2785

Test Name: SOCIAL INTERDEPENDENCE SCALE

Purpose: To measure teenagers' attitudes toward cooperative, competitive, and individualistic learning situations.

Number of Items: 22

Format: Items rated on 7-point response categories.

Reliability: Alphas ranged from .84 to .97 across subscales.

Author: Norem-Hebeisen, A., et al.

Article: Predictors and concomitants of changes in drug use patterns among teenagers.

Journal: *Journal of Social Psychology,* October 1984, *124*(first half), 43–50.

Related Research: Johnson, D. W., & Norem-Hebeisen, A. (1977). Attitudes toward interdependence among persons and psychological health. *Psychological Reports, 109,* 253–261.

■ ■ ■

2786

Test Name: STATISTICS ATTITUDE SURVEY

Purpose: To measure student attitudes toward statistics.

Number of Items: 34

Format: At least one third of the items measure student success in solving statistics problems or success in understanding statistics concepts.

Reliability: Coefficient alpha values were approximately .94.

Author: Wise, S. L.

Article: The development and validation of a scale measuring attitudes toward statistics.

Journal: *Educational and Psychological Measurement,* Summer 1985, *45*(2), 401–405.

Related Research: Roberts, D. M., & Bilderback, E. W. (1980). Reliability and validity of a statistics attitude survey. *Educational and Psychological Measurement, 40,* 235–238.

■ ■ ■

2787

Test Name: STEREOTYPE SURVEY

Purpose: To measure attitudes toward the roles of males and females.

Number of Items: 25

Format: Subjects answer *true* or *false* to each item. All items are presented.

Reliability: Kuder-Richardson formula 21 produced a coefficient of .88.

Validity: Correlation with the Attitude Toward Women Scale was .75 (*N* = 100).

Author: Wilson, J., and Daniel, R.

Article: The effects of a career-option workshop on social and vocational stereotypes.

Journal: *Vocational Guidance Quarterly,* June 1981, *29*(4), 341–349.

■ ■ ■

2788

Test Name: STUDENT DEVELOPMENT INVENTORY

Purpose: To document college students' present attitudes and possible changes in attitudes associated with counseling, remediation, and general educational programs.

Number of Items: 70

Format: Includes the following subscales: self-confidence in mathematics, enjoyment of mathematics, smooth communication, self-confidence with superiors, self-confidence with peers, self-confidence in writing, and enjoyment of writing. Responses are made on a 5-point scale from *almost always characteristic of me* (5) to *never characteristic of me* (1).

Reliability: Coefficient alphas for the seven subscales ranged from .82 to .93.

Author: Jackson, L. M., et al.

Article: Reliability and factorial validity of the Student Development Inventory.

Journal: *Educational and Psychological Measurement,* Autumn 1985, *45*(3), 671–677.

Related Research: Chickering, A. W. (1972). *Education and identity.* San Francisco: Jossey-Bass Publishers.

■ ■ ■

2789

Test Name: STUDENT FEES AND SERVICES QUESTIONNAIRE

Purpose: To measure student attitudes about fees and services made available by fees.

Number of Items: 31

Format: Items rated on a 3-point rating scale of importance, 2-point use scale (*yes–no*), and 2-point provision scale (*should provide–should not provide*).

Reliability: Cronbach's alphas: usage (.75), importance (.95), provision (.93).

Author: Matross, R.

Article: An analysis of student attitudes toward cocurricular services and fees.

Journal: *Journal of College Student Personnel,* September 1981, *22*(5), 424–428.

Related Research: Matross, R., & Barnett, R. (1978). The 1978 survey on Twin Cities Campus student service fees. *Office for Student Affairs Research Bulletin, 18*(10).

■ ■ ■

2790

Test Name: SUBSTANCE-USE SCALE

Purpose: To measure attitudes toward substance use.

Number of Items: 4 vignettes.

Format: Items rated on a 5-point Likert scale (*strongly disapprove* to *strongly approve*). All items are presented.

Reliability: Alpha was .72. Item-to-scale correlations ranged between .72 and .76.

Author: Gary, L. E., and Berry, G. L.

Article: Some determinants of attitudes toward substance use in an urban ethnic community.

Journal: *Psychological Reports,* April 1984, *54*(2), 539–545.

Related Research: Giovannoni, J. M., & Becerra, R. M. (1979). *Defining child abuse.* New York: Free Press.

■ ■ ■

2791

Test Name: TEST ATTITUDE SURVEY

Purpose: To identify children's attitudes toward tests and the test-taking situation.

Number of Items: 12

Format: Items were answered either *yes* or *no,* indicating agreement or disagreement with the statement. Examples are presented.

Reliability: Kuder-Richardson formula 20 was .78 and .76.

Author: Scruggs, T. E., et al.

Article: Attitudes of behaviorally disordered students toward tests.

Journal: *Perceptual and Motor Skills,* April 1985, *60*(2), 467–470.

Related Research: Taylor, C., & Scruggs, T. E. (1983). Research in progress: Improving the test-taking skills of LD and BD elementary students. *Exceptional Children, 50,* 277.

2792

Test Name: TEST ATTITUDE SURVEY

Purpose: To measure students' feelings toward tests.

Number of Items: 22

Format: Responses to each item were *yes* or *no*. Examples are presented.

Reliability: Kuder-Richardson formula 20 was .75.

Author: Tolfa, D., et al.

Article: Attitudes of behaviorally disordered students toward tests: A replication.

Journal: *Perceptual and Motor Skills,* December 1985, *61*(3, Part 1), 963–966.

Related Research: Scruggs, T. E., et al. (1985). Attitudes of behaviorally disordered students toward tests. *Perceptual and Motor Skills, 60,* 467–470.

• • •

2793

Test Name: TEST OF SCIENCE RELATED ATTITUDES

Purpose: To measure science related attitudes.

Number of Items: 70

Format: Includes seven scales.

Reliability: Subscale reliability (Cronbach's alpha) ranged from .68 to .91. Reliability for the whole test was .95.

Author: Schibeci, R. A., and McGaw, B.

Article: Empirical validation of the conceptual structure of a test of science-related attitudes.

Journal: *Educational and Psychological Measurement,* Winter 1981, *41*(4), 1195–1201.

Related Research: Fraser, B. J. (1978). Development of a test of

science-related attitudes. *Science Education, 62,* 509–515.

• • •

2794

Test Name: TUTORING ATTITUDE QUESTIONNAIRE

Purpose: To measure attitudes toward tutoring.

Number of Items: 24

Format: Items rated in 9-point Likert format.

Reliability: Cronbach's alpha was .93 (internal consistency was .88 or above on three subscales).

Validity: Correlations between subscales ranged from .28 to .68.

Author: Bierman, K. L., and Furman, W.

Article: Effects of role and assignment rationale on attitudes formed during peer tutoring.

Journal: *Journal of Educational Psychology,* February 1981, *73*(1), 33–40.

• • •

2795

Test Name: VALUE OF MATHEMATICS SCALE

Purpose: To measure attitude toward mathematics.

Number of Items: 10

Format: Employs a 5-point Likert-style format from 0 (*strongly disagree*) to 4 (*strongly agree*). All items are presented.

Reliability: Coefficient alpha was .68.

Validity: Correlations with other variables ranged from −.016 to .146.

Author: Watson, J. M.

Article: The Aiken attitude to mathematics scales: Psychometric data on reliability and

discriminant validity.

Journal: *Educational and Psychological Measurement,* Winter 1983, *43*(4), 1247–1253.

Related Research: Aiken, L. R. (1974). Two scales of attitude toward mathematics. *Journal for Research in Mathematics Education, 5,* 67–71.

• • •

2796

Test Name: WOMEN AS MANAGERS SCALE

Purpose: To measure attitudes towards women as managers.

Number of Items: 21

Format: 7-point rating scales (*strongly agree* to *strongly disagree*). Sample item presented.

Reliability: Alpha was .90.

Author: Beutell, N. J.

Article: Correlates of attitudes toward American women as managers.

Journal: *Journal of Social Psychology,* October 1984, *124*(first half), 57–63.

Related Research: Peters, L. H., et al. (1974). Women as Managers Scale (WAMS): A measure of attitudes toward women in management positions. *JSAS Catalog of Selected Documents in Psychology, 27*(MS No. 585).

• • •

2797

Test Name: WORK INVOLVEMENT ATTITUDE SCALES

Purpose: To measure work involvement.

Number of Items: 16

Format: Items rated in 5-point Likert format. All items presented.

Reliability: Alphas ranged from .68 and .81 across subscales.

Validity: Two of three subscales discriminate between subjects who select *same* or *different* employment areas.

Author: Jans, N. A.

Article: The nature and measurement of work involvement.

Journal: *Journal of Occupational Psychology,* March 1984, *55*(1), 57–67.

Related Research: Saleh, S. D., & Hosek, J. (1976). Job involvement: Concepts and measurement. *Academy of Management Journal, 19,* 213–224.

• • •

2798

Test Name: WORLD MINDEDNESS SCALE

Purpose: To measure attitude toward nations and tolerance toward foreigners.

Number of Items: 32

Format: Likert. Sample items presented.

Reliability: Odd–even reliability was .87 (corrected Spearman-Brown = .93). Test–retest reliability was .93 (over 28 days).

Author: Crawford, J. C., and Lamb, C. W., Jr.

Article: Effect of worldmindedness among professional buyers upon their willingness to buy foreign products.

Journal: *Psychological Reports,* 1982, *50*(3, part 1), 859–862.

Related Research: Sampson, D. L., & Smith, H. P. (1957). A scale to measure worldmindedness attitudes. *Journal of Social Psychology, 45,* 99–106.

CHAPTER 8
Behavior

2799

Test Name: ACHENBACH CHILD BEHAVIOR CHECKLIST

Purpose: To measure problem behavior in children.

Number of Items: 118

Format: Checklist format.

Reliability: Interparent reliability was .84; intraclass reliability was .98; test–retest (1 week) reliability was .95.

Author: Webster-Stratton, C.

Article: Randomized trial of two-parent programs for families with conduct-disordered children.

Journal: *Journal of Consulting and Clinical Psychology,* August 1984, *52*(4), 666–678.

Related Research: Achenbach, T. M., & Edelbrock, C. S. (1981). Behavioral problems and competencies reported by parents of normal and disturbed children aged four through sixteen. *Monographs of the Society for Research in Child Development, 46,* 1–82.

· · ·

2800

Test Name: AGGRESSIVE ACT REPORT

Purpose: To measure subjects' experience with aggression.

Number of Items: 303

Format: Items represent specific aggressive acts designed to sample three types of aggression: direct active physical aggression, direct active verbal aggression, and indirect physical aggression. Examples are presented.

Reliability: Cronbach's alpha was .97.

Validity: Correlations with Buss-Durkee Hostility-Guilt Inventory was .43 (*N* = 45).

Author: Driscoll, J. M.

Article: Effects of perceiver's experience with aggression on attributions about aggressors.

Journal: *Perceptual and Motor Skills,* June 1985, *60*(3), 815–826.

Related Research: Driscoll, J. M. (1982). Perception of an aggressive interaction as a function of the perceiver's aggression. *Perceptual and Motor Skills, 54,* 1123–1154.

· · ·

2801

Test Name: AGGRESSION, MOODINESS, LEARNING PROBLEMS SCALE (AML)

Purpose: To measure problems of aggression, moodiness, and learning of preschoolers as perceived by teachers.

Number of Items: 11

Format: A 5-point adjustment scale for each item.

Reliability: Test–retest reliability ranged between .73 and .86 across subscales and ages of children.

Author: Handal, P. J., and Hopper, S.

Article: Relationship of sex, social class, and rural/urban locale to preschoolers' AML scores.

Journal: *Psychological Reports,* December 1985, *57*(3, I), 707–713.

Related Research: Cowen, E. L., et al. (1973). The AML: A quick screening device for early identification of school adaptation. *American Journal of Community Psychology, 1,* 12–35.

· · ·

2802

Test Name: ALCOHOL ABUSE SCALE OF THE PIPS

Purpose: To identify alcohol abusers.

Number of Items: 12

Format: *Yes–no* format. Sample items are presented.

Validity: Scale correctly classified 88% of women and 82% of men as alcoholics or non-alcoholics.

Author: Vincent, K. R., and Williams, W.

Article: Alcohol abuse scale of the Psychological Inventory of Personality and Symptoms: A cross-validation.

Journal: *Psychological Reports,* December 1985, *57*(3, II), 1077–1078.

Related Research: Vincent, K. R. (1985). The Psychological Inventory of Personality and Symptoms (PIPS): A new test of psychopathology based on DSM-III. *The Journal: Houston International Hospital, 3,* 20–27.

· · ·

2803

Test Name: ASSERTIVE FRIEND CARTOON TEST

Purpose: To measure the ability to refuse.

Number of Items: 4

Time Required: 15 minutes.

Format: Four prompting lines are paired with empty word balloons respondents fill in. Sample measure for smoking marijuana presented.

Reliability: Interrater reliability .90 or greater.

Author: Bobo, J. K., et al.

Article: Assessment of refusal skill in minority youth.

Journal: *Psychological Reports,* December 1985, *57*(3, II), 1187–1191.

■ ■ ■

2804

Test Name: ATTRIBUTION INTERFERENCE CODING SYSTEM

Purpose: To measure teachers' tendency to attribute cause of problem classroom behavior to students or to situation, or to both.

Number of Items: 24 vignettes.

Format: Vignettes are short descriptions of problem behavior to which teachers respond by stating strategies they would use. All vignettes presented along with coding system.

Reliability: Percent exact agreement was 76%.

Author: Brophy, J. E., and Rohrkemper, M. M.

Article: The influence of problem ownership on teachers' perceptions and strategies for coping with problem students.

Journal: *Journal of Educational Psychology,* June 1981, *73*(3), 295–311.

Related Research: Rohrkemper, M. M., & Brophy, J. E. (1979). *Classroom strategy study: Investigating teacher strategies with problem students.* (Research Series No. 50). Michigan State University, Institute for Research on Teaching.

■ ■ ■

2805

Test Name: AUTHORITY BEHAVIOR INVENTORY (ABI)

Purpose: To measure behavior relating to acceptance of authority.

Number of Items: 16

Format: Score 1 (*never*) to 5 (*very frequently*). Sample items are presented.

Reliability: Alpha was .78.

Validity: Correlated .76 with General Attitude to Institutional Authority Scale. Correlated –.11 with Ray Directiveness Scale.

Author: Rigby, K.

Article: Acceptance of authority and directiveness as indicators of authoritarianism: A new framework.

Journal: *Journal of Social Psychology,* April 1984, *122*(second half), 171–180.

■ ■ ■

2806

Test Name: AUTONOMY-CONTROL SCALE

Purpose: To measure role autonomy-control in children and adolescents.

Number of Items: 14 childhood and 16 adolescence items.

Format: Items rated on a 5-point scale form. Items taken from existing scales.

Reliability: Test–retest reliability was .91 (2-month, new sample, $N = 41$).

Validity: Significant correlations found between autonomy-control scores and separate family ratings ($N = 50$).

Author: DeMan, A. F.

Article: Autonomy-control variation in child-rearing and self-image disparity in young adults.

Journal: *Psychological Reports,* December 1982, *51*(3, II), 1039–1044.

Related Research: Koch, H. L., et al. (1934). A scale for measuring attitudes toward the question of children's freedom. *Child Development, 5,* 253–266.

Itkin, W. (1982). Some relationships between intra-family attitudes and pre-parental attitudes toward children. *Journal of Genetic Psychology, 112,* 71–78.

■ ■ ■

2807

Test Name: BEHAVIOR PROBLEM CHECKLIST

Purpose: To assess problem behavior.

Number of Items: 55

Format: Informed observers check problems they observe in the subject.

Reliability: Test–retest reliability ranged from .79 to .83. Interrater reliability ranged from .67 to .78.

Author: Szapocznik, J., et al.

Article: Conjoint versus one-person family therapy: Some evidence for the effectiveness of conducting family therapy through one person.

Journal: *Journal of Consulting and Clinical Psychology,* December 1983, *51*(6), 889–899.

Related Research: Quay, H. C., & Paterson, D. R. (1979). *Behavior Problem Checklist.* Graduate School of Applied and Professional Psychology, Rutgers State University.

2808

Test Name: BEHAVIOR RATING INDEX FOR CHILDREN

Purpose: To provide a prothetic measure of children's behavior problems.

Number of Items: 13

Format: Each item is rated on a 5-point Likert scale from 1 (*rarely or never*) to 5 (*most or all of the time*). All items are presented.

Reliability: Coefficient alphas ranged from .60 to .86. Test–retest reliability ranged from .50 to .89. Intraclass correlation coefficients ranged from .71 to .92.

Validity: Correlation with the Child Behavior Checklist was .76.

Author: Stiffman, A. R., et al.

Article: A brief measure of children's behavior problems: The Behavior Rating Index for Children.

Journal: *Measurement and Evaluation in Counseling and Development,* July 1984, *17*(2), 83–90.

■ ■ ■

2809

Test Name: BEHAVIORAL INDECISION SCALE

Purpose: To measure behavioral indecision.

Number of Items: 22

Format: Thurstone format.

Reliability: Cronbach's alpha was .66; Test–retest reliability was .57.

Validity: Correlates .62 with Career Decision Scale; .59 with Identity Scale; .27 with A-State Anxiety; .35 with A-Trait Anxiety; and .13 with Locus of Control.

Author: Fuqua, D. R., and Hartman, B. W.

Article: A behavioral index of career indecision for college students.

Journal: *Journal of College Student Personnel,* November 1983, *24*(6), 507–512.

■ ■ ■

2810

Test Name: BEHAVIORAL RATING SCALES

Purpose: To measure duration, intimacy, and nonverbal affective behavior in dyads and triads.

Number of Items: 9

Format: Observer-coders rate interaction on 9 behaviors. All items presented.

Reliability: Ranged between $r = .75$ and $r = .90$ across subscales.

Author: Solano, C. H., and Dunnam, M.

Article: Two's company: Self-disclosure and reciprocity in triads versus dyads.

Journal: *Social Psychology Quarterly,* June 1985, *48*(2), 183–187.

Related Research: Taylor, R. B., et al. (1979). Sharing secrets: Disclosure and discretion in dyads and triads. *Journal of Personality and Social Psychology, 37,* 1196–1203.

■ ■ ■

2811

Test Name: BEHAVIORAL STYLE QUESTIONNAIRE

Purpose: To assess children's temperament or behavioral style.

Number of Items: 100

Format: Parents rate their child on a 6-point scale. Includes three factors: (a) intensity of affective expression such as intensity, mood, activity, and threshold; (b) flexibility–rigidity such as adaptability, persistence, and distractability; and (c) approach–

withdrawal such as dimension, activity, persistence, and sensory thresholds.

Validity: Correlations with neonatal noncrying movements per hour ranged from .04 to .30. Correlations with neonatal median amplitude of movements per day ranged from .01 to .09.

Author: Korner, A. F., et al.

Article: The relation between neonatal and later activity and temperament.

Journal: *Child Development,* February 1985, *56*(1), 38–42.

Related Research: McDevitt, S. C., and Carey, W. B. (1978). The measurement of temperament in 3 to 7 year old children. *Journal of Child Psychology and Psychiatry, 19,* 245–253.

Field, T., & Greenberg, R. (1982). Temperament ratings by parents and teachers of infants, toddlers and preschool children. *Child Development, 53*(1), 160–163.

■ ■ ■

2812

Test Name: BODY SENSATIONS QUESTIONNAIRE

Purpose: To measure body sensation associated with autonomic arousal.

Number of Items: 17

Format: Items are rated on a 5-point scale.

Reliability: Item-total ranged from .44 to .79 in agoraphobic sample and from −.09 to .88 in normal sample.

Validity: Correlated .36 with Beck Depression Inventory; correlated .21 with Trait Anxiety–STAI; correlated .67 with Agoraphobic Cognition.

Author: Chambliss, D. L., et al.

Article: Assessment of fear in agoraphobics: The Body

Sensations Questionnaire and the Agoraphobic Cognitions Questionnaire.

Journal: *Journal of Consulting and Clinical Psychology*, December 1984, *52*(6), 1090–1097.

■ ■ ■

2813

Test Name: BULIMIA TEST

Purpose: To measure symptoms of bulimia.

Number of Items: 32

Format: Self-report, multiple-choice format. All items presented.

Reliability: Test–retest reliability was .87 ($p < .0001$).

Validity: Correlated .82 (point-biserial) with bulimic and control group subjects. Correlated .93 with binge scale and .68 with the EAT scale (Garner & Garfinkel, 1979).

Author: Smith, M. C., and Thelen, M. H.

Article: Development and validation of a test for bulimia.

Journal: *Journal of Clinical and Consulting Psychology*, October 1984, *52*(5), 863–872.

■ ■ ■

2814

Test Name: CAREER ACTIVITIES SURVEY

Purpose: To assess information-seeking activities.

Number of Items: 30

Format: A behavioral checklist.

Reliability: Coefficient alpha was .64.

Author: Robbins, S. B., et al.

Article: Attrition behavior before career development workshops.

Journal: *Journal of Counseling Psychology*, April 1985, *32*(2), 232–238.

Related Research: Miller, M. (1982). Interest pattern structure and personality characteristics of clients who seek career information. *Vocational Guidance Quarterly, 31*, 28–35.

■ ■ ■

2815

Test Name: CHILD ABUSE POTENTIAL INVENTORY

Purpose: To screen individuals suspected of abuse.

Number of Items: 160

Format: Forced-choice format.

Reliability: Kuder-Richardson formula 20 ranged from .92 to .96; Test–retest reliability was .94 (1 day) and .90 (1 week).

Author: Ellis, R. H., and Milner, J. S.

Article: Child abuse and locus of control.

Journal: *Psychological Reports*, April 1981, *48*(2), 507–510.

Related Research: Milner, J. S., & Wimberly, R. C. (1979). An inventory for the identification of child abusers. *Journal of Clinical Psychology, 35*, 95–100.

■ ■ ■

2816

Test Name: CHILD BEHAVIOR PROFILE–TEACHER VERSION

Purpose: To obtain teachers' reports of problem behavior of children.

Number of Items: 118

Format: Items rated on 5- and 7-point rating scales. Sample item presented.

Reliability: Test–retest reliability was .89; 2–4 month stability ranged from .64 to .77.

Author: Edelbrock, C., and Achenbach, T. M.

Article: The teacher version of the Child Behavior Profile: I. Boys aged 6–11.

Journal: *Journal of Consulting and Clinical Psychology*, April 1984, *52*(1), 207–217.

Related Research: Achenbach, T. M., & Edelbrock, C. The Child Behavior Profile: II. Boys aged 12–16 and girls aged 6–11 and 12–16. *Journal of Consulting and Clinical Psychology, 47*, 223–233.

■ ■ ■

2817

Test Name: CHILD TEMPERAMENT QUESTIONNAIRE

Purpose: To measure child behavior in an educational setting.

Number of Items: 23

Format: Items rated in 6-point Likert format.

Validity: LISREL revealed the same three temperament variables across five grade levels.

Author: Cadwell, J., and Pullis, M.

Article: Assessing changes in the meaning of children's behavior: Factorial invariance of teachers' temperament ratings.

Journal: *Journal of Educational Psychology*, August 1983, *75*(4), 553–560.

Related Research: Keogh, B. K., et al. (1982). A short form of the Teacher Temperament Questionnaire. *Journal of Educational Measurement, 19*, 323–329.

■ ■ ■

2818

Test Name: CHILDREN'S COERCIVE BEHAVIOR SCALE

Purpose: To measure coercive behavior in children.

Number of Items: 16

Format: Observed behavior

recorded as a rate per minute for child, mother, and father. All items presented are taken from Toobert et al., MOSAIC.

Reliability: Interobserver agreement ranged from .57 to .75.

Author: Loeber, R., and Dishion, T. J.

Article: Boys who fight at home and school: Family conditions influencing cross-setting consistency.

Journal: *Journal of Consulting and Clinical Psychology,* October 1984, *52*(5), 759–768.

Related Research: Toobert, D. J., et al. (1980). *Measure of social adjustment in children: MOSAIC.* Unpublished manuscript.

■ ■ ■

2819

Test Name: CHILDREN'S DRUG-USE SURVEY

Purpose: To measure drug-use of children.

Number of Items: 16

Format: How often, when, and where alcohol, marijuana, and inhalants are used is asked.

Reliability: Internal consistency ranged from .87 to .94.

Validity: Item clusters correlated positively.

Author: Oetting, E. R.

Article: Reliability and discriminant validity of the Children's Drug-Use Survey.

Journal: *Psychological Reports,* June 1985, *56*(3), 751–756.

■ ■ ■

2820

Test Name: CLASSROOM ADJUSTMENT RATING SCALE

Purpose: To measure problem classroom behaviors.

Number of Items: 41

Format: Items rated on a 5-point severity scale.

Validity: Test–retest reliability exceeded .85 on all subscales.

Author: Weissberg, R. P., et al.

Article: The primary mental health project: Seven consecutive years of program outcome research.

Journal: *Journal of Consulting and Clinical Psychology,* February 1983, *51*(1), 100–107.

Related Research: Lorion, R. P., et al. (1975). Normative and parametric analyses of school maladjustment. *American Journal of Community Psychology, 3,* 293–301.

■ ■ ■

2821

Test Name: CLASSROOM BEHAVIOR OBSERVATION

Purpose: To measure behavior of LD children and nondisabled children in six categories: inattentive behavior, off-task verbalizations/vocalizations; nonacademic/nondisruptive behavior; impulse behavior; disruptive behavior; inappropriate location of activities.

Time Required: Observations made at 10-second intervals for 6 minutes.

Reliability: Interobserver agreements ranged from 79% to 100%. Stability coefficients ranged from .43 to 1.00.

Validity: Behaviors supplied by teachers of LD children.

Author: Gettinger, M., and Fayne, H. R.

Article: Classroom behavior during small group instruction and learning performance in learning disabled and nondisabled children.

Journal: *Journal of Educational Research,* January/February 1982, *75*(3), 182–187.

Related Research: Brophy, J. E., et al. (1975). Classroom observation scales: Stability across time and context and relationships with student learning gains. *Journal of Educational Psychology, 67,* 873–881.

■ ■ ■

2822

Test Name: CLASSROOM INAPPROPRIATE BEHAVIOR SCALE

Purpose: To measure inappropriate classroom behavior.

Number of Items: 8

Format: Raters observe classroom in 30-minute sessions, divided into 10-second intervals. (8 seconds observation, 2 seconds recording.)

Reliability: Interrater reliability was 82–99% (median 94%).

Author: Witt, J. C., and Elliott, S. N.

Article: The response cost lottery: A time efficient and effective classroom intervention.

Journal: *Journal of School Psychology,* 1982, *20*(2), 155–161.

Related Research: Madsen, C. H., et al. (1968). Rules, praise and ignoring: Elements of elementary classroom control. *Journal of Applied Behavior Analysis, 1,* 139–150.

■ ■ ■

2823

Test Name: CLASSROOM INTERACTION ANALYSIS

Purpose: To assess patterns of action in classrooms between students and teachers.

Number of Items: 47

Format: The 47 items are grouped into five major categories (types) of interaction that trained raters observe on tapescripts. All items presented.

Reliability: Interrater reliability ranged from 95% to 99%.

Author: Thomas, E. C., and Holcomb, H.

Article: Nurturing productive thinking in able students.

Journal: *Journal of General Psychology,* January 1981, *104*(first half), 67–79.

Related Research: Aschner, M. J., et al. (1965). *A system for classifying thought processes in the context of classroom verbal interaction.* Unpublished manuscript, University of Illinois, Urbana.

■ ■ ■

2824

Test Name: CODE FOR INSTRUCTIONAL STRUCTURE AND STUDENT ACADEMIC RESPONSE

Purpose: To measure behavior of students.

Number of Items: 53 events in six areas.

Time Required: 10 seconds for three areas.

Format: Behavior recorded on code sheets.

Reliability: Interobserver agreement exceeded 85%.

Author: Thurlow, M., et al.

Article: Student reading during reading class: The lost activity in reading instruction.

Journal: *Journal of Educational Research,* May/June 1984, *77*(5), 267–272.

Related Research: Greenwood, C. R., et al. (1978). *Code for instructional structure and student academic response: CISSAR.* Kansas City, KS: Juniper Gardens

Children's Project, Bureau of Child Research, University of Kansas.

■ ■ ■

2825

Test Name: COMBAT EXPOSURE SCALE

Purpose: To measure combat involvement from hospital records of veterans' military experience.

Number of Items: 7

Format: Guttman. All items presented.

Reliability: Coefficient of reproducibility was .93.

Validity: Correlated .86 with Egendorf et al., Combat Scale.

Author: Foy, D. W., et al.

Article: Etiology of post-traumatic stress disorder in Vietnam veterans: Analysis of premilitary, military and combat exposure influences.

Journal: *Journal of Consulting and Clinical Psychology,* February 1984, *52*(1), 79–87.

■ ■ ■

2826

Test Name: COMPETITION KNOWLEDGE TEST

Purpose: To measure competitive behavior.

Number of Items: 60

Format: Multiple-choice test. All items are presented.

Reliability: Internal consistency, split-half was .89 (*N* = 178). Test–retest was .88 (*N* = 130).

Author: Kildea, A. E.

Article: The Competition Knowledge Test.

Journal: *Perceptual and Motor Skills,* April 1985, *60*(2), 477–478.

Related Research: Kildea, A. E., & Kukulka, G. (1984). Reliability of

the Competition Knowledge Test. *Psychological Reports, 54,* 957–958.

■ ■ ■

2827

Test Name: CONNERS TEACHER RATING SCALE

Purpose: To screen for hyperactivity in children.

Number of Items: 39

Reliability: Alphas ranged from .61 to .94 across subscales (all but one alpha was below .76).

Validity: Coefficients of congruence of factor structure ranged from .42 to .91 across studies; from .86 to .99 across whole versus random half and across random half samples.

Author: Trites, R. L., et al.

Article: Factor analysis of the Conners Teacher Rating Scale based on a large normative sample.

Journal: *Journal of Consulting and Clinical Psychology,* October 1982, *50*(5), 615–623.

Related Research: Conners, C. K. (1969). A teacher rating scale for use in drug studies with children. *American Journal of Psychiatry, 126,* 884–888.

■ ■ ■

2828

Test Name: CONNERS TEACHER RATING SCALE—REVISED

Purpose: To enable teachers to rate pupils' classroom behavior.

Number of Items: 28

Format: Includes three subscales: conduct problems, hyperactivity, and inattentive–passive. Also 5 miscellaneous items were included.

Reliability: Intraclass reliability coefficient was .758.

Author: Conger, A. J., et al.

Article: A generalizability study of the Conners Teacher Rating Scale—Revised.

Journal: *Educational and Psychological Measurement,* Winter 1983, *43*(4), 1019–1031.

Related Research: Goyette, C. H., et al. (1978). Normative data on revised Conners parent and teacher rating scales. *Journal of Abnormal Child Psychology, 6,* 221–238.

• • •

2829

Test Name: CONSUMPTION EXPERIENCES SCALE

Purpose: To assess what kinds of activities are approached in terms of cause and effect, involvement, escape, or learning experience.

Number of Items: 14

Format: Checklist format.

Reliability: Kuder-Richardson formula 20 ranged from .71 to .77 across subscales.

Author: Hirschman, E. C.

Article: Sexual identity and the acquisition of rational, absorbing, escapist and modelling experiences.

Journal: *Journal of Social Psychology,* February 1985, *125*(1), 63–73.

Related Research: Swanson, G. E. (1978). Travels through inner space: Family structure and openness to absorbing experience. *American Journal of Sociology, 83,* 890–919.

Tellegren, A., and Atkinson, B. (1974). Openness to absorbing and self-altering experiences. *Journal of Abnormal Psychology, 38,* 268–277.

Hirschman, E. C. (1983). On the acquisition of aesthetic, escapist and agentic experiences. *Empirical Studies of the Arts, 1,* 153–168.

2830

Test Name: COPING STRATEGIES INVENTORY

Purpose: To measure cognitive and behavioral strategies people use to confront stressful situations.

Number of Items: 76

Format: Items rated in 5-point Likert format.

Reliability: Cronbach's alpha ranged from .76 to .93 across subscales.

Author: Ritchey, K. M., et al.

Article: Problem-solving appraisal versus hypothetical problem solving.

Journal: *Psychological Reports,* December 1984, *55*(3), 815–818.

Related Research: Tobin, D. L., et al. (1982). *The assessment of coping: Psychometric development of coping strategies inventory.* Unpublished manuscript, Ohio University, Athens.

• • •

2831

Test Name: DAILY CHILD BEHAVIOR CHECKLIST

Purpose: To assess child behavior problems initially and to serve as a measure of change that occurs with treatment.

Number of Items: 65

Format: A checklist containing pleasing and displeasing behaviors. All items are presented.

Reliability: Test–retest (2 weeks) correlations ranged from –.189 to .665.

Validity: Correlations with the Parent Attitude Test ranged from –.855 to .581.

Author: Furey, W., and Forehand, R.

Article: The Daily Child Behavior Checklist.

Journal: *Journal of Behavioral Assessment,* June 1983, *5*(2), 83–95.

• • •

2832

Test Name: DELINQUENCY SCALES

Purpose: To measure delinquency through self-report.

Number of Items: 31

Format: Items rated on 6-point frequency scales.

Reliability: Alpha ranged from .52 to .78 across subscales.

Author: McCarthy, J. D., and Hoge, D. R.

Article: The dynamics of self-esteem and delinquency.

Journal: *American Journal of Sociology,* September 1984, *90*(2), 396–400.

Related Research: Short, J. F., & Nye, E. I. (1957). Reported behavior as a criterion of deviant behavior. *Social Problems, 5,* 207–213.

• • •

2833

Test Name: DISORDERED EATING TEST

Purpose: To measure disordered eating.

Number of Items: 10

Format: True–false. Sample item presented.

Reliability: Cronbach's alpha was .70.

Validity: Correlated .60 with shortened version of the Eating Attitude Test.

Author: Segal, S. A., and Figley, C. R.

Article: Bulimia: Estimate of incidence and relationship to shyness.

Journal: *Journal of College Student Personnel,* May 1985, *26*(3), 240–244.

Related Research: Garner, D. M., & Garfinkel, P. E. (1979). The Eating Attitude Test: An index of the symptoms of anorexia nervosa. *Psychological Medicine, 9,* 273–281.

■ ■ ■

2834

Test Name: FUNCTIONAL BEHAVIOR SURVEY

Purpose: To provide a behavior rating scale of mental impairment.

Number of Items: 20

Format: Instrument is completed by two independent observers. Each item is rated on a 5-point scale from 1 (*hardly ever*) to 5 (*nearly always*). All items are presented.

Validity: Correlation with Competence Index was –.65; Impairment Index was –.78; Memory Check was .71.

Author: Tobacyk, J., et al.

Article: Two brief measures for assessing mental competence in the elderly.

Journal: *Journal of Personality Assessment,* December 1983, *47*(6), 648–655.

Related Research: Dixon, J. C. (1965). Cognitive structure in senile conditions with some suggestions for developing a brief screening test of mental status. *Journal of Gerontology, 20,* 41–49.

■ ■ ■

2835

Test Name: HEALTH AND DAILY LIVING FORM

Purpose: To assess health status.

Number of Items: 38

Format: Consists of three lists: medical conditions, physical symptoms, and medications. Subjects check whether each item in each list was experienced during the past 12 months.

Reliability: Cronbach's alphas ranged from .30 to .80.

Validity: Correlations with loneliness scores ranged from –.04 to .54.

Author: Schmitt, J. P., and Kurdek, L. A.

Article: Age and gender differences in and personality correlates of loneliness in different relationships.

Journal: *Journal of Personality Assessment,* October 1985, *49*(5), 485–496.

Related Research: Moos, R. H., et al. (1983). *The Health and Daily Living Form Manual.* Unpublished manuscript, Stanford University.

■ ■ ■

2836

Test Name: HOLISTIC LIVING INVENTORY

Purpose: To measure frequency of activities that indicate a holistic style of life.

Number of Items: 20

Format: Multiple-choice. Sample items presented.

Reliability: Split-half ranged from .08 to .91 across subscales.

Validity: Nonalcoholics score higher than alcoholics on physical scale. People without medical problems score higher than those with, and exercisers score higher than nonexercisers (all $ps < .01$).

Author: Stoudenomice, J., et al.

Article: Validation of a Holistic Living Inventory.

Journal: *Psychological Reports,* August 1985, *57*(1), 303–311.

2837

Test Name: HOLT INTIMACY DEVELOPMENT INVENTORY

Purpose: To measure behaviors in closest relationships.

Number of Items: 66

Format: Likert type.

Reliability: Guilford's *R* ranged from .67 to .84 across three subscales.

Author: Prager, K. J.

Article: Development of intimacy in young adults: A multidimensional view.

Journal: *Psychological Reports,* June 1983, *52*(3), 751–756.

Related Research: Holt, M. L. (1977). *Human intimacy in young adults: An experimental development scale.* Unpublished doctoral dissertation, University of Georgia.

■ ■ ■

2838

Test Name: IJR BEHAVIOR CHECKLIST FOR PARENTS, TEACHERS AND CLINICIANS

Purpose: To measure behavior syndromes for diagnostic evaluations.

Number of Items: 597

Time Required: Takes 1 month for parent and teacher form. Single interview for clinician.

Format: Frequency rating scale for each item.

Reliability: Alpha ranged from .66 to .90 across subscales and across forms.

Author: Lessing, E. E., et al.

Article: Parallel forms of the IJR Behavior Checklist for Parents, Teachers and Clinicians.

Journal: *Journal of Consulting and Clinical Psychology,* February 1981, *49*(1), 34–50.

Related Research: Lessing, E. E., et al. (1973). Differentiating children's symptoms checklist items on the basis of the judged severity of psychopathology. *Genetic Psychology Monographs,* *88,* 329–350.

• • •

2839

Test Name: ILLNESS BEHAVIOR INVENTORY

Purpose: To provide a self-report measure of illness behavior.

Number of Items: 20

Format: Responses are made to each item on a 6-point Likert scale ranging from *strong agreement* to *strong disagreement.* Includes two dimensions: work-related illness behavior and social illness behavior. All items are presented.

Reliability: Coefficient alphas were .88 and .89. Test–retest (2 weeks) reliability coefficients for each item ranged from .82 to 1.00 (*N* = 32).

Validity: Correlations with other illness behavior measures ranged from .32 to .48. Predictive validity coefficients ranged from .30 to .38 (*N* = 63).

Author: Turkat, I. D., and Pettegrew, L. S.

Article: Development and validation of the Illness Behavior Inventory.

Journal: *Journal of Behavioral Assessment,* March 1983, *5*(1), 35–47.

• • •

2840

Test Name: INFANT BEHAVIOR QUESTIONNAIRE

Purpose: To provide an assessment of infant temperament.

Number of Items: 87

Format: Includes 6 scales: activity level, smiling and laughter, fear, distress of limitations, soothability, duration of orienting.

Reliability: Coefficient alpha ranged from .67 to .85.

Author: Rothbart, M. K.

Article: Measurement of temperament in infancy.

Journal: *Child Development,* June 1981, *52*(2), 569–578.

Related Research: Thomas, A., et al. (1963). *Behavioral individuality in early childhood.* New York: New York University Press.

• • •

2841

Test Name: INGRATIATION TACTICS SCALE

Purpose: To measure extent of use of ingratiating behavior by self report.

Number of Items: 35

Format: Items rated on 5-point response categories (*completely true* to *completely false*). Sample items are presented.

Reliability: Alphas ranged from .46 to .76 across subscales.

Author: Bohra, K. A., and Pandey, J.

Article: Ingratiation toward strangers, friends, and bosses.

Journal: *Journal of Social Psychology,* April 1984, *122*(second half), 217–222.

Related Research: Bohra, K. A. (1981). *The effects of social power, need dimension and incentive on ingratiation.* Doctoral dissertation, University of Allahabad, India.

• • •

2842

Test Name: INITIATING STRUCTURE SCALE

Purpose: To measure a supervisor's behavior to initiate structured activity.

Number of Items: 10

Format: Items given. Response categories not given, but would appear to be Likert scales. Items taken from the Leadership Behavior Description Questionnaire Form XII.

Reliability: .87

Author: Markham, S. E., and Scott, K. D.

Article: A component factor analysis of the Initiating Structure Scale of the Leadership Behavior Description Questionnaire.

Journal: *Psychological Reports,* 1983, *52*(1), 71–77.

Related Research: Schriesheim, C., & Stogdill, R. (1975). Differences in factor structure across three versions of the Ohio State Leadership Scales. *Personnel Psychology, 28,* 189–206.

• • •

2843

Test Name: LEADER BEHAVIOR DESCRIPTION SCALE

Purpose: To provide a behavior description.

Number of Items: 27

Format: Response to each item is made on an 8-point scale from *very true of him* to *not at all true of him.* Some examples are given.

Reliability: Cronbach's alpha was .91.

Validity: Correlations with other scales ranged from .38 to .75.

Author: Vecchio, R. P.

Article: A further test of leadership effects due to between-group variation and within-group variation.

Journal: *Journal of Applied Psychology,* April 1982, *67*(2), 200–208.

Related Research: Rice, R. W., & Chemers, M. M. (1975). Personality and situational determinants of leader behavior. *Journal of Applied Psychology, 60,* 20–27.

■ ■ ■

2844

Test Name: LEADERSHIP INVENTORY

Purpose: To measure leadership characteristics of elementary and secondary gifted students.

Number of Items: 19

Format: Items rated on 4-point Likert categories.

Reliability: .69 when items reduced to 18 by Spearman-Brown formula. Guttman split-half reliability was .68.

Author: Chauvin, J. C., and Karnes, F. A.

Article: Reliability of a leadership inventory used with gifted students.

Journal: *Psychological Reports,* December 1982, *51*(3, Part 1), 770.

Related Research: Stacy, M. (1979). *Leadership inventory.* Yakima, WA: Yakima Public Schools.

■ ■ ■

2845

Test Name: LEADERSHIP STYLE SCALE

Purpose: To measure executives' perception of their own leadership styles.

Number of Items: 45

Format: Items rated on a 5-point Likert scale. Sample items are presented.

Reliability: Split-half ranged from .67 to .75 across subscales.

Validity: Authoritarian subscale correlated .27 with nurturant task

subscale and −.18 with participative subscale. Participative and nurturant subscales correlated .88 (all *p*s < .05).

Author: Sinha, J. B. P., and Ghowdhary, G. P.

Article: Perception of subordinates as a moderator of leadership effectiveness in India.

Journal: *Journal of Social Psychology,* February 1981, *113*(first half), 115–121.

■ ■ ■

2846

Test Name: LIE SCALE

Purpose: To detect lying on Child Abuse Potential Inventory.

Number of Items: 18

Format: Agree–disagree. All items presented.

Reliability: Kuder-Richardson formula 20 ranged from .64 to .79.

Validity: No significant correlations between the lie scale and the abuse scales.

Author: Milner, J. S.

Article: Development of a lie scale for the Child Abuse Potential Inventory.

Journal: *Psychological Reports,* 1982, *50*(3, Part 1), 871–874.

Related Research: Milner, J. S. (1980). *The Child Abuse Inventory: Manual.* Webster, NC: Psytec.

■ ■ ■

2847

Test Name: MAZE TEST

Purpose: To measure stimulus-seeking behavior.

Number of Items: 5 presentations of a maze.

Format: Paper-and-pencil maze presented five times. Contains no blind alleys and all routes are of

equal distance from start to goal. Score is based upon number of different traversions from preceding traversions.

Reliability: Cronbach's alpha was .81.

Validity: Correlations with which-to-discuss test was −.06.

Author: Silverstein, A. B., et al.

Article: Psychometric properties of two measures of intrinsic motivation.

Journal: *Perceptual and Motor Skills,* October 1981, *53*(2), 655–658.

Related Research: Howard, K. I. (1961). A test of stimulus-seeking behavior. *Perceptual and Motor Skills, 13,* 416.

■ ■ ■

2848

Test Name: MOTION SICKNESS QUESTIONNAIRE

Purpose: To measure susceptibility to motion sickness.

Number of Items: 5

Format: The entire questionnaire is presented.

Reliability: Test–retest correlations were .81 and .65.

Validity: Correlation with number of chair rotations was −.45.

Author: Mirabile, C. S., Jr., and Ford, M. R.

Article: A clinically useful polling technique for assessing susceptibility to motion sickness.

Journal: *Perceptual and Motor Skills,* June 1982, *54*(3, Part 1), 987–991.

■ ■ ■

2849

Test Name: MULTI-ALCOHOLIC PERSONALITY INVENTORY SCALE

Purpose: To measure alcohol dependency.

Number of Items: 20

Format: A paper-and-pencil self-report questionnaire involving *yes* and *no* responses. Includes four factors: drinking pattern, psychological, stress, personality. All items are presented.

Reliability: Test–retest (2 weeks) reliability coefficients ranged from .89 to .95. Alpha coefficient was .95.

Validity: Concurrent validity established by means of the two group discriminant function in which alcoholics' overall mean was 14.29 and that of nonalcoholics was 2.10, the difference being significant beyond the 0.001 level.

Author: Kim, Y. C.

Article: Development of a behavioral scale via factor analysis.

Journal: *Journal of Experimental Education*, Spring 1984, *52*(3), 163–167.

• • •

2850

Test Name: NOISE SENSITIVITY SCALE

Purpose: To measure general reactivity to noise among college students.

Number of Items: 21

Format: Responses are made on a 6-point scale ranging from *agree strongly* (1) to *disagree strongly* (6).

Reliability: Kuder-Richardson reliability ranged from .84 to .87. Test–retest (9 weeks) reliability was .75 ($N = 72$). Cronbach's alpha was .76 ($N = 150$).

Author: Topf, M.

Article: Personal and environmental predictors of

patient disturbance due to hospital noise.

Journal: *Journal of Applied Psychology*, February 1985, *70*(1), 22–28.

Related Research: Weinstein, N. (1978). Individual differences in reactions to noise: A longitudinal study in a college dormitory. *Journal of Applied Psychology, 63*, 458–466.

• • •

2851

Test Name: ORGANIZATIONAL CITIZENSHIP BEHAVIOR SCALE

Purpose: To measure helpful but not necessarily required employee behavior.

Number of Items: 16

Format: Employees are rated in 16 behaviors on a 5-point scale. All items are presented.

Reliability: Alpha ranged from .85 to .88 across two subscales (factors).

Validity: Two factors, altruism and generalized compliance, were identified by factor analysis (oblique rotation). Factors correlated .43.

Author: Smith, C. A., et al.

Article: Organizational citizenship behavior: Its nature and antecedents.

Journal: *Journal of Applied Psychology*, November 1983, *68*(4), 653–663.

• • •

2852

Test Name: OVEREXCITABILITY QUESTIONNAIRE

Purpose: To assess five forms of overexcitability.

Number of Items: 21

Format: Subjects' responses to each item written at their leisure were rated independently by two raters using a scale of intensity from 0 (*no overexcitability*) to 3 (*rich and intense expression*).

Reliability: Interrater correlation coefficients ranged from .60 to .95.

Author: Piechowski, M. M., et al.

Article: Comparison of intellectually and artistically gifted on five dimensions of mental functioning.

Journal: *Perceptual and Motor Skills*, April 1985, *60*(2), 539–549.

Related Research: Lysy, K. Z., & Piechowski, M. M. (1983). Personal growth: An empirical study using Jungian and Dabrowskian measures. *Genetic Psychology Monographs, 108*, 267–320.

• • •

2853

Test Name: OZAWA BEHAVIORAL RATING SCALE

Purpose: To assess attention deficit disorder (DSM III) in learning disabled children.

Number of Items: 15

Format: Employs a Likert format in which each item is assigned a value of 1 (*optimal attentive behavior*) to 5 (*optimal inattentive behavior*). The test provides 3 scores: impulsivity, distractability, and total score. Examples are presented.

Reliability: Coefficient alpha was .952 ($N = 52$).

Validity: Correlations with the WISC-R and the Matching Familiar Figures Test ranged from .18 to .50.

Author: Ozawa, J. P., and Michael, W. B.

Article: The concurrent validity of a behavioral rating scale for assessing attention deficit disorder (DSM III) in learning disabled children.

Journal: *Educational and Psychological Measurement,* Summer 1983, *43*(2), 623–632.

■ ■ ■

2854

Test Name: PAIN BEHAVIOR SCALE

Purpose: To provide a scale for rating pain behavior.

Number of Items: 10

Format: Items include: verbal, nonverbal, downtime, grimace, posture, mobility, body language, equipment use, stationary movement, medications. Items are rated 0 (*none*), .5 (*occasional*), or 1 (*frequent*).

Reliability: Three trained raters produced interrater reliabilities ranging from .94 to .96. Test–retest reliability over 2 consecutive days was .89.

Author: Feuerstein, M., et al.

Article: The Pain Behavior Scale: Modification and validation for outpatient use.

Journal: *Journal of Psychopathology and Behavioral Assessment,* December 1985, *7*(4), 301–305.

Related Research: Richards, J. S., et al. (1982). Assessing pain behavior: The UAB pain behavior scale. *Pain, 14,* 393–398.

■ ■ ■

2855

Test Name: PARENTAL BEHAVIOR SCALE

Purpose: To assess maternal and grandmaternal child-rearing activity.

Number of Items: 30

Format: Includes four parental

behaviors: supporting, demanding, controlling, and punishing. Examples are presented.

Reliability: Mean internal consistency for all subscales was .63. Mean factor-score reliability was .76.

Author: Wilson, M. N.

Article: Mothers' and grandmothers' perceptions of parental behavior in three-generational Black families.

Journal: *Child Development,* August 1984, *55*(4), 1333–1339.

Related Research: Devereux, E. C., et al. (1969). Child-rearing in England and the United States: A cross-national campaign. *Journal of Marriage and the Family, 31,* 257–270.

■ ■ ■

2856

Test Name: PARENT CHECKLIST OF CHILD BEHAVIOR

Purpose: To rate behaviors of children during the prior month.

Number of Items: 53

Format: *Never true* to *always true* response categories.

Reliability: Alphas ranged from .58 to .83 over subscales. Total alpha was .88.

Author: Hodges, W. F., et al.

Article: The cumulative effect of stress on preschool children of divorced and intact families.

Journal: *Journal of Marriage and the Family,* August 1984, *46*(3), 611–617.

Related Research: Hodges, W. F., et al. (1983). Parent–child relationships and adjustment in preschool children in divorced and intact families. *Journal of Divorce, 7,* 43–58.

2857

Test Name: PEDIATRIC PAIN QUESTIONNAIRE

Purpose: To elicit children's description of pain.

Number of Items: 45

Format: All items are presented. Items include short answer responses.

Reliability: Test–retest (72-hour time span, $N = 97$ children grades 4 to 7) produced 70% agreement between first and second sets of responses.

Author: Tesler, M., et al.

Article: Developing an instrument for eliciting children's description of pain.

Journal: *Perceptual and Motor Skills,* February 1983, *56*(1), 315–321.

Related Research: Melzack, R. (1975). The McGill questionnaire: Major properties and scoring methods. *Pain, 1,* 277–299.

■ ■ ■

2858

Test Name: PEJORATIVE EPITHET SCALE

Purpose: To measure the aggressiveness and frequency of aggressive use of epithets.

Number of Items: 316

Format: Subjects were to indicate how much aggression a word implied if used against them and how often it has been used in general (on TV, in print media, and so on).

Reliability: Repeated words reliability was .95 ($p < .01$; correlation between first and second ratings).

Validity: Aggressiveness and frequency of use ratings correlated .59 ($p < .001$).

Author: Driscoll, J. M.

Article: Aggressiveness and frequency of aggressive-use ratings for pejorative epithets by Americans.

Journal: *Journal of Social Psychology,* June 1981, *114*(first half), 111–126.

■ ■ ■

2859

Test Name: PERCEPTIONS OF STUDENT MISBEHAVIOR SCALE

Purpose: To measure perceived reasons for student problem behavior.

Number of Items: 26

Format: Likert response categories for each of 26 reasons (*very important* to *not important*). All items presented.

Reliability: Interjudge reliability of 26 reasons: 87.6%.

Author: Guttman, J.

Article: Pupils', teachers', and parents' causal attributions for problem behavior at school.

Journal: *Journal of Educational Research,* September/October 1982, *76*(1), 14–21.

Related Research: Weiner, B. (Ed.). (1974). *Achievement motivation and attribution theory.* Morristown, NJ: General Learning Press.

■ ■ ■

2860

Test Name: PHYSICAL HEALTH LOG

Purpose: To measure frequency and duration of acute and chronic physical illness by self-report.

Number of Items: 45

Format: Individuals are asked how many episodes of 28 diseases they experienced and how long they lasted (over past 12 months).

Reliability: Test–retest ranged between .66 and .91 for various items.

Validity: No sex differences in reliabilities were found.

Author: Blotcky, A. D., et al.

Article: Reliability of retrospective self-reports of physical illness.

Journal: *Psychological Reports,* February 1984, *54*(1), 179–182.

■ ■ ■

2861

Test Name: PLAY BEHAVIORS OBSERVATION SYSTEM

Purpose: To measure play behaviors in children.

Number of Items: 8

Format: Eight cognitive play categories (all described) are rated by trained observers.

Reliability: Interobserver agreement per 30-s time units ranged from .74 to 1.00 (M = .90; Mdn = .88).

Author: Rooparine, J. L.

Article: Peer play interaction in a mixed-age preschool setting.

Journal: *Journal of General Psychology,* April 1981, *101*(second half), 161–166.

Related Research: Parten, M. B. (1932). Social participation among preschool children. *Journal of Abnormal and Social Psychology,* 1932, *27*, 243–269.

Smilansky, S. (1975). *The effects of sociodramatic play on disadvantaged preschool children.* New York: Wiley.

■ ■ ■

2862

Test Name: PLAY REPORT

Purpose: To measure the degree of social complexity present in play choices.

Number of Items: 4

Format: For each question, two play choices were requested and the children were to circle with whom they played, that is, by themselves, with grownups, with friends, or on a team. All items are presented.

Reliability: Ranged from .43 to .88 (boys) and .24 to .77 (girls).

Validity: .75 (boys) and .64 (girls).

Author: Sleet, D. A.

Article: Differences in the social complexity of children's play choices.

Journal: *Perceptual and Motor Skills,* February 1985, *60*(1), 283–287.

Related Research: Seagoe, M. V. (1970). An instrument for the analysis of children's play as an index of degree of socialization. *Journal of School Psychology, 8,* 139–143.

■ ■ ■

2863

Test Name: PRACTICAL TRAINING OBSERVATION SCHEDULE

Purpose: To measure behavior of instructors and trainees in the metalworking industry.

Number of Items: 18 (behavior categories).

Format: Behavior coded on observation sheet in linear time structure. All items presented. Code sheet illustrated.

Reliability: Interobserver agreement was .91.

Author: Jungermann, H., et al.

Article: Observation of interaction in practical training.

Journal: *Journal of Occupational Psychology,* December 1981, *54*(4), 233–245.

Related Research: Flanders, N. A.

(1970). *Analyzing teaching behavior*. Reading, MA: Addison-Wesley.

• • •

2864

Test Name: PREVENTIVE HEALTH BEHAVIOR INVENTORY

Purpose: To assess extent of preventive health care behavior.

Number of Items: 41 behaviors.

Format: Items rated on a 5-point frequency scale (*always* to *never*).

Reliability: Kuder-Richardson formula 20 was .79. Test–retest (3-day interval) reliability was .84.

Author: Price, J. H., et al.

Article: Preventive health behaviors related to the ten leading causes of mortality of health-fair attenders and non-attenders.

Journal: *Psychological Reports*, February 1985, *56*(1), 131–135.

Related Research: Baur, K. G., & Wilson, R. W. (1981). The challenge of prevention: Are America's greatest health burdens avoidable? *HCFA Form, 5,* 16–25.

• • •

2865

Test Name: PROBLEM BEHAVIOR RATING SCALE

Purpose: To assess teachers' perceptions of problem classroom behavior.

Number of Items: 20

Format: Items rated on a 5-point rating scale. All items presented.

Reliability: Alpha was .80.

Author: Safran, S. P., and Safran, J. S.

Article: Classroom context and teachers' perceptions of problem behaviors.

Journal: *Journal of Educational Psychology*, February 1985, *77*(1), 20–28.

Related Research: Gropper, G., et al. (1968). Training teachers to recognize and manage social and emotional problems in the classroom. *Journal of Teacher Education, 19,* 477–485.

• • •

2866

Test Name: PROBLEM INVENTORY FOR ADOLESCENT GIRLS

Purpose: To measure the competence of the behavior of adolescent girls.

Number of Items: 52

Format: Subjects respond to 52 situations by explaining what they would do. Raters then judge the competence of the response on a 5-point scale. Sample situations are presented.

Reliability: Interrater alphas .70 or larger.

Validity: Classified 85% of subjects into delinquent/nondelinquent categories.

Author: Gaffney, L. R., and McFall, R. M.

Article: A comparison of social skills in delinquent and non-delinquent girls using a behavioral role-playing inventory.

Journal: *Journal of Consulting and Clinical Psychology*, December 1981, *49*(6), 959–967.

• • •

2867

Test Name: PROCEDURE BEHAVIOR CHECKLIST

Purpose: To assess behavioral manifestations of pain.

Number of Items: 8

Format: Each behavior is rated by observers on a 1–5 scale of pain severity. All categories presented.

Reliability: Interrater correlations ranged from .16 to .86 across pain types and three time periods. Of 9 total correlations only one was nonsignificant ($p < .05$ or $p < .01$).

Author: LeBaron, S., and Zeltzer, L.

Article: Assessment of acute pain and anxiety in children and adolescents by self-reports, observer reports, and a behavior checklist.

Journal: *Journal of Consulting and Clinical Psychology*, October 1984, *52*(5), 729–738.

Related Research: Katz, E. R., et al. (1981). Behavioral distress in children with cancer undergoing medical procedures: Developmental considerations. *Journal of Consulting and Clinical Psychology, 49,* 470–471.

• • •

2868

Test Name: PROCRASTINATION LOG

Purpose: To measure clients' perceptions of their current levels of procrastination, their effort to change, and their satisfaction with those levels.

Number of Items: 22

Format: Includes four scales: procrastination behavior, procrastination satisfaction, effort to change, and effort satisfaction. Responses were made on 7-point scales.

Reliability: Test–retest reliabilities ranged from .50 to .62. Internal consistency reliabilities ranged from .63 to .78.

Author: Claiborn, C. D., et al.

Article: Effects of congruence between counselor interpretations and client beliefs.

Journal: *Journal of Counseling*

Psychology, March 1981, *28*(2), 101–109.

Related Research: Strong, S. R., et al. (1979). Motivational and equipping functions of interpretation in counseling. *Journal of Counseling Psychology, 26*, 98–107.

■ ■ ■

2869

Test Name: PROCRASTINATION LOG

Purpose: To measure procrastination behavior and satisfaction with that behavior.

Number of Items: 11

Format: Self-report form including two subscales.

Reliability: Internal consistency reliabilities were .63 and .77.

Author: Damstreegt, D. C., and Christofferson, J.

Article: Objective self-awareness as a variable in counseling process and outcome.

Journal: *Journal of Counseling Psychology*, July 1982, *29*(4), 421–424.

Related Research: Strong, S. R., et al. (1979). Motivational and equipping functions of interpretation in counseling. *Journal of Counseling Psychology, 26*, 98–107.

■ ■ ■

2870

Test Name: PUPIL RATING FORM

Purpose: To measure behavior and personality of students by quantifying information in school records.

Time Required: 15 minutes.

Format: Teachers rate 28 dimensions on a 1-to-5 rating scale.

Reliability: Test–retest ranged from .63 to .95 (*Mdn* = .84). Interjudge reliability ranged from .41 to .82 (*Mdn* = .70).

Validity: Correlations with observational data ranged from .26 to .69 (*Mdn* = .48).

Author: Watt, N. F., et al.

Article: Social, emotional and intellectual behavior at school among children at high risk for schizophrenia.

Journal: *Journal of Consulting and Clinical Psychology*, April 1982, *50*(2), 171–181.

Related Research: Watt, N. F., et al. (1970). School adjustment and behavior of children hospitalized for schizophrenia as adults. *American Journal of Orthopsychiatry, 40*, 637–657.

■ ■ ■

2871

Test Name: RATIONAL BEHAVIOR INVENTORY

Purpose: To measure the rationality–irrationality continuum.

Number of Items: 37

Format: Agreement or disagreement indicated on a 5-point scale.

Reliability: Correlation between pre- and posttest scores ranged between .32 and .69 (10-week interval).

Author: Thyer, B. A., et al.

Article: Cognitive belief systems and their persistence: Test–retest reliability of the Rational Behavior Inventory.

Journal: *Psychological Reports*, December 1983, *53*(3, Part 1), 915–918.

Related Research: Shorkey, C., & Whiteman, V. (1977). Development of the Rational Behavior Inventory: Initial

validity and reliability. *Educational and Psychological Measurement, 37*, 527–534.

■ ■ ■

2872

Test Name: SCHOOL LEADERSHIP INVENTORY

Purpose: To measure leadership styles in schools.

Number of Items: 20

Format: Multiple-choice.

Reliability: Split-half reliability was .89.

Author: Cummings, O. W., and Nall, R. L.

Article: Counselor burnout and school leadership style: A connection.

Journal: *The School Counselor*, January 1982, *29*(3), 190–195.

Related Research: Likert, R. (1967). *The human organization: Its management and value.* New York: McGraw-Hill.

■ ■ ■

2873

Test Name: SELF-CONTROL SCHEDULE

Purpose: To measure learned resourcefulness.

Number of Items: 36

Format: Items rated on a 6-point self-rating scale.

Reliability: Test–retest (4 weeks) reliability was .96; alpha ranged from .78 to .86.

Author: Rosenbaum, M., and Palmon, N.

Article: Helplessness and resourcefulness in coping with epilepsy.

Journal: *Journal of Consulting and Clinical Psychology*, April 1984, *52*(2), 244–253.

Related Research: Rosenbaum, M.

(1980). A schedule for assessing self-control behaviors: Preliminary findings. *Behavior Therapy, 11,* 109–121.

■ ■ ■

2874

Test Name: SELF REPORT DELINQUENCY SCALE

Purpose: To measure delinquency.

Number of Items: 6

Format: Open-ended frequency scales. All items presented.

Reliability: Alpha was .78.

Author: Hagan, J., et al.

Article: The class structure of gender and delinquency: Toward a power-control theory of common delinquent behavior.

Journal: *American Journal of Sociology,* May 1986, *90*(3), 1151–1178.

Related Research: Hirschi, T. (1969). *Causes of delinquency.* Berkeley and Los Angeles: University of California Press.

■ ■ ■

2875

Test Name: SEXUAL EXPERIENCES SURVEY

Purpose: To measure sexual aggression and victimization.

Number of Items: 10

Format: Yes–no format.

Reliability: Alpha was .74 (women); .89 (men). Test–retest agreement over 2 weeks was 93%.

Validity: Self-report correlated .73 (women) and .61 (men) with report to an interviewer (both $ps < .01$).

Author: Koss, M. P., and Gidycz, C. A.

Article: Sexual experiences survey: Reliability and validity.

Journal: *Journal of Consulting and*

Clinical Psychology, June 1985, *53*(3), 422–423.

Related Research: Koss, M. P., & Oros, C. J. (1982). The sexual experiences survey: A research instrument for investigating sexual aggression and victimization. *Journal of Consulting and Clinical Psychology, 50,* 455–457.

■ ■ ■

2876

Test Name: SEXUAL FANTASY QUESTIONNAIRE

Purpose: To measure intensity of sexual fantasies.

Number of Items: 34

Format: Frequency indicated in Likert format: occasion of fantasy indicated by noting masturbation or intercourse. Items presented.

Reliability: Cronbach's alpha was .79; test–retest (2-day interval) reliability was .84.

Author: Price, J. H., and Miller, P. A.

Article: Sexual fantasies of Black and of White college students.

Journal: *Psychological Reports,* June 1984, *54*(3), 1007–1014.

Related Research: Shanor, K. (1977). *The fantasy files.* New York: Times Books.

■ ■ ■

2877

Test Name: SLEEP QUESTIONNAIRE

Purpose: To provide a subjective assessment of sleep.

Number of Items: 55

Format: Includes 7 factors: depth of sleep, difficulties in waking up, quality and latency of sleep, negative-affect dreams, length of sleep, dream recall and vividness, and sleep irregularity. Responses are made on a 5-point Likert scale.

Sample items are presented.

Reliability: Test–retest (10 weeks) reliability coefficients ranged from .68 to .96 ($N = 45$); Cronbach's alpha ranged from .53 to .88 ($N = 88$).

Author: Domino, G., et al.

Article: Subjective assessment of sleep by sleep questionnaire.

Journal: *Perceptual and Motor Skills,* August 1984, *59*(1), 163–170.

Related Research: Domino, G., & Fogl, A. (1980). Sleep patterns in college students. *Psychology, 17,* 7–14.

■ ■ ■

2878

Test Name: STONY BROOK SCALE

Purpose: To assess hyperactivity and aggression in hyperactive children.

Number of Items: 92

Format: Judges use 5- or 6-point scale to rate children.

Validity: Correlations between the Stony Brook Scale and the Connors Teacher-Rating Scale and Peterson-Quay Behavior Problem Checklist confirm validity through factor structure of responses on the latter two scales.

Author: O'Leary, S., and Steen, P. L.

Article: Subcategorizing hyperactivity: The Stony Brook Scale.

Journal: *Journal of Consulting and Clinical Psychology,* June 1982, *50*(3), 426–432.

Related Research: Loney, J., et al. (1978). An empirical basis for subgrouping the hyperkinetic/ minimal brain dysfunction syndrome. *Journal of Abnormal Psychology, 87,* 431–441.

2879

Test Name: STUDENT ACTIVIST SCALE

Purpose: To measure activist behavior.

Number of Items: 3

Format: Guttman.

Reliability: Reproducibility .90 or greater. Scalability .60 or greater.

Author: Green, J. J., et al.

Article: College activism reassessed: The development of activists and non-activists from successive cohorts.

Journal: *Journal of Social Psychology*, October 1984, *124*(first half), 105–113.

■ ■ ■

2880

Test Name: STUDENT BEHAVIOR OBSERVATION INSTRUMENT

Purpose: To measure types of behavior in classrooms.

Number of Items: 19

Format: Behavior recorded for one student at a time for 6 minutes over 10 days. Procedure involved 5 seconds of observation and 7 seconds of recording.

Reliability: Cohen's Kappa was .91.

Author: Howe, A. C., et al.

Article: Pupil behaviors and interactions in desegregated urban junior high activity-centered science classrooms.

Journal: *Journal of Educational Psychology*, February 1985, *75*(1), 97–103.

Related Research: Power, C. N., & Tisher, R. P. (1974). *Interaction patterns and their relationship with outcomes in Australian science education project classrooms*. Paper presented at the annual meeting of the National Association for Research in Science Teaching, Chicago, April.

■ ■ ■

2881

Test Name: STUDENT BEHAVIORS QUESTIONNAIRE

Purpose: To measure desirability of student behavior as assessed by faculty members.

Number of Items: 57

Format: Items rated on 5-point Likert response categories. All items presented.

Reliability: Internal consistency was .81.

Author: Brozo, W. G., and Schmelzer, R. V.

Article: Faculty perceptions of student behaviors: A comparison of two universities.

Journal: *Journal of College Student Personnel*, May 1985, *26*(3), 229–234.

Related Research: Williams, V. G., & Winkworth, J. M. (1974). The faculty looks at student behaviors. *Journal of College Student Personnel, 15,* 305–310.

■ ■ ■

2882

Test Name: STUDENT OBSERVATION FORM

Purpose: To measure observed student behavior in the classroom.

Number of Items: 5 variables each with 2 to 7 categories.

Time Required: 55-second observation cycles.

Format: 10 observations per subject per 55-minute class period. Coded variables are presented.

Reliability: Interrater reliability was .78.

Author: Seifert, E. H., and Beck, J. J., Jr.

Article: Relationships between task time and learning gains in secondary schools.

Journal: *Journal of Educational Research,* September/October 1984, *78*(1), 5–10.

■ ■ ■

2883

Test Name: STUDY SKILLS QUESTIONNAIRE

Purpose: To measure time management, concentration, listening, note-taking, text-reading, and test preparation.

Number of Items: 36

Format: Respondents are asked to indicate how representative an item is of their behavior. Sample items are presented.

Reliability: Test–retest (over 2 weeks) reliability was .82 ($N = 72$).

Author: Scott, K. J., and Robbins, S. B.

Article: Goal instability: Implications for academic performance among students in learning skills courses.

Journal: *Journal of College Student Personnel*, March 1985, *26*(2), 129–133.

Related Research: Kochenour, E., et al. (1983). *Developing a model of academic success: An empirical analysis*. Paper presented at the American College Personnel Association Convention, Houston, March.

■ ■ ■

2884

Test Name: SUPPORTIVE LEADERSHIP BEHAVIOR SCALE

Purpose: To measure leader supportiveness.

Number of Items: 17

Format: Includes 10 items from Form XII of the Ohio State Leader

Behavior Description Questionnaire and 7 items pertaining to other leader behavior dimensions.

Reliability: Coefficient alpha was .86.

Validity: Correlations with other variables ranged from −.33 to .26.

Author: Smith, C. A., et al.

Article: Organizational citizenship behavior: Its nature and antecedents.

Journal: *Journal of Applied Psychology,* November 1983, *68*(4), 653–663.

Related Research: House, R. J., & Dressler, G. (1974). The path-goal theory of leadership: Some post hoc and a priori tests. In J. G. Hunt & L. L. Larson (Eds.), *Contingency approaches to leadership.* Carbondale: Southern Illinois University Press.

■ ■ ■

2885

Test Name: SURVEY OF HETEROSOCIAL INTERACTIONS

Purpose: To measure approach behavior.

Number of Items: 20

Format: Taps interactive ability in specific heterosexual-social situations.

Validity: Correlations with Heterosocial Assessment Inventory for Women ranged from .51 to .78.

Author: Kolko, D. J.

Article: The Heterosocial Assessment Inventory for Women: A psychometric and behavioral evaluation.

Journal: *Journal of Psychopathology and Behavioral Assessment,* March 1985, *7*(1), 49–64.

Related Research: Twentyman,

C. T., & McFall, R. M. (1975). Behavioral training of social skills in shy males. *Journal of Consulting and Clinical Psychology, 43,* 384–395.

■ ■ ■

2886

Test Name: SUSTAINING FANTASY QUESTIONNAIRE— SHORT FORM

Purpose: To measure sustaining functions of fantasies.

Number of Items: 88

Format: Includes 10 factors: aesthetics, use of God, power and revenge, admiration of self, dying and illness, withdrawal and protection, love and closeness, suffering, competition, restitution. Responses to each item are made on a 5-point Likert-scale from 1 (*hardly at all*) to 5 (*extremely*). All items are presented.

Reliability: Cronbach's alpha for each scale ranged from .67 to .90.

Validity: Correlations with MMPI scores ranged from −.33 to .52.

Author: Zelin, M. L., et al.

Article: The Sustaining Fantasy Questionnaire: Measurement of sustaining functions of fantasies in psychiatric inpatients.

Journal: *Journal of Personality Assessment,* August 1983, *47*(4), 427–439.

■ ■ ■

2887

Test Name: TEACHER BEHAVIOR SCALE

Purpose: To measure teacher classroom behavior.

Number of Items: 19

Time Required: 80 minutes (ten 8-minute periods).

Format: Test consists of 8 minutes of observation in 10-second

blocks. Examples of behavior are presented for all 19 behaviors.

Reliability: Number of Agreement/ Total Agreement + Disagreements = .79.

Author: Hoskins, R., et al.

Article: Teacher and student behavior in high and low ability groups.

Journal: *Journal of Educational Psychology,* December 1983, *75*(6), 865–876.

■ ■ ■

2888

Test Name: TEACHER CLASSROOM BEHAVIOR SCALE

Purpose: To measure anger, praise, instruction-giving, and encouragement of students.

Number of Items: 17

Format: Observations done in half-day sessions using a tally-system. All 17 behaviors presented with examples.

Reliability: Ranged from .67 to 1.00 across items.

Author: Ascione, F. R., and Borg, W. R.

Article: A teacher-training program to enhance mainstreamed handicapped pupils' self-concepts.

Journal: *Journal of School Psychology,* 1983, *21*(4), 297–301.

Related Research: Borg, W. F. (1977). Changing teacher and pupil performance with protocols. *Journal of Experimental Education, 45,* 9–18.

■ ■ ■

2889

Test Name: TEACHER LEADERSHIP BEHAVIOR SCALE

Purpose: To measure student

perceptions of teacher leadership behavior.

Number of Items: 5

Format: Items rated on a 5-point scale from *a very little extent* to *a very great extent*. All items presented.

Reliability: Alpha was .90.

Author: Peterson, M. F., and Cooke, R. A.

Article: Attitudinal and contextual variables explaining teachers' leadership behavior.

Journal: *Journal of Educational Psychology,* February 1983, *75*(1), 50–62.

Related Research: Taylor, J. C., & Bowers, D. G. (1972). *Survey of organizations.* Ann Arbor, MI: Institute for Social Research, University of Michigan.

■ ■ ■

2890

Test Name: TEACHER RATING SCALE

Purpose: To measure teachers' ratings of children on misbehavior and academic concentration.

Number of Items: 73

Format: Items rated on a 5-point (*always–never*) scale.

Reliability: Internal consistency was .98.

Author: Forness, S. R., and MacMillan, D. L.

Article: Influences on the sociometric ratings of mildly handicapped children: A path analysis.

Journal: *Journal of Educational Psychology,* February 1983, *75*(1), 63–74.

Related Research: Agard, J. A., et al. (1978). *Teacher Rating Scale: An Instrument of the PRIME Instrument Battery.* Unpublished manuscript: U.S. Office of

Education/Bureau for Education of the Handicapped.

■ ■ ■

2891

Test Name: TEACHER'S SELF-CONTROL RATING SCALE

Purpose: To enable teachers to rate children on self-control.

Number of Items: 15

Format: Items rated on a 5-point rating scale (1 = *never,* 5 = *very often*). All items are presented.

Reliability: Test–retest (2-week) reliability was .94. Reliability was .88 to .93 across two subscales.

Validity: A total of 24 out of 30 correlation coefficients correlated significantly with Child Behavior Rating Scale (significant correlations ranged from .30 to .81; $p < .05$).

Author: Humphrey, L. L.

Article: Children's and teachers' perspectives on children's self-control: The development of two rating scales.

Journal: *Journal of Consulting and Clinical Psychology,* October 1982, *50*(5), 624–633.

Related Research: Kendall, P. C., & Wilcox, L. E. (1979). Self-control in children: Development of a rating scale. *Journal of Consulting and Clinical Psychology, 47,* 1020–1029.

■ ■ ■

2892

Test Name: TEACHER TREATMENT INVENTORY

Purpose: To measure teacher behavior toward high or low achieving students (both male and female).

Number of Items: 43

Format: Items rated on a 4-category response scale (*always, often, sometimes, never*). All items

are presented.

Reliability: Alpha ranged from .71 to .80 across subscales.

Author: Weinstein, R. S., et al.

Article: Student perceptions of differential treatment in open and traditional classrooms.

Journal: *Journal of Educational Psychology,* October 1982, *74*(5), 678–692.

Related Research: Weinstein, R. S., and Middlestodt, S. E. (1979). Student perceptions of teacher interactions with male high and low achievers. *Journal of Educational Psychology, 71,* 421–431.

■ ■ ■

2893

Test Name: TEACHING BEHAVIOR SCALE FOR CHILD TUTORS

Purpose: To measure teaching behavior of children as tutors.

Number of Items: 11

Time Required: 10-minute tutoring session.

Format: Verbal transcripts coded by raters. All items presented.

Reliability: Percentage of observer agreement ranged from 88% to 96% across items.

Author: Ludeke, R. J., and Hartup, W. W.

Article: Teaching behaviors of 9- and 11-year-old girls in mixed-age and same-age dyads.

Journal: *Journal of Educational Psychology,* December 1983, *75*(6), 908–914.

2894

Test Name: UNION MEMBERSHIP AND BEHAVIOR SCALE

Purpose: To measure extent of union membership and behavior for university faculty members.

Number of Items: 6

Format: Yes–no format.

Reliability: Internal consistency was .57.

Author: Zalesny, M. D.

Article: Comparison of economic and non-economic factors in predicting faculty vote preference in a union representation election.

Journal: *Journal of Applied Psychology*, May 1985, *70*(2), 243–256.

Related Research: Terborg, J. R., et al. (1982). *University faculty dispositions toward unionization: A test of Triand's model.* Paper presented at the American Psychological Association Meeting, Washington, DC.

■ ■ ■

2895

Test Name: VALENCE SCALE

Purpose: To assess desirability,

importance, attractiveness, and influence of actions.

Number of Items: 4

Format: Items rated on a 5-point Likert scale.

Reliability: Alpha was .80.

Author: Campbell, D. J.

Article: The effects of goal-contingent payment on the performance of a complex task.

Journal: *Personnel Psychology*, Spring 1984, *37*(2), 23–40.

Related Research: Campbell, D. J. (1976). *A critical examination and comparison of instrumentality and social exchange theories.* Unpublished doctoral dissertation, Purdue University.

■ ■ ■

2896

Test Name: WILE GROUP LEADERSHIP QUESTIONNAIRE

Purpose: To measure alternative

leaders' behavior.

Number of Items: 21 group situations are described.

Format: For each situation, 19 alternative behaviors are listed. Respondents choose which one most closely resembles their own styles.

Reliability: Ranged from .50 to .86 over the 19 scales.

Author: Gardner, K. G., et al.

Article: Toward a comprehensive assessment of leadership behavior in groups.

Journal: *Psychological Reports*, December 1982, *51*(3, Part 1), 991–998.

Related Research: Wile, D. B. (1972). Non-experimental uses of the Group Leadership Questionnaire (GTO-C). In J. W. Pfeiffer & J. E. Jones (Eds.), *The 1972 annual handbook for group facilitators* (pp. 36–67). Iowa City: University Associates.

CHAPTER 9
Communication

2897

Test Name: ADOLESCENT COMMUNICATION INVENTORY

Purpose: To elicit the child's perception of satisfaction of communication with his or her parents.

Number of Items: 33

Format: Children address the questions twice: first with reference to mother and again in reference to father.

Reliability: Test–retest (2 to 3 weeks) reliability coefficients ranged from .78 to .88. Split-half reliability coefficient was .86.

Validity: Correlations with Coopersmith Self-Esteem Inventory were .74 and .14 ($N=$ 60).

Author: Omizo, M. M., et al.

Article: The Coopersmith Self-Esteem Inventory as a predictor of feelings and communication satisfaction toward parents among learning disabled, emotionally disturbed and normal adolescents.

Journal: *Educational and Psychological Measurement,* Summer 1985, *45*(2), 389–395.

Related Research: Bienvenu, M. J. (1970). Measurement of marital communication. *Family Coordinator, 18,* 26–31.

•••

2898

Test Name: ADOLESCENT GOAL ATTAINMENT SCALE

Purpose: To measure and evaluate

goal attainment of individual counseling.

Number of Items: Can contain one to five goals.

Format: Items rated on a 5-point scale ranging from best anticipated success to most likely unfavorable outcome. Ratings made independently by student and counselor.

Reliability: Weighted kappas averaged between .42 and .82 with all but one showing significant pupil–counselor agreement.

Validity: Correlation was .48 between goal attainment scores and teacher ratings of satisfaction with students.

Author: Maher, C. A., and Barbrack, C. R.

Article: Evaluating individual counseling of conduct problem adolescents: The goal attainment scaling method.

Journal: *Journal of School Psychology,* 1984, *22*(3), 285–297.

Related Research: Kiresuk, T. J., & Sherman, R. E. (1968). Goal attainment scaling: A general method for evaluating mental health programs. *Community Mental Health Journal, 4,* 443–453.

•••

2899

Test Name: BARRETT-LEONARD RELATIONSHIP INVENTORY

Purpose: To measure development of client–counselor relationship.

Number of Items: 64

Format: Multiple-choice for positive and negative items pertaining to core therapeutic conditions.

Reliability: Test–retest reliability was .92.

Author: Lawe, C. F., et al.

Article: Effects of pretraining procedures for clients in counseling.

Journal: *Psychological Reports,* August 1983, *53*(1), 327–334.

Related Research: Lin, T. (1964). Counseling relationship as a function of counselor's self-confidence. *Journal of Counseling Psychology, 20,* 293–297.

Hill, C. E., et al. (1981). Nonverbal communication and counseling outcome. *Journal of Counseling Psychology, 28*(3), 203–212.

Curtis, J. M. (1981). Effect of therapist's self-disclosure on patients' impressions of empathy, competence and trust in analogue of a psychotherapeutic interaction. *Psychological Reports, 48*(1), 127–136.

Chippaone, D., et al. (1981). Relationship of client-perceived facilitative conditions on outcome of behaviorally oriented assertive training. *Psychological Reports, 49*(1), 251–256.

•••

2900

Test Name: BARRETT-LEONARD RELATIONSHIP INVENTORY—REVISED

Purpose: To measure the client's

perception of the counselor.

Number of Items: 36

Format: Includes 5 dimensions: empathic understanding, unconditionality of regard, level of regard, congruence, and resistance.

Reliability: Reliability coefficients corrected by the Spearman-Brown formula ranged from .82 to .93.

Author: Bacorn, C. N., and Dixon, D. N.

Article: The effects of touch on depressed and vocationally undecided clients.

Journal: *Journal of Counseling Psychology,* October 1984, *31*(4), 488–496.

Related Research: Mann, B., & Murphy, K. C. (1975). Timing of self-disclosure, reciprocity of self-disclosure and reactions to an initial interview. *Journal of Counseling Psychology, 22,* 304–308.

Claiborn, C. D., et al. (1983). Effects of intervention discrepancy for negative emotions. *Journal of Counseling Psychology, 30*(2), 164–171.

■ ■ ■

2901

Test Name: BARRETT-LEONARD RELATIONSHIP INVENTORY—REVISED

Purpose: To measure counselor effectiveness.

Number of Items: 85

Format: Includes the following: empathy, genuineness, unconditionality of regard, level of regard, and resistance. Examples are presented.

Reliability: Internal consistency reliabilities ranged from .73 to .92. Test–retest (2-week to 12-month intervals) reliability ranged from .80 to .90.

Author: Ponterotto. J. G., and Furlong, M. J.

Article: Evaluating counselor effectiveness: A critical review of rating scale instruments.

Journal: *Journal of Counseling Psychology,* October 1985, *32*(4), 597–616.

Related Research: Claiborn, C. D., et al. (1983). Effects of intervention discrepancy for negative emotions. *Journal of Counseling Psychology, 30*(2), 164–171.

■ ■ ■

2902

Test Name: CARLETON UNIVERSITY RESPONSIVENESS TO SUGGESTION SCALE (CURSS)

Purpose: To assess responsiveness to test suggestions associated with hypnosis.

Number of Items: 7

Format: Subjects rate extent to which they experience what is suggested by each item on a 4-point scale.

Reliability: Item-total correlations ranged from .43 to .98.

Validity: Coefficients of reproducibility ranged from .86 to .89 over subscales.

Author: Spanos, N. P., et al.

Article: The Carleton University Responsiveness to Suggestion Scale: Normative data and psychometric properties.

Journal: *Psychological Reports,* October 1983, *53*(2), 523–535.

Related Research: Spanos, N. P., et al. (1983). The Carleton University Responsiveness to Suggestion Scale: Relationship with other measures of hypnotic susceptibility, expectancies and absorption. *Psychological Reports, 53,* 723–734.

2903

Test Name: CLIENT RATING SCALE

Purpose: To measure therapists' ratings of client.

Number of Items: 11

Format: Items rated on a 7-point scale.

Reliability: Interrater reliability ranged from .83 to .91 across items.

Validity: Face validity judged acceptable.

Author: Genschaft, J. L.

Article: The effects of race and role preparation on therapeutic interaction.

Journal: *Journal of College Student Personnel,* January 1982, *23*(1), 33–35.

■ ■ ■

2904

Test Name: COMMUNICATION SATISFACTION QUESTIONNAIRE

Purpose: To measure satisfaction with communication in organizations.

Number of Items: 42

Format: Items rated on a 7-point Likert rating scale. All items are presented.

Reliability: Alpha ranged between .76 and .86 across 8 subscales.

Author: Crino, M. D., and White, M. C.

Article: Satisfaction in communication: An examination of the Downs-Hazen Measure.

Journal: *Psychological Reports,* 1981, *49*(3), 831–837.

Related Research: Downs, C., & Hazen, M. (1977). A factor analytic study of communication satisfaction. *Journal of Business Communication, 14,* 63–73.

2905

Test Name: COMMUNICATION SCALE

Purpose: To assess accurate conveyance of thoughts and feelings and ability to transmit expectations in dyads.

Number of Items: 18

Format: Responses are made on a 5-point scale from 1 (*never*) to 5 (*always*).

Reliability: Reliability coefficients were .75 (older parents) and .94 (children).

Validity: Correlations with other variables ranged from −.192 to .693.

Author: Quinn, W. H.

Article: Personal and family adjustment in later life.

Journal: *Journal of Marriage and the Family*, February 1983, *45*(1), 57–73.

Related Research: Bienvenu, M. J. (1970). Measurement of marital communication. *Family Coordinator, 19*, 26–31.

■ ■ ■

2906

Test Name: COMPLIANCE WITH INTERVIEWER REQUESTS SCALE

Purpose: To measure importance and willingness to give information to interviewer.

Number of Items: 26

Time Required: 10 minutes.

Format: Items rated on a 5-point rating scale for willingness and importance.

Reliability: Cronbach's alphas were .70 (importance) and .75 (willingness).

Author: Siegfried, W. D. (Jr)., and Wood, K.

Article: Reducing college student's

compliance with inappropriate interviewer requests: An educational approach.

Journal: *Journal of College Student Personnel*, January 1983, *24*(1), 66–71.

■ ■ ■

2907

Test Name: CONFIDENCE SCALE

Purpose: To measure information-processing confidence.

Number of Items: 10

Format: Likert format.

Reliability: Test–retest reliability was .69; alpha was .43.

Author: Evans, R. H.

Article: Innovativeness and information processing confidence.

Journal: *Psychological Reports*, April 1985, *56*(2), 557–558.

Related Research: Wright, P. (1975). Factors affecting cognitive resistance to advertising. *Journal of Consumer Research, 2*, 1–9.

■ ■ ■

2908

Test Name: CONTEXTUAL UNCERTAINTY SCALE

Purpose: To assess agreement and disagreement with second-order outcome links.

Number of Items: 5

Format: Items rated on a 5-point Likert format. All items presented.

Reliability: Alpha was .74.

Author: Ashford, S. J., and Cummings, L. L.

Article: Proactive feedback seeking: The instrumental use of the information environment.

Journal: *Journal of Occupational Psychology*, March 1985, *58*(1), 67–79.

Related Research: Heslin, R., et al. (1972). Information search as a function of stimulus uncertainty and the importance of the response. *Journal of Personality and Social Psychology, 23*, 333–339.

Tybout, A., & Scott, C. (1982). *When self-perception occurs: Certainty and informativeness of behaviors as mediators of processing.* Unpublished manuscript, Northwestern University.

■ ■ ■

2909

Test Name: COUNSELING APPROPRIATENESS CHECKLIST

Purpose: To measure appropriateness of discussing problems with counselors.

Number of Items: 66

Format: Items rated on 5-point Likert scales.

Reliability: Test–retest reliability was .88.

Validity: Five-member panel judged items to be valid.

Author: Miles, G. B., and McDavis, R. J.

Article: Effects of four orientation approaches on disadvantaged Black freshmen students' attitudes toward the counseling center.

Journal: *Journal of College Student Personnel*, September 1982, *23*(5), 413–418.

Related Research: Warman, R. (1969). Differential perceptions of counseling role. *Journal of Counseling Psychology, 7*, 269–274.

■ ■ ■

2910

Test Name: DECISION-MAKING POLICY SCALE

Purpose: To measure perceived influence in decision-making.

Number of Items: 4

Format: Items rated on a 5-point scale (*never true* to *always true*). Items are a subscale of Newman's PWE Scale.

Reliability: Alpha was .59.

Author: Jackson, S. E.

Article: Participation in decision-making as a strategy for reducing job-related stress.

Journal: *Journal of Applied Psychology*, February 1983, *68*(1) 3–19.

Related Research: Newman, J. E. (1977). Development of a measure of perceived work environment (PWE). *Academy of Management Journal, 20,* 520–534.

■ ■ ■

2911

Test Name: DYADIC INTERACTION SCALE

Purpose: To measure student-teacher interaction.

Number of Items: 11 categories of interaction.

Time Required: 40 minutes.

Format: Three observers record teacher–student interaction in classrooms.

Reliability: Interobserver agreement ranged from .80 to 1.00.

Author:. Irvine, J. J.

Article: Teacher communication patterns as related to the race and sex of the student.

Journal: *Journal of Educational Research,* July/August 1985, *78*(6), 338–345.

Related Research: Good, T., & Brophy, J. (1978). *Looking in classrooms.* New York: Harper & Row.

2912

Test Name: GROUP DECISION-MAKING SCALE

Purpose: To measure extent to which individuals perceive their work group as having decision-making responsibilities.

Number of Items: 13

Format: Items rated on a 5-point response format. Sample items are presented.

Reliability: Alpha was .82.

Author: Kemp, N. J., et al.

Article: Autonomous work groups in a Greenfield site: A comparative study.

Journal: *Journal of Occupational Psychology,* December 1983, *56*(4), 271–288.

Related Research: Gulowsen, J. (1972). A measure of work group autonomy. In L. E. Davis & J. C Taylor (Eds.), *Design of jobs.* London: Penguin.

■ ■ ■

2913

Test Name: INTERACTION CODING SYSTEM

Purpose: To assess speaker and listener skills.

Number of Items: 12 categories.

Format: Raters code responses that are homogeneous in content without regard to duration and syntactical structure. Sample items are presented for each of the 12 categories.

Reliability: Alpha ranged from .85 to .99 (verbal codes) and from .52 to .82 (nonverbal codes).

Author: Hahlweg, K., and Revenstorf, D.

Article: Effects of behavior marital therapy in couples' communication and problem-solving skills.

Journal: *Journal of Consulting and Counseling Psychology,* August 1984, *52*(4), 553–566.

Related Research: Wegener, C., et al. (1979). Empirical analysis of communication in distressed couples. *Behavior Analysis Modification, 3,* 178–188.

■ ■ ■

2914

Test Name: INTERPERSONAL TRUST SCALE

Purpose: To measure the generalized expectancy that oral and written statements can be relied upon.

Number of Items: 25

Reliability: Test–retest reliability was .58 and .68. Split-half reliability was .76. Cronbach's alpha was .79.

Validity: Correlations with other variables ranged from –.17 to .14.

Author: Cutler, B. L., and Wolfe, R. N.

Article: Construct validity of the Concern for Appropriateness Scale.

Journal: *Journal of Personality, Assessment,* June 1985, *49*(3), 318–323.

Related Research: Rotter, J. B. (1980). Interpersonal trust, trustworthiness and gullibility. *American Psychologist, 35,* 1–7.

■ ■ ■

2915

Test Name: LEADER–MEMBER EXCHANGE SCALE—REVISED

Purpose: To assess the quality of supervisor–subordinate interaction.

Number of Items: 5

Format: A 1-to-5 response format was employed.

Reliability: Coefficient alpha was .83.

Validity: Correlations with: average leadership style was .68, .48; turnover was −.19, −.44.

Author: Ferris, G. R.

Article: Role of leadership in the employee withdrawal process: A constructive replication.

Journal: *Journal of Applied Psychology,* November 1985, *70*(4), 777–781.

Related Research: Graen, G., et al. Role of leadership in the employee withdrawal process. *Journal of Applied Psychology, 67,* 868–872.

• • •

2916

Test Name: LEADER–MEMBER EXCHANGE SCALE—MEMBER FORM

Purpose: To measure the quality of exchange between supervisors and subordinates.

Number of Items: 7

Format: Response to each item was made on 4–point scales. All items were presented.

Reliability: Cronbach's alphas were .86 and .84. Test–retest correlation (6 months) was .67.

Author: Scandura, T. A., and Graen, G. B.

Article: Moderating effects of initial leader-member exchange status on the effects of a leadership intervention.

Journal: *Journal of Applied Psychology,* August 1984, *69*(3), 428–436.

Related Research: Liden, R., & Graen, G. (1980). Generalizability of the vertical dyad linkage model of leadership. *Academy of Management Journal, 23,* 451–465.

2917

Test Name: MEASURE OF ELEMENTARY COMMUNICATION APPREHENSION

Purpose: To measure communication apprehension.

Number of Items: 20

Format: Likert statements employing smiling and frowning faces. All items are presented.

Reliability: Test–retest reliability was .80. Split-half reliabilities ranged from .64 to .77.

Author: Harris, K. R., and Brown, R. D.

Article: Cognitive behavior modification and informed teacher treatments for shy children.

Journal: *Journal of Experimental Education,* Spring 1982, *50*(3), 137–143.

Related Research: Garrison, J. P., & Garrison (Harris), K. R. (1979). Measurement of communication apprehension among children: A factor in the development of basic speech skills. *Communication Education, 28,* 119–128.

• • •

2918

Test Name: NEGOTIATING LATITUDE SCALES

Purpose: To measure member-reported and leader-reported negotiating latitude.

Number of Items: 8 (4 member and 4 leader).

Format: Likert and multiple-choice formats. All items presented.

Reliability: Cronbach's alpha ranged from .62 to .68 across scales.

Author: Rosse, J. G., and Kraut, A. I.

Article: Reconsidering the vertical

dyad linkage model of leadership.

Journal: *Journal of Occupational Psychology,* March 1983, *56*(1), 63–71.

Related Research: Graen, G., & Schiemann, W. (1978). Leader–member agreement: A vertical dyad approach. *Journal of Applied Psychology, 63,* 206–212.

• • •

2919

Test Name: ORGANIZATIONAL COMMUNICATION SCALE

Purpose: To measure frequency of communication levels of organizational personnel.

Number of Items: 8

Format: 12-point frequency rating scale (daily to never). Sample items presented.

Reliability: Alpha ranged from .67 to .75 across three subscales.

Validity: Items factored into three dimensions corresponding to Hall's interpersonal, organizational, and interorganizational communication types.

Author: Hoffman, E.

Article: The effect of race-ratio composition on the frequency of organizational communication.

Journal: *Social Psychology Quarterly,* March 1985, *48*(1), 17–26.

Related Research: Hall, R. H. (1982). *Organizations: Structure and process.* Englewood Cliffs, NJ: Prentice-Hall.

• • •

2920

Test Name: PEAK COMMUNICATIONS EXPERIENCES SCALES

Purpose: To measure "great

moments" in interpersonal communication.

Number of Items: 19

Format: Items rated on 6-point Likert response categories. All items presented.

Validity: Six factors extracted. Women rated peak experiences higher than men ($p < .02$).

Author: Gordon, R. D.

Article: Dimensions of peak communications experiences: An exploratory study.

Journal: *Psychological Reports,* December 1985, *57*(3, Part 1), 824–826.

Related Research: Gordon, R., & Dulaney, E. (1983). Peak communication experiences: Concept, structure and sex differences. ERIC Research Document No. 221931.

■ ■ ■

2921

Test Name: PRIMARY COMMUNICATION INVENTORY

Purpose: To measure the frequency of both verbal and nonverbal communication.

Number of Items: 50

Format: Includes 25 verbal and nonverbal communications for which couples rate the frequency of occurrence between them.

Reliability: Test–retest reliability was .73.

Author: Tucker, C. M., and Horowitz, J. E.

Article: Assessment of factors in marital adjustment.

Journal: *Journal of Behavioral Assessment,* December 1981, *3*(4), 243–252.

Related Research: Navran, L. (1967). Communication and adjustment in marriage. *Family Process, 6,* 173–184.

■ ■ ■

2922

Test Name: RATING OF ALTER-COMPETENCE

Purpose: To measure partner's communicative competence in a particular episode.

Number of Items: 27

Format: Items assess the degree to which other was cooperative, trustworthy, disclosing, assertive, expressive, attentive, and so forth.

Reliability: Cronbach's alpha reliability coefficient was .95.

Validity: Correlations with other variables ranged from .48 to .79.

Author: Spitzberg, B. H., and Cupach, W. R.

Article: Conversational skill and locus of perception.

Journal: *Journal of Psychopathology and Behavioral Assessment,* September 1985, *7*(3), 207–220.

Related Research: Cupach, W. R., & Spitzberg, B. H. (1981). *Relational competence: Measurement and validation.* Paper presented at the Western Speech Communication Association Convention, San Jose, CA.

■ ■ ■

2923

Test Name: REFERENTIAL COMMUNICATIONS TEST

Purpose: To measure effectiveness of referential communication.

Number of Items: 10 pretest, 10 posttest, and 10 follow-up items.

Format: Items are word-pairs in which one is underlined. Children must create clues communicating which word is underlined to another child who must select between the two words. All pairs presented.

Reliability: Judges reach 80% agreement on quality of clues.

Author: Asher, S. R., and Wigfield, A.

Article: Influence and comparison training on children's referential communication.

Journal: *Journal of Educational Psychology,* April 1981, *73*(2), 232–241.

Related Research: Rosenberg, S., & Cohen, B. D. (1966). Referential processes of speakers and listeners. *Psychological Reports, 73,* 208–231.

■ ■ ■

2924

Test Name: SELF-RATED COMPETENCE

Purpose: To measure self's communicative competence in a particular episode.

Format: Items assess the degree to which self was cooperative, trustworthy, disclosing, assertive, expressive, attentive, and so forth.

Reliability: Cronbach's alpha reliability coefficient was .84.

Validity: Correlations with other variables ranged from .51 to .65.

Author: Spitzberg, B. H., and Cupach, W. R.

Article: Conversational skill and locus of perception.

Journal: *Journal of Psychopathology and Behavioral Assessment,* September 1985, *7*(3), 207–220.

Related Research: Cupach, W. R., & Spitzberg, B. H. (1981). *Relational competence: Measurement and validation.* Paper presented at the Western Speech Communication Association Convention, San Jose, CA.

2925

Test Name: SOCIAL REINFORCEMENT ORIENTATION CHECKLIST

Purpose: To measure the extent of use of smiling and other behavior in daily interaction.

Number of Items: 50

Format: Items rated on 3-point response categories indicating the extent of use. All items are presented.

Reliability: Test–retest reliability ranged from .65 to .78. Split-half reliability was .75.

Validity: Correlated .29 ($p < .05$) with extroversion and .37 ($p < .05$) with the F scale.

Author: Ibrahim, A.

Article: Social reinforcement orientation approach to personality.

Journal: *Psychological Reports,* June 1985, *56*(3), 743–750.

■ ■ ■

2926

Test Name: VERTICAL EXCHANGE SCALE

Purpose: To measure leader–member exchange.

Number of Items: 12

Format: Included: approachability and flexibility of supervisor toward the newcomer, supervisor's willingness to use authority to help the newcomer solve problems, clarity of the supervisor's expectations and feedback to the newcomer, the newcomer's latitude to influence the supervisor to change his or her role situation, and the opportunity of newcomers to share after-hours social and leisure activities.

Reliability: Cronbach's alpha ranged from .87 to .92; test–retest correlation coefficients ranged from .37 to .80.

Validity: Correlation with other variables ranged from −.18 to .36.

Author: Wakabayashi, M., and Graen, G. B.

Article: The Japanese career progress study: A 7-year follow-up.

Journal: *Journal of Applied Psychology,* November 1984, *69*(4), 603–614.

Related Research: Wakabayashi, M. (1980). *Managerial career progress in a Japanese organization.* Ann Arbor, MI: UMI Research Press.

CHAPTER 10
Concept Meaning

2927

Test Name: AUTOMATIC WORD PROCESSING TASK

Purpose: To measure the automaticity of word processing.

Number of Items: 20 (line drawings).

Format: Items are line drawings of an easily pictured noun of one syllable. Time for naming pictures appearing alone is subtracted from the time of name in Stroop condition. The difference is the measure of automatic word processing.

Reliability: SB ranged from .74 to .75.

Author: DeSoto, J. L., and DeSoto, C. B.

Article: Relationship of reading achievement to verbal processing abilities.

Journal: *Journal of Educational Psychology,* February 1983, *75*(1), 116–127.

Related Research: Rosinski, R. R., et al. (1975). Automatic semantic processing in a picture-word interference task. *Child Development, 46,* 247–253.

...

2928

Test Name: COMPETITION KNOWLEDGE TEST

Purpose: To measure the ability to distinguish between competition and other associated constructs.

Number of Items: 60

Format: Multiple-choice.

Reliability: Internal consistency ranged from .78 to .92. Kuder-Richardson formula 20 was .91.

Author: Kildea, A. E., and Kukulka, G.

Article: Reliability of the Competition Knowledge Test.

Journal: *Psychological Reports,* June 1984, *54*(3), 957–958.

Related Research: Kildea, A. E. (1983). Competition: A model for conception. *Quest, 35,* 169–181.

...

2929

Test Name: CONCEPT ATTAINMENT SCALE

Purpose: To measure concept attainment in science courses.

Number of Items: 12 items for each of 5 concepts.

Format: Multiple-choice. Sample concepts and items presented.

Reliability: Kuder-Richardson formula 20 was .89.

Validity: Validated by a panel of science educators.

Author: Rollins, M. M., et al.

Article: Attainment of selected earth science concepts by Texas high school seniors.

Journal: *Journal of Educational Research,* November/December 1983, *77*(2), 81–88.

Related Research: Frayer, D. A., et al. (1969). *A schema for testing the level of concept mastery* (Working Paper No. 16). Madison: Wisconsin Research and Development Center for Cognitive Learning.

...

2930

Test Name: CONCEPT DEFINITION AND APPLICATION TEST

Purpose: To measure student success at learning and applying concepts.

Number of Items: 20

Format: 10 "definition" and 10 "application" questions each with 5 multiple-choice responses.

Validity: Kuder-Richardson formula 20 was .78 (*N* = 68).

Author: Ross, S., et al.

Article: Field experiences as meaningful contexts for learning about learning.

Journal: *Journal of Educational Research,* November/December 1981, *75*(2), 103–107.

Related Research: Ross, S. M., & Bush, A. J. (1980). Effects of abstract and educationally oriented learning contexts on achievement and attitudes of preservice teachers. *Journal of Educational Research, 74,* 19–23.

...

2931

Test Name: IDEA INVENTORY

Purpose: To measure the rationality–irrationality cognitive dimension.

Number of Items: 33

Format: Items rated on a 3-point

agree–disagree scale. Sample items are presented.

Reliability: Test–retest reliability was .81 or more over two test occasions and for men and women.

Author: Vestre, N. D.

Article: Test–retest reliability of the idea inventory.

Journal: *Psychological Reports,* June 1984, *54*(3), 873–874.

Related Research: Kassinove, H. (et al). (1977). Developmental trends in rational thinking: Implications for rational emotive school mental health programs. *Journal of Community Psychology, 5,* 266–274.

■ ■ ■

2932

Test Name: INTERNAL SCANNING SCALE

Purpose: To measure breadth of association.

Number of Items: 73

Format: Free associations obtained for each of 73 words (items) that have no popular responses. Scores obtained by averaging the normative frequencies of responses.

Reliability: Split-half reliability was .93.

Author: Heilbrun, A. B., Jr.

Article: Cognitive defenses and life stress: An information-processing analysis.

Journal: *Psychological Reports,* February 1984, *54*(1), 3–17.

Related Research: Heilbrun, A. B., Jr. (1972). Style of adaptation to perceived aversive maternal control and internal scanning behavior. *Journal of Consulting and Clinical Psychology, 39,* 15–21.

2933

Test Name: NEGATION ELICITATION SCALE

Purpose: To measure negative language constructions.

Number of Items: 24

Format: Items were objects with something missing (wheels from small cars, for example). Children are asked what is wrong with objects. All items described.

Reliability: Interobserver agreement was 95%.

Validity: Correct constructions increase with age (3 to 6 years) for both monolingual and bilingual children.

Author: Madrid, D., and Garcia, E. E.

Article: Development of negation in bilingual Spanish/English and monolingual English speakers.

Journal: *Journal of Educational Psychology,* October 1981, *73*(5), 624–631.

■ ■ ■

2934

Test Name: PARAGRAPH COMPLETION METHOD

Purpose: To measure the degree of integrative complexity relative to interpersonal stimuli.

Number of Items: 5

Time Required: 2 minutes.

Format: A semi-projective measure, whereby subjects complete each stem by adding at least two additional sentences within a 2-minute time limit. Items are presented.

Reliability: Interrater reliability was .83.

Author: Strohmer, D. C., et al.

Article: Cognitive style and synchrony in measures of anxiety.

Journal: *Measurement and Evaluation in Guidance,* April 1983, *16*(1), 13–17.

Related Research: Harvey, O. J., et al. (1961). *Conceptual systems and personality organization.* New York: Wiley.

■ ■ ■

2935

Test Name: RECEPTIVE LANGUAGE MEASURE

Purpose: To measure infants' receptive language.

Number of Items: 34

Format: The infant is required to correctly identify the picture in each pair labeled by the experimenter.

Author: Ungerer, J. A., and Sigman, M.

Reliability: Test–retest reliabilities were .87 and .94. Kuder-Richardson coefficient was .91.

Article: The relation of play and sensorimotor behavior to language in the second year.

Journal: *Child Development,* August 1984, *55*(4), 1448–1455.

Related Research: Beckwith, L., & Thompson, S. (1976). Recognition of verbal labels of pictured objects and events by 17-to-30 month old infants. *Journal of Speech and Hearing Research, 19,* 690–699.

■ ■ ■

2936

Test Name: RELATIONSHIP JUDGEMENT TEST

Purpose: To measure the perceived relationship between pairs of concepts.

Number of Items: 20

Time Required: 15 minutes.

Format: Degree of relationship indicated on a 9-point scale.

Reliability: Test–retest (10-minute interval with concept pairs reversed) reliability was .67. (This is the mean correlation between test and retest for all respondents.)

Validity: Individual reliability correlated significantly with a multiple-choice exam over the same material ($r = .43$, $p < .001$).

Author: Diekhoff, G. M.

Article: Testing through relationship judgments.

Journal: *Journal of Educational Psychology,* April 1983, *75*(2), 227–233.

■ ■ ■

2937

Test Name: SIGHT WORD VOCABULARY TEST

Purpose: To measure sight word vocabulary.

Number of Items: 178 words for preprimer through second grade.

Format: List presented to students.

Reliability: Kuder-Richardson formula 21 was .97.

Author: Reifman, B., et al.

Article: Effects of work bank instruction on sight word acquisition: An experimental note.

Journal: *Journal of Educational Psychology,* January/February 1981, *74*(3), 175–178.

Related Research: Mangieri, J. (1978). Dolch list revisited. *Reading World, 18,* 91–95.

■ ■ ■

2938

Test Name: SIMILE APPRECIATION SCALE

Purpose: To measure appreciation of figurative language usage.

Number of Items: 36

Time Required: 60–90 minutes.

Format: Paired-comparisons. Sample items presented. Students are asked to choose the "best" of two similes.

Validity: Verbal IQ related to appreciation for sixth and third graders, and figured-fluency and originality related to appreciation for kindergartners.

Author: Malgady, R. G.

Article: Metric distance models of creativity and children's appreciation of figurative language.

Journal: *Journal of Educational Psychology,* December 1981, *73*(6), 866–871.

2939

Test Name: TEST OF NUMBER CONCEPTS

Purpose: To assess young children's number development.

Number of Items: 59

Format: Includes nine subtests: rational counting; choosing more; just after, before, and between; counting on and back; equalizing two sets of counters; identity; equivalence conservation; verbal word problems; concrete word problems.

Reliability: Coefficient alphas were .95 (pretest) and .97 (posttest).

Author: Clements, D., et al.

Article: Relationship between pretraining knowledge and learning.

Journal: *Child Study Journal,* 1985, *15*(1), 57–70.

Related Research: Carpenter, T. P., & Moser, J. M. (1982). The development of addition and subtraction problem solving skills. In T. P. Carpenter, et al. (Eds.), *Addition and subtraction: A cognitive perspective.* Hillsdale, NJ: Erlbaum.

CHAPTER 11
Creativity

2940

Test Name: CREATIVE ACTIVITIES CHECKLIST

Purpose: To identify creative activities of children.

Number of Items: 65

Format: Includes seven domains of items: art, writing, science, performing arts, crafts, music, and public presentation. An example is presented.

Reliability: Coefficient alpha was .94.

Author: Runco, M. A., and Albert, R. S.

Article: The reliability and validity of ideational originality in the divergent thinking of academically gifted and nongifted children.

Journal: *Educational and Psychological Measurement,* Autumn 1985, *45*(3), 483–501.

Related Research: Hocevar, D. (1978). Studies in the evaluation of tests of divergent thinking. *Dissertation Abstracts International, 35,* 4658A–4686A. (University Microfilms No. 78–69)

2941

Test Name: REMOTE ASSOCIATES TEST

Purpose: To measure creativity.

Number of Items: 30

Format: Respondents write a word that has something in common with three listed words.

Reliability: Kuder-Richardson formula was .53.

Author: Shaw, G. A.

Article: The use of imagery by intelligent and by creative school children.

Journal: *Journal of General Psychology,* April 1985, *112*(2), 153–171.

Related Research: Mednick, S. A. (1962). The associative basis of the creative process. *Psychological Review, 69,* 220–232.

2942

Test Name: TEACHER'S EVALUATION OF STUDENT'S CREATIVITY

Purpose: To enable teachers to evaluate their students' creativity.

Number of Items: 25

Format: Each item is a behavioral descriptor which the teacher rates on a 7-point Likert scale from (1) *rarely* to (7) *extremely*. An example is provided.

Reliability: Coefficient alpha was .96.

Author: Runco, M. A., and Albert, R. S.

Article: The reliability and validity of ideational originality in the divergent thinking of academically gifted and nongifted children.

Journal: *Educational and Psychological Measurement,* Autumn 1985, *45*(3), 483–501.

Related Research: Runco, M. A. (1984). Teachers' judgments of creativity and social validation of divergent thinking tests. *Perceptual and Motor Skills, 59,* 711–717.

CHAPTER 12
Development

2943

Test Name: ADULT DEVELOPMENT SCALE

Purpose: To measure the dimensions of early adult development.

Number of Items: 16

Format: Raters coded interview responses to 16 items as (1) developmentally young, (3) developmentally advanced, and (2) unable to determine. Items presented.

Reliability: Interrater reliability ranged from .31 to .93, and averaged .68.

Validity: Significant relationships to age were found for 11 of the 16 items.

Author: Kuh, G. D., and Thomas, M. L.

Article: The use of adult development theory with graduate students.

Journal: *Journal of College Student Personnel*, January 1983, *24*(1), 12–19.

Related Research: Thomas, M. L., & Kuh, G. D. (1982). A composite framework for understanding development during the early adult years. *Personnel and Guidance Journal, 61*, 14–17.

...

2944

Test Name: ADULT VOCATIONAL MATURITY ASSESSMENT INTERVIEW

Purpose: To measure vocational maturity in adults with delayed career development.

Number of Items: 120

Format: Numerical response scales of varying ranges, all with a definition of scoring. Sample item included.

Reliability: Alphas ranged from .52 to .82 across subscales. Total reliability was .91.

Validity: Subscales were more highly related to total measure than to each other. Scales responded to career development intervention.

Author: Manuele, C. A.

Article: The development of a measure to assess vocational maturity in adults with delayed career development.

Journal: *Journal of Vocational Behavior*, August 1983, *23*(1), 45–63.

...

2945

Test Name: CHILD BEHAVIOR RATING SCALE

Purpose: To evaluate children's psychosocial development.

Number of Items: 28

Format: Combines items from Classroom Adjustment Rating Scale and the Health Resources Inventory.

Reliability: Test–retest reliability ranged from .72 to .92.

Author: Humphrey, L. L.

Article: Children's and teachers' perspectives on children's self-control: The development of two rating scales.

Journal: *Journal of Consulting and Clinical Psychology*, October 1982, *50*(5), 624–633.

Related Research: Rochester Social Problem Solving Core Group, 1980. *The Child Behavior Rating Scale.* Unpublished manuscript, University of Rochester.

Lorion, R. P., et al. (1975). Normative and parametric analysis of school maladjustment. *American Journal of Community Psychology, 3*, 291–301.

Gesten, E. L. (1976). A health resources inventory: The development of a measure of the personal and social competence of primary grade children. *Journal of Consulting and Clinical Psychology, 44*, 775–786.

...

2946

Test Name: CLASSIFICATION AND SERIATION TEST

Purpose: To measure acquisition of classification and seriation as logical operations.

Number of Items: 50 operations.

Format: All operations described.

Reliability: Alphas were .90 (pretest) and .92 (posttest).

Validity: Consistent, moderate, and positive correlations between classification and seriation scores and scores of number concepts test were reported. Correlations ranged from .07 to .69 (13 of 14 significant).

Author: Clements, D. H.

Article: Training effects on the development and generalization of Piagetian logical operations and knowledge of numbers.

Journal: *Journal of Educational Psychology,* October 1984, *76*(5), 766–776.

■ ■ ■

2947

Test Name: CONTENT ANALYSIS SCALES OF PSYCHOSOCIAL MATURITY

Purpose: To measure positive and negative constructs used at each of Erikson's eight stages.

Number of Items: 16

Format: Key self-descriptive statements for each construct are presented.

Reliability: Interjudge reliability ranged from .80 to .95.

Author: Viney, L. L., and Tych, A. M.

Article: Content analysis scales measuring psychosocial maturity in the elderly.

Journal: *Journal of Personality Assessment,* June 1985, *49*(3), 311–317.

Related Research: Viney, L. L., & Tych, A. M. (1982). *Content analysis scales to measure psychosocial maturity: A set of research tools.* Unpublished paper: The University of Wollongong.

■ ■ ■

2948

Test Name: EGO DEVELOPMENT TEST (SHORT VERSION)

Purpose: To measure ego development.

Number of Items: 12

Format: Sentence completion. Items from Loevinger and Wessler's 36-item scale.

Reliability: Alpha was .69; interrater reliability was .91.

Author: Hansell, S.

Article: Ego development and peer friendship networks.

Journal: *Sociology of Education,* January 1981, *54*(1), 51–63.

Related Research: Loevinger, J., & Wessler, R. (1970). *Measuring ego development: Volume 1.* San Francisco: Jossey-Bass.

■ ■ ■

2949

Test Name: EGO IDENTITY SCALE

Purpose: To reflect the degree of successful or unsuccessful resolution of each of the first six of Erikson's eight stage crises within a theory of psychosocial development.

Number of Items: 72

Format: Respondents agree or disagree with each item.

Reliability: Split-half (corrected) reliability coefficients were .849 (*N* = 70) and .85 (*N* = 70).

Author: Caillet, K. C., and Michael, W. B.

Article: The construct validity of three self-report instruments hypothesized to measure the degree of resolution for each of the first six stage crises in Erikson's developmental theory of personality.

Journal: *Educational and Psychological Measurement,* Spring 1983, *43*(1), 197–209.

Related Research: Rasmussen, J. E. (1964). Relationship of ego identity to psychosocial

effectiveness. *Psychological Reports, 15,* 815–825.

■ ■ ■

2950

Test Name: EGO IDENTITY SCALE

Purpose: To measure progress toward ego-identity achievement.

Number of Items: 12

Format: Each item pairs two statements in a forced-choice format to minimize effects of social desirability. Sample items presented.

Reliability: Split-half reliability was .68.

Validity: Correlates negatively with dogmatism and positively with internal locus of control, intimacy, personally derived values and political, moral, and occupational commitment.

Author: Savickas, M. L.

Article: Identity in vocational development.

Journal: *Journal of Vocational Behavior,* December 1985, *27*(3), 329–337.

Related Research: Tan, A. L., et al. (1977). A short measure of Eriksonian ego identity. *Journal of Personality Assessment, 41,* 279–284.

■ ■ ■

2951

Test Name: EGO STAGE DEVELOPMENT INVENTORY

Purpose: To reflect the degree of successful or unsuccessful resolution of each of the first six of Erikson's eight stage crises within a theory of psychosocial development.

Number of Items: 144

Format: Twelve items represent

each of the positive resolutions and 12 items represent each of the negative resolutions for each of the first six stage crises.

Reliability: Coefficient alphas ranged from .68 to .90.

Author: Caillet, K. C., and Michael, W. B.

Article: The construct validity of three self-report instruments hypothesized to measure the degree of resolution for each of the first six stage crises in Erikson's developmental theory of personality.

Journal: *Educational and Psychological Measurement,* Spring 1983, *43*(1), 197–209.

Related Research: Caillet, K. C. (1980). *Ego Stage Development Inventory.* Unpublished self-report inventory. (Available from author, California State University, Long Beach, CA.)

■ ■ ■

2952

Test Name: EMOTIONAL MATURITY SCALE

Purpose: To measure emotional empathy.

Number of Items: 33

Format: Each item is scored from +4 (*very strong agreement*) to –4 (*very strong disagreement*).

Reliability: Split-half reliability was .84.

Author: Hanson, R. A., et al.

Article: Age and gender differences in empathy and moral reasoning among adolescents.

Journal: *Child Study Journal,* 1985, *15*(3), 181–188.

Related Research: Mehrabian, A., & Epstein, N. (1972). A measure of emotional empathy. *Journal of Personality, 40,* 525–543.

2953

Test Name: INTELLECTUAL/ ACADEMIC DEVELOPMENT SCALE

Purpose: To measure satisfaction with intellectual/academic development of freshmen.

Number of Items: 7

Format: Likert scale.

Reliability: Alpha was .74.

Author: Pascarella, E. T., and Terenzini, P. T.

Article: Contextual analysis as a method for assessing resident group effects.

Journal: *Journal of College Student Personnel,* March 1982, *23*(2), 108–114.

Related Research: Pascarella, E. T., & Terenzini, P. T. (1980). Predicting persistence and voluntary dropout decisions from a theoretical model. *Journal of Higher Education, 51,* 60–75.

■ ■ ■

2954

Test Name: INTELLECTUAL AND PERSONAL DEVELOPMENT

Purpose: To measure intellectual and personal development.

Number of Items: 11

Format: Items rated on a 4-point response scale.

Reliability: For intellectual development alpha was .74; for personal development alpha was .80.

Author: Pascarella, E. T., and Terenzini, P. T.

Article: Residence arrangement, student/faculty relationships and freshmen-year educational outcomes.

Journal: *Journal of College*

Student Personnel, March 1981, *22*(2), 147–156.

Related Research: Pascarella, E., & Terenzini, P. (1978). Student–faculty informal relationships and freshmen-year educational outcomes. *Journal of Educational Research, 71,* 183–189.

■ ■ ■

2955

Test Name: INVENTORY OF PSYCHOSOCIAL DEVELOPMENT

Purpose: To reflect the degree of successful or unsuccessful resolution of each of the first six of Erikson's eight stage crises within a theory of psychosocial development.

Number of Items: 60

Format: Five items reflect successful and 5 reflect unsuccessful resolutions of each of Erikson's first six stages of psychosocial development. Subjects respond to each item on a 7-point scale from *definitely most characteristic of you* (7) to *definitely most uncharacteristic of you* (1).

Reliability: Test–retest reliability ranged from .45 to .81 (6-week interval).

Author: Caillet, K. C., and Michael, W. B.

Article: The construct validity of three self-report instruments hypothesized to measure the degree of resolution for each of the first six stage crises in Erikson's developmental theory of personality.

Journal: *Educational and Psychological Measurement,* Spring 1983, *43*(1), 197–209.

Related Research: Constantinople, A. (1969). An Eriksonian measure of personality development in college students. *Developmental Psychology, 1,* 357–372.

■ ■ ■

2956

Test Name: MENTAL DEVELOPMENT SCALES

Purpose: To assess developmental levels of children from birth to three years of age in a familiar setting.

Number of Items: Six scales whose readings come from assessments of drawing, playing, object exploration, and other characteristics.

Format: Observations obtained in a semistructured mode.

Reliability: Guttman reproducibility ranged from .938 to .997. Scalability ranged from .667 to .984.

Validity: Correlations of six scales ranged from .508 to .954 with Bayley Scales of Infant Development and Stanford-Binet Intelligence Scale.

Author: Wagner, B.

Article: Reliability, scalability and validity of an instrument to assess developmental levels of children from birth to three years of age.

Journal: *Psychological Reports,* February 1983, *52*(1), 217–218.

■ ■ ■

2957

Test Name: MORAL DEVELOPMENT SCALE

Purpose: To assess overall level of children's moral reasoning within a Piagetian framework.

Number of Items: 15

Format: Consists of six stories concerned with moral realism and nine concerned with justice. Stick figure cartoons depicting each

story are presented while each story is read. Responses are scored on the basis of moral choice and justification for the choice. Examples are presented.

Reliability: Coefficient alpha was .83 ($N = 112$). Test–retest reliability was .82 ($N = 32$).

Validity: Correlations with a composite measure of verbal and math reasoning ability were .31 and .29.

Author: Kurtines, W., and Pimm, J. B.

Article: The Moral Development Scale: A Piagetian measure of moral judgment.

Journal: *Educational and Psychological Measurement,* Spring 1983, *43*(1), 89–105.

Related Research: Kurtines, W., & Pimm, J. (1978). *The Moral Development Scale Manual.* Unpublished manuscript. (Available from William M. Kurtines, Department of Psychology, Florida International University, Miami, FL 33199.)

■ ■ ■

2958

Test Name: SCALE OF INTELLECTUAL DEVELOPMENT

Purpose: To measure intellectual–ethical development in undergraduates.

Number of Items: 86

Format: Items rated on a 4-choice Likert scale. Sample items are presented.

Reliability: Cronbach's alphas were .81 (dualism), .70 (relativism), .76 (commitment), and .73 (empathy).

Validity: Correlations with Erwin Identity Scale were generally negative, except for SID

Commitment Scale, which were positive. Correlations with perceived self scale were generally negative and low (a total of 48 correlations are presented).

Author: Erwin, T. D.

Article: The Scale of Intellectual Development.

Journal: *Journal of College Student Personnel,* January 1983, *24*(1), 6–12.

Related Research: Perry, W. G., Jr. (1970). *Forms of intellectual and ethical development in the college years.* New York: Holt, Rinehart & Winston.

■ ■ ■

2959

Test Name: SENTENCE COMPLETION TEST

Purpose: To measure ego development.

Number of Items: 36

Format: Items are incomplete sentences to be completed. An example is presented.

Reliability: Cronbach's alpha was .89.

Author: Browning, D. L., and Quinlan, D. M.

Article: Ego development and intelligence in a psychiatric population: Wechsler subtest scores.

Journal: *Journal of Personality Assessment,* June 1985, *49*(3), 260–263.

Related Research: Loevinger, J., et al. (1970). *Measuring ego development* (Vol. 2). San Francisco: Jossey-Bass.

Swensen, C. H., et al. (1981). Stage of family life cycle, ego development and the marriage relationship. *Journal of Marriage and the Family, 43*(4), 841–853.

2960

Test Name: SOCIAL SCIENCES PIAGETIAN INVENTORY

Purpose: To measure performance on a variety of concrete and formal operational tasks.

Number of Items: 30

Format: Multiple-choice items: Examples are presented.

Reliability: Kuder-Richardson formula 20 reliability coefficients cluster around .80. Test–retest coefficient was .87 ($N = 141$ fifth through ninth graders with 1-week interval).

Validity: Correlation with Otis-Lennon Mental Ability Test was .54.

Author: Carter, K. R., and Ormrod, J. E.

Article: Acquisition of formal operations by intellectually gifted children.

Journal: *Gifted Child Quarterly,* Summer 1982, *26*(3), 110–115.

■ ■ ■

2961

Test Name: TESTS OF SPECIFIC COGNITIVE ABILITIES FOR 3-YEAR-OLDS

Purpose: To measure specific mental abilities in preschool children as young as three years of age.

Number of Items: 60

Format: Includes 4 subtests: vocabulary, recognition memory, form discrimination, and hidden animals.

Reliability: Test–retest reliability coefficients ranged from .57 to .82 ($N = 48$).

Validity: Correlation with the Stanford-Binet was .64 ($N = 50$).

Author: Singer, S., et al.

Article: The development and validation of a test battery to measure differentiated cognitive abilities in three-year-old children.

Journal: *Educational and Psychological Measurement,* Autumn 1984, *44*(3), 703–713.

CHAPTER 13
Family

2962

Test Name: ABBREVIATED DYADIC ADJUSTMENT SCALE

Purpose: To measure marital adjustment.

Number of Items: 7

Format: All items are presented.

Reliability: Alpha reliability coefficient was .76.

Author: Sharpley, C. F., and Rogers, H. J.

Article: Preliminary validation of the abbreviated Spanier Dyadic Adjustment Scale: Some psychometric data regarding a screening test of marital adjustment.

Journal: *Educational and Psychological Measurement,* Winter 1984, *44*(4), 1045–1049.

Related Research: Spanier, G. B. (1976). Measuring dyadic adjustment: New scales for assessing the quality of marriage and similar dyads. *Journal of Marriage and the Family, 38,* 15–38.

Sharpley, C. F., & Cross, D. G. (1982). A psychometric evaluation of the Spanier Dyadic Adjustment Scale. *Journal of Marriage and the Family, 44,* 739–741.

■ ■ ■

2963

Test Name: ACCEPTANCE OF MARITAL TERMINATION SCALE

Purpose: To identify a range of feelings about marital termination.

Number of Items: 11

Format: Responses are made on a 4-point scale: *not at all, slightly, somewhat, very much.* All items are presented.

Reliability: Cronbach's alpha was .90.

Validity: Correlations with other variables ranged from –.50 to .28 (men) and from –.45 to .26 (women).

Author: Thompson, L., and Spanier, G. B.

Article: The end of marriage and acceptance of marital termination.

Journal: *Journal of Marriage and the Family,* February 1983, *45*(1), 103–113.

Related Research: Kitson, G. C. (1982). Attachment to the spouse and divorce: A scale and its application. *Journal of Marriage and the Family, 44,* 379–393.

■ ■ ■

2964

Test Name: ADOLESCENT ABUSE INVENTORY

Purpose: Measures parental attitudes toward maltreatment and the likelihood that they would act in abusive manners given provocative adolescent behavior.

Number of Items: 26

Format: Items consist of hypothetical situations. A sample item is presented.

Reliability: Overall coefficient alpha reliabilities for mothers ranged from .607 to .877 and for fathers they ranged from .644 to .881.

Author: Garbarino, J., et al.

Article: Families at risk for destructive parent–child relations in adolescence.

Journal: *Child Development,* February 1984, *55*(1), 174–183.

Related Research: Sebes, J. M. (1983). *Determining risk for abuse in families with adolescents: The development of a criterion measure.* Unpublished doctoral dissertation, Pennsylvania State University.

■ ■ ■

2965

Test Name: AFFECTIVE INTIMACY INDEX

Purpose: To measure one's perception of closeness and emotional bonding in an intimate relationship.

Number of Items: 10

Format: Subjects agree or disagree with each item on a 7-point scale. Scores range from 10 (least intimate) to 70.

Reliability: Coefficient alpha was .78.

Validity: Correlations with other variables ranged from –.64 to .74.

Author: Tolstedt, B. E., and Stokes, J. P.

Article: Relation of verbal, affective and physical intimacy to marital satisfaction.

Journal: *Journal of Counseling Psychology,* October 1983, *30*(4), 573–580.

Related Research: Walster, E., et

al. (1978). *Equity: Theory, and research.* Boston: Allyn & Bacon.

■ ■ ■

2966

Test Name: AREAS OF CHANGE QUESTIONNAIRE

Purpose: To measure spouse's presenting complaints in areas of marital change.

Number of Items: 34

Format: Multiple-choice and 7-point Likert scales. All items presented.

Reliability: Internal consistency was .89.

Validity: Correlated −.70 with Marital Adjustment Scale. Correlated from −.02 to +.44 on subscales of Spouse Observation Checklist.

Author: Margolin, G., et al.

Article: Areas of Change Questionnaire: A practical approach to marital assessment.

Journal: *Journal of Consulting and Clinical Psychology,* December 1983, *51*(6), 920–931.

Related Research: Weiss, R. L., & Birchler, G. R. (1975). *Areas of change.* Unpublished manuscript, University of Oregon, Eugene, Department of Psychology.

Witkin, S., et al. (1983). Group training in marital communication: A comparative study. *Journal of Marriage and the Family, 45*(3), 661–669.

■ ■ ■

2967

Test Name: ATTITUDE TOWARD NONMATERNAL CARE RATING

Purpose: To measure degree to which a mother believes others can take care of her child.

Number of Items: 1

Format: 9-point rating scale.

Reliability: Interrater reliability was .88.

Author: Morgan, K. C., and Hock, E.

Article: A longitudinal study of the psychosocial variables affecting the career patterns of women with young children.

Journal: *Journal of Marriage and the Family,* May 1984, *46*(2), 383–390.

Related Research: Hock, E. (1976). *Alternative approaches to child rearing and their effects on the mother-infant relationship.* (ED 122943.) Urbana, IL: Educational Resources Information Center/Early Childhood Education.

■ ■ ■

2968

Test Name: BARRIERS TO MARITAL DISSOLUTION SCALE

Purpose: To measure perceptions of barriers to dissolution of marriage.

Number of Items: 11

Format: Items rated in 5-point Likert format.

Reliability: Alpha was .74.

Author: Sabatelli, R. M., and Cecil-Pigo, E. F.

Article: Relational interdependence and commitment in marriage.

Journal: *Journal of Marriage and the Family,* November 1985, *47*(4), 931–937.

Related Research: Levinger, G. (1974). A three-level approach to attraction: Toward an understanding of pair relatedness. In T. L. Huston (Ed.), *Foundations of interpersonal attraction.* New York: Academic Press.

2969

Test Name: CALDWELL INVENTORY OF HOME STIMULATION

Purpose: To measure several dimensions of the child's environment in a structured interview.

Number of Items: 45

Format: The scale is administered during a home visit, includes six subscales: maternal responsiveness, avoid restriction/punishment, organization of environment, provision of play materials, maternal involvement, variety of stimulation.

Reliability: .90

Validity: Correlations with Bayley and Reynell Scales ranged from .06 to .40.

Author: Siegal, L. S.

Article: Infant tests as predictors of cognitive and language development at two years.

Journal: *Child Development,* June 1981, *52*(2), 545–557.

Related Research: Elardo, R., et al. (1975). The relation of infants' home environment to mental tests performance from six to thirty six months: A longitudinal analysis. *Child Development, 46,* 71–76.

van Dourninck, W. J., et al. (1981). The relationship between twelve-month home stimulation and school achievement. *Child Development, 52*(8), 1080–1083.

■ ■ ■

2970

Test Name: CHANGES IN SELF-PERCEPTION SCALE

Purpose: To measure a woman's feelings about herself after having a baby.

Number of Items: 17

Format: Items rated on 5-point adjective rating scales. Sample items are presented.

Reliability: Alpha ranged from .79 to .85 across two subscales.

Author: Pistrang, N.

Article: Women's work involvement and experience of new motherhood.

Journal: *Journal of Marriage and the Family*, May 1984, *46*(2), 433–447.

Related Research: Steffensmeier, R. H. (1982). A role model of the transition to parenthood. *Journal of Marriage and the Family, 44*, 319–334.

■ ■ ■

2971

Test Name: CHILD'S REPORT OF PARENTAL BEHAVIOR INVENTORY

Purpose: To assess parental child-rearing behaviors.

Number of Items: 108

Format: Includes 18 subscales. Responses to each item are recorded on a 3-point scale of *like, somewhat like,* and *not like.*

Reliability: The mean internal consistency was .71. The mean interrater agreement was .30.

Author: Schwarz, J. C., et al.

Article: Assessing child-rearing behaviors: A comparison of ratings made by mother, father, child and sibling on the CRPBI.

Journal: *Child Development,* April 1985, *56*(2), 462–479.

Related Research: Schludermann, E., & Schludermann, S. (1970). Replicability of factors in children's report of parent (CRPBI). *Journal of Psychology, 76*, 239–249.

2972

Test Name: COMMUNICATIONS SKILLS TEST

Purpose: To measure interaction in married couples.

Format: Observation scale. Observers rate statements made by couples on a 5-point scale. Examples of the rating protocol presented.

Reliability: Interobserver agreement averaged .82 (range .71 to .95).

Validity: Mean scores at pre-assessment comparable. Intervention increased scores, control group scores decreased slightly. Correlates .30 ($p < .01$) with communication box ratings.

Author: Floyd, F. J., and Markman, H. J.

Article: An economical observational measure of couples' communication skill.

Journal: *Journal of Consulting and Clinical Psychology,* February 1984, *52*(1), 97–103.

■ ■ ■

2973

Test Name: CONFLICT TACTICS SCALE

Purpose: To measure marital conflict.

Number of Items: 18

Format: Items rated on a 7-point frequency scale (*never* to *more than 20 times per year*).

Reliability: Interspousal reliability ranged from –.07 to 1.00.

Author: Jouriles, E. N., and O'Leary, K. D.

Article: Interspousal reliability of reports of marital violence.

Journal: *Journal of Consulting and Clinical Psychology,* June 1985,

53(3), 419–421.

Related Research: Hornung, C. A., et al. (1981). Status relationships in marriage: Risk factors in spouse abuse. *Journal of Marriage and the Family, 43*, 675–692.

Straus, M. A. (1979). Measuring intrafamily conflict and violence: The Conflict Tactics (CT) Scale. *Journal of Marriage and the Family, 6*, 131–149.

■ ■ ■

2974

Test Name: COPING STRATEGIES AND RESOURCES INVENTORY

Purpose: To identify coping strategies and resources of wives divorced or widowed.

Number of Items: 45

Format: The perceived efficacy of coping strategies was rated on a 4-point scale from *not at all helpful* to *very helpful*. Six factors are included.

Reliability: Coefficient alphas ranged from .675 to .793.

Author: Berman, W. H., and Turk, D. C.

Article: Adaptation to divorce: Problems and strategies.

Journal: *Journal of Marriage and the Family,* February 1981, *43*(1), 179–189.

Related Research: McCubbin, H. I., et al. (1976). Coping repertories of families adapting to prolonged war-induced separations. *Journal of Marriage and the Family, 38*, 461–472.

■ ■ ■

2975

Test Name: COPING WITH SEPARATION INVENTORY— REVISED

Purpose: To measure wives' coping behavior upon separation.

Number of Items: 30

Format: Items rated on a 3-point helpfulness rating scale.

Reliability: Alphas ranged from .71 to .85 across subscales.

Author: Patterson, J. M., and McCubbin, H. I.

Article: Gender roles and coping.

Journal: *Journal of Marriage and the Family*, February 1984, *46*(1), 95–104.

Related Research: McCubbin, H., et al. (1980). Developing family invulnerability to stress: Coping patterns and strategies wives employ in managing family separations. In J. Trost (Ed.), *The family in change*. Västeraos, Sweden: International Library.

• • •

2976

Test Name: DIVORCE POTENTIAL INDEX

Purpose: To measure marital satisfaction.

Number of Items: 5

Format: Respondents are asked to report specific behaviors considered indicative of potential for divorce. Scores are obtained on a scale with a mean of 50 and a standard deviation of 10.

Reliability: Coefficient alpha was .73.

Validity: Correlations with other variables ranged from −.54 to −.80.

Author: Tolstedt, B. E., and Stokes, J. P.

Article: Relation of verbal, affective, and physical intimacy to marital satisfaction.

Journal: *Journal of Counseling Psychology*, October 1983, *30*(4), 573–580.

2977

Test Name: DIVORCE REACTION INVENTORY

Purpose: To measure postseparation attachment.

Number of Items: 46

Format: A few sample items are presented.

Reliability: Cronbach's alphas were .97 and .99; split-half (odd–even) was .98.

Validity: Correlation with self-rated adjustment was −.75.

Author: Brown, S. D., and Reimer, D. A.

Article: Assessing attachment following divorce: Development and psychometric evaluation of the divorce reaction inventory.

Journal: *Journal of Counseling Psychology*, October 1984, *31*(4), 521–531.

Related Research: Bowlby, J. (1980). *Attachment and loss, III: Loss.* New York: Basic Books.

• • •

2978

Test Name: DYADIC ADJUSTMENT SCALE

Purpose: To measure the process of marital adjustment.

Number of Items: 32

Format: Yields a total score of dyadic adjustment from well adjusted to maladjusted.

Reliability: Internal consistency of .76 (husbands) and .73 (wives).

Author: Belsky, J., and Isabella, R. A.

Article: Marital and parent–child relationships in family of origin and marital change following the birth of a baby: A retrospective analysis.

Journal: *Child Development*, April 1985, *56*(2), 342–349.

Related Research: Spanier, G. (1976). Measuring dyadic adjustment: New scale for assessing the quality of marriage and similar dyads. *Journal of Marriage and the Family, 38,* 15–28.

Nice, D. S., et al. (1981). The families of U. S. Navy prisoners of war from Vietnam five years after reunion. *Journal of Marriage and the Family, 43*(2), 431–437.

Houseknecht, S. K., & Macke, A. S. (1981). Combining marriage and career: The marital adjustment of professional women. *Journal of Marriage and the Family, 43,* 651–661.

Filsinger, E. E., & Lamke, L. K. (1983). The lineage transmission of interpersonal competence. *Journal of Marriage and the Family, 45,* 75–80.

Davidson, B., et al. (1983). Affective self-disclosure and marital adjustment: A test of equity theory. *Journal of Marriage and the Family, 45,* 93–102.

Norton, R. (1983). Measuring marital quality: A critical look at the dependent variable. *Journal of Marriage and the Family, 45,* 141–151.

Sullaway, M., & Christensen, A. (1983). Assessment of dysfunctional interaction patterns in couples. *Journal of Marriage and the Family, 45,* 653–660.

King, C. E., & Christensen, A. (1983). The relationship events scale: A Guttman scaling of progress in courtship. *Journal of Marriage and the Family, 45,* 671–678.

• • •

2979

Test Name: DYADIC PARENT–CHILD INTERACTION CODING SYSTEM

Purpose: To measure parent–child interaction.

Number of Items: 31

Time Required: 2 days.

Reliability: Interrater reliability was .91 for parent behaviors and .92 for child behaviors.

Validity: Significant differences between normal and problem children were reported.

Author: Robinson, E. A., and Eyberg, S. M.

Article: The dyadic parent–child interaction coding system: Standardization and validation.

Journal: *Journal of Consulting and Clinical Psychology*, April 1981, *49*(2), 245–250.

Related Research: Eyberg, S. M. (1974). *Manual for coding dyadic parent-child interactions.* Unpublished manuscript.

■ ■ ■

2980

Test Name: EDMONDS MARITAL CONVENTIONALIZATION SCALE

Purpose: To measure tendency of people to report socially desirable levels of marital adjustment.

Number of Items: 5 (plus 3 filler items).

Format: True–false. Sample items presented.

Reliability: Cronbach's alpha ranged from .59 to .85.

Author: Schumm, W. R., et al.

Article: Marital conventionalization revisited.

Journal: *Psychological Reports,* 1981, *49*(2), 607–615.

Related Research: Edmonds, V. H. (1967). Marital conventionalization: Definition and measurement. *Journal of*

Marriage and the Family, 29, 681–688.

■ ■ ■

2981

Test Name: EXPERIENCES AS A MOTHER SCALE

Purpose: To measure pleasures and frustrations of new mothers.

Number of Items: 17

Format: Items rated on a 5-point rating scale.

Reliability: Alpha ranged from .74 to .84 across two subscales.

Author: Pistrang, N.

Article: Women's work involvement and experience of new motherhood.

Journal: *Journal of Marriage and the Family,* May 1984, *46*(2), 433–447.

Related Research: Westbrook, M. T. (1979). Socioeconomic differences in coping with childbearing. *American Journal of Community Psychology, 7,* 397–412.

■ ■ ■

2982

Test Name: FACES

Purpose: To measure how family members perceive their families as social systems.

Number of Items: 111

Format: Yields two primary dimensions: adaptability and cohesion.

Reliability: Internal consistency (alpha) reliability was .75 for adaptability and .83 for cohesion.

Author: Garbarino, J., et al.

Article: Families at risk for destructive parent–child relations in adolescence.

Journal: *Child Development,* February 1984, *55*(1), 174–183.

Related Research: Olson, D. H., et al. (1979). Circumplex model of marital and family system II: Empirical studies and clinical intervention. In J. Vincent (Ed.), *Advances in family intervention, assessment and theory.* Greenwich, CT: JAI.

■ ■ ■

2983

Test Name: FACES SCALES— REVISED

Purpose: To measure family dynamics.

Number of Items: 50

Format: Includes four factors: social desirability, togetherness, rules, and autonomy. Responses are made on a 5-point Likert scale from *strongly disagree* to *strongly agree.*

Reliability: Kuder-Richardson formula 20 reliabilities ranged from .48 to .91.

Author: Kunce, J. T., and Priesmeyer, M. L.

Article: Measuring family dynamics.

Journal: *Journal of Counseling Psychology,* January 1985, *32*(1), 40–46.

Related Research: Olson, D. H., et al. (1983). Circumplex model of marital and family systems: VI. Theoretical update. *Family Process, 22,* 69–83.

■ ■ ■

2984

Test Name: FAMILY COPING INVENTORY—SHORT FORM

Purpose: To determine usefulness of various coping behaviors to new parents.

Number of Items: 28

Format: Responses are made on a

4-point scale: *not helpful, a little helpful, fairly helpful, very helpful.*

Reliability: Coefficient alpha was .85.

Author: Ventura, J. N., and Bass, P. G.

Article: The Family Coping Inventory applied to parents with new babies.

Journal: *Journal of Marriage and the Family,* November 1983, *45*(4), 867–875.

Related Research: McCubbin, H., et al. (1979). *Family Coping Inventory.* (Instrument available from University of Minnesota Family Social Sciences, 290 McNeal Hall, St. Paul, MN 55108.)

■ ■ ■

2985

Test Name: FAMILY ENVIRONMENT SCHEDULE

Purpose: To measure the learning environment of families.

Number of Items: 38

Format: Multiple-choice. Sample items presented.

Reliability: Theta reliabilities all greater than .75 across subscales.

Author: Marjoribanks, K.

Article: Occupational status, family environments and adolescents' aspirations: The Laosa Model.

Journal: *Journal of Educational Psychology,* August 1984, *76*(4), 690–700.

Related Research: Marjoribanks, K. (1979). *Families and their learning environments.* London: Routledge and Kegan Paul.

■ ■ ■

2986

Test Name: FAMILY INVOLVEMENT SCALE

Purpose: To measure commitment to satisfaction with and involvement in family life.

Number of Items: 11

Format: Items rated on 5-point Likert response categories. All items are presented. Items modeled after Lodahl and Kejner work involvement items.

Reliability: Alpha was .80.

Author: Yogev, S., and Brett, J.

Article: Patterns of work and family involvement among single and dual-earner couples.

Journal: *Journal of Applied Psychology,* November 1985, *70*(4), 754–768.

Related Research: Lodahl, T. M., & Kejner, M. (1965). The definition and measurement of job involvement. *Journal of Applied Psychology, 49,* 24–33.

■ ■ ■

2987

Test Name: FAMILY MATERIAL WELL-BEING SCALES

Purpose: To measure family material well-being.

Number of Items: 49

Format: Includes two scales: family ownership and family economizing.

Reliability: Coefficient alphas were: .85 (economizing) and .83 (ownership).

Validity: Correlations with other variables ranged from –.24 to .60.

Author: Fergusson, D. M., et al.

Article: The measurement of family material well-being.

Journal: *Journal of Marriage and the Family,* August 1981, *43*(3), 715 725.

Related Research: Department of Social Welfare, New Zealand. *Survey of persons aged 65 years and over: Report of results relating to social security benefit rates.* Wellington: New Zealand Government Printer.

■ ■ ■

2988

Test Name: FAMILY RESOURCE QUESTIONNAIRE

Purpose: To measure social support after stroke.

Number of Items: 17

Format: Items rated on 4-point Likert response categories. All items are presented. Items administered in an interview setting.

Reliability: Interrater reliability was .91.

Validity: Correlates .65 ($p < .01$) with Social Ties Checklist (Starr, Robinson & Price, 1983).

Author: Pomeroy, S., et al.

Article: Family Resource Questionnaire: Reliability and validity of a social support measure for families of stroke patients.

Journal: *Psychological Reports,* April 1985, *56*(2), 411–414.

■ ■ ■

2989

Test Name: FAMILY VIGNETTES

Purpose: To assess probable presence and duration of maltreatment.

Number of Items: 9

Format: Interviewers decide which of nine 58–62 word sample family descriptions rank ordered from severe long-term maltreatment, through more recent, less severe maltreatment to positive parenting represents the family being assessed.

Reliability: Pearson product–moment correlations among

interviewer ratings ranged from .52 to .93.

Author: Garbarino, J., et al.

Article: Families at risk for destructive parent–child relations in adolescence.

Journal: *Child Development,* February 1984, *55*(1), 174–183.

Related Research: Sebes, J. M. (1983). *Determining risk for abuse in families with adolescents: The development of a criterion measure.* Unpublished doctoral dissertation, Pennsylvania State University.

■ ■ ■

2990

Test Name: FILIAL EXPECTANCY SCALE— ADAPTED

Purpose: To measure obligation adult children feel toward their elderly parents.

Number of Items: 5

Format: Subjects indicate degree of agreement with each item by responding on a 5-point scale with high scores indicating greater filial responsibility.

Reliability: Cronbach's alpha was .73.

Author: Cicirelli, V. G.

Article: Adult children's attachment and helping behavior to elderly parents: A path model.

Journal: *Journal of Marriage and the Family,* November 1983, *45*(4), 815–825.

Related Research: Seelbach, W., & Saver, W. (1977). Filial responsibility, expectations and morale among aged persons. *Gerontologist, 17,* 421–425.

■ ■ ■

2991

Test Name: FILIAL EXPECTATIONS MEASURE

Purpose: To assess parents' expectations of their children's involvement with them across content areas.

Number of Items: 10

Format: Areas covered are contact, sentiment, caretaking, and accessibility. Responses are made on a scale from 1 (*strongly disagree*) to 4 (*strongly agree*).

Reliability: Reliability coefficient was .74.

Validity: Correlations with other variables ranged from −.198 to .082.

Author: Quinn, W. H.

Article: Personal and family adjustment in later life.

Journal: *Journal of Marriage and the Family,* February 1983, *45*(1), 57–73.

Related Research: Seelbach, W. C. (1978). Correlates of aged parents' filial responsibility expectations and realizations. *Family Coordinator, 27,* 341–350.

■ ■ ■

2992

Test Name: FILIAL RESPONSIBILITY MEASURE

Purpose: To assess children's attitudes regarding the extent of responsibility they hold for their parents across content areas.

Number of Items: 10

Format: Areas covered are: contact, sentiment, caretaking, and accessibility. Responses are made on a scale from 1 (*strongly disagree*) to 4 (*strongly agree*).

Reliability: Reliability coefficient was .88 (adult children).

Validity: Correlations with other variables ranged from −.091 to .437.

Author: Quinn, W. H.

Article: Personal and family adjustment in later life.

Journal: *Journal of Marriage and the Family,* February 1983, *45*(1), 57–73.

Related Research: Seelbach, W. C. (1978). Correlates of aged parents' filial responsibility expectations and realizations. *Family Coordinator, 27,* 341–350.

■ ■ ■

2993

Test Name: HENDERSON ENVIRONMENTAL LEARNING PROCESS SCALE—MODIFIED

Purpose: To measure the intellectual environment of the home.

Number of Items: 34

Format: Items rated on a 5-point (*high–low*) scale.

Reliability: Carmines and Zeller reliability was .80.

Author: Valencia, R. R.

Article: Family status, family constellation, and home environmental variables as predictors of cognitive performance of Mexican-American children.

Journal: *Journal of Educational Psychology,* June 1984, *77*(3), 323–331.

Related Research: Henderson, R. W., et al. (1982). Development and validation of the Henderson Environmental Learning Process Scale. *Journal of Social Psychology, 88,* 185–196.

■ ■ ■

2994

Test Name: HOME EDUCATIONAL ENVIRONMENT INDEX

Purpose: To evaluate the educational environment of the home.

Number of Items: 39

Format: Includes four dimensions: parent's knowledge and interest in school-related activities; parent's support of academic activities; opportunities for and quality of the interaction between parent and child on school-related activities; and parent's belief in the use of schooling for the child's future.

Reliability: Coefficient alpha ranged from .71 to .80. Test–retest coefficient was .76 (4 weeks, $N=$ 40).

Validity: Correlation with the Dave structured interview was .61. Correlations with standardized reading achievement ranged from .51 to .63.

Author: Dolan, L.

Article: The prediction of reading achievement and self-esteem from an index of home educational environment: A study of urban elementary schools.

Journal: *Measurement and Evaluation in Guidance*, July 1983, *16*(2), 86–94.

Related Research: Dolan, L. J. (1980). Home, school and pupil attitudes. *Evaluation in Education: An International Review Series, 4,* 265–358.

■ ■ ■

2995

Test Name: HOMEMAKERS SATISFACTION QUESTIONNAIRE

Purpose: To measure homemaker's "job" satisfaction.

Number of Items: 13

Format: Items taken from 20-item Minnesota Satisfaction Questionnaire. Items rated on a 5-point Likert response categories. Items are presented.

Reliability: Alpha was .83.

Author: Ivancevich, J. M., and Matteson, M. T.

Article: Occupational stress, satisfaction, physical well-being and coping: A study of homemakers.

Journal: *Psychological Reports,* 1982, *50*(3, Part 1), 995–1005.

Related Research: Weiss, D. J., et al. (1967). *Manual for the Minnesota Satisfaction Questionnaire: Minnesota studies in vocational rehabilitation XXII.* Minneapolis: Industrial Relations Center, University of Minnesota.

■ ■ ■

2996

Test Name: HOMEMAKING COMMITMENT SCALE

Purpose: To assess how much a person values family and home-related activities.

Number of Items: 8

Format: Items are rated on a 5-point scale.

Reliability: Coefficient alpha was .81.

Author: Koski, L. K., and Subich, L. M.

Article: Career and homemaking choices of college preparatory and vocational education students.

Journal: *Vocational Guidance Quarterly,* December 1985, *34*(2), 116–123.

Related Research: Farmer, H. (1983). Career and homemaking plans for high school youth. *Journal of Counseling Psychology, 30,* 40–45.

CHAPTER 13 Family 343Super, D. E., et al. (1978). *The Work Salience Inventory* (mimeo). New York: Columbia University, Teachers College.

2997

Test Name: HOME OBSERVATION FOR MEASUREMENT OF THE ENVIRONMENT

Purpose: To provide a measure of environmental stimulation.

Number of Items: 45

Format: A checklist for marking whether present or absent in the home. Includes six subscales: emotional and verbal responsivity; avoidance of restriction and punishment; organization of the environment; provision of appropriate play materials; maternal involvement with child; and opportunities for variety in daily stimulation.

Reliability: Stability for total scores over first two years of life was .79. Stability of subscales ranged from .44 to .66. Internal consistency coefficients ranged from .44 to .89.

Author: Mitchell, S. K., and Gray, C. A.

Article: Developmental generalizability of the HOME Inventory.

Journal: *Educational and Psychological Measurement,* Winter 1984, *41*(4), 1001–1010.

Related Research: Bradley, R. H., & Caldwell, B. M. (1976). The relation of infants' home environments to mental test performance at 54 months: A follow-up study. *Child Development, 47,* 1172–1174.

■ ■ ■

2998

Test Name: HOME OBSERVATION FOR MEASUREMENT OF THE ENVIRONMENT INVENTORY

Purpose: To provide a preschool scale for assessing environmental processes of Black children.

Number of Items: 55

Format: Includes 8 subscales: toys, games, and reading materials; language stimulation; physical environment; pride, affection, and warmth; stimulation of academic behavior; encouraging social maturity; variety of stimulation; and physical punishment.

Validity: Correlations with elementary school achievement tests ranged from −.03 to .50.

Author: Bradley, R. H., and Caldwell, B. M.

Article: The Home Inventory: A validation of the preschool scale for Black children.

Journal: *Child Development*, June 1981, *52*(2), 708–710.

Related Research: Bradley, R., & Caldwell, B. (1979). Home Observation for Measurement of the Environment: A revision of the preschool scale. *American Journal of Mental Deficiency, 84*, 235–244.

• • •

2999

Test Name: INDEX OF ACHIEVEMENT VALUES

Purpose: To assess the mother's general valuation of achievement and independence within the family.

Number of Items: 7

Format: Items rated on a 5-choice scale.

Validity: Correlation with Traditional Family Ideology was .54.

Author: McGowan, R. J., and Johnson, D. L.

Article: The mother–child relationship and other antecedents of childhood intelligence: A causal analysis.

Journal: *Child Development*, June 1984, *55*(3), 810–820.

Related Research: Strodtbeck, F. (1958). Family interaction, value, and achievement. In D. C. McClelland (Ed.), *Talent and society*. New York: Van Nostrand.

• • •

3000

Test Name: INDEX OF SPOUSE ABUSE

Purpose: To measure extent of abuse inflicted upon a woman by her spouse or partner.

Number of Items: 30

Format: Includes two types of abuse: physical and nonphysical. Responses are made on a 5-point scale from 1 (*never*) to 5 (*very frequently*). All items are presented.

Reliability: Coefficient alphas were .903 and .942 (physical abuse) and .912 and .969 (nonphysical abuse).

Validity: Coefficient of discriminant validity was .73 (physical abuse) and .80 (nonphysical abuse).

Author: Hudson, W. W., and McIntosh, S. R.

Article: The assessment of spouse abuse: Two quantifiable dimensions.

Journal: *Journal of Marriage and the Family*, November 1981, *43*(4), 873–885.

• • •

3001

Test Name: INFLUENCE ON PARENTS SCALE

Purpose: To measure the extent to which early adolescents feel they influence their parents' decision making.

Number of Items: 30

Format: Includes two subscales for identifying influence on mother and on father. Responses are

made on a 6-point Likert scale. Examples are presented.

Reliability: Cronbach's alphas ranged from .749 to .859.

Author: Thornburg, H. D., and Shinn, J. M.

Article: Early adolescents' perceived influence on parental behavior.

Journal: *Child Study Journal*, 1982, *12*(1), 21–26.

Related Research: Baranowski, M. D. (1978). Adolescents' attempted influences on parental behavior. *Adolescence, 13*, 585–604.

• • •

3002

Test Name: INTERACTION STRAIN QUESTIONNAIRE

Purpose: To measure role conflict.

Number of Items: 12

Format: Items rated on *true, don't know,* and *untrue* response categories.

Reliability: Alpha was .75.

Author: Barling, J., and VanBart, D.

Article: Mothers' subjective employment experiences and the behavior of their nursery school children.

Journal: *Journal of Occupational Psychology*, March 1984, *57*(1), 49–56.

Related Research: Parry, G., & Warr, P. (1980). The measurement of mother's work attitudes. *Journal of Occupational Psychology, 53*, 245–252.

• • •

3003

Test Name: INTERPARENTAL CONFLICT SCALES

Purpose: To assess amount of conflict in family settings.

Number of Items: 37

Format: The parents and adolescents rate the amount of conflict in family settings across such domains as finances, child rearing, and so forth.

Reliability: Test–retest reliability was .91.

Author: Garbarino, J., et al.

Article: Families at risk for destructive parent–child relations in adolescence.

Journal: *Child Development,* February 1984, *55*(1), 174–183.

Related Research: Schwartz, J. C., & Zuroff, D. C. (1979). Family structure and depression in female college students: Effects of parental conflict, decision-making power and inconsistence of love. *Journal of Abnormal Psychology, 80,* 398–406.

■ ■ ■

3004

Test Name: INTIMACY SCALE

Purpose: To measure general intimacy or affection of mothers and daughters.

Number of Items: 17

Format: Individual scores are produced by summing and averaging the items. All items are presented.

Reliability: Cronbach's alphas ranged from .91 to .97.

Author: Walker, A. J., and Thompson, L.

Article: Intimacy and intergenerational aid and contact among mothers and daughters.

Journal: *Journal of Marriage and the Family, 45*(4), 841–849.

Related Research: Walker, A. J. (1979). *The social networks of young marrieds: Distinguishing among relationship types.*

Unpublished dissertation, Pennsylvania State University.

■ ■ ■

3005

Test Name: INVENTORY OF FAMILY RELATIONSHIPS

Purpose: To measure parent–child interaction in the family by questioning children.

Number of Items: 26

Format: Rating scale format.

Reliability: Alpha ranged from .66 to .84 across subscales.

Author: Howell, F. M., and McBroom, L. W.

Article: Social relations at home and at school: An analysis of the correspondence principle.

Journal: *Sociology of Education,* January 1982, *55*(1), 40–52.

Related Research: Bachman, J. G. (1970). The impact of family background and intelligence on tenth grade boys. *Youth in transition* (Vol. 1). Ann Arbor, MI: Institute for Social Research.

■ ■ ■

3006

Test Name: JEALOUSY SCALE

Purpose: To measure jealousy in marriage.

Number of Items: 8

Format: Subjects respond, on an 11-point scale, how they would feel about their mates' behavior in 8 situations. All items presented.

Reliability: Alpha was .65.

Author: Hansen, G.

Article: Perceived threats and marital jealousy.

Journal: *Social Psychology Quarterly,* September 1985, *48*(3), 262–268.

Related Research: Mathes, E. W.,

et al. (1982). A convergent validity study of six jealousy scales. *Psychological Reports, 50,* 1143–1147.

■ ■ ■

3007

Test Name: KANSAS MARITAL SATISFACTION SCALE

Purpose: To measure marital satisfaction.

Number of Items: 3

Format: Items are of the "how satisfied are you with …?" format followed by 7 numbered response categories (*extremely dissatisfied* to *extremely satisfied*).

Reliability: Alphas ranged from .93 to .98.

Validity: Correlated with marital social desirability (.41, $p < .0001$), but not with individual social desirability (.05).

Author: Schumm, W. R., et al.

Article: Characteristics of responses to the Kansas Marital Satisfaction Scale by a sample of 84 married mothers.

Journal: *Psychological Reports,* October 1983, *53*(2), 567–572.

Related Research: Mitchell, S. E., et al. (1983). Test–retest reliability of the Kansas Marital Satisfaction Scale. *Psychological Reports, 53*(2), 545–546.

Schumm, W. R. (1983). Characteristics of the Kansas Marital Satisfaction Scale in a sample of 79 married couples. *Psychological Reports, 53*(2), 583–588.

■ ■ ■

3008

Test Name: KANSAS PARENTAL SATISFACTION SCALE

Purpose: To measure parental satisfaction with children and parenting.

Number of Items: 3

Format: Items rated in 7-point Likert format.

Reliability: Alpha ranged from .78 to .84.

Validity: Significantly correlated with self-esteem (.38 to .68).

Author: James, D. E., et al.

Article: Characteristics of the Kansas Parental Satisfaction Scale among two samples of married parents.

Journal: *Psychological Reports,* August 1985, *57*(1), 163–169.

■ ■ ■

3009

Test Name: LIFE CHANGES SCALE

Purpose: To measure how much a mother's life changes after the birth of a child.

Number of Items: 8

Format: Items rated on 5-point response scales. Sample items are presented.

Reliability: Alpha was .88.

Author: Pistrang, N.

Article: Women's work involvement and experience of new motherhood.

Journal: *Journal of Marriage and the Family,* May 1984, *46*(2), 433–447.

Related Research: Hoffman, L. W. (1978). Effects of the first child on the woman's role. In W. B. Miller & L. F. Newman (Eds.), *The first child and family formation.* Chapel Hill, NC: Carolina Population Center.

■ ■ ■

3010

Test Name: LITTLE PARENTAL VALUING STYLES SCALE

Purpose: To evaluate attitudes and

behaviors expressed by parents toward problem children.

Number of Items: 52

Format: Items rated on a 6-point Likert format.

Reliability: Internal consistency was .50 to .79.

Author: Little, L. F., and Thompson, R.

Article: Truancy: How parents and teachers contribute.

Journal: *The School Counselor,* March 1983, *30*(4), 285–291.

Related Research: Little, L. F. (1981). The impact of Gestalt group psychotherapy on parents' perceptions of children identified as problematic. Doctoral dissertation, 1980, University of Kentucky. *Dissertation Abstracts International, 42.* (University Microfilms No. 8116912)

■ ■ ■

3011

Test Name: LOCKE WALLACE SHORT MARITAL ADJUSTMENT TEST

Purpose: To measure marital dissatisfaction.

Number of Items: 14

Format: Multiple-choice items with a high score representing a high level of marital dissatisfaction.

Validity: With Ryder's Lovesickness Scale, $r = .54$ (husbands), and $r = .53$ (wives). With individual locus of control, $r = -.03$ (husbands), and $r = .19$ (wives).

Author: Doherty, W. J.

Article: Locus of control differences and marital dissatisfaction.

Journal: *Journal of Marriage and the Family,* May 1981, *43*(2), 369–377.

Related Research: Locke, H. J., & Wallace, K. M. (1959). Short marital adjustment and prediction tests: Their reliability and validity. *Marriage and Family Living, 21,* 251–255.

■ ■ ■

3012

Test Name: LOVESICKNESS SCALE

Purpose: To measure marital dissatisfaction relative to one's partner not being sufficiently loving or attentive.

Number of Items: 32

Format: Responses either *true, partly true,* or *false.* A sample item is presented.

Reliability: Cronbach's alpha was .89 (husbands) and .91 (wives).

Validity: With Locke Wallace Short Marital Adjustment Test, $r = .54$ (husbands) and $r = .53$ (wives). With individual locus of control, $r = -.02$ (husbands) and $r = .17$ (wives).

Author: Doherty, W. J.

Article: Locus of control differences and marital dissatisfaction.

Journal: *Journal of Marriage and the Family,* May 1981, *43*(2), 369–377.

Related Research: Ryder, R. G. (1973). Longitudinal data relating marriage satisfaction and having a child. *Journal of Marriage and the Family, 35,* 604–608.

■ ■ ■

3013

Test Name: MARITAL ACTIVITIES INVENTORY

Purpose: To discriminate between distressed and nondistressed couples.

Number of Items: 85

Format: Contains an inventory of common recreational, self-enhancing, affectional, and utilitarian activities.

Reliability: Test–retest (11 weeks) reliability coefficients were .71 and .87 ($N = 12$).

Author: Stein, S. J., et al.

Article: The interrelationships and reliability of a multilevel behavior-based assessment package for distressed couples.

Journal: *Journal of Behavioral Assessment*, December 1982, *4*(4), 343–360.

Related Research: Weiss, R. L., et al. (1973). A framework for conceptualizing marital conflict, a technology for altering it, some data for evaluating it. In L. A. Hamerlynck et al. (Eds.), *Behavior change: Methodology concepts and practice* (pp. 309–342). Champaign, IL: Research Press.

■ ■ ■

3014

Test Name: MARITAL ADJUSTMENT SCALE

Purpose: To measure marital adjustment.

Number of Items: 7

Format: Three agreement items, three frequency of occurrence items, and one global happiness item.

Reliability: Alpha was .77.

Author: Hansen, G.

Article: Perceived threats and marital jealousy.

Journal: *Social Psychology Quarterly*, September 1985, *48*(3), 262–268.

Related Research: Spanier, G. B. (1976). Measuring dyadic adjustment. New scales for assessing the quality of marriage and similar dyads. *Journal of*

Marriage and the Family, 38, 15–38.

Sharpley, C. F., & Cross, D. G. (1982). A psychometric evaluation of the Spanier Dyadic Adjustment Scale. *Journal of Marriage and the Family, 44*, 39–41.

■ ■ ■

3015

Test Name: MARITAL ADJUSTMENT TEST

Purpose: To provide an index of marital adjustment.

Number of Items: 15

Format: A score of 100 is the cutoff between nondistressed (above 100) and distressed (below 100).

Reliability: Split-half coefficient was .90.

Author: Volkin, J. I., and Jacob, T.

Article: The impacts of spouse monitoring on target behavior and recorder satisfaction.

Journal: *Journal of Behavioral Assessment*, June 1981, *3*(2), 99–109.

Related Research: Locke, H. J., & Wallace, K. M. (1957). Short marital adjustment and prediction tests: Their reliability and validity. *Marriage and Family Living, 21*, 251–255.

■ ■ ■

3016

Test Name: MARITAL ALTERNATIVE SCALE

Purpose: To measure frequency of marital alternatives if separation or divorce were to occur.

Number of Items: 11

Format: Possible alternatives to marriage followed by 4-point scale (*impossible* to *certain*). Sample items are presented.

Reliability: Alpha was .78.

Author: Hansen, G.

Article: Perceived threats and marital jealousy.

Journal: *Social Psychology Quarterly*, September 1985, *48*(3), 262–268.

Related Research: Udry, J. R. (1981). Marital alternatives and marital disruption. *Journal of Marriage and the Family, 43*, 889–897.

■ ■ ■

3017

Test Name: MARITAL COMMUNICATION INVENTORY

Purpose: To measure marital communication.

Number of Items: 46

Format: Self-report. Items are given.

Reliability: Internal consistency reliabilities ranged from .73 to .95.

Author: Schumm, W. R., et al.

Article: Dimensionality of the Marital Communication Inventory and marital conventionalization: A third report.

Journal: *Psychological Reports*, February 1981, *48*(1), 163–171.

Related Research: Schumm, W. R., et al. (1979). Dimensionality of the Marital Communication Inventory: A preliminary factor analytic study. *Psychological Reports, 45*, 123–128.

■ ■ ■

3018

Test Name: MARITAL COMPARISON LEVEL INDEX

Purpose: To measure evaluations of marital relationships.

Number of Items: 32

Format: Items rated on 7-point scales expressing a comparison of current experiences with current expectations.

Reliability: Alpha was .93.

Author: Sabatelli, R. M., and Cecil-Pigo, E. F.

Article: Relational interdependence and commitment in marriage.

Journal: *Journal of Marriage and the Family*, November 1985, *47*(4), 931–937.

Related Research: Sabatelli, R. M. (1984). The Marital Comparison Level Index: A measure for assessing outcomes relative to expectations. *Journal of Marriage and the Family, 46*, 651–662.

■ ■ ■

3019

Test Name: MARITAL CONVENTIONALIZATION SCALE

Purpose: To measure marital conventionalization.

Number of Items: 15

Format: There are two formats: (a) Respondents mark either *true* or *false* for each item. (b) Respondents select one statement from a pair of statements in a forced-choice format. All items are presented.

Reliability: Alpha reliability was .83 (*N* = 205) for true–false format and .90 (*N* = 160) for forced-choice format.

Validity: Correlations with marital adjustment ranged from .629 to .787.

Author: Hansen, G. L.

Article: Marital adjustment and conventionalization: A reexamination.

Journal: *Journal of Marriage and the Family*, November 1981, *43*(4), 855–863.

Related Research: Edmonds, V. H. (1967). Marital

conventionalization: Definition and measurement. *Journal of Marriage and the Family, 29*, 681–688.

■ ■ ■

3020

Test Name: MARITAL DISAFFECTION AND DISHARMONY SCALES

Purpose: To measure marital disaffection and disharmony (items from Marital Satisfaction Inventory).

Number of Items: 44

Format: True–false. All items presented.

Reliability: Internal consistency ranged from .87 to .95. Test–retest reliability ranged from .83 to .89.

Validity: A total of 29 behavioral correlations ($p < .05$) ranged from .22 to .41.

Author: Snyder, D. K., and Regts, J. M.

Article: Factor scales for measuring marital disharmony and disaffection.

Journal: *Journal of Consulting and Clinical Psychology*, October 1982, *50*(5), 736–743.

Related Research: Snyder, D. K. (1979). *Marital Satisfaction Inventory*. Los Angeles, CA: Western Psychological Services.

■ ■ ■

3021

Test Name: MARITAL GOAL-ORIENTATION SCALE

Purpose: To assess intentionality that couples employ to improve their marriages.

Number of Items: 7

Format: Multiple-choice (1 = *once in a while* to 5 = *almost always*).

Reliability: Alpha ranged from .86 to .89. Test–retest reliability

ranged from .76 to .87.

Validity: Correlated .51 to .90 with marital conflict.

Author: Eggeman, K., et al.

Article: Assessing spouses' perceptions of Gottman's Temporal Form in marital conflict.

Journal: *Psychological Reports*, August 1985, *57*(1), 171–181.

■ ■ ■

3022

Test Name: MARITAL HAPPINESS SCALE

Purpose: To measure marital happiness.

Number of Items: 10

Format: Areas include: household responsibilities; occupational progress; sex; spouse independence; other marital dimensions; and general happiness. Responses are made on a 10-point scale.

Reliability: Reliability coefficients ranged from .66 to .89 (*N* = 12).

Validity: Correlations with other variables ranged from −.30 to .78 (*N* = 46).

Author: Stein, S. J., et al.

Article: The interrelationships and reliability of a multilevel behavior-based assessment package for distressed couples.

Journal: *Journal of Behavioral Assessment*, December 1982, *4*(4), 343–360.

Related Research: Azrin, N., et al. (1973). Reciprocity counseling: A rapid learning based procedure for marital counseling. *Behavior Research Therapy, 11*, 365–382.

■ ■ ■

3023

Test Name: MARITAL INSTABILITY INDEX

Purpose: To measure instability in marriage.

Number of Items: 12

Format: Yes–no format.

Reliability: Internal consistency was .93.

Author: Booth, A., and Edwards, J. N.

Article: Age at marriage and marital instability.

Journal: *Journal of Marriage and the Family*, February 1985, *47*(1), 67–75.

Related Research: Booth, A., et al. (1983). Measuring marital instability. *Journal of Marriage and the Family, 40*, 387–394.

■ ■ ■

3024

Test Name: MARITAL INTERACTION CODING SYSTEM

Purpose: To measure interaction between married couples.

Number of Items: 28

Format: Observers code behavior every 30 seconds in 10-minute exchanges. Sample types of behavior presented.

Reliability: Mean interobserver correlation was .81. Point-by-point reliability ranged from .57 to .74.

Author: Margolin, G., and Wampold, B. E.

Article: Sequential analysis of conflict and accord in distressed and non-distressed marital partners.

Journal: *Journal of Consulting and Clinical Psychology*, August 1981, *49*(4), 554–567.

Related Research: Hops, H., et al. (1972). *Marital Interaction Coding System.* Unpublished manuscript.

University of Oregon and Oregon Research Institute.

■ ■ ■

3025

Test Name: MARITAL INTERACTION SATISFACTION SCALE

Purpose: To measure satisfaction with marital interaction.

Number of Items: 14

Format: Items rated on a 7-point desired frequency scale. Sample items presented.

Reliability: Alpha averaged .73 across husbands and wives and across three time periods.

Author: Belsky, J., et al.

Article: Stability and change in marriage across the transition to parenthood: A second study.

Journal: *Journal of Marriage and the Family*, November 1985, *47*(4), 855–865.

Related Research: Huston, T. (1983). *The topography of marriage: A longitudinal study of change in husband-wife relationships over the first year.* Plenary address: International Conference on Personal Relationships, Madison, WI.

■ ■ ■

3026

Test Name: MARITAL QUALITY SCALE

Purpose: To measure marital quality.

Number of Items: 27

Format: A Likert scale composed of five parts.

Reliability: Cronbach's alpha was .91.

Author: Bowen, G. L., and Orthner, D. K.

Article: Sex-role congruency and marital quality.

Journal: *Journal of Marriage and the Family*, February 1983, *45*(1), 223–230.

Related Research: Powers, W. G., & Hutchinson, K. (1979). The measurement of communication apprehension in the marriage relationship. *Journal of Marriage and the Family, 41*, 89–95.

■ ■ ■

3027

Test Name: MARITAL SATISFACTION QUESTIONNAIRE

Purpose: To measure marital satisfaction of wives.

Number of Items: 36

Format: Includes three parts: general issues, issues of agreement with husband, and extent of satisfaction of handling issues with husbands.

Reliability: Cronbach's alpha was .95.

Validity: Correlation with interviewer's perception of respondent's marital satisfaction was .64.

Author: Madden, M. E., and Janoff-Bulman, R.

Article: Blame, control, and marital satisfaction: Wives' attributions for conflict in marriage.

Journal: *Journal of Marriage and the Family*, August 1981, *43*(3), 663–674.

Related Research: Locke, H. J. (1968). *Predicting adjustment in marriage.* Westport, CT: Greenwood Press.

■ ■ ■

3028

Test Name: MARITAL SATISFACTION SCALE

Purpose: To measure marital satisfaction.

Number of Items: 10

Format: Items rated on 5-point frequency scales. Sample items presented.

Reliability: Alpha was .80.

Author: Farrell, J., and Markides, K. S.

Article: Marriage and health: A three-generational study of Mexican-Americans.

Journal: *Journal of Marriage and the Family,* November 1985, *47*(4), 1029–1036.

Related Research: Gilford, R., & Bengston, V. (1979). Measuring marital satisfaction in three generations: Positive and negative dimensions. *Journal of Marriage and the Family, 41,* 387–398.

■ ■ ■

3029

Test Name: OBJECTIVE MARITAL DEPENDENCY MEASURE

Purpose: To provide an index of wives' objective dependency.

Number of Items: 3

Format: Includes three dichotomous variables: women working, children age 5 or younger, husband earned 75% of couples' income.

Reliability: Cronbach's alpha was .598

Validity: Correlation with wives' subjective marital dependency was .147.

Author: Kalmuss, D. S., and Straus, M. A.

Article: Wife's marital dependency and wife abuse.

Journal: *Journal of Marriage and the Family,* May 1982, *44*(2), 277–286.

3030

Test Name: PARENT– ADOLESCENT RELATIONSHIPS SCALE

Purpose: To measure closeness to parents.

Number of Items: 21

Format: Items rated on 5-point closeness response categories. Sample items presented.

Reliability: Alpha ranged from .71 to .78 across two subscales.

Author: Bell, N. J., and Avery, A. W.

Article: Family structure and parent–adolescent relationships: Does family structure really make a difference?

Journal: *Journal of Marriage and the Family,* May 1987, *47*(2), 503– 508.

Related Research: Rundquist, E. A., & Sletto, R. F. (1936). *Personality in the Depression.* Minneapolis: University of Minnesota Press.

■ ■ ■

3031

Test Name: PARENTAL ACCEPTANCE–REJECTION QUESTIONNAIRE

Purpose: To measure parental warmth.

Number of Items: 60

Format: A self-report questionnaire on which children are asked to reflect upon the warmth, hostility, neglect, and undifferentiated rejection they experienced in their families. Responses are made on a 4-point Likert scale ranging from *almost always true* to *almost never true.* Examples are presented.

Reliability: Coefficient alphas ranged from .72 to .90.

Author: Rohner, R. P., and Pattengill, S. M.

Article: Perceived parental acceptance–rejection and parental control among Korean adolescents.

Journal: *Child Development,* April 1985, *56*(2), 524–528.

Related Research: Rohner, R. P. (1984). *Handbook for the study of parental acceptance and rejection* (Rev. ed.). Storrs, CT: Center for the Study of Parental Acceptance and Rejection, University of Connecticut.

■ ■ ■

3032

Test Name: PARENT ATTITUDE SURVEY (PAS)

Purpose: To measure parents' child-rearing attitudes.

Number of Items: 77

Format: Likert format.

Reliability: Split-half ranged from .68 to .86.

Author: Williams, R. E., et al.

Article: Effects of STEP on parental attitudes and locus of control of their learning disabled children.

Journal: *The School Counselor,* November 1984, *32*(2), 126–133.

Related Research: Hereford, C. F. (1963). *Changing parental attitudes through group discussion.* Austin: University of Texas Press.

■ ■ ■

3033

Test Name: PARENT–CHILD RELATION QUESTIONNAIRE— SHORT FORM II

Purpose: To measure adults' retrospective reports of parental behavior.

Number of Items: 50

Format: Items rated on a 5-point response scale (*very true* to *very untrue*).

Reliability: Cronbach's alpha ranged from .64 to .90 across scales, by sex.

Author: Tzuriel, D., and Haywood, H. C.

Article: Locus of control and child-rearing practices in intrinsically motivated and extrinsically motivated children.

Journal: *Psychological Reports,* December 1985, *57*(3, Part 1), 887–894.

Related Research: Roe, A., & Siegelman, M. (1963). A parent–child relation questionnaire. *Child Development, 34,* 335–369.

■ ■ ■

3034

Test Name: PARENT–CHILD RELATIONSHIP SURVEY

Purpose: To assess the quality of parent–child relationships.

Number of Items: 48 (24 for mothers, 24 for fathers).

Format: Likert items.

Reliability: .96 for father scale and .94 for mother scale.

Author: Worley, S. M., and Shwebel, A. I.

Article: The parent–child relationship survey: An examination of its psychometric properties.

Journal: *Psychological Reports,* August 1985, *57*(1), 155–161.

Related Research: Fine, M. A., et al. (1983). Long-term effects of divorce on parent–child relationships. *Developmental Psychology, 19,* 703–713.

3035

Test Name: PERCEIVED MARITAL SATISFACTION INDEX

Purpose: To measure marital satisfaction.

Number of Items: 5

Format: Respondents indicate the degree to which they are happy or satisfied with their marriage. Scores range from 5 to 35.

Reliability: Coefficient alpha was .88.

Validity: Correlations with other variables ranged from −.80 to .74.

Author: Tolstedt, B. E., and Stokes, J. P.

Article: Relation of verbal, affective, and physical intimacy to marital satisfaction.

Journal: *Journal of Counseling Psychology,* October 1983, *30*(4), 573–580.

Related Research: Locke, H. J., & Wallace, K. M. (1959). Short marital adjustment and prediction tests: Their reliability and validity. *Marriage and Family Living, 21,* 251–255.

■ ■ ■

3036

Test Name: PERCEIVED PATERNAL PARENTING SCALES

Purpose: To measure perceived paternal parenting.

Number of Items: 19

Format: Includes four scales: nurturance, instrumental companionship, affective punishment, and sex-role enforcement.

Reliability: Internal reliability coefficients ranged from .66 to .81.

Author: Devlin, P. K., and Cowan, G. A.

Article: Homophobia, perceived fathering and male intimate relationships.

Journal: *Journal of Personality Assessment,* October 1985, *49*(5), 467–473.

Related Research: McDonald, M. P. (1971). Internal–external locus of control: Parental antecedents. *Journal of Consulting and Clinical Psychology, 37,* 141–147.

Spence, J., & Helmreich, R. L. (1978). *Masculinity and femininity. Their psychological dimensions, correlates and antecedents.* Austin: University of Texas Press.

■ ■ ■

3037

Test Name: PERCEIVED SECURITY SCALE

Purpose: To measure mothers' perceptions of children's fear, anxiety, and sorrow in daily separations and in unfamiliar surroundings.

Number of Items: 11

Format: Items rated on 4- and 5-point rating scales. All items are presented.

Reliability: Cronbach's alpha was .84.

Validity: When subjects were divided into A1 + A2, B1 + B2 + B3, and B4 + C groups on Ainsworth's Strange Situation (1978), the means differed significantly ($F = 7.01, p < .01$) with the B4 + C scoring considerably less secure than the other groups.

Author: Van Ijzendoorn, M. H., et al.

Article: How B is B4? Attachment and security of Dutch children in Ainsworth's Strange Situation and at home.

Journal: *Psychological Reports,* June 1983, *52*(3), 683–691.

■ ■ ■

3038

Test Name: PERSONAL HISTORY INVENTORY FOR CHILDREN

Purpose: To measure parental support systems of children as perceived by teachers.

Number of Items: 14

Format: Yes–no. All items presented.

Reliability: Test–retest (1 month) reliability ranged from .80 (divorced parents) to .90 (intact families).

Validity: Correlates significantly with evaluations of self, mothers' evaluations, and fathers' evaluations ($p < .05$). Significant correlations ranged in magnitude from .18 to .41.

Author: Parish, T. S., and Wigle, S. E.

Article: Discerning functionality of children's support systems through use of the Personal History Inventory for children.

Journal: *Psychological Reports,* August 1985, *57*(1), 32–34.

■ ■ ■

3039

Test Name: PHYSICAL INTIMACY MEASURE

Purpose: To measure physical intimacy.

Number of Items: 15

Format: Items deal with: attractiveness of spouse, a variety of physical and sexual activities, and pleasure derived from those physical and sexual activities.

Reliability: Coefficient alpha was .89.

Validity: Correlations with other variables ranged from –.54 to .66.

Author: Tolstedt, B. E., and Stokes, J. P.

Article: Relation of verbal, affective and physical intimacy to marital satisfaction.

Journal: *Journal of Counseling Psychology,* October 1983, *30*(4), 573–580.

■ ■ ■

3040

Test Name: PSYCHOLOGICAL SEPARATION INVENTORY

Purpose: To measure adolescent psychological separation from parents.

Number of Items: 138

Format: Includes four scales of independence: functional, emotional, conflictual, and attitudinal. Examples of each are presented. Responses are made on a 5-point Likert scale ranging from *not at all true of me* (0) to *very true of me* (4).

Reliability: Cronbach's coefficient alpha ranged from .84 to .92. Test–retest (2 to 3 weeks) reliability coefficients ranged from .49 to .94 for 26 male responders and from .70 to .96 for 28 female responders.

Validity: Correlations with other variables ranged from –.37 to .30 for male responders and from –.38 to .41 for female responders.

Author: Hoffman, J. A.

Article: Psychological separation of late adolescents from their parents.

Journal: *Journal of Counseling Psychology,* April 1984, *31*(2), 170–178.

Related Research: Sherman, A. W. (1946). Emancipation status of college students. *Journal of Genetic Psychology, 68,* 171–180.

■ ■ ■

3041

Test Name: REWARDINGNESS SCALE

Purpose: To measure how rewarding marriage is.

Number of Items: 7

Format: Likert format.

Reliability: Alpha was .86.

Author: Hansen, G.

Article: Perceived threats and marital jealousy.

Journal: *Social Psychology Quarterly,* September 1985, *48*(3), 262–268.

Related Research: Cate, R. M., et al. (1982). Fairness and reward level as predictors of relationship satisfaction. *Social Psychology Quarterly, 45,* 177–181.

■ ■ ■

3042

Test Name: ROLLINS CHILD-REARING SCALE

Purpose: To measure parental behavior with children.

Number of Items: 78

Format: Children rate parents on each item. Items available from B. Rollins and D. Thomas, Department of Child Development, Brigham Young University, Provo, Utah 84602.

Reliability: Alpha ranged from .66 to .86 across subscales.

Validity: Items yielded similar factors in cross-cultural comparisons.

Author: Jenson, L., et al.

Article: Maternal behavior and the development of empathy in preschool children.

Journal: *Psychological Reports,* June 1981, *48*(3), 879–884.

Related Research: Thomas, P. L. (1977). *Validity in parent–child research: A comparison of self-report and behavioral observations.* Paper presented to the annual meeting of the Council of Family Relations.

■ ■ ■

3043

Test Name: SCALES FOR INVESTIGATION OF DUAL-CAREER FAMILY—REVISED

Purpose: To assess relevant information about dual-career women.

Number of Items: 44

Format: Includes 6 scales: Marriage type, domestic responsibility, satisfaction, self-image, career line, and career salience. All items are presented.

Reliability: Coefficient alphas for the scales ranged from .29 to .74.

Validity: Correlations with PRF ANDRO SCALES ranged from −.38 to .43.

Author: Gaddy, C. D., et al.

Article: A study of the Scales for Investigation of the Dual-Career Family.

Journal: *Measurement and Evaluation in Counseling and Development,* October 1985, *18*(3), 120–127.

Related Research: Pendleton, B. F., et al. (1980). Scales for investigation of the dual-career family. *Journal of Marriage and the Family, 42,* 269–276.

■ ■ ■

3044

Test Name: SIBLING RELATIONSHIP QUESTIONNAIRE

Purpose: To assess children's perceptions of the qualities of their sibling relationships.

Number of Items: 51

Format: Measures the following qualities: intimacy, prosocial behavior, companionship, similarity, nurturance by sibling, nurturance of sibling, admiration by sibling, admiration of sibling, affection, dominance by sibling, dominance over sibling, quarreling, antagonism, competition, parental partiality, general relationship evaluation.

Reliability: Test–retest (10 days) reliabilities ranged from .58 to .86 ($N = 84$).

Validity: Mean correlation with Children's Social Desirability Questionnaire was .14.

Author: Furman, W., and Buhrmester, D.

Article: Children's perceptions of the qualities of sibling relationships.

Journal: *Child Development,* April 1985, *56*(2), 448–461.

■ ■ ■

3045

Test Name: SPOUSE ADJECTIVE TEST

Purpose: To measure spouses' descriptions of self and partner.

Number of Items: 45

Format: Spouse checks adjectives that apply to self and on identical list for those that apply to spouse. Examples are presented. Provides 4 scores.

Validity: Correlations with locus of control ranged from −.37 to .26 (husbands) and from −.48 to .32 (wives).

Author: Doherty, W. J.

Article: Locus of control differences and marital dissatisfaction.

Journal: *Journal of Marriage and the Family,* May 1981, *43*(2), 369–377.

Related Research: Ryder, R. G. (1971). Dimensional structure of SPAT (The Spouse Adjective Test). *Catalog of Selected Documents in Psychology, 1,* 17.

■ ■ ■

3046

Test Name: SUBJECTIVE MARITAL DEPENDENCY SCALE

Purpose: To assess perceptions of wives concerning who would be hurt more in each of five areas by a marriage break up.

Number of Items: 5

Format: Includes 5 areas: financial, sexual, loss of friends, angry relatives, and loneliness.

Reliability: Coefficient alpha was .35.

Validity: Correlation with wives' objective marital dependency was .147.

Author: Kalmuss, D. S., and Straus, M. A.

Article: Wife's marital dependency and wife abuse.

Journal: *Journal of Marriage and the Family,* May 1982, *44*(2), 277–286.

■ ■ ■

3047

Test Name: TRADITIONAL FAMILY IDEOLOGY

Purpose: To measure the mother's attitude toward traditional versus modern family behavior.

Number of Items: 12

Format: Employs a 5-choice rating scale.

Validity: Correlation with the Index of Achievement Values was .54.

Author:. McGowan, R. J., and Johnson, D. L.

Article: The mother–child relationship and other antecedents of childhood intelligence: A causal analysis.

Journal: *Child Development,* June 1984, *55*(3), 810–820.

Related Research: Levinson, D., & Huffman, P. (1955). Traditional family ideology and its relation to personality. *Journal of Personality, 23,* 251–273.

■ ■ ■

3048

Test Name: TRANSITION TO PARENTHOOD MEASURE

Purpose: To measure the degree of difficulty of the transition to parenthood.

Number of Items: 25

Format: Includes three factors: parental responsibilities and restrictions, parental gratifications, and marital intimacy and stability. All items are presented.

Reliability: Reliability coefficients for the three factors were .751, .822, and .762.

Validity: Correlations with other variables ranged from –.334 to .394.

Author: Steffensmeier, R. H.

Article: A role model of the transition to parenthood.

Journal: *Journal of Marriage and the Family,* May 1982, *44*(2), 319–334.

Related Research: Steffensmeier, R. H. (1977). *A role analysis of the transition to parenthood: Research continuities and further development.* Unpublished doctoral dissertation, University of Iowa.

CHAPTER 14
Institutional Information

3049

Test Name: ADJECTIVE RATING SCALE

Purpose: To measure student expectations and perceptions of academic program and nonacademic life.

Number of Items: 24 adjectives, plus 2 statements.

Format: Four-point response scale per adjective. Sample adjective presented. Statements also presented.

Reliability: Internal consistency was .83 for program and .94 for nonacademic life on a factorially derived subscale.

Author: Pascarella, E. T., and Terenzini, P. T.

Article: Residence arrangement, student/faculty relationships and freshman year educational outcomes.

Journal: *Journal of College Student Personnel*, March 1981, *22*(2), 147–156.

Related Research: Kelly, E., et al. (1978). The development and use of the Adjective Rating Scale: A measure of attitude toward causes and programs. *Journal of Selected Abstracts in Science, 8,* 19–20.

■ ■ ■

3050

Test Name: AGENCY CLIMATE QUESTIONNAIRE

Purpose: To measure organization in six dimensions: structure, support, concern, autonomy, morale, and conflict.

Number of Items: 80

Format: Items rated on a 5-point scale.

Reliability: Internal consistency across scales ranged from .53 to .83.

Author: Heller, R. M., et al.

Article: Convergent and discriminant validity of psychological and objective indices of organizational climate.

Journal: *Psychological Reports,* 1982, *51*(1), 183–195.

Related Research: Schneider, B., & Bartlett, C. J. (1968). Individual differences and organizational climate: Research plan and questionnaire development. *Personnel Psychology, 21,* 323–333.

■ ■ ■

3051

Test Name: AUTONOMY SCALE

Purpose: To measure job autonomy and influence.

Number of Items: 9

Format: Items rated on a 5-point scale (*never true* to *always true*). Taken from Moos and Insel's Work Environment Scale.

Reliability: Alpha was .62.

Author: Jackson, S. E.

Article: Participation in decision-making as a strategy for reducing job-related stress.

Journal: *Journal of Applied Psychology,* February 1983, *68*(1), 3–19.

Related Research: Moos, R. H., &

Insel, P. M. (1984). *Work environment scale (Form R).* Palo Alto, CA: Consulting Psychologists Press.

■ ■ ■

3052

Test Name: BEHAVIOR CODES FOR JOB ENVIRONMENT

Purpose: To measure, by observation, job behavior.

Number of Items: 133 behaviors.

Format: Observers enter codes on a Datamyte 900 data collector. All categories of work are presented.

Reliability: Levels of agreement (Spearman rank-order correlation) ranged from .76 to .97 after observers had been trained 6 hours per week for 18 weeks.

Author: Ruggiero, M., and Steinberg, L. D.

Article: The empirical study of teenage work: A behavioral code for the assessment of adolescent job environments.

Journal: *Journal of Vocational Behavior,* August 1981, *19*(2), 163–174.

Related Research: Torgerson, L. (1977). Datamyte 900. *Behavior Research Methods and Instrumentation, 9*(5), 405–406.

■ ■ ■

3053

Test Name: BOUNDARY-SPANNING ROLES QUESTIONNAIRE

Purpose: To measure the extent of boundary-spanning roles in school psychologists' jobs.

Number of Items: 13

Format: Items rated on 5-point Likert response categories.

Reliability: Cronbach's alpha was .89.

Author: Jerrell, J. M.

Article: Boundary-spanning functions served by rural school psychologists.

Journal: *Journal of School Psychology*, 1984, *22*(3), 259–271.

Related Research: Jemison, D. B. (1980). *An empirical identification of interorganizational boundary-spanning roles.* Paper presented at the Academy of Management Annual Conference, San Diego.

■ ■ ■

3054

Test Name: BRANCH BANK CLIMATE FOR SERVICE SURVEY

Purpose: To measure perceptions of the service-related practices of the branch bank.

Number of Items: 28

Format: Includes four climate for service dimensions: branch management, systems support, customer attention/retention, and logistics support. Examples are presented.

Reliability: Coefficient alphas ranged from .53 to .85.

Validity: Correlations with other variables ranged from –.28 to .64.

Author: Schneider, B., and Bowen, D. E.

Article: Employee and customer perceptions of service in banks: Replication and extension.

Journal: *Journal of Applied Psychology*, August 1985, *70*(3), 423–433.

Related Research: Katz, K., & Kahn, R. L. (1978). *The social*

psychology of organizations (2nd ed.). New York: Wiley.

■ ■ ■

3055

Test Name: CHILDREN'S PERCEPTIONS OF EVERYDAY SCHOOLING CONVENTIONS

Purpose: To measure children's "perceived reality" at their schools.

Number of Items: 35

Format: Semistructured interview. Sample items presented.

Reliability: 98.5% agreement among raters of interview responses.

Validity: 98.1% correspondence between children's values and values implicit in several "value" items.

Author: Lee, P. C., et al.

Article: Elementary school children's perceptions of their actual and ideal school experience: A developmental study.

Journal: *Journal of Educational Psychology*, December 1983, *75*(6), 838–847.

■ ■ ■

3056

Test Name: CLASSROOM BEHAVIOR SCALE

Purpose: To measure classroom context.

Number of Items: 12 discreet behaviors monitored.

Time Required: 15 minutes per day for 4 days per child.

Format: 10-s observation followed by 10-s recording in each 15-min period. Behavior categories presented.

Reliability: .94 across all behaviors. Range was .60 to 1.00.

Author: Low, B. P., and Clement, P. W.

Article: Relationships of race and socioeconomic status to classroom behavior, academic achievement and referral for special education.

Journal: *Journal of School Psychology*, 1982, *20*(2), 103–112.

■ ■ ■

3057

Test Name: CLASSROOM ENVIRONMENT INDEX

Purpose: To measure psychological environment or press of the classroom.

Number of Items: 300

Reliability: Kuder-Richardson formula 20 ranged from .32 to .80 across 30 subscales.

Validity: Differentiates between grades, subjects, classrooms, and levels.

Author: Walker, W. J., and Richman, J.

Article: Dimensions of classroom environmental press.

Journal: *Psychological Reports*, October 1984, *55*(2), 555–562.

Related Research: Stern, G. G. (1970). *People in context.* New York: Wiley.

■ ■ ■

3058

Test Name: CLASSROOM LIFE INSTRUMENT

Purpose: To measure aspects of classroom life in 15 dimensions.

Number of Items: 67

Format: Items rated on a 5-point *truth–falsity* scale.

Reliability: Alpha ranged from .51 to .85 across subscales.

Validity: Factor analysis confirms 15 factors.

Author: Johnson, D. W., and Johnson, R. T.

Article: Social interdependence

and perceived academic and personal support in the classroom.

Journal: *Journal of Social Psychology*, June 1983, *120*(first half), 77–82.

■ ■ ■

3059

Test Name: CLIENT SATISFACTION SCALE

Purpose: To measure satisfaction with psychiatric treatment services.

Number of Items: 28

Format: Yes–no format. All items presented.

Validity: Two factors were extracted in a factor analysis: General satisfaction and satisfaction with activities and hospital environment.

Author: Distefano, M. K., et al.

Article: Factor structure of a clients' satisfaction scale with psychiatric patients.

Journal: *Psychological Reports*, December 1983, *53*(3, Part 2), 1155–1159.

Related Research: Glenn, R. N. (1978). Measuring patient opinions about hospitalization using the Client Satisfaction Scale. *Hospital and Community Psychiatry, 29*(3), 158–161.

■ ■ ■

3060

Test Name: COMMUNITY SATISFACTION SCALE— REVISED

Purpose: To measure community satisfaction.

Number of Items: 34

Reliability: Cronbach's alpha was .89.

Validity: A factor analysis revealed 8 interpretable factors in which

social and physical variables were intermingled.

Author: Bardo, J. W., and Bardo, D. J.

Article: A re-examination of substantive components of community satisfaction in a British new town.

Journal: *Journal of Social Psychology*, June 1983, *120*(first half), 35–45.

Related Research: Bardo, J. W. (1976). Dimensions of community satisfaction in a British new town. *Multivariate Experimental Clinical Research, 2*, 129–134.

■ ■ ■

3061

Test Name: COMPREHENSIVE JOB EVALUATION TECHNIQUE

Purpose: To provide an instrument for job evaluation.

Number of Items: 75

Format: Includes 15 scales of 5 items each: education, time to proficiency, previous experience, mental effort, physical effort, supervisory responsibility, financial responsibility, responsibility for the safety of others, surroundings, hazards, dexterity, monotony, visual effort, social interaction involving teaching and counseling, and social interaction involving negotiating and influencing.

Reliability: Correlations between raters equalled or exceeded .70.

Author: Doverspike, D., and Barrett, G. V.

Article: An internal bias analysis of a job evaluation instrument.

Journal: *Journal of Applied Psychology*, November 1984, *69*(4), 648–662.

Related Research: Treiman, D. J. (1979). *Job evaluation: An*

analytic review. Washington: National Academy of Sciences.

■ ■ ■

3062

Test Name: CONGREGATION SATISFACTION QUESTIONNAIRE

Purpose: To measure satisfaction with eight aspects of a religious congregation: leaders, members, facilities, services, education, rules, special programs, and clergy.

Number of Items: 79

Format: Multiple-choice. Sample items presented.

Reliability: Alphas ranged from .67 to .90 across subscales. Test–retest ranged from .62 to .82 across subscales.

Validity: Multitrait-multimethod matrix of CSQ and single-item criterion measures yielded support of validity in two of three Campbell and Fiske criteria.

Author: Silverman, W. H., et al.

Article: Measuring member satisfaction with the church.

Journal: *Journal of Applied Psychology*, November 1983, *68*(4), 664–677.

■ ■ ■

3063

Test Name: COUNSELING EVALUATION INVENTORY

Purpose: To measure counseling climate, comfort, and satisfaction with counseling.

Number of Items: 19

Format: Each item is rated on a 5-point scale.

Reliability: Test–retest reliability ranged from .62 to .83.

Validity: Correlations with congruence measures ranged from −.16 to .38.

Author: Hill, C. E., et. al.

Article: Nonverbal communication and counseling outcome.

Journal: *Journal of Counseling Psychology,* May 1981, *28*(3), 203–212.

Related Research: Linden, J. D., et al. (1965). Development and evaluation of an inventory for rating counselors, *Personnel and Guidance Journal, 43,* 267–276.

■ ■ ■

3064

Test Name: COURSE EVALUATION SCALES

Purpose: To measure student perceptions of college courses.

Number of Items: 31

Format: Seven-point Likert type items with appropriate anchor adjectives.

Reliability: Cronbach's alpha ranged from .50 to .80 across subscales.

Validity: Eight factors extracted, of which three significantly discriminated between dropping or not dropping a course (they were: student performance, motivation, and impression of instructor).

Author: Reed, J. G.

Article: Dropping a college course: Factors influencing students' withdrawal decisions.

Journal: *Journal of Educational Psychology,* June 1981, *73*(3), 376–385.

■ ■ ■

3065

Test Name: COURSE RATING SCALE FOR ORGANIZATIONAL BEHAVIOR

Purpose: To measure importance of topics in organizational behavior courses (in 13 dimensions).

Number of Items: 56

Format: Items rated on a 7-point scale ranging from *important topics* to *quite unimportant topics.* All items are presented.

Reliability: Cronbach's alpha ranged from .69 to .90 across dimensions.

Author: Rahim, A.

Article: Organizational behavior courses for graduate students in business administration: Views from the tower and battlefield.

Journal: *Psychological Reports,* 1981, *49*(2), 583–592.

■ ■ ■

3066

Test Name: CUSTOMER SERVICE-RELATED PRACTICES SURVEY

Purpose: To measure attitudes about service quality provided to customers.

Number of Items: 24

Format: Includes five dimensions: courtesy/competency; utility/security; adequate staff; employee morale; branch administration. Sample items are presented.

Reliability: Coefficient alphas ranged from .41 to .88

Validity: Correlations with other variables ranged from −.41 to .72.

Author: Schneider, B., and Bowen, D. E.

Article: Employee and customer perceptions of service in banks: Replication and extension.

Journal: *Journal of Applied Psychology,* August 1985, *70*(3), 423–433.

■ ■ ■

3067

Test Name: DEPARTMENTAL QUALITY SCALE

Purpose: To measure quality of college departments.

Number of Items: 11

Format: Items rated on a 5-point bipolar response scale. Items presented in abbreviated form.

Reliability: Horst reliability ranged from .17 to .94 across items in separate student and alumni samples.

Validity: Students scored higher than alumni on 3 instruction and classroom items. Alumni scored higher on vocational guidance item ($p < .01$).

Author: Wise, S. L., et al.

Article: Alumni ratings as an indicator of departmental quality.

Journal: *Journal of Educational Psychology,* February 1981, *73*(1), 71–77.

■ ■ ■

3068

Test Name: EDUCATIONAL GOALS SCALE

Purpose: To assess student and parental beliefs about the importance of and how well schools are meeting goals.

Number of Items: 12

Format: Rating scale format. All items presented.

Reliability: Alpha ranged from .91 (parents) to .95 (students).

Author: Grandjean, B. D., and Vaughn, E. S., III.

Article: Client perceptions of school effectiveness: A reciprocal causation model for students and their parents.

Journal: *The Sociology of Education,* October 1981, *54*(4), 275–290.

Related Research: Grandjean, B. D., & Bernal, H. H. (1979). Sex and centralization in a semiprofession. *Sociology of Work and Occupations, 6,* 84–102.

■ ■ ■

3069

Test Name: EFFECTANCE TEST

Purpose: To measure the production of effects upon the environment.

Number of Items: 80

Format: Includes three subscales: effect on self, effect on objects, and effect on people.

Reliability: Kuder-Richardson formula 20 reliabilities ranged from .71 to .86 ($N = 609$).

Validity: Correlations with other scales ranged from −.25 to .54 ($N = 82$ men) and from −.41 to .61 ($N = 110$ women).

Author: Lamont, D. J.

Article: A three-dimensional test for White's effectance motive.

Journal: *Journal of Personality Assessment,* February 1983, *47*(1), 91–99.

■ ■ ■

3070

Test Name: ENVIRONMENTAL CHECKLIST

Purpose: To measure geographical environments such as cities, neighborhoods, and college campuses.

Number of Items: 140

Format: Respondents checked adjectives that describe a specified place.

Reliability: Phi coefficient was .82 (test–retest, 21-day interval).

Validity: Correlates .58 with number of positive urban items checked on the McKechnie's urbanity scale (1975).

Author: Domino, G.

Article: Measuring geographical

environments through adjectives: The environmental checklist.

Journal: *Psychological Reports,* August 1984, *55*(1), 151–160.

■ ■ ■

3071

Test Name: ENVIRONMENTAL STRESS SCALE

Purpose: To measure environmental stress.

Number of Items: 10

Format: Employs a 5-point answer scale. A sample question is presented.

Reliability: Cronbach's alpha was .84.

Author: Frese, M., and Okonek, K.

Article: Reasons to leave shiftwork and psychological and psychosomatic complaints of former shiftworkers.

Journal: *Journal of Applied Psychology,* August 1984, *69*(3), 509–514.

Related Research: Semmer, N. (1982). Stress at work, stress in private life, and psychological well-being. In W. Bachmann et al. (Eds.), *Mental load and stress in activity: European approaches.* Berlin: Deutscher Verlag der Wissenschaften, and Amsterdam: North Holland.

■ ■ ■

3072

Test Name: ENVIRONMENTAL UNCERTAINTY SCALE

Purpose: To measure perceived level of environmental uncertainty.

Number of Items: 12

Format: Items rated on a 6-point frequency scale (*never* to *always*) indicated how often respondent encountered each of 12 situations in the job.

Reliability: Alpha was .56.

Author: Anderson, T. N. (Jr)., and Kida, T. E.

Article: The effect of environmental uncertainty on the association of expectancy attitudes, effort and performance.

Journal: *Journal of Social Psychology,* October 1985, *125*(5), 631–636.

Related Research: Duncan, R. B. (1972). Characteristics of organizational environments and perceived environmental uncertainty. *Administrative Science Quarterly, 17,* 313–327.

■ ■ ■

3073

Test Name: GLOBAL JOB CLASSIFICATION SCALE

Purpose: To classify jobs by global assessments of supervisors and incumbents in place of more time-consuming and costly task approaches.

Number of Items: 28

Time Required: 10–15 minutes.

Format: All possible pairs of 8 jobs rated on a 7-point similarity scale.

Validity: Correlation between global and task methods was .84. Correlation between supervisor and incumbent ratings was .94.

Author: Sackett, P. R.

Article: A comparison of global judgement vs. task-oriented approaches to job classification.

Journal: *Personnel Psychology,* Winter 1981, *34*(4), 791–804.

■ ■ ■

3074

Test Name: GROUP ATMOSPHERE SCALE

Purpose: To measure group atmosphere.

Number of Items: 10

Format: Semantic differential.

Reliability: Alpha was .91.

Author: Vecchio, R. P.

Article: A further test of leadership effects due to between-group variation and within-group variation.

Journal: *Journal of Applied Psychology,* April 1982, *67*(2), 200–208.

Related Research: Fiedler, F. E. (1967). *A theory of leadership effectiveness.* New York: McGraw-Hill.

■ ■ ■

3075

Test Name: HASSLES SCALE

Purpose: To measure irritants of daily living.

Number of Items: 117

Format: Checklist.

Reliability: Test–retest was .68 (4-month interval).

Author: Nowack, K. M.

Article: Type A behavior, family health history and psychological distress.

Journal: *Psychological Reports,* December 1985, *57*(3, Part 1), 799–806.

Related Research: Kanner, A. D., et al. (1979). Comparison of two modes of stress measurement: Daily hassles and uplifts versus major life events. *Journal of Behavioral Medicine, 4,* 41–51.

■ ■ ■

3076

Test Name: HENDERSON ENVIRONMENTAL LEARNING PROCESS SCALE

Purpose: To measure stimulation, parental guidance, modes, reinforcement, and aspiration.

Number of Items: 51 (of 55 original items).

Format: All items presented. Each is a "how often" question.

Reliability: Average item interitem correlation ranged from .14 to .22 using alternative methods.

Validity: Factors do not correspond to those extracted by Henderson.

Author: Silverstein, A. B., et al.

Article: Factor structure of the Henderson Environmental Learning Process Scale.

Journal: *Psychological Reports,* 1982, *50*(3, Part 1), 856–858.

Related Research: Henderson, R. W. (1972). Development and validation of the Henderson Environmental Learning Process Scale. *Journal of Social Psychology, 88,* 185–196.

■ ■ ■

3077

Test Name: HUMAN RESOURCES PRACTICES SURVEY

Purpose: To measure perceptions of the organization's human resources practices.

Number of Items: 40

Format: Includes five dimensions: work facilitation, supervision, organizational career facilitation, organizational status, new employee socialization. Examples are presented.

Reliability: Coefficient alphas ranged from .54 to .91.

Validity: Correlations with other variables ranged from .01 to .56.

Author: Schneider, B., and Bowen, D. E.

Article: Employee and customer perceptions of service in banks: replication and extension.

Journal: *Journal of Applied Psychology,* August 1985, *70*(3), 423–433.

■ ■ ■

3078

Test Name: INDIVIDUALIZED CLASSROOM ENVIRONMENT QUESTIONNAIRE

Purpose: To measure environmental perceptions of classrooms.

Number of Items: 50

Format: Includes five subscales: personalization, participation, independence, investigation, and differentiation.

Reliability: Alpha reliability coefficients for the subscales ranged from .74 to .92.

Validity: Correlation with other scales ranged from .16 to .37.

Author: Fraser, B. J.

Article: Development of short forms of several classroom environment scales.

Journal: *Journal of Educational Measurement,* Fall 1982, *19*(3), 221–227.

Related Research: Rentoul, A. J., & Fraser, B. J. (1979). Conceptualization of enquiry-based or open classroom learning environments. *Journal of Curriculum Studies, 11,* 233–245.

■ ■ ■

3079

Test Name: JOBS-CAREER KEY

Purpose: To measure four domains of job information (economic, education-training, job parts, and worker relationships).

Number of Items: 157

Format: Multiple-choice.

Reliability: Internal consistency ranged from .43 to .91. Test–retest

(N = 19) reliability was .62 (4-month interval).

Author: Yanico, B. J., and Mihlbauer, T. C.

Article: Students' self-estimated and actual knowledge of gender traditional and nontraditional occupation.

Journal: *Journal of Vocational Behavior,* June 1983, *22*(3), 278–287.

Related Research: Blank, J. R. (1978). Job-Career Key: A test of occupational information. *Vocational Guidance Quarterly, 27,* 6–17.

■ ■ ■

3080

Test Name: JOB CHARACTERISTICS INVENTORY

Purpose: To measure workers' perceptions of eight core job characteristics.

Number of Items: 24

Format: Characteristics assessed include: variety, autonomy, feedback, significance, identity, challenge, dealing with others, and friendship opportunities. Employs a Likert scale.

Reliability: Internal consistency estimates ranged from .24 to .76.

Author: Abush, R., and Burkhead, E. J.

Article: Job stress in midlife working women: Relationships among personality type, job characteristics and job tension.

Journal: *Journal of Counseling Psychology,* January 1984, *31*(1), 36–44.

Related Research: Sims, H. P., Jr., et al. (1976). The measurements of job characteristics. *Academy of Management Journal, 19,* 195–212.

3081

Test Name: JOB COMPONENTS INVENTORY

Purpose: A job analysis technique to measure physical and perceptual requirements, mathematical requirements, communication requirements, and decision-making/responsibility requirements.

Number of Items: 26 tools-use categories, 23 perceptual/physical items, 27 mathematical items, 22 communication items, 9 decision-making items.

Format: Paper-and-pencil and physical testing formats.

Reliability: Kendal's tau ranged between .21 and .85 across subscales for supervisor–jobholder pairing.

Validity: Scales discriminated occupational area (clerical vs. engineering) and job title (8 titles). Ten of 12 F ratios were significant at $p < .001$. Discriminated between organization less well. Three of six Fs were significant at $p < .05$.

Author: Banks, M. H.

Article: The Job Components Inventory and the analysis of jobs requiring limited skill.

Journal: *Personnel Psychology,* Spring 1983, *36*(1), 57–66.

■ ■ ■

3082

Test Name: JOB COMPONENTS INVENTORY II

Purpose: To measure the characteristics of work.

Time Required: 40 minutes to 53 minutes.

Format: Interview format.

Reliability: Interoffice correlation was .80; interrater agreement was .75.

Validity: Supervisor–job holder agreement was .72.

Author: Banks, M. H., and Miller, R. L.

Article: Reliability and convergent validity of the Job Components Inventory.

Journal: *Journal of Occupational Psychology,* September 1984, *57*(3), 181–184.

Related Research: Banks, M. H., et al. (1983). The Job Components Inventory and the analysis of jobs requiring limited skill. *Personnel Psychology, 36,* 57–66.

■ ■ ■

3083

Test Name: JOB FEEDBACK SURVEY

Purpose: To assess the amount and type of feedback information available to individuals at work.

Number of Items: 95

Format: Various formats. All items presented.

Reliability: Alphas ranged from .68 to .90 across 15 subscales.

Validity: A total of 9 subscales discriminated two feedback environments (a utility and a hospital), $p < .05$.

Author: Herold, D. M., and Parsons, C. K.

Article: Assessing the feedback environment in work organizations: Development of the Job Feedback Survey.

Journal: *Journal of Applied Psychology,* May 1985, *70*(2), 290–305.

Related Research: Herold, D. M., & Greller, M. M. (1977). Feedback: The definition of a construct. *Academy of Management Journal, 20,* 142–147.

3084

Test Name: JOB STRUCTURE PROFILE

Purpose: To describe the structure of jobs.

Number of Items: 248

Format: Trained interviewer prompts job raters.

Reliability: Interrater reliability was .95. Single-rater reliability was .71. Test–retest reliability was .76.

Author: Patrick, J., and Moore, A. K.

Article: Development and reliability of a job analysis technique.

Journal: *Journal of Occupational Psychology*, June 1985, *58*(2), 149–158.

Related Research: McCormick, E. K., et al. (1972). A study of characteristics and job dimensions as based on the Position Analysis Questionnaire (PAQ). *Journal of Applied Psychology, 56*, 347–368.

■ ■ ■

3085

Test Name: JOB TREATMENT INDEX

Purpose: To measure perceptions of job-related sex discrimination.

Number of Items: 11

Format: Men and women are asked to respond to each item by comparing their own treatment to that of the opposite sex (*worse than, same as, better than*).

Reliability: Alpha was .92.

Author: Graddick, M. M., and Farr, J. L.

Article: Professionals in scientific disciplines: Sex-related differences in working life commitments.

Journal: *Journal of Applied Psychology*, November 1983, *68*(4), 641–645.

Related Research: Connolly, T., et al. (1976). *The woman professional in science and engineering: An empirical study of key decisions.* New York: National Science Foundation.

■ ■ ■

3086

Test Name: LECTURE EVALUATION INSTRUMENT

Purpose: To measure qualities that make a good mathematics lecture.

Number of Items: 63

Format: Items rated on 5-point response categories (*very poor* to *very good*).

Reliability: Alphas ranged from .70 to .94 across subscales.

Author: Clarkson, P. C.

Article: Papua New Guinea students: Perceptions of mathematics lecturers.

Journal: *Journal of Educational Psychology*, December 1984, *76*(6), 1386–1395.

Related Research: Marsh, H. W. (1981). Students' evaluation of tertiary instruction: Testing the applicability of American surveys in an Australian setting. *Australian Journal of Education, 25,* 177–193.

■ ■ ■

3087

Test Name: LIVING ENVIRONMENT SCALE

Purpose: To measure living environment.

Number of Items: 6

Format: Includes assessment of satisfaction with privacy, transportation, feelings of security, housing, neighborhood, and proximity of supportive relationships. Responses are made on a scale from 1 (*very dissatisfied*) to 4 (*very satisfied*).

Reliability: Reliability coefficient was .64 (older parents).

Validity: Correlations with other variables ranged from −.070 to .210.

Author: Quinn, W. H.

Article: Personal and family adjustment in later life.

Journal: *Journal of Marriage and the Family,* February 1983, *45*(1), 57–73.

Related Research: Johnson, E. S. (1978). Good relationships between older mothers and their daughters: A causal model. *The Gerontologist, 18,* 301–308.

■ ■ ■

3088

Test Name: MECHANISTIC STRUCTURAL JOB CHARACTERISTICS SCALES

Purpose: To measure mechanistic structural job characteristics.

Number of Items: 20

Format: Includes the following scales: job codification, job specificity, hierarchy of authority, and lack of participation. Sample items are presented.

Reliability: Coefficient alphas ranged from .62 to .83.

Author: Marino, K. E., and White, S. E.

Article: Departmental structure, locus of control and job stress: The effect of a moderator.

Journal: *Journal of Applied Psychology*, November 1985, *70*(4), 782–784.

Related Research: Hage, G., & Aiken, M. (1969). Routine technology, social structure, and organizational goals.

Administrative Science Quarterly,
14, 366–376.

■ ■ ■

3089

Test Name: MEDICAL SCHOOLS
LEARNING ENVIRONMENT
SURVEY

Purpose: To measure students'
perceptions of their medical
school.

Number of Items: 55

Format: Includes a 4-point
response scale (*seldom,*
occasionally, fairly often, very
often). Items made up seven
subscales: flexibility, student–
student interaction, emotional
climate, supportiveness,
meaningful learning experience,
organization, and breadth of
interest. Some items are presented.

Reliability: Coefficient alphas
ranged from .56 to .94.

Author: Feletti, G. I., and Clark,
R. M.

Article: Construct validity of a
learning environment survey for
medical schools.

Journal: *Educational and*
Psychological Measurement,
Autumn 1981, *41*(3), 875–882.

Related Research: Marshall, R. E.
(1978). Measuring the medical
school learning environment.
Journal of Medical Education, 53,
98–104.

■ ■ ■

3090

Test Name: MINNESOTA
THERAPY RATING SCALE

Purpose: To identify differences
between two forms of therapy used
in treatment of depression.

Number of Items: 48

Format: Items rated in 9-point
Likert format. Raters view tapes of
sessions and rate them on 9-point

scales. All items are presented.

Reliability: Modal item reliability
was .70. Reliabilities of subscales
ranged from .46 to .90.

Validity: Classification of 12
sample tapes with 18 variable
discriminant functions yielded
perfect classification.

Author: DeRubeis, R. J., et al.

Article: Can psychotherapies for
depression be discriminated? A
systematic investigation of
cognitive therapy and
interpersonal therapy.

Journal: *Journal of Consulting and*
Clinical Psychology, October
1982, *50*(5), 744–756.

Related Research: Young, J.
(1981). *The development of the*
Cognitive Therapy Scale.
Unpublished manuscript, Center
for Cognitive Therapy,
Philadelphia.

■ ■ ■

3091

Test Name: MOTIVATING
POTENTIAL SCORE

Purpose: To measure job
complexity.

Number of Items: 15

Format: Includes five job
characteristics: skill variety,
autonomy, task identity, task
significance, and feedback from
the job itself. Items rated on 5-
point response scales.

Reliability: Alpha coefficient was
.89 (*N* = 166).

Validity: Correlations with other
variables ranged from .04 to .45.

Author: Tharenou, P., and
Harker, P.

Article: Moderating influence of
self-esteem on relationship
between job complexity,
performance, and satisfaction.

Journal: *Journal of Applied*

Psychology, November 1984,
69(4), 623–632.

Related Research: Hackman,
J. R., & Oldham, G. R. (1974).
The Job Diagnostic Survey: An
instrument for the diagnosis of
jobs and the evaluation of redesign
projects (Tech. Rep. No. 4). New
Haven, CT: Yale University,
Department of Administrative
Sciences.

■ ■ ■

3092

Test Name: MULTIMETHOD JOB
DESIGN QUESTIONNAIRE

Purpose: To permit an
examination of job design.

Number of Items: 70

Format: Includes four sections:
motivational, mechanistic,
biological, and perceptual/motor.
Sample items are presented.

Reliability: Interrater reliabilities
ranged from .89 to .93.

Validity: Correlations with
theoretical job outcome composites
ranged from −.77 to .54.

Author: Campion, M. A., and
Thayer, P. W.

Article: Development and field
evaluation of an interdisciplinary
measure of job design.

Journal: *Journal of Applied*
Psychology, February 1983, *70*(1),
29–43.

■ ■ ■

3093

Test Name: MY CLASS
INVENTORY

Purpose: To measure actual
classroom environment.

Number of Items: 38

Format: Subjects respond to each
item on a yes–no format. Includes
five scales: satisfaction, friction,
competitiveness, difficulty, and
cohesiveness.

Reliability: Alpha reliability coefficients for the subscales ranged from .73 to .88.

Validity: Correlation with other scales ranged from .13 to .30.

Author: Fraser, B. J.

Article: Development of short forms of several classroom environment scales.

Journal: *Journal of Educational Measurement*, Fall 1982, *19*(3), 221–227.

Related Research: Fisher, D. L., & Fraser, B. J. (1981). Validity and use of My Class Inventory. *Science Education, 65*, 145–156.

■ ■ ■

3094

Test Name: MY CLASS INVENTORY

Purpose: To measure primary classroom climate.

Number of Items: 45

Format: Includes five scale dimensions: satisfaction, friction, competitiveness, difficulty, and cohesion. Employs a yes–no format.

Reliability: Scale reliabilities ranged from .54 to .77.

Validity: Correlations with sex-bias scores ranged from –.61 to .84.

Author: Prawat, R. S., and Solomon, D. J.

Article: Validation of a classroom climate inventory for use at the early elementary level.

Journal: *Educational and Psychological Measurement,* Summer 1981, *41*(2), 567–573.

Related Research: Anderson, G. J., & Walberg, H. J. (1974). Learning environments. In H. J. Walberg (Ed.), *Evaluating educational performance.* Berkeley, CA: McCutcheon.

3095

Test Name: NARRATIVE JOB DESCRIPTION CLASSIFICATION SYSTEM

Purpose: To describe key characteristics of jobs and similarities and differences between jobs.

Number of Items: 121

Format: Narrative job descriptions taken from U. S. Civil Service Commission Qualification Standards (1978).

Reliability: Intraclass correlations of PAQ Job Dimensions for 121 jobs ranged between .20 and .90. Average pairings correlations ranged from .36 to .88.

Validity: PAQ job dimensions for the 121 descriptions demonstrated multiple correlations of .51 to .85 with ability requirement estimates from the Dictionary of Occupational Titles.

Author: Jones, A. P., et al.

Article: Narrative job descriptions as potential sources of job analysis ratings.

Journal: *Personnel Psychology,* Winter 1982, *35*(4), 813–828.

Related Research: McCormick, E. J., et al. (1972). A study of job characteristics and job dimensions as based on the Position Analysis Questionnaire (PAQ). *Journal of Applied Psychology, 56,* 347–368.

■ ■ ■

3096

Test Name: OCCUPATION ANALYSIS INVENTORY

Purpose: To rate jobs and occupations.

Number of Items: 617

Format: The items are referred to as "work elements," which are descriptions of work activities and conditions. Examples are given.

Reliability: The mean element reliability coefficient was .53.

Author: Cunningham, J. W., et al.

Article: Systematically derived work dimensions: Factor analysis of the Occupational Analysis Inventory.

Journal: *Journal of Applied Psychology,* May 1983, *68*(2), 232–251.

Related Research: Cunningham, J. W., et al. (1974). The development of the Occupation Analysis Inventory: An "ergometric" approach to an educational problem. *JSAS Catalog of Selected Documents in Psychology, 4,* 144 (Ms. No. 803).

■ ■ ■

3097

Test Name: ORGANIZATIONAL CLIMATE QUESTIONNAIRE

Purpose: To measure working conditions.

Number of Items: 30

Format: Items rated on 4-point agreement scales. All items are presented. Items were modified from Litwin and Stringer Organizational Climate Scale.

Validity: Subscales correlate significantly ($p < .01$) with intrinsic, extrinsic, and social job satisfaction.

Author: Schnake, M. E.

Article: An empirical assessment of the effects of affective response in the measurement of organizational climate.

Journal: *Personnel Psychology,* Winter 1983, *36*(4), 791–807.

Related Research: Litwin, G. H., & Stringer, R. A. (1968). *Motivation and organizational climate.* Boston: Harvard University.

3098

Test Name: ORGANIZATIONAL CLIMATE QUESTIONNAIRE—REVISED

Purpose: To measure 7 dimensions of organizational climate.

Number of Items: 34

Format: Items rated on a 7-point Likert scale. Sample items are presented.

Reliability: All alphas were .69 or greater ($M = .78$).

Author: Mossholder, K. W., et al.

Article: An examination of intraoccupational differences: Personality, perceived work climate and outcome preferences.

Journal: *Journal of Vocational Behavior*, April, 1985, *26*(2), 164–176.

Related Research: Litwin, G. H., & Stringer, R. A. (1968). *Motivation and organizational climate.* Boston: Harvard University.

■ ■ ■

3099

Test Name: ORGANIZATIONAL CLIMATE SCALE

Purpose: To assess the perceptions of workers and employers regarding organizational climate.

Number of Items: 18

Format: Items deal with the following climate dimensions: leadership, motivation, communication, decisions, goals, and control.

Validity: Item correlations between workers and employers ranged from −.84 to .73.

Author: Narayanan, S., and Venkatachalam, R.

Article: Perception of organizational climate.

Journal: *Perceptual and Motor Skills*, August 1982, *55*(1), 15–18.

Related Research: Likert, R. (1967). *The human organization.* New York: McGraw-Hill.

■ ■ ■

3100

Test Name: ORIGIN CLIMATE QUESTIONNAIRE

Purpose: To assess classroom climate.

Number of Items: 24

Format: Items rated on a Likert scale that includes measures of the students' perceptions of teachers' behaviors directed toward developing goal-setting, goal-directed behavior, accurate perceptions of reality, internal control, personal responsibility, and self-confidence among students. The items are split between positive and negative wording.

Validity: Correlations with attributed responsibility for success were .254 (grade 8) and .345 (grade 11); failure were .185 (grade 8) and .448 (grade 11). Correlations with grades were .204 (grade 8) and .198 (grade 11).

Author: Sadowski, C. J., and Woodward, H. R.

Article: Relationship between origin climate, perceived responsibility and grades.

Journal: *Perceptual and Motor Skills*, August 1981, *53*(1), 259–261.

Related Research: DeCharms, R. (1976). *Enhancing motivation: Changes in the classroom.* New York: Irvington.

■ ■ ■

3101

Test Name: PLEASANT EVENTS SCHEDULE

Purpose: To measure potentially reinforcing events by behavioral self-report.

Number of Items: 320

Format: Items rated on a 3-point rating scale (*not happened, happened a few times, happened often*). All items are presented.

Reliability: Test–retest reliability ranged from .50 to .88 with 1-, 2-, and 3-month intervals.

Validity: Validity ranged from .22 to .77 (multitrait, multimethod). Extensive validity data was reported.

Author: MacPhillamy, D. J., and Lewinsohn, P. M.

Article: The Pleasant Events Schedule: Studies on reliability, validity and scale intercorrelation.

Journal: *Journal of Consulting and Clinical Psychology*, June 1982, *50*(3), 363–380.

Related Research: MacPhillamy, D. J., & Lewinsohn, P. M. (1972). *Pleasant Events Schedule.* Unpublished manuscript, University of Oregon.

■ ■ ■

3102

Test Name: PREFERRED ORGANIZATIONAL CLIMATES SCALE

Purpose: To measure how well hypothetical organizations satisfy personality needs and vocational interests of individuals.

Number of Items: 9 (organizational types).

Format: Items rated on 9-point Likert scales. All nine organizational climates are presented.

Reliability: Alpha ranged from .89 to .95.

Author: Burke, R. J., and Deszca, E.

Article: Preferred organizational climates of Type A individuals.

Journal: *Journal of Vocational*

Behavior, August 1982, *21*(1), 50–59.

Related Research: Rothstein, M., & Rush, J. C. (1980). *Organizational choice as a means of satisfying individual needs and interests.* Unpublished working paper, School of Business Administration, University of Western Ontario, London, Ontario.

■ ■ ■

3103

Test Name: PROJECT COMPLEXITY CHECKLIST

Purpose: To measure the dimensions of project complexity.

Number of Items: 11

Format: Item stems followed by three to seven responses, any or all of which can be checked. All items presented in an appendix. Projects rated were validated at national or state levels and offered to schools for adoption.

Reliability: Interrater reliability of five raters was .96.

Validity: Content validity assessed by a panel of four experts.

Author: Humphries, J., and Newfield, J.

Article: Identifying and measuring dimensions of project complexity.

Journal: *Journal of Educational Research,* March/April 1982, *75*(4), 248–253.

Related Research: Goodlad, J. I., & Klein, M. F. (1974). *Looking behind the classroom door.* Worthington, OH: Charles A. Jones.

3104

Test Name: POSITION DESCRIPTION QUESTIONNAIRE—SHORT FORM

Purpose: To provide a vehicle for

analyzing managerial positions.

Number of Items: 54

Format: Includes nine dimensions of managerial behavior: strategic planning, product/service activities, controlling, monitoring business indicators, supervising, coordinating, customer relations/marketing, external contact, and consulting.

Reliability: Median internal consistency was .73. Median alternate form reliability coefficient was .71. Coefficient alphas ranged from .69 to .91.

Author: Colarelli, S. M., et al.

Article: Cross-validation of a short form of the position description questionnaire.

Journal: *Educational and Psychological Measurement,* Winter 1982, *42*(4), 1279–1283.

Related Research: Page, R. C., & Gomez, L. R. (1979). *The development and application of job evaluation and staffing systems using the Position Description Questionnaire* (Personal Research Report No. 162–79). Minneapolis, MN: Control Data Corporation.

■ ■ ■

3105

Test Name: PUPIL CONTROL IDEOLOGY FORM

Purpose: To measure the pupil control ideology of schools.

Number of Items: 20

Format: Likert items with responses scored from 5 (*strongly agree*) to 1 (*strongly disagree*).

Reliability: Split-half corrected reliability coefficients were .95 (*N* = 170) and .91 (*N* = 55).

Validity: Correlations with self-concept as a learner ranged from –.29 to –.51 (for 35 students), and –.12 to –.51 (for 35 teachers).

Author: Lunenburg, F. C.

Article: Pupil control ideology and self-concept as a learner.

Journal: *Educational Research Quarterly,* 1983, *8*(3), 33–39.

Related Research: Willower, D. J., et al. (1967). *The school and pupil control ideology.* University Park: Pennsylvania State University.

■ ■ ■

3106

Test Name: REACTION INVENTORY

Purpose: To identify specific stimulus situations which lead to anger.

Number of Items: 76

Format: Responses to each item are made on a 5-point scale ranging from *not at all* to *very much.*

Reliability: Test–retest reliability coefficient was .70.

Author: Biaggio, M. K., et al.

Article: Reliability and validity of four anger scales.

Journal: *Journal of Personality Assessment,* December 1981, *45*(6), 639–648.

Related Research: Evans, D. R., & Strangeland, M. (1971). Development of the Reaction Inventory to measure anger. *Psychological Reports, 29,* 412–414.

■ ■ ■

3107

Test Name: ROBUSTNESS SEMANTIC DIFFERENTIAL SCALE

Purpose: To measure school principals' job robustness.

Number of Items: 10

Format: Includes polar adjectives and a 7-point response scale. Examples are presented.

Reliability: Test–retest (4 weeks)

reliabilities were .77 and .78.

Validity: Correlations with other variables ranged from .21 to .59.

Author: Eisenhauer, J. E., et al.

Article: Role conflict, role ambiguity and school principals' job robustness.

Journal: *Journal of Experimental Education,* Winter 1984/85, *53*(2), 86–90.

Related Research: Licata, J. W., & Willower, D. J. (1978). Toward an operational definition of environmental robustness. *Journal of Educational Research, 71,* 218–222.

■ ■ ■

3108

Test Name: SCHOOL CLIMATE QUESTIONNAIRE

Purpose: To measure qualities such as openness and cohesiveness of staff.

Number of Items: 14

Format: Likert format.

Reliability: Internal consistency was .81.

Author: Nagy, S., and Davis, L.

Article: Burnout: A comparative analysis of personality and environmental variables.

Journal: *Psychological Reports,* December 1985, *57*(3, Part 2), 1319–1326.

Related Research: Fielding, M. (1982). Personality and situational correlates of teacher stress and burnout. *Dissertation Abstracts International, 43,* 400-A.

■ ■ ■

3109

Test Name: SCHOOL LEARNING ENVIRONMENT SCHEDULE

Purpose: To assess adolescents' perceptions of their school learning environment.

Number of Items: 20

Format: Likert items dealing with contexts identified as regulative, instructional, imaginative or innovative, and interpersonal. Examples are presented.

Validity: Correlations with aspirations ranged from .16 to .41.

Author: Marjoribanks, K.

Article: Families, schools and aspirations: Ethnic group differences.

Journal: *Journal of Experimental Education,* Spring 1985, *53*(3), 141–147.

Related Research: Bernstein, B. (1977). Social class, language and socialization. In J. Karabel & A. H. Halsey (Eds.), *Power and ideology in education.* New York: Oxford University Press.

■ ■ ■

3110

Test Name: SENSITIVITY TO NOISE SCALE

Purpose: To measure reactivity to noise.

Number of Items: 21

Format: Items rated in 6-point Likert format.

Reliability: Test–retest reliability was .75 (N = 72). Alpha was .76 (N = 150).

Author: Topf, M.

Article: Personal and environmental predictors of patient disturbance due to hospital noise.

Journal: *Journal of Applied Psychology,* February 1985, *70*(1), 22–28.

Related Research: Weinstein, N. (1978). Individual differences in reactions to noise: A longitudinal study in a college dormitory. *Journal of Applied Psychology, 63,* 458–466.

3111

Test Name: SOUTH AFRICAN LIFE EVENT SCALE

Purpose: To measure exposure and seriousness of life events among South African Whites.

Number of Items: 92

Format: Multiple-choice.

Reliability: Test–retest varied between .83 and .93.

Author: Chalmers, B.

Article: Types of life events and factors influencing their seriousness rating.

Journal: *Journal of Social Psychology,* December 1983, *121*(second half), 283–295.

Related Research: Antononsky, A. (1974). Conceptual and methodological problems in the study of resistance resources and stressful life events. In B. S. Dohrenwend & B. P. Dohrenwend (Eds.), *Stressful life events: Their nature and effects* (pp. 245–258). New York: Wiley.

Chalmers, B. (1981). Development of a life event scale for pregnant, White South African women. *South African Journal of Psychology, 11,* 74–79.

■ ■ ■

3112

Test Name: STAFF DEVELOPMENT EVALUATION QUESTIONNAIRE

Purpose: To measure clinical staffs perceptions and valuations of in-service programs.

Number of Items: 16

Format: Six-point Likert scale. (1 = *strongly disagree* to 6 = *strongly agree.*) Sample items presented.

Reliability: Cronbach's alpha was .83. Test–retest reliability was .81.

Validity: Face validity (by experts

in adult learning and continuing education).

Author: Abraham, I. L., and Hagerty, B. K.

Article: Development and internal reliability testing of an instrument to measure attitudes toward in-service programming among psychiatric hospital staff.

Journal: *Psychological Reports,* October 1983, *53*(2), 589–590.

■ ■ ■

3113

Test Name: STAFF DEVELOPMENT QUESTIONNAIRE

Purpose: To measure factors productive of knowledge use in staff development.

Number of Items: 52

Format: Likert items. Sample items presented.

Reliability: Ranged from .20 to .78 on various items and scales.

Author: Walberg, H. J., and Genova, W. J.

Article: Staff, school, and workshop influences on knowledge use in educational improvement efforts.

Journal: *Journal of Educational Research,* November/December 1982, *76*(2), 69–80.

Related Research: Genova, W. J., & Walberg, H. J. (1979). *Promoting student integration in city high schools: A research study and improvement guide for practitioners.* Washington, DC: NIE.

■ ■ ■

3114

Test Name: STUDENT LEARNING ENVIRONMENT QUESTIONNAIRE

Purpose: To measure motivation to learn, quality of instruction, class

environment, and home, peer and media environment.

Number of Items: 5 to 7 items on each of seven subscales.

Format: Items rated in 5-point Likert format. Sample items are presented.

Reliability: Internal consistency ranged from .35 to .64 (*M* = .52).

Validity: Items as measures of the subscales were assessed by LISREL.

Author: Parkerson, J. A., et al.

Article: Exploring causal models of educational achievement.

Journal: *Journal of Educational Psychology,* August 1984, *76*(4), 638–646.

■ ■ ■

3115

Test Name: TASK COMPLEXITY SCALE

Purpose: To measure complexity of tasks.

Number of Items: 7

Format: Semantic differential. Sample adjective pairs presented.

Reliability: Alpha was .71.

Author: Huber, V. L.

Article: Effects of task difficulty, goal setting and strategy on performance of a heuristic task.

Journal: *Journal of Applied Psychology,* August 1985, *70*(3), 492–504.

Related Research: Scott, W. E. (1967). Activation theory and task design. *Organizational Behavior and Human Performance, 1,* 3–30.

■ ■ ■

3116

Test Name: TEACHER ASSESSMENT OF STUDENT SCALE

Purpose: To measure the qualities of a "good class."

Number of Items: 3

Format: Multiple-choice. All items presented.

Reliability: Alpha was .80.

Validity: Correlates with student assessments of their own standards (*r* = .41, *p* < .01).

Author: Peterson, M. F., and Cooke, R. A.

Article: Attitudinal and contextual variables explaining teachers' leadership behavior.

Journal: *Journal of Educational Psychology,* February 1983, *75*(1), 50–62.

■ ■ ■

3117

Test Name: TEACHER OCCUPATIONAL STRESS FACTOR QUESTIONNAIRE

Purpose: To identify occupational stress factors perceived by public school teachers.

Number of Items: 30

Format: Factors include: administration support, working with students, financial security, relationships with teachers, and task overload.

Reliability: Cronbach's alpha reliabilities ranged from .85 to .91.

Author: Moracco, J. C., et al.

Article: Comparison of perceived occupational stress between teachers who are contented and discontented in their career choices.

Journal: *Vocational Guidance Quarterly,* September 1983, *32*(1), 44–51.

Related Research: Moracco, J. C., et al. (1981). The factorial validity of the Teacher Occupational Stress Questionnaire. *Educational and*

Psychological Measurement, 42, 275–283.

•••

3118

Test Name: UNION AS A MECHANISM FOR CHANGE SCALE

Purpose: To measure the value of union representation in the organization.

Number of Items: 6

Format: A 6-point scale was used to respond to each item. All items are presented.

Reliability: Estimate of internal consistency was .80.

Validity: Correlation with other variables ranged from −.21 to .18. Correlation with direct questions about the instrumentality of the union as a mechanism for changing conditions of employment and company policy was .56.

Author: Hammer, T. H., et al.

Article: Absenteeism when workers have a voice: The case of employee ownership.

Journal: *Journal of Applied Psychology,* October 1981, *66*(5), 561–573.

Related Research: Hammer, T. H., & Stern, R. M. (1980). Employee ownership implications for the organizational distribution of power. *Academy of Management Journal, 23,* 78–100.

•••

3119

Test Name: VANDERBILT NEGATIVE INDICATORS SCALE (VNIS)

Purpose: To measure factors negatively related to therapeutic outcome.

Number of Items: 42

Format: A rating scale ranging from 0 to 5 reflects judgments by raters of therapeutic interaction.

Reliability: Alpha ranged from .26 to .84 across subscales. Interrater reliability ranged from .73 to .93 across subscales.

Validity: Canonical correlation between VNIS and six outcome variables was .95. Subscale correlations ranged from −.34 to −.59 across outcome measures.

Author: Sachs, J. S.

Article: Negative factors in brief psychotherapy: An empirical assessment.

Journal: *Journal of Consulting and Clinical Psychology,* August 1983, *51*(4), 557–564.

Related Research: Strupp, H. H., et al. (1981). *Vanderbilt Negative Indicators Scale: An instrument for the identification of deterrents to progress in time-limited dynamic psychotherapy.* Unpublished manuscript, Vanderbilt University.

•••

3120

Test Name: WARD ATMOSPHERE SCALE— SHORT FORM

Purpose: To conceptualize and evaluate the psychiatric treatment environment with particular attention to the therapeutic milieux.

Number of Items: 40

Format: Includes three major dimensions and 10 subscales.

Reliability: Overall internal consistency was .93. Internal consistency coefficients for major dimensions ranged from .80 to .85. Subscale internal consistency coefficients ranged from .45 to .79.

Author: Abraham, I. L., and Foley, T. S.

Article: The Work Environment Scale and the Ward Atmosphere Scale (short forms): Psychometric data.

Journal: *Perceptual and Motor Skills,* February 1984, *58*(1), 319–322.

Related Research: Moos, R. H., & Moos, B. S. (1983). Adaptation and the quality of life in work and family settings. *Journal of Community Psychology, 11*(2), 158–170.

•••

3121

Test Name: WEATHER BELIEFS INVENTORY

Purpose: To obtain ratings of the weather's influence on affective states and overt behaviors.

Number of Items: 158

Format: Includes 50 preselected affective states and 108 overt behaviors. Half of the items in each category have positive value and half negative. A 5-point scale is employed.

Validity: Correlations with weather superstitiousness ranged from .26 to .35.

Author: Jorgenson, D. O.

Article: Superstition and the perceived causal influence of the weather.

Journal: *Perceptual and Motor Skills,* February 1981, *52*(1), 111–114.

Related Research: Jorgenson, D. O. (1981). Perceived causal influence of the weather as a function of actor–observer perspective, affect-behavior locus, affect–behavior evaluation and locus of control. *Environment and Behavior, 13*(2), 239–256.

3122

Test Name: WORK EXPECTATIONS SCALE

Purpose: To measure expectation for expanding work role beyond working hours.

Number of Items: 4

Format: Items rated on 7-point response scales. All items presented.

Reliability: Alpha was .88.

Validity: Correlates with perceived work overload ($r = .21$, $p < .01$) and with interrole conflict ($r = .25$, $p < .01$).

Author: Cooke, R. A., and Rousseau, D. M.

Article: Stress and strain from family roles and work-role expectations.

Journal: *Journal of Applied Psychology*, May 1984, *69*(2), 252–260.

Related Research: Quinn, R. P., & Staines, G. L. (1979). *The Quality of Employment Survey*. Ann Arbor, MI: Institute for Social Research.

· · ·

CHAPTER 15
Motivation

3123

Test Name: ACADEMIC MOTIVATION SCALE

Purpose: To measure academic motivation.

Number of Items: 46

Format: A 19-point rating scale on 38 items. Seriated responses on 4 items.

Reliability: Cronbach's alpha was .88.

Validity: Significant correlations presented with high school class rank, first semester GPA, and self-assessed academic self-adjustment.

Author: Baker, R. W., and Siryk, B.

Article: Measuring academic motivation of matriculating college freshmen.

Journal: *Journal of College Student Personnel*, September 1984, *25*(5), 459–464.

Related Research: Topkin, W. E. (1967). *Commitment and academic performance in college freshmen.* Unpublished doctoral dissertation, Clark University.

· · ·

3124

Test Name: ACHIEVEMENT MOTIVATION SCALE

Purpose: To measure achievement motivation.

Number of Items: 20

Format: Ten of the items are positive and ten are negative. All items are presented.

Reliability: Reliability was .87.

Validity: Correlations with: prediction of rated actual life achievement was .405; occupation was .315; rated success orientation was .394; rated task orientation was .094; rated achievement orientation was .342; rated fear of failure was .254; rated need for achievement was .295.

Author: Ray, J. J.

Article: Measuring achievement motivation by immediate emotional reactions.

Journal: *Journal of Social Psychology*, February 1981, *113*(first half), 85–93.

· · ·

3125

Test Name: ACHIEVEMENT MOTIVATION SCALE

Purpose: To measure achievement motivation.

Number of Items: 6

Format: Items are rated on a scale from 1 (*disagree*) to 5 (*agree*).

Validity: Correlations with other variables ranged from −.05 to .39.

Author: Tepper, M. E., and Powers, S.

Article: Prediction of high school algebra achievement with attributional, motivational, and achievement measures.

Journal: *Perceptual and Motor Skills*, August 1984, *59*(1), 120–122.

Related Research: Myers, A. E. (1965). Risk taking and academic success and their relation to an objective measure of achievement motivation. *Educational and Psychological Measurement, 25*, 355–363.

· · ·

3126

Test Name: ACHIEVEMENT ORIENTATION—REVISED

Purpose: To measure achievement motivation.

Number of Items: 20

Reliability: Alpha was .68.

Validity: Correlation with Directiveness Scale was .021.

Author: Ray, J. J.

Article: Authoritarianism and achievement motivation in India.

Journal: *Journal of Social Psychology*, August 1982, *117*(second half), 171–182.

Related Research: Ray, J. J. (1980). The comparative validity of Likert, projective and forced-choice indices of achievement motivation. *Journal of Social Psychology, 111*, 63–72.

· · ·

3127

Test Name: CHILDREN'S ACADEMIC INTRINSIC MOTIVATION INVENTORY

Purpose: To measure intrinsic motivation for school learning.

Number of Items: 122

Format: Items rated on 5-point Likert response categories. Sample items are presented.

Reliability: Alphas ranged from .67 to .93 across subscales. Test–retest reliability ranged from .66 to .76.

Validity: Shared variance of subscales average 15%. Factor analysis supported distinctions between subscales: reading, math, social studies, sciences, and general.

Author: Gottfried, A. E.

Article: Academic intrinsic motivation in elementary and junior high school students.

Journal: *Journal of Educational Psychology,* October 1985, *77*(5), 631–645.

Related Research: Gottfried, A. E. (1982). Relationships between academic intrinsic motivation and anxiety in children and young adolescents. *Journal of School Psychology, 20*(3), 205–215.

■ ■ ■

3128

Test Name: DATING MOTIVE SCALE

Purpose: To measure motives for dating member of the opposite sex.

Number of Items: 15

Format: Items rated on a 7-point importance scale. Sample items are presented.

Reliability: Alpha ranged from .73 to .88 across subscales.

Validity: Four-factor structure of items was similar for men and women. Factor intercorrelations were similar for men and women.

Author: White, G. L.

Article: Jealousy and partner's perceived motives for attraction to a rival.

Journal: *Social Psychology Quarterly,* March 1981, *44*(1), 24–30.

■ ■ ■

3129

Test Name: DESIRE FOR SOCIAL POWER SCALE

Purpose: To measure desire for social power.

Number of Items: 28

Format: Items rated on 6-point Likert response categories. All items presented.

Reliability: Test–retest reliability was .88. Alpha was .89.

Author: Booth, R. Z., et al.

Article: Social power need and gender among college students.

Journal: *Psychological Reports,* August 1984, *55*(1), 243–246.

Related Research: Good, L. R., & Good, K. C. (1972). An objective measure of the motive to attain social power. *Psychological Reports, 30,* 247–251.

■ ■ ■

3130

Test Name: DESIRE TO HAVE PAID EMPLOYMENT SCALE

Purpose: To measure desire to have paid employment.

Number of Items: 6

Format: Items rated on a 5-point agreement scale.

Reliability: Alpha was .82.

Author: Warr, P., and Jackson, P.

Article: Men without jobs: Some correlates of age and length of employment.

Journal: *Journal of Occupational Psychology,* March 1984, *57*(1), 77–85.

Related Research: Warr, P., et al. (1979). Scales for the measurement of some work attitudes and aspects of psychological well-being. *Journal of Occupational Psychology, 52,* 129–148.

■ ■ ■

3131

Test Name: GHISELLI SELF-DESCRIPTION INVENTORY

Purpose: To measure initiative.

Number of Items: 64

Format: Forced-choice.

Validity: Multitrait–multimethod evaluation shows clear support for convergent validity.

Author: Schippman, J. S., and Prien, E. P.

Article: The Ghiselli self-description inventory: A psychosomatic appraisal.

Journal: *Psychological Reports,* December 1985, *53*(3, Part 2), 1171–1177.

Related Research: Ghiselli, E. E. (1955). A scale for the measurement of initiative. *Personnel Psychology, 8,* 157–164.

■ ■ ■

3132

Test Name: GOOD AND GOOD SOCIAL POWER MOTIVATION SCALE

Purpose: To measure social power motivation.

Number of Items: 28

Format: True–false responses.

Reliability: Kuder-Richardson formula 20 estimate for internal consistency reliability was .89.

Author: Golden, S. B., Jr., and Royal, E. G.

Article: A construct validation of the Good and Good Measure of Social Power Motivation.

Journal: *Educational and Psychological Measurement,* Winter 1982, *42*(4), 1219–1226.

Related Research: Good, L. R., & Good, K. C. (1972). An objective measure of the motive to attain social power. *Psychological Reports, 30,* 247–251.

■ ■ ■

3133

Test Name: INDEX OF NOVELTY SEEKING

Purpose: To measure internal and external cognition seeking.

Number of Items: 20

Format: Self-report scales scored in a dichotomous manner.

Reliability: Internal consistency ranged from .71 to .79.

Author: Hirschman, E.

Article: Psychological sexual identity and hemispheric orientation.

Journal: *Journal of General Psychology,* April 1983, *108*(second half), 153–168.

Related Research: Pearson, P. (1970). Relationships between global and specified measures of novelty seeking. *Journal of Consulting and Clinical Psychology, 32,* 199–204.

■ ■ ■

3134

Test Name: INSTRUMENT OF ALTRUISTIC MOTIVATION

Purpose: To measure altruistic motivation in two dimensions: altruism and anti-utilitarianism.

Number of Items: 10

Format: Respondents indicate on a 4-point scale how much ten activities are enjoyed. All items are presented.

Reliability: Cronbach's alphas were .69 (altruism) and .67 (anti-utilitarianism).

Author: Yogev, A., and Ronen, R.

Article: Cross-age tutoring: Effects on tutors' attitudes.

Journal: *Journal of Educational Research,* May/June 1982, *75*(5), 261–268.

Related Research: Vizeltir, V. (1974). *Evaluation of altruistic motivations as intrinsic or extrinsic by men and women.* Master's thesis, Tel Aviv University (in Hebrew).

3135

Test Name: INTRACEPTION SCALE

Purpose: To measure interest in and response to specific needs, motives, and experiences of others and how these social meanings are used to understand behavior.

Number of Items: 30

Format: Adjective checklist.

Reliability: Alpha ranged from .77 to .79.

Author: Heilbrun, A. B., Jr.

Article: Cognitive factors in social effectiveness.

Journal: *Journal of Social Psychology,* August 1983, *120*(second half), 235–243.

Related Research: Gough, H. G., & Heilbrun, A. B. (1965). *Manual for the Adjective Checklist.* Palo Alto, CA: Consulting Psychologists Press.

■ ■ ■

3136

Test Name: INTRINSIC MOTIVATION SCALE

Purpose: To measure intrinsic (job) motivation.

Number of Items: 4

Format: Items rated in 5-point Likert format.

Reliability: Internal consistency was .71.

Author: Blau, G. J.

Article: A multiple study investigation of the dimensionality of job involvement.

Journal: *Journal of Vocational Behavior,* August 1985, *27*(1), 19–36.

Related Research: Lawler, E., & Hall, D. (1970). Relationship of job characteristics to job involvement satisfaction and

intrinsic motivation. *Journal of Applied Psychology, 54,* 305–312.

■ ■ ■

3137

Test Name: INTRINSIC TASK INTEREST SCALE

Purpose: To measure intrinsic task motivation, interest, and satisfaction.

Number of Items: 15

Format: Items rated in 7-point Likert format. Sample items are presented.

Reliability: Alphas ranged from .85 to .94 across subscales.

Author: Phillips, J. S., and Freedman, S. M.

Article: Contingent pay and intrinsic task interest: Moderating effects of work values.

Journal: *Journal of Applied Psychology,* May 1985, *70*(2), 306–313.

Related Research: Mayo, R. J. (1977). The development and construct validation of a measure of intrinsic motivation. *Dissertation Abstracts International, 37,* 5417B–5418B. (University Microfilms No. 77-7491, 103)

■ ■ ■

3138

Test Name: JOB MOTIVATION SCALES

Purpose: To measure intrinsic, social, and service motivation.

Number of Items: 9

Format: "How important is this reward to you?" followed by 9 work rewards. Respondents rate rewards on a 7-point importance scale.

Reliability: Alphas ranged from .69 to .77 across subscales.

Author: Pearce, J. L.

Article: Job attitude and motivation differences between volunteers and employees from comparable organizations.

Journal: *Journal of Applied Psychology,* November 1983, *68*(4), 646–652.

Related Research: Pearce, J. L. (1983). Participation in voluntary associations: How membership in formal organizations changes the rewards of participation. In D. H. Smith & J. Van Til (Eds.), *International Perspective on Voluntary Action Research.* Washington, DC: University Press of America.

■ ■ ■

3139

Test Name: LEVEL OF MOTIVATION FOR RETRAINING SCALE

Purpose: To measure motivation for vocational retraining.

Number of Items: 23 (descriptions of subject).

Format: Items rated on 5-point bipolar scales ranging from *highly correct* to *highly incorrect.* All items presented.

Reliability: Test–retest reliability ranged from .68 to .74 across subscales.

Validity: Internalization subscale correlated with locus of control (.33, $p < .01$), and vocational maturity (.47, $p < .01$).

Author: Schwarzwald, J., and Shoham, M.

Article: A trilevel approach to motivators for retraining.

Journal: *Journal of Vocational Behavior,* June 1981, *18*(3), 265–276.

■ ■ ■

3140

Test Name: MAYO TASK REACTION QUESTIONNAIRE— MODIFIED

Purpose: To measure intrinsic motivation.

Number of Items: 8

Format: Responses are made on a 7-point Likert scale. Sample items are presented.

Reliability: Coefficient alpha was .94.

Validity: Correlation with performance was .32.

Author: Phillips, J. S., and Freedman, S. M.

Article: Contingent pay and intrinsic task interest: Moderating effects of work values.

Journal: *Journal of Applied Psychology,* May 1985, *70*(2), 306–313.

Related Research: Mayo, R. J. (1977). The development and construct validity of a measure of intrinsic motivation. *Dissertation Abstracts International, 37,* 5417B–5418B. (University Microfilms No. 77-7491, 103)

■ ■ ■

3141

Test Name: MEHRABIAN AND BANK ACHIEVEMENT QUESTIONNAIRE

Purpose: To measure achievement motivation.

Number of Items: 38

Format: Items rated on 9-point agreement scales.

Reliability: Kuder-Richardson formula 20 was .91.

Validity: Correlates .74 with Jackson's (1967) scale.

Author: Waddell, F. T.

Article: Factors affecting choice, satisfaction and success in the female self-employed.

Journal: *Journal of Vocational Behavior,* December 1983, *23*(3), 294–304.

Related Research: Mehrabian, A., & Bank, L. (1969). A questionnaire measure of individual differences in achieving tendency. *Educational and Psychological Measurement, 29,* 445–461.

■ ■ ■

3142

Test Name: NACH NAFF SCALE

Purpose: To measure achievement motivation.

Number of Items: 30

Format: Forced-choice questionnaire on which the subject selects either an achievement- or an affiliation-oriented response from each pair of self-descriptive adjectives.

Reliability: Split-half corrected reliability is estimated to be .80.

Validity: Correlations with: grade-point average .27 (68 female students) and .49 (30 male students); psychology quiz grades .21 (106 female students) and –.10 (56 male students); Strong Vocational Interest Blank Scales ranged from –.24 to .37 (56 male students) and –.33 to .41 (107 female students); California Psychological Inventory Scales ranged from –.24 to .29 (49 male students) and –.32 to .34 (86 female students).

Author: Sid, A. K. W., and Lindgren, H. C.

Article: Achievement and affiliation motivation and their correlates.

Journal: *Educational and Psychological Measurement,* Winter 1982, *42*(4), 1213–1218.

Related Research: Lindgren, H. C. (1976). Measuring need to achieve by Nach Naff Scale—A forced-choice questionnaire. *Psychological Reports, 39,* 907–910.

3143

Test Name: NEED SATISFACTION SCALE

Purpose: To measure job-derived need and fulfillment.

Number of Items: 10

Format: Multiple-choice.

Reliability: Alphas ranged from .69 to .89.

Author: Lefkowitz, J., et al.

Article: The role of need level and/or need salience as moderators of the relationship between need satisfaction and work alienation–involvement.

Journal: *Journal of Vocational Behavior*, April 1984, *24*(2), 142–158.

Related Research: Porter, L. W. (1961). A study in perceived need satisfaction in bottom and middle management jobs. *Journal of Applied Psychology, 45*, 1–10.

■ ■ ■

3144

Test Name: REWARD LEVEL SCALE

Purpose: To assess love, status, services, goods, money, and information as rewards.

Number of Items: 7

Format: Items rated in 9-point Likert format.

Reliability: Alpha was .90.

Author: Cate, R. M., et al.

Article: The effect of equity, equality and reward level on the stability of students' premarital relationships.

Journal: *Journal of Social Psychology*, December 1985, *125*(6), 715–721.

Related Research: Foa, U. G., & Foa, E. G. (1974). *Societal structures of the mind.*

Springfield, IL: Charles C Thomas.

Cate, R. M., et al. (1982). Fairness and reward level as predictors of relationship satisfaction. *Journal of Social Psychology, 45*(3), 177–181.

■ ■ ■

3145

Test Name: SARNOFF SURVEY OF ATTITUDES TOWARD LIFE

Purpose: To measure motivation for upward mobility.

Number of Items: 18

Format: Items rated on 6-point agreement scales.

Reliability: Alpha was .67.

Author: Howard, A., et al.

Article: Motivation and values among Japanese and American managers.

Journal: *Personnel Psychology*, Winter 1983, *36*(4), 883–898.

Related Research: Bray, D. W., et al. (1979). *Formative years in business: A long-term AT&T study of managerial lives.* New York and Melbourne, FL: Robert E. Krieger.

■ ■ ■

3146

Test Name: SENSATION SEEKING SCALE

Purpose: To measure "optimum stimulation level."

Number of Items: 22

Format: Forced-choice format requires respondents to choose between two events.

Reliability: Split-half reliability ranged from .68 to .74.

Author: Miller, A., and Cooley, E.

Article: Moderator variables for the relationship between life cycle change and disorders.

Journal: *Journal of General Psychology*, April 1981, *104*(second half), 223–233.

Related Research: Zuckerman, M., et al. (1964). Development of sensation seeking scale. *Journal of Consulting Psychology, 28*, 477–482.

■ ■ ■

3147

Test Name: SENSATION SEEKING SCALE FORM VI

Purpose: To measure sensation seeking.

Number of Items: 128

Format: Includes four subscales: Experience—thrill and adventure seeking; Experience—disinhibition; Intention—thrill and adventure seeking; Intention—disinhibition.

Reliability: Coefficient alphas ranged from .62 ($N = 38$) to .94 ($N = 38$). Test–retest (7 weeks) reliability ranged from .84 to .93 ($N = .49$).

Author: Zuckerman, M.

Article: Experience and desire: A new format for sensation seeking scales.

Journal: *Journal of Behavioral Assessment*, June 1984, *6*(2), 101–114.

Related Research: Zuckerman, M., et al. (1978). Sensation seeking in England and America: Cross-cultural, age and sex comparisons. *Journal of Consulting and Clinical Psychology, 46*, 139–149.

■ ■ ■

3148

Test Name: SENTENCE COMPLETION SCALE

Purpose: To measure the motivation to manage and to predict managerial performance.

Number of Items: 40

Format: Sentence completion format.

Reliability: Interscorer reliabilities ranged from .61 to .91 with an average of .83.

Author: Bartal, K. M., et al.

Article: Sex and ethnic effects on motivation to manage among college business students.

Journal: *Journal of Applied Psychology,* February 1981, *66*(1), 40–44.

Related Research: Miner, J. B. (1965). *Studies in management education.* New York: Springer.

Miner, J. B. (1978). The Miner Sentence Completion Scale: A reappraisal. *Academy of Management Journal, 21,* 283–294.

■ ■ ■

3149

Test Name: TASK AROUSAL SCALE

Purpose: To measure task-specific arousal.

Number of Items: 7

Format: Semantic differential. Sample adjective pairs presented.

Reliability: Alpha was .87.

Author: Huber, V. L.

Article: The effects of task difficulty, goal setting, and strategy on performance of a heuristic task.

Journal: *Journal of Applied Psychology,* August 1985, *70*(3), 492–504.

Related Research: Scott, W. E., & Rowland, K. M. (1970). The generality and significance of semantic differential scales as measures of "morale."

Organizational Behavior and Human Performance, 5, 576–591.

■ ■ ■

3150

Test Name: TEACHER EFFECTANCE MOTIVATION RATING

Purpose: To measure effectance motivation.

Number of Items: 30

Format: Includes a rating checklist describing student characteristics to which the teacher responds on a 7-point scale to indicate the extent to which each student is described by the characteristic. Sample items are presented.

Reliability: Reliability coefficients (alpha) were .96 and .95.

Author: Pearlman, C.

Article: The effects of level of effectance motivation, IQ, and a penalty/reward contingency on the choice of problem difficulty.

Journal: *Child Development,* April 1984, *55*(2), 537–542.

Related Research: Pearlman, C. (1982). The measurement of effectance motivation. *Educational and Psychological Measurement, 42*(1), 49–56.

■ ■ ■

3151

Test Name: WELLS-BLEDSOE MOTIVATION CHECKLIST

Purpose: To measure adolescents' school motivation.

Number of Items: 51

Format: Includes two factors. All items are presented.

Reliability: Cronbach's alphas were .83 and .82.

Validity: Correlations with Iowa Test of Basic Skills ranged from –.17 to .30. Correlations with Otis-Lennon Quick Scoring Test ranged from –.22 to .33.

Author: Wells, G. R., and Bledsoe, J. C.

Article: Development and validation of the Wells-Bledsoe Motivation Checklist.

Journal: *Perceptual and Motor Skills,* August 1984, *59*(1), 243–248.

■ ■ ■

3152

Test Name: WHICH-TO-DISCUSS TEST

Purpose: To measure curiosity.

Number of Items: 20

Format: Each item includes a pair of geometric figures and symbols with one of each pair being more balanced than the other. Subjects indicate which one they would choose if they could hear a story about only one of them.

Reliability: Cronbach's alpha was .90.

Validity: Correlation with Maze test was –.06.

Author: Silverstein, A. B., et al.

Article: Psychometric properties of two measures of intrinsic motivation.

Journal: *Perceptual and Motor Skills,* October 1981, *53*(2), 655–658.

Related Research: Maw, W. H., & Maw, E. W. (1961). Nonhomeostatic experiences as stimuli of children with high curiosity. *California Journal of Educational Research, 12,* 57–61.

CHAPTER 16
Perception

3153

Test Name: ACADEMIC SELF-CONCEPT SCALE

Purpose: To measure general academic self-concept.

Number of Items: 40

Format: Subjects indicate one of four levels of agreement to each item. Examples are presented.

Reliability: Internal consistency estimate of reliability was .91.

Validity: Correlations with the Dimensions of Self-Concept measure ranged from –.37 to .34 ($N = 202$). Correlation with GPA was .52 ($N = 589$).

Author: Halote, B., and Michael, W. B.

Article: The construct and concurrent validity of two college-level academic self-concept scales for a sample of primarily Hispanic community college students.

Journal: *Educational and Psychological Measurement,* Winter 1984, *44*(4), 993–1007.

Related Research: Reynolds, W. M., et al. (1980). Initial development and validation of the Academic Self-Concept Scale. *Educational and Psychological Measurement, 40,* 1013–1016.

■ ■ ■

3154

Test Name: ACADEMIC SELF-ESTEEM SCALE

Purpose: To measure academic self-esteem.

Number of Items: 11

Format: Yes–no. Sample items presented.

Reliability: Alpha was .72.

Author: Rosenfield, D., et al.

Article: Classroom structure and prejudice in desegregated schools.

Journal: *Journal of Educational Psychology,* February 1981, *73*(1), 17–26.

Related Research: Vitale, M. (1974). *Evaluation of the Title III Dallas junior high school career education project: 1973–1974.* (Report No. 74-291). Dallas Independent School District, Department of Research and Evaluation.

■ ■ ■

3155

Test Name: ACADEMIC SELF-SCHEMA

Purpose: To measure academic self-esteem.

Number of Items: 26 of 58 from Coopersmith Self-Esteem Inventory.

Format: Sample items presented.

Reliability: Pretest alpha was .73.

Author: Corno, L., and Mandinach, E. B.

Article: Using existing classroom data to explore relationships in a theoretical model of academic motivation.

Journal: *Journal of Educational Research,* September/October 1983, *77*(1), 33–42.

Related Research: Coopersmith, S. (1967). Coopersmith Self-Esteem Inventory. In S. Coopersmith (Ed.), *The antecedents of self esteem.* San Francisco: Freeman.

■ ■ ■

3156

Test Name: ACHIEVABILITY OF FUTURE GOALS SCALE

Purpose: To measure optimism.

Number of Items: 8

Format: Items rated on a 7-point Likert scale. Sample items are presented.

Reliability: Alpha was .73.

Author: Wolf, F. M., and Savickas, M. L.

Article: Time perspective and causal attributions for achievement.

Journal: *Journal of Educational Psychology,* August 1985, *77*(4), 471–480.

Related Research: Heimberg, L. (1961). *Development and construct validation of an inventory for the measurement of future time perspectives.* Unpublished master's thesis, Vanderbilt University.

Savickas, M. L., et al. (1984). Time perspective in vocational maturity and career decision making. *Journal of Vocational Behavior, 25*(3), 258–269.

■ ■ ■

3157

Test Name: ACHIEVEMENT ATTRIBUTION SCALE

Purpose: To measure attributions for achievement (subscale of multidimensional–multi-attributional causality scale).

Number of Items: 24

Format: Items rated on 5-point Likert scales. Sample items are presented.

Reliability: Alpha ranged from .47 to .71 over subscales.

Author: Wolf, F. M., and Savickas, M. L.

Article: Time perspective and causal attributions for achievement.

Journal: *Journal of Educational Psychology*, August 1985, *77*(4), 471–480.

Related Research: Lefcourt, H. M., et al. (1979). The Multidimensional–Multi-attributional Causality Scale. *Canadian Journal of Behavioral Science, 11*, 286–304.

■ ■ ■

3158

Test Name: AFFECTIVE ENTRY QUESTIONNAIRE

Purpose: To measure expectations of course, instructor, and subject matter at the beginning of a semester.

Number of Items: 52

Format: Likert format.

Reliability: Internal consistency was .85.

Validity: In this use of the scale large proportions of respondents (87%) reported "no basis for judgment" on 5 items; 60% made that response to all 15 questions measuring instructor characteristics.

Author: Barké, C. R., et al.

Article: Relationship between course entry attitudes and end-of-course ratings.

Journal: *Journal of Educational*

Psychology, February 1983, *75*(1), 75–85.

■ ■ ■

3159

Test Name: ALCOHOL EXPECTANCY QUESTIONNAIRE

Purpose: To measure perceived effects of alcohol consumption.

Number of Items: 90

Format: Agree–disagree format.

Reliability: Alpha ranged from .28 to .95 across subscales (five of six scales had alphas of .79 or greater).

Author: Brown, S. A., et al.

Article: Do alcohol expectancies mediate drinking patterns of adults?

Journal: *Journal of Consulting and Clinical Psychology*, August 1985, *53*(4), 512–519.

Related Research: Brown, S. A. (1985). Expectancies versus background in the prediction of college drinking patterns. *Journal of Consulting and Clinical Psychology, 53*, 123–130.

■ ■ ■

3160

Test Name: ALCOHOL EXPECTANCY QUESTIONNAIRE FOR ADOLESCENTS

Purpose: To measure expectancies associated with alcohol consumption.

Number of Items: 100

Format: True–false.

Reliability: Alpha was .90.

Validity: Two-factor solutions were produced at all age levels–one revealed alcohol as a positive transforming agent and one

revealed alcohol to be a negative transforming agent.

Author: Christiansen, B. A., et al.

Article: Development of alcohol-related expectancies in adolescents: Separating pharmacological from social-learning influences.

Journal: *Journal of Consulting and Clinical Psychology*, June 1982, *50*(3), 336–344.

Related Research: Brown, S. A., et al. (1980). Expectations of reinforcement from alcohol: Their domain and relation to drinking patterns. *Journal of Consulting and Clinical Psychology, 48*, 419–426.

■ ■ ■

3161

Test Name: AMOUNT OF INVESTED MENTAL EFFORT SCALE

Purpose: To measure the perceived effort required to understand material presented on film and in print.

Number of Items: 4

Format: Items rated in 4-category multiple-choice format. All items are presented.

Reliability: Cronbach's alpha was .81.

Author: Soloman, G.

Article: Television is "easy" and print is "tough": The differential investment of mental effort in learning as a function of perceptions and attributions.

Journal: *Journal of Educational Psychology*, August 1984, *76*(4), 647–658.

Related Research: Kunkle, D. (1981). *Answering the AIME: An empirical analysis of the relationship between mental effort and learning from TV.*

Unpublished manuscript, University of Southern California.

■ ■ ■

3162

Test Name: APPRAISAL INTERVIEW ASSESSMENT SCALE

Purpose: To measure subordinates perceptions of the most recent appraisal interview.

Number of Items: 23

Format: Items rated on 7-point *very true* to *very false* response scales.

Reliability: Alphas ranged from .79 to .87 across subscales.

Author: Ivancevich, J. M.

Article: Subordinates' reactions to performance appraisal interviews: A test of feedback and goal-setting techniques.

Journal: *Journal of Applied Psychology*, October 1982, *67*(5), 581–587.

Related Research: Greller, M. M. (1978). The nature of subordinate participation in the appraisal interview. *Academy of Management Journal, 21*, 646–658.

■ ■ ■

3163

Test Name: ARTICULATION SURVEY

Purpose: To measure importance of the problem of articulation of community college and 4-year colleges and universities.

Number of Items: 41

Format: Items rated on 6-point response categories, ranging from *not a problem* to *problem of major significance.*

Reliability: Intercorrelations were .71 to 1.00 (*p* < .05) for 38 of 41 items.

Validity: Items reviewed by a panel of expert articulation professionals.

Author: Remley, T. P., Jr., and Stripling, R. O.

Article: Perceptions of transfer problems experienced by community college graduates.

Journal: *Journal of College Student Personnel*, January 1981, *24*(1), 43–50.

■ ■ ■

3164

Test Name: ATTRIBUTION QUESTIONNAIRE

Purpose: To assess degree to which people believe that obtaining or not obtaining a job is due to internal or external factors.

Number of Items: 12

Format: Responses to items ranged from *always true* to *never true*. All items are presented.

Reliability: Alpha ranged from .51 to .54. Interitem correlations ranged from −.24 to .54.

Validity: Factor analysis revealed a general external and a general internal factor plus a situational factor.

Author: Gurney, R. M.

Article: Leaving school, facing unemployment and making attributions about the causes of unemployment.

Journal: *Journal of Vocational Behavior*, February 1981, *18*(1), 79–91.

■ ■ ■

3165

Test Name: ATTRIBUTIONAL STYLE QUESTIONNAIRE

Purpose: To assess the general attributional style of clients.

Number of Items: 12

Format: Each item is an event with either good or bad outcomes. The subject is asked to list the major cause of the event and then to rate the internality, stability, and globality of the cause on a 7-point continuum.

Reliability: Coefficient alphas ranged from .46 to .69. Test–retest reliabilities ranged from .57 to .69.

Author: Claiborn, C. D., and Dowd, E. T.

Article: Attributional interpretations in counseling: Content versus discrepancy.

Journal: *Journal of Counseling Psychology*, April 1985, *32*(2), 197–205.

Related Research: Peterson, C., et al. (1982). The Attributional Style Questionnaire. *Cognitive Therapy and Research, 6*, 188–196.

■ ■ ■

3166

Test Name: ATTRIBUTIONAL TENDENCY SCALE

Purpose: To measure if attributions in the classroom represent high or low locus of control.

Number of Items: 5

Format: Guttman.

Reliability: Reproducibility was .92. Scalability was .56.

Author: Oren, D. L.

Article: Evaluation systems and attributional tendencies in the classroom: A sociological approach.

Journal: *Journal of Educational Research*, May/June 1983, *76*(5), 307–312.

Related Research: Massey, G. C., & Dornbusch, S. M. (1977). *Self-enhancement, self-consistency and distinctiveness of feedback in a field study of academic self-*

concept: *Attribution processes in inner-city high schools* (Tech. Rep. No. 49). Center for Research and Development in Education, Stanford University.

■ ■ ■

3167

Test Name: AUSTRALIAN SEX-ROLE SCALE

Purpose: To measure masculine and feminine characteristics.

Number of Items: 30

Format: Items rated on a 7-point scale (1 = *never or almost never true*, 7 = *always or almost always true*).

Reliability: Alpha ranged from .14 to .80 over subscales on Forms A and B.

Author: Hong, S.-M., et al.

Article: Factor structure of the Australian Sex-Role Scale.

Journal: *Psychological Reports,* October 1983, *53*(2), 499–505.

Related Research: Antill, J. K., et al. (1981). An Australian Sex-Role Scale. *Australian Journal of Psychology, 33,* 169–183.

■ ■ ■

3168

Test Name: AUTONOMY–CONTROL SCALE

Purpose: To measure autonomy–control variation.

Number of Items: 40

Format: Items rated on a 5-point response scale.

Reliability: Test–retest reliability was .91 (*N* = 41, 2 months).

Author: DeMan, A. F.

Article: Autonomy–control variation in child-rearing and anomie in young adults.

Journal: *Psychological Reports,* 1982, *51*(1) 7–10.

Related Research: DeMan, A. F. (1982). Autonomy–control variation and self-esteem: Additional findings. *Journal of Psychology, 111,* 9–13.

■ ■ ■

3169

Test Name: AUTOSTEREOTYPE HETEROSTEREOTYPE SCALE

Purpose: To measure stereotypes among managers of different nationalities.

Number of Items: 18

Format: Adjectival pairs scored from 1 to 7. All pairs (items) are presented along with instructions to respondents.

Validity: Two factors identified by method of principal components. Comparability coefficient for respondents of different nationalities was .96.

Author: Stening, B. W., et al.

Article: Mutual perception of managerial performance and style in multinational subsidiaries.

Journal: *Journal of Occupational Psychology,* December 1981, *54*(4), 255–263.

Related Research: Triandis, H. C. (1972). *The analysis of subjective culture.* New York: Wiley.

■ ■ ■

3170

Test Name: AWARENESS OF COMPREHENSION FAILURE TEST

Purpose: To measure children's ability to monitor and detect their own cognitive processes.

Number of Items: 18

Format: Children are asked questions concerning their awareness that information is lacking. Sample questions presented.

Reliability: Test–retest reliability was .73.

Author: Clements, D. H., and Gullo, D. F.

Article: Effects of computer programming on young children's cognition.

Journal: *Journal of Educational Psychology,* December 1984, *76*(6), 1051–1058.

Related Research: Markman, E. M. (1977). Realizing you don't understand: A preliminary investigation. *Child Development, 48,* 986–992.

■ ■ ■

3171

Test Name: BEHAVIOROID INTERNAL–EXTERNAL SCALE

Purpose: To measure relationships between verbalized beliefs and behavior by keying on behavioral attributes on the internal and external end of the Rotter I-E Scale.

Number of Items: 26

Format: All items are presented.

Reliability: Test–retest reliability was .78. Kuder-Richardson formula 20 was .83. Spearman-Brown split-half reliability ranged from .72 to .93.

Validity: Correlated .19 with Blame Attribution and .16 with Social Desirability.

Author: Russell, G. M.

Article: Development of a behavioroid I-E locus of control scale.

Journal: *Psychological Reports,* December 1982, *51*(3, Part 2), 1095–1099.

■ ■ ■

3172

Test Name: BELIEF IN LUNAR EFFECTS SCALE

Purpose: To assess beliefs in lunar effects.

Number of Items: 9

Format: Items rated on a 3-point agreement scale. All items are presented.

Reliability: Cronbach's alpha was .85.

Validity: Correlates .47 ($p < .001$) with reported positive influence of a full moon. Correlates significantly with logical ability (−.17) and with various paranormal scales (.19 to .39).

Author: Rotton, J., and Kelly, I. W.

Article: A scale for assessing belief in lunar effects: Reliability and concurrent validity.

Journal: *Psychological Reports,* August 1985, *57*(1), 239–245.

■ ■ ■

3173

Test Name: BELL REALITY TESTING INVENTORY

Purpose: To assess the perceptions of reality.

Number of Items: 45

Format: True–false format.

Reliability: Alphas ranged from .82 to .87. Split-half reliability ranged from .77 to .85.

Validity: 92% correct classification with inpatient schizophrenics. Age unrelated to subscales. Other validity data presented.

Author: Bell, M. D., et al.

Article: Scale for the assessment of reliability testing: Reliability, validity and factorial invariance.

Journal: *Journal of Consulting and Clinical Psychology,* August 1985, *53*(4), 506–511.

Related Research: Bell, M., et al. (1980). *Reality testing–object relations assessment scale:*

Reliability and validity studies. Paper presented at the meeting of the American Psychological Association, Montreal.

■ ■ ■

3174

Test Name: BLOOD DONOR SALIENCE SCALE

Purpose: To assess if donor role is part of a person's self-concept.

Number of Items: 5

Format: Items rated on a 9-point agreement scale. All items presented.

Reliability: Alpha was .81.

Validity: Salience of donor role ranked third behind work and religion.

Author: Callero, P.

Article: Role-identity salience.

Journal: *Social Psychology Quarterly,* June 1985, *48*(3), 203–215.

Related Research: Jackson, S. (1981). Measurement of commitment to role identities. *Journal of Personality and Social Psychology, 40,* 138–146.

■ ■ ■

3175

Test Name: BODY CATHEXIS SCALE—MODIFIED

Purpose: To assess the degree of satisfaction or dissatisfaction felt about parts and processes of the body.

Number of Items: 40

Format: Subjects evaluate body characteristics on a 5-point Likert scale ranging from 1 *(strongly negative)* to 5 *(strongly positive).*

Reliability: Test–retest reliability was .87.

Author: Tucker, L. A.

Article: Internal structure, factor

satisfaction and reliability of the Body Cathexis Scale.

Journal: *Perceptual and Motor Skills,* December 1981, *53*(3), 891–896.

Related Research: Secord, P. F., & Jourard, S. M. (1953). The appraisal of body-cathexis: Body cathexis and the self. *Journal of Consulting Psychology, 17,* 343–347.

■ ■ ■

3176

Test Name: BODY-ESTEEM SCALE

Purpose: To measure children's affective evaluation of their bodies.

Number of Items: 24

Format: Subjects respond to each item by *yes* or *no.* High esteem has an equal number of *yes* and *no* responses. All items are presented.

Reliability: Split-half reliability was .85.

Validity: Correlation with self-body was .67; relative weight was −.55; self-esteem was .68; self-rest was .62.

Author: Mendelson, B. K., and White, D. R.

Article: Relation between body-esteem and self-esteem of obese and normal children.

Journal: *Perceptual and Motor Skills,* June 1982, *54*(3, Part 1), 899–905.

■ ■ ■

3177

Test Name: BODY PARTS SATISFACTION SCALE

Purpose: To assess satisfaction with body.

Number of Items: 24

Format: Items rated on 6-point Likert satisfaction scales.

Reliability: Alpha was .89.

Author: Noles, S. W., et al.

Article: Body image, physical attractiveness, and depression.

Journal: *Journal of Consulting and Clinical Psychology,* February 1985, *53*(1), 88–94.

Related Research: Bohrnstedt, G. W. (1977). *On measuring body satisfaction.* Unpublished manuscript, Indiana University.

Berscheid, E., et al. (1973, November). The happy American body: A survey report. *Psychology Today,* pp. 119–131.

■ ■ ■

3178

Test Name: BRIEF LOCUS OF CONTROL SCALE

Purpose: To measure locus of control.

Number of Items: 6

Format: Likert format applied to Rotter items. All items presented.

Reliability: Alpha was .68.

Validity: Correlates .25 with life satisfaction; –.13 with perceived risk; –.32 with not coping; .22 with good health; and .19 with activity (all *p*s < .001).

Author: Lumpkin, J. R.

Article: Validity of a brief locus of control scale for survey research.

Journal: *Psychological Reports,* October 1985, *57*(2), 655–659.

■ ■ ■

3179

Test Name: CANADIAN SELF-ESTEEM INVENTORY FOR ADULTS

Purpose: To measure self-esteem.

Number of Items: 40

Format: Dichotomous scoring categories.

Reliability: Internal consistency coefficients ranged from .20 to .76 across subscales.

Author: Blau, G. J., and Lenihan, M.

Article: Note on internal consistency of Canadian Self-Esteem Inventory for Adults.

Journal: *Psychological Reports,* 1981, *49*(1), 81–82.

Related Research: Battle, J. (1980). Relationship between self-esteem and depression among high school students. *Perceptual and Motor Skills, 51,* 157–158.

■ ■ ■

3180

Test Name: CAREER DECISION-MAKING SELF-EFFICACY SCALE

Purpose: To measure self-efficacy expectations related to a variety of tasks or behaviors associated with career decision-making.

Number of Items: 50

Format: Includes five subscales. Responses to each item are made on a 10-point Likert scale.

Reliability: Average alpha for all subscales is .88.

Author: Robbins, S. B.

Article: Validity estimates for the Career Decision-Making Self-Efficacy Scale.

Journal: *Measurement and Evaluation in Counseling and Development,* July 1985, *18*(2), 64–71.

Related Research: Taylor, K. M., & Betz, N. M. (1983). Application of self-efficacy theory to the understanding and treatment of career indecision. *Journal of Vocational Behavior, 22,* 63–81.

■ ■ ■

3181

Test Name: CAUSAL DIMENSION SCALE

Purpose: To measure how individuals perceive causes.

Number of Items: 9

Format: Includes three subscales, one of which is controllability: the degree to which loneliness could be altered by someone. The higher the score the greater the possibility.

Reliability: Coefficient alpha was .88 for each subscale.

Author: Conoley, C. W., and Garber, R. A.

Article: Effects of reframing and self-control directives on loneliness, depression, and controllability.

Journal: *Journal of Counseling Psychology,* January 1985, *32*(1), 139–142.

Related Research: Russell, D. (1982). The Causal Dimension Scale: A measure of individuals' perceived causes. *Journal of Personality and Social Psychology, 42,* 1137–1145.

Abraham, I. L. (1985). Causal attributions of depression: Reliability of the "Causal Dimension Scale" in research on clinical inference. *Psychological Reports, 56*(2), 415–418.

■ ■ ■

3182

Test Name: CHILDREN'S LOCUS OF CONTROL SCALE

Purpose: To measure locus of control.

Number of Items: 26

Format: Yes–no format.

Reliability: Test–retest was .68 (1-week interval).

Author: Thomson-Rountree, P., and Woodruff, A. E.

Article: An examination of project aware: The effects on children's attitudes toward themselves, others and school.

Journal: *Journal of School Psychology*, 1982, *20*(1), 20–31.

Related Research: Bradley, R. H., & Teeter, T. A. (1977). Perceptions of control over social outcomes and student behavior. *Psychology in the Schools, 14,* 230–235.

Thomson-Rountree, P., et al. (1981). An examination of the relationship between role-taking and social competence. *Child Study Journal, 71*(4), 253–264.

■ ■ ■

3183

Test Name: CHILDREN'S NOWICKI-STRICKLAND INTERNAL–EXTERNAL CONTROL SCALE

Purpose: To measure generalized locus of control orientation.

Number of Items: 40

Format: Yes–no format.

Reliability: Test–retest (6-week interval) ranged from .63 to .71 across grade levels.

Author: Piotrowski, C., and Dunham, F. Y.

Article: Locus of control orientation and perception of "hurricane" in fifth graders.

Journal: *Journal of General Psychology*, July 1983, *109*(first half), 119–127.

Related Research: Nowicki, S., Jr., & Strickland, B. R. (1973). A locus of control scale for children. *Journal of Consulting and Clinical Psychology, 40,* 148–154.

■ ■ ■

3184

Test Name: CHILDREN'S OWN PERCEPTIONS AND EXPERIENCES OF STRESSORS

Purpose: To measure children's perceptions of stressors in their lives and their experiences and emotional reactions to those stressors.

Number of Items: 60

Format: A 5-point Likert scale from 1 (*not upsetting at all*) to 5 (*extremely upsetting*) is used to determine how upsetting each item is. Also the children are asked whether the event ever happened to them and if so, whether it upset or worried them. Seven factors are identified. All items are presented.

Reliability: The average coefficient alpha for the factors was .84.

Author: Colton, J. A.

Article: Childhood stress: Perceptions of children and professionals.

Journal: *Journal of Psychopathology and Behavioral Assessment*, June 1985, *17*(2), 155–173.

Related Research: Chandler, L. A. (1981). The source of stress inventory. *Psychology in the Schools, 18,* 164–168.

■ ■ ■

3185

Test Name: CHILDREN'S PERCEIVED SELF-CONTROL SCALE

Purpose: To measure children's perception of self-control.

Number of Items: 11

Format: Children respond to items either by choosing *usually yes* or *usually no*. All items presented.

Reliability: Test–retest (2-week interval) was .71 (from .18 to .63 across 4 subscales).

Validity: Five of 40 correlations with Child Behavior Rating Scale were significant (significant correlations ranged from .39 to .49, *p* < .05).

Author: Humphrey, L. L.

Article: Children's and Teachers' perspectives on children's self-control: The development of two rating scales.

Journal: *Journal of Consulting and Clinical Psychology*, October 1982, *50*(5), 624–633.

■ ■ ■

3186

Test Name: CHILDREN'S PERSONAL ATTRIBUTES INVENTORY

Purpose: To measure evaluative-affective aspects of self-concept.

Number of Items: 48

Format: Checklist format. Respondents mark the 15 adjectives on the list of 48 that best describes themselves.

Reliability: Split-half reliability was .83.

Validity: Correlates .66 with Piers-Harris measure of self-concept.

Author: Verna, G. B., and Runion, K. B.

Article: The effects of contextual dissonance on the self-concept of youth from a high versus low socially valued group.

Journal: *Journal of Social Psychology*, August 1985, *125*(4), 449–458.

Related Research: Parish, T. S., & Taylor, J. (1978). The Personal Attribute Inventory for Children: A report on its validity and reliability. *Educational and Psychological Measurements, 38,* 565–569.

■ ■ ■

3187

Test Name: CHILDREN'S SELF-PERCEPTION SCALE

Purpose: To measure self-perception of children.

Number of Items: 17

Format: Items rated on 5-point Likert response categories. Sample items are presented.

Reliability: Alpha was .82.

Validity: Perceived ability correlates with grades (.11) and teacher's judgment of achievement (.10). Perceived effort and perceived conduct correlated with grades (.17; in all cases, $p < .001$).

Author: Pintrich, P. R., and Blumenfield, P. C.

Article: Classroom experience and children's self-perceptions of ability, effort and conduct.

Journal: *Journal of Educational Psychology,* October 1985, *77*(5), 646–657.

■ ■ ■

3188

Test Name: CHILDREN'S SEX-ROLE TEST

Purpose: To measure masculinity and femininity.

Number of Items: 24

Format: Items rated on a 4-point rating scale. All items presented.

Reliability: Split-half and test–retest reliabilities were .79 or above.

Validity: Boys scored significantly higher on masculinity than girls.

Author: Moore, S. M.

Article: The Children's Sex-Role Test.

Journal: *Psychological Reports,* October 1985, *57*(2), 586.

■ ■ ■

3189

Test Name: CLASS CONSCIOUSNESS SCALE

Purpose: To measure awareness of social class among children.

Number of Items: 18 drawings.

Format: Children match drawings of upper, middle, and lower class mothers, fathers, children, houses, and automobiles into families. All drawings presented.

Reliability: Split-half reliability was .77.

Validity: Correlates .91 with age of child.

Author: Mookherjee, H. N., and Hogan, H. W.

Article: Class consciousness among young rural children.

Journal: *Journal of Social Psychology,* June 1981, *114*(first half), 91–98.

■ ■ ■

3190

Test Name: CLIENT BELIEFS INVENTORY

Purpose: To measure beliefs about problems with negative emotions and the prospects for change.

Number of Items: 32

Format: Includes four scales: expectation to change, motivation to change, self-control, and understanding.

Reliability: Alpha coefficients ranged from .39 to .83.

Author: Claiborn, C. D., et al.

Article: Effects of intervention discrepancy in counseling for negative emotions.

Journal: *Journal of Counseling Psychology,* April 1983, *30*(2), 164–171.

Related Research: Strong, S. R., et al. (1979). Motivational and equipping functions of interpretation in counseling. *Journal of Counseling Psychology, 26*, 98–107.

■ ■ ■

3191

Test Name: CLIENT EXPECTANCY QUESTIONNAIRE

Purpose: To measure clients' expectations for counseling sessions.

Number of Items: 14

Format: Items rated in 6-point Likert format.

Reliability: Cronbach's alpha was .88.

Author: Friedlander, M. L., and Kaul, J. J.

Article: Preparing clients for counseling: Effect of role induction on counseling process and outcome.

Journal: *Journal of College Student Personnel,* 1983, *24*(3), 207–214.

Related Research: Howard, K., et al. (1970). Patients' satisfactions in psychotherapy as a function of patient–therapist pairing. *Psychotherapy: Theory, Research and Practice, 7*, 130–134.

Friedlander, M. L. (1982). Expectations and perceptions of counseling: Changes over time and in relation to verbal behavior. *Journal of College Student Personnel, 23*(5), 402–408.

■ ■ ■

3192

Test Name: COGNITIVE ERROR QUESTIONNAIRE (GENERAL AND LOWER BACK PAIN VERSIONS)

Purpose: To measure cognitive error (cognitive distortion).

Number of Items: 24 items in each version.

Format: Vignettes are presented to subjects, after which they respond to cognitions that reflect one of four cognitive errors (responses are made on a 5-point scale). Sample items presented.

Reliability: Test–retest reliability ranged from .80 to .85. Alternate forms ranged from .76 to .82.

Internal consistency ranged from .89 to .92.

Validity: Correlated .53 to .60 with Hammen and Krantz Depressed–Distorted Questionnaire.

Author: Lefebvre, M. F.

Article: Cognitive distortion and cognitive errors in depressed psychiatric and low back pain patients.

Journal: *Journal of Consulting and Clinical Psychology*, August 1981, *49*(4), 517–525.

Related Research: Lefebvre, M. F. (1980). Cognitive distortion in depressed psychiatric and low back pain patients. Doctoral dissertation, University of Vermont. *Dissertation Abstracts International*, *41*, 693B. (University Microfilms No. 80-17, 652)

■ ■ ■

3193

Test Name: COGNITIVE PROCESS SURVEY

Purpose: To assess imaginal life, orientation toward imaginal life, and defensiveness.

Number of Items: 30

Format: Subjects respond to each item on a 5-point scale from *strongly agree* to *strongly disagree*. Examples are presented.

Reliability: Subscale coefficient alphas ranged from .72 to .78 (*N* = 350).

Validity: Correlations with other variables ranged from −.33 to .65 (*N* = 222).

Author: Martinetti, R. F.

Article: Cognitive antecedents of dream recall.

Journal: *Perceptual and Motor Skills*, April 1985, *60*(2), 395–401.

Related Research: Martinetti, R. F. (1983). Dream recall,

imaginal processes and short-term memory: A pilot study. *Perceptual and Motor Skills*, *57*, 718.

■ ■ ■

3194

Test Name: COLLEGE STUDENT ACADEMIC LOCUS OF CONTROL SCALE

Purpose: To predict a wide range of relevant college students' behaviors.

Number of Items: 28

Format: True–false response is made to each item. All items are presented.

Reliability: Test–retest (5 weeks) reliability was .92. Kuder-Richardson formula 20 internal consistency was .70.

Validity: Correlations with other variables ranged from .50 to −.38.

Author: Trice, A. D.

Article: An academic locus of control scale for college students.

Journal: *Perceptual and Motor Skills*, December 1985, *61*(3, Part 2), 1043–1046.

■ ■ ■

3195

Test Name: CONNECTICUT NEEDS ASSESSMENT SURVEY

Purpose: To assess the counselor's role.

Number of Items: 24

Format: Items rated in 4-point Likert format. All items presented.

Reliability: Alpha ranged from .66 to .76 across subscales.

Author: Helms, B. J., and Ibrahim, F. A.

Article: A comparison of counselor and parent perceptions of the role and function of the secondary school counselor.

Journal: *The School Counselor*, March 1985, *32*(4), 266–274.

Related Research: Ibrahim, F. A. (1981). *Design and methodology for the development of a model school counselor education curriculum*. Paper presented at the annual convention of the American Personnel and Guidance Association, St. Louis, MO.

■ ■ ■

3196

Test Name: CONTINGENT–NONCONTINGENT EXPECTANCY SCALE

Purpose: To measure locus of control for academic achievement by distinguishing whether one's academic success will be contingent or noncontingent with one's actions or attributes.

Number of Items: 32

Format: Items rated on a 10-point Likert format. Sample items are presented.

Reliability: Cronbach's alpha ranged from .74 to .90 over five subscales.

Validity: Significant correlations with ability, effort, worry, emotionality, extrinsic–intrinsic motivation, and other measures reported for various subscales were in the predicted direction.

Author: Palenzuela, D. L.

Article: Critical evaluation of locus of control: Towards a reconceptualization of the construct and its measurement.

Journal: *Psychological Reports*, June 1984, *54*(3), 683–709.

■ ■ ■

3197

Test Name: COOPERSMITH SELF-ESTEEM INVENTORY

Purpose: To measure self-esteem in various contexts.

Number of Items: 58

Format: True–false items with eight items constituting a "lie" scale.

Reliability: Test–retest reliability was .88 (50 items over 5 weeks) and .70 (over 3 years).

Author: Miller, L. B., and Bizzell, R. P.

Article: Long-term effects of four preschool programs: ninth- and tenth-grade results.

Journal: *Child Development,* August 1984, *55*(4), 1570–1587.

Related Research: Coopersmith, S. (1967). *Antecedents of self-esteem.* San Francisco: Freeman.

Halpin, G., et al. (1981). Locus of control and self-esteem among American Indians and Whites: A cross-cultural comparison. *Psychological Reports, 48*(1), 91–98.

■ ■ ■

3198

Test Name: COUNSELING EXPECTATION INVENTORY

Purpose: To describe possible outcomes clients might hope to accomplish through counseling.

Number of Items: 14

Format: Items are rated twice: first to indicate the probability that an item can be accomplished through counseling, a 0 (*not at all likely*) to 10 (*completely likely*) scale is used; second to rate the importance of each outcome, a 1 (*extremely unimportant*) to 7 (*extremely important*) scale is used. The product of each pair of ratings is added for all items. Items are presented.

Reliability: Coefficient alphas were .93 (200 clients) and .92 (200 counselors).

Author: Turner, C. J., and Schwartzbach, H.

Article: A construct validation study of the counseling expectation inventory.

Journal: *Measurement and Evaluation in Guidance,* April 1983, *16*(1), 18–24.

Related Research: Schwartzbach, H. (1981). *The development and validation of the prognostic expectation inventory for use with a college counseling population.* Unpublished doctoral dissertation, Rutgers–The State University.

■ ■ ■

3199

Test Name: COUNSELOR FUNCTION INVENTORY

Purpose: To provide counselors' perceptions of the role of the school counselor.

Number of Items: 77

Format: Includes 7 areas of counselor service: placement, counseling, follow-up, orientation, student data, information, and miscellaneous.

Reliability: Test–retest reliability was .96. Odd–even split-half reliability was .86.

Author: Brown, D. R., and Hartman, B.

Article: Differential effects of incentives on response error, response rate and reliability of a mailed questionnaire.

Journal: *Measurement and Evaluation in Guidance,* April 1980, *13*(1), 20–28.

Related Research: Shumate, G. F., & Oelke, M. C. (1967). Counselor function inventory. *School Counselor, 15,* 130–133.

■ ■ ■

3200

Test Name: COUNSELOR PERCEPTION QUESTIONNAIRE

Purpose: To measure counselor's perceptions of counseling sessions.

Number of Items: 14

Format: Items rated in 6-point Likert format.

Reliability: Cronbach's alpha was .94.

Author: Friedlander, M. L., and Kaul, T. J.

Article: Preparing clients for counseling: Effect of role induction on counseling process and outcome.

Journal: *Journal of College Student Personnel,* 1983, *24*(3), 207–214.

Related Research: Howard, K., et al. (1970). Patients' satisfactions in psychotherapy as a function of patient-therapist pairing. *Psychotherapy: Theory, Research and Practice, 7,* 130–134.

■ ■ ■

3201

Test Name: COVERT THOUGHTS QUESTIONNAIRE

Purpose: To assess self-statements.

Number of Items: 26

Format: Includes an equal number of positive and negative self-statements to which subjects respond on a scale from 1 (*never had the thought*) to 5 (*very often had the thought*).

Reliability: Cronbach's alphas were .81 (positive items) and .87 (negative items).

Validity: Correlations with other variables ranged from −.47 to .53.

Author: Bruch, M. A., et al.

Article: Relationships of cognitive components of test anxiety to test performance: Implications for assessment and treatment.

Journal: *Journal of Counseling Psychology,* October 1983, *30*(4), 527–536.

Related Research: Galassi, J. P., et al. (1981). Behavior of high, moderate and low test-anxious students during an actual test situation. *Journal of Consulting and Clinical Psychology, 49,* 51–62.

■ ■ ■

3202

Test Name: DEVIANT ROLE/ IDENTITY SCALE

Purpose: To measure role/ identities of deviant individuals.

Number of Items: 11 adjective pairs.

Format: Semantic differential (all adjective pairs presented).

Validity: MMPI *Pd* Scale: subjects with delinquent self-concepts described themselves as having more deviant feelings and behavior than subjects with disturbed or popular self-concepts.

Author: Chassin, L., et al.

Article: Identifying with a deviant label: The validation of a methodology.

Journal: *Social Psychology Quarterly,* March 1981, *44*(1), 31–36.

Related Research: Burke, P., & Tully, J. (1977). The measurement of role identity. *Social Forces, 55,* 881–897.

■ ■ ■

3203

Test Name: EDUCATIONAL ATTRIBUTION SCALE

Purpose: To measure role of attributional processes in educational outcomes (i.e., locus of control).

Number of Items: 3

Format: Items rated on 9-point rating scales. All items presented

(one each for distinctiveness, consistency, and consensus).

Validity: Low scores on test are made by students who are high in external attribution.

Author: Forsyth, D. R., and McMillan, J. H.

Article: The attribution cube and reaction to educational outcomes.

Journal: *Journal of Educational Psychology,* October 1981, *73*(5), 632–641.

Related Research: Kelly, H. H. (1981). *Attribution in social interaction.* Morristown, NJ: General Learning Press.

■ ■ ■

3204

Test Name: EFFICACY TO INFLUENCE CHANGE SCALE

Purpose: To measure perceived collective efficacy to influence change in university policy and to change the present situation.

Number of Items: 18

Format: Responses were scored as indicating either positive or negative outcome.

Reliability: Internal consistency reliability was .88.

Validity: Correlations with other variables ranged from −.72 to .78.

Author: Zalesny, M. D.

Article: Comparison of economic and noneconomic factors in predicting faculty vote preference in a union representation election.

Journal: *Journal of Applied Psychology,* May 1985, *70*(2), 243–256.

■ ■ ■

3205

Test Name: EFFORT VERSUS ABILITY VERSUS EXTERNAL SCALE

Purpose: To assess children's causal attributions for academic difficulties.

Number of Items: 30

Format: For each of five failure situations children choose one of three causes of failure, and for each selected cause of failure children select two of three attributions.

Reliability: Test–retest ranged from .56 to .82. Internal consistency ranged from .63 to .77.

Validity: Correlations with Intellectual Achievement Responsibility Scale (Crandall et al., 1965) ranged from .59 to .63.

Author: Licht, B. G., et al.

Article: Causal attributions of learning disabled children: Individual differences and their implications for persistence.

Journal: *Journal of Educational Psychology,* April 1985, *77*(2), 208–216.

■ ■ ■

3206

Test Name: EGO-STRENGTH AND SELF-ESTEEM MEASURE

Purpose: To measure levels of ego-strength and self-esteem (ability to share feelings, personal adequacy, sense of reality, alienation, loneliness, self-confidence).

Number of Items: 80

Format: True–false.

Reliability: Alphas ranged from .62 to .67 across subscales.

Author: Fry, P. S., and Addington, J.

Article: Comparison of social problem solving of children from open and traditional classrooms: A two-year longitudinal study.

Journal: *Journal of Educational*

Psychology, April 1984, *76*(2), 318–329.

Related Research: Barron, F. (1953). An ego-strength scale which predicts response to psychotherapy. *Journal of Consulting Psychology, 17,* 327–333.

Helmreich, R., & Stapp, J. (1974). Short forms of the Texas Social Behavior Inventory (TSBI), an objective measure of self-esteem. *Bulletin of the Psychonomic Society, 4,* 473–475.

■ ■ ■

3207

Test Name: ESTIMATE OF SELF-COMPETENCE SCALE

Purpose: To measure generalized expectancy of task success.

Number of Items: 12

Reliability: Internal consistency reliability estimate was .78. Test–retest estimate was .86.

Validity: Correlations with other variables ranged from –.40 to .51.

Author: Motowidlo, S. J.

Article: Construct validity for a measure of generalized expectancy of task success.

Journal: *Educational and Psychological Measurement,* Winter 1981, *41*(4), 963–972.

Related Research: Motowidlo, S. J. (1979). Development of a measure of generalized expectancy of task success. *Educational and Psychological Measurement, 39,* 69–80.

■ ■ ■

3208

Test Name: EXPECTATIONS ABOUT COUNSELING QUESTIONNAIRE

Purpose: To measure clients' expectations about counseling prior to entering counseling.

Number of Items: 35

Format: Includes 17 scales and employs a Likert format with 7 response alternatives (1 = *not true* to 7 = *definitely true*).

Reliability: Internal consistency estimates for the 17 scales ranged from .71 to .89.

Author: Heesacker, M., and Heppner, P. P.

Article: Using real client perceptions to examine psychometric properties of the Counselor Rating Form.

Journal: *Journal of Counseling Psychology,* April 1983, *30*(2), 180–187.

Related Research: Heppner, P. P., & Heesacker, M. (1983). Perceived counselor characteristics, client expectations and client satisfaction with counseling. *Journal of Counseling Psychology, 30,* 31–39.

■ ■ ■

3209

Test Name: EXPECTATIONS ABOUT COUNSELING—SHORT FORM

Purpose: To measure expectations about counseling.

Number of Items: 53

Format: Responses to each item are made on a 7-point continuum from *definitely do not expect this to be true* (1) to *definitely do expect this to be true* (7).

Reliability: Reliabilities ranged from .69 to .81.

Author: Hardin, S. I., and Subich, L. M.

Article: A methodological note: Do students expect what clients do?

Journal: *Journal of Counseling Psychology,* January 1985, *32*(1), 131–134.

Related Research: Tinsley, H. E. A.,

et al. (1980). Factor analysis of the domain of client expectancies about counseling. *Journal of Counseling Psychology, 27,* 561–570.

■ ■ ■

3210

Test Name: EXPECTATIONS ABOUT COUNSELING QUESTIONNAIRE—REVISED

Purpose: To measure clients' expectations about counseling prior to entering counseling.

Number of Items: 45

Format: Includes six scales: client openness, motivation, counselor acceptance, expertness, attractiveness, and trustworthiness. Likert format with 7 response alternatives.

Reliability: Internal consistency for the six scales ranged from .84 to .95.

Validity: Correlation with other variables ranged from –.33 to .35.

Author: Heppner, P. P., and Heesacker, M.

Article: Perceived counselor characteristics, client expectations and client satisfaction with counseling.

Journal: *Journal of Counseling Psychology,* January 1983, *30*(1), 31–39.

Related Research: Tinsley, H. E. A., et al. (1980). Factor analysis of the domain of client expectancies about counseling. *Journal of Counseling Psychology, 27,* 561–570.

■ ■ ■

3211

Test Name: EXTRAORDINARY BELIEF INVENTORY

Purpose: To survey belief in paranormal phenomena.

Number of Items: 30

Format: Items rated in 7-point Likert format. Sample items are presented.

Reliability: Alpha ranged from .68 to .92 across subscales.

Validity: Mean correlation between subscales was .48.

Author: Otis, L. P., and Alcock, J. E.

Article: Factors affecting extraordinary belief.

Journal: *Journal of Social Psychology,* October 1982, *118*(first half), 77–85.

■■■

3212

Test Name: FEELINGS OF INADEQUACY SCALE

Purpose: To measure self-esteem.

Number of Items: 19

Format: Multiple-choice. All items presented.

Reliability: Alpha ranged from .68 to .88 across subscales.

Validity: Correlated .40 to .82 with Rosenberg Self-Esteem Scale.

Author: O'Brien, E. J.

Article: Global self-esteem scales: Unidimensional or multidimensional.

Journal: *Psychological Reports,* October 1985, *57*(2), 383–389.

Related Research: Eagly, A. H. (1967). Involvement as a determinant of response to favorable and unfavorable information. *Journal of Personality and Social Psychology, 7*(3, Whole No. 643).

■■■

3213

Test Name: FLORIDA KEY OF LEARNER SELF-CONCEPT— REVISED

Purpose: To measure self-concept.

Number of Items: 22

Format: Uses behavioral ratings of student self-concept and includes the factors relating, asserting, investing, and coping.

Reliability: Ranged from .84 to .93.

Validity: Correlation with Behavioral Academic Self-Esteem was .90.

Author: Benner, E. H., et al.

Article: A construct validation of academic self-esteem for intermediate grade-level children.

Journal: *Measurement and Evaluation in Guidance,* October 1983, *16*(3), 127–134.

Related Research: Purkey, W. W., et al. (1973). The Florida Key: A scale to infer learner self-concept. *Educational and Psychological Measurement, 33,* 979–984.

■■■

3214

Test Name: GENDER POWER SCALES

Purpose: To measure perceived power of persons.

Number of Items: 17

Format: Bipolar scales with a 7-point range. All items presented.

Reliability: Alpha on subscales ranged from .43 to .89.

Author: Molm, L. D.

Article: Gender and power use: An experimental analysis of behavior and perceptions.

Journal: *Social Psychology Quarterly,* December 1985, *48*(4), 285–300.

Related Research: Bovermon, I. K., et al. (1972). Sex-role stereotypes: A current appraisal. *Journal of Social Issues, 28,* 59–78.

3215

Test Name: GENERALIZED EXPECTANCY OF SPORT SUCCESS SCALE

Purpose: To measure athlete's expectation of future athletic success.

Number of Items: 20

Format: Bipolar adjectives rated on 5-point scale.

Reliability: Test–retest reliability was .90. Internal consistency was .95.

Author: Horn, T. S.

Article: Coaches' feedback and changes in children's perceptions of their physical competence.

Journal: *Journal of Educational Psychology,* April 1985, *77*(2), 174–186.

Related Research: Coulson, H. M., & Cobb, R. (1979). *Assessment of a scale to measure generalized expectancy of sport success.* Paper presented at the Annual Meeting of the American Alliance for Health, Physical Education, and Health, New Orleans.

■■■

3216

Test Name: GENERALIZED SELF-EFFICACY SCALE

Purpose: To measure one's expectations to perform across broad range of challenging activities that require effort and perseverance.

Number of Items: 27

Format: Responses to each item are made on a 7-point Likert scale ranging from *strongly agree* to *strongly disagree.* Examples are provided.

Validity: Correlation with the Goal Attainment Scale was .37.

Author: Tipton, T. M., and Worthington, E. L., Jr.

Article: The measurement of generalized self-efficacy: A study of construct validity.

Journal: *Journal of Personality Assessment,* October 1984, *48*(5), 545–548.

Related Research: Tipton, R. M., et al. (1980). Faith and locus of control. *Psychological Reports, 46,* 1151–1154.

■ ■ ■

3217

Test Name: HEALTH LOCUS OF CONTROL SCALE

Purpose: To measure the extent to which individuals perceive themselves to be in control of their own personal health.

Number of Items: 11

Format: Includes two factors: one with items worded in an internal direction, the other factor with items worded in an external direction.

Reliability: Coefficient alphas were .70 and .67 (for Factors 1 and 2, respectively).

Validity: Correlations with the Marlowe-Crowne Social Desirability Scale were –.009 (Factor 1) and –.13 (Factor 2).

Author: Gutkin, T. B., et al.

Article: The Health Locus of Control Scale: Psychometric properties.

Journal: *Educational and Psychological Measurement,* Summer 1985, *45*(2), 407–409.

Related Research: Wallston, B. S., et al. (1976). Development of validation of the Health Locus of Control (HLC) scale. *Journal of Consulting and Clinical Psychology, 44,* 580–585.

Keller, R. T. (1983). Predicting absenteeism from prior absenteeism, attitudinal factors, and nonattitudinal factors.

Journal of Applied Psychology, 68(3), 536–540.

■ ■ ■

3218

Test Name: HEALTH LOCUS OF CONTROL SCALE

Purpose: To measure perceived patient control over health in a hospital setting.

Number of Items: 6

Format: Two-option forced-choice items. All items presented.

Reliability: Test–retest reliability was .81.

Validity: Medical care givers scored more highly internal than patients.

Author: Tadmor, C. S., and Hofman, J. E.

Article: Measuring locus of control in a hospital setting.

Journal: *Psychological Reports,* April 1985, *56*(2), 525–526.

■ ■ ■

3219

Test Name: HEART DISEASE LOCUS OF CONTROL SCALE

Purpose: To assess locus of control relating to heart disease.

Number of Items: 20

Format: Items rated on 6-point Likert agreement response categories.

Reliability: Test–retest reliability was .83. Cronbach's alpha ranged from .76 to .86 across subscales.

Validity: Subscales correlated significantly with Multidimensional Health Scale subscales (significant correlations ranged from .27 to .73 in absolute value).

Author: O'Connell, J. K., and Price, J. H.

Article: Development of a heart disease locus of control scale.

Journal: *Psychological Reports,* February 1985, *56*(1), 159–164.

■ ■ ■

3220

Test Name: ILLNESS BEHAVIOR INVENTORY

Purpose: To assess perceived illness behavior of one's mother, father, and oneself as a child.

Number of Items: 20

Format: Each item is rated on a Likert scale from 1 to 6.

Reliability: Test–retest reliabilities ranged from .77 to 1.0 (2 weeks).

Author: Turkat, I. D., and Guise, B. J.

Article: Test of reliability of perception of parental and childhood illness behavior.

Journal: *Perceptual and Motor Skills,* August 1983, *57*(1), 101–102.

Related Research: Turkat, I. D., & Pettegrew, L. S. (1983). Development and validation of the Illness Behavior Inventory. *Journal of Behavioral Assessment, 5,* 35–47.

■ ■ ■

3221

Test Name: INSTRUCTIONAL OBJECTIVES EXCHANGE SELF-APPRAISAL INVENTORY

Purpose: To measure self-concept.

Number of Items: 36

Format: Yes–no. Inventory is read to children who after each question respond on an answer sheet.

Reliability: Test–retest (total) reliability was .70 (.29 to .58 across subscales). Kuder-Richardson formula 20 internal consistency (total) = .37 (.50 to .60 across subscales).

Author: Soule, J. C., et al.

Article: Dimensions of self-concept for children in kindergarten and grades 1 and 2.

Journal: *Psychological Reports,* February 1981, *48*(1), 83–88.

Related Research: UCLA. (1972). *Measures of self-concept K-12* (Rev. ed.). Los Angeles: University of California, Instructional Objectives Exchange.

▪ ▪ ▪

3222

Test Name: INTELLECTUAL ACHIEVEMENT RESPONSIBILITY SCALE

Purpose: To measure perceived locus of control in intellectual and academic activities.

Number of Items: 34

Format: Forced-choice.

Reliability: Test–retest ranged from .66 to .74 over grade levels.

Author: Tzuriel, D., and Haywood, H. C.

Article: Locus of control and child-rearing practices in intrinsically motivated and extrinsically motivated children.

Journal: *Psychological Reports,* December 1985, *57*(3, Part 1), 887–894.

Related Research: Crandall, V. C., et al. (1965). Children's beliefs in their own control of reinforcements in intellectual-academic situations. *Child Development, 36,* 90–108.

Halpin, G., et al. (1981). Locus of control and self-esteem among American Indians and Whites: A cross-cultural comparison. *Psychological Reports, 48*(1), 91–98.

Benner, E. H., et al. (1983). A construct validation of academic self-esteem for intermediate grade-level children. *Measurement and*

Evaluation in Guidance, 16(3), 127–134.

▪ ▪ ▪

3223

Test Name: INTERNAL CONTROL INDEX

Purpose: To measure locus of control in adults.

Number of Items: 28

Format: Responses are made on a 5-point scale from (A) *rarely* to (E) *usually*. All items are presented.

Reliability: Reliability coefficient alpha was .84 and .85.

Validity: Correlation with Mirels' Factor I of Rotter's I-E Scale was –.385.

Author: Duttweiler, P. C.

Article: The Internal Control Index: A newly developed measure of locus of control.

Journal: *Educational and Psychological Measurement,* Summer 1984, *44*(2), 209–221.

▪ ▪ ▪

3224

Test Name: I-E SCALE

Purpose: To measure internal or external locus of control.

Number of Items: 45 (including 13 buffer items).

Format: Forced-choice. Modification of Rotter I-E Scale.

Reliability: Test–retest reliability was .76.

Author: Hood, J., et al.

Article: Locus of control as a measure of ineffectiveness in anorexia nervosa.

Journal: *Journal of Consulting and Clinical Psychology,* February 1982, *50*(1), 3–13.

Related Research: Ried, D. W., & Ware, E. E. (1973).

Multidimensionality of internal–external control: Implications for past and future research. *Canadian Journal of Behavioral Science, 5,* 264–271.

▪ ▪ ▪

3225

Test Name: I-E LOCUS OF CONTROL SCALE

Purpose: To measure locus of control.

Number of Items: 23

Format: Includes six nonreactive filler items to make it more difficult to identify the test's purpose.

Reliability: Internal consistency coefficient (Kuder-Richardson) was .70 ($N = 400$). Test–retest reliability coefficient was .72 ($N = 60$, 1 month), and .55 ($N = 117$, 2 months).

Validity: Correlations with Marlowe-Crowne Social Desirability Scale ranged from –.34 to –.42.

Author: Harris, R. M., and Salomone, P. R.

Article: Toward an abbreviated internal–external locus of control.

Journal: *Measurement and Evaluation in Guidance,* January 1981, *13*(4), 229–234.

Related Research: Roller, J. B. (1966). Generalized expectancies for internal versus external control of reinforcement. *Psychological Monographs, 80*(Whole No. 609).

▪ ▪ ▪

3226

Test Name: IRRATIONAL BELIEFS TEST

Purpose: To assess degree of irrational beliefs.

Number of Items: 100

Format: Items rated on 5-point Likert agreement scales.

Reliability: Test–retest ranged from .61 to .80. Alphas ranged from .35 to .73.

Author: Lohr, J. M., and Rea, R. G.

Article: A disconfirmation of the relationship between fear of public speaking and irrational beliefs.

Journal: *Psychological Reports,* June 1981, *48*(3), 795–798.

Related Research: Lohr, J. M., & Bonge, D. (1980). Retest reliability of the Irrational Beliefs Test. *Psychological Reports, 47,* 1314.

■ ■ ■

3227

Test Name: IRRATIONAL PERSONALITY TRAIT INVENTORY SCALE REVISED

Purpose: To measure irrational beliefs and perceptions.

Number of Items: 52

Format: Consists of clinically derived items. Examples are presented. Responses are recorded on a 5-point Likert scale. Scores ranged from 52 to 260. Higher scores reflect irrational self-thoughts.

Reliability: Cronbach's alpha was .95.

Validity: Correlations with other variables ranged from .50 to .73.

Author: Thompson, D. G., and Hudson, G. R.

Article: Values clarification and behavioral group counseling with ninth grade boys in a residential school.

Journal: *Journal of Counseling Psychology,* July 1982, *29*(4), 394–399.

Related Research: Ross, G. R. (1977). *Reducing irrational personality traits, trait anxiety,*

and intra-interpersonal needs in high school students. Paper presented at the annual meeting of the Florida Educational Research Association, St. Petersburg Beach.

■ ■ ■

3228

Test Name: ITALIAN STEREOTYPE SCALE

Purpose: To measure respondent's involvement with a set of Italian behaviors.

Number of Items: 21

Format: Respondent estimated frequency of each behavior for nine target persons on a 5-point (*never–always*) scale.

Reliability: Cronbach's alpha was .83.

Validity: Factor analysis revealed four interpretable factors: Socio-Cultural Activities, Family, In-Group, and Tradition.

Author: Caltabiano, N. J.

Article: Perceived differences in ethnic behavior: A pilot study of Italo-Australian Canberra residents.

Journal: *Psychological Reports,* December 1984, *55*(3), 867–873.

■ ■ ■

3229

Test Name: JANIS-FIELD FEELINGS OF INADEQUACY SCALE

Purpose: To measure self-esteem.

Number of Items: 20

Format: Responses are made on a 5-point Likert scale.

Validity: Correlations with the Irrational Beliefs Test ranged from −.59 to .16 (*N*= 251).

Author: Daly, M. J., and Burton, R. L.

Article: Self-esteem and irrational beliefs: An exploratory investigation with implications for counseling.

Journal: *Journal of Counseling Psychology,* July 1983, *30*(3), 361–366.

Related Research: Eagly, A. H. (1967). Involvement as a determinant of response to favorable and unfavorable information. *Journal of Personality and Social Psychology Monographs, 7*(3, Whole No. 643).

■ ■ ■

3230

Test Name: LEVENSON LOCUS OF CONTROL QUESTIONNAIRE

Purpose: To measure locus of control.

Number of Items: 24

Format: Items rated on a 6-point Likert rating scale.

Validity: Previously reported factor structure not found in these data from Australian high school students, although the findings indicate multidimensionality.

Author: Hong, S.-M., and Bartenstein, C.

Article: Dimensions of Levenson's locus of control with Australian high school students.

Journal: *Psychological Reports,* 1982, *51*(2), 395–400.

Related Research: Walkey, F. H. (1979). Internal control, powerful others and chance: A confirmation of Levenson's factor structure. *Journal of Personality Assessment, 43,* 532–535.

Levenson, H. (1974). Activism and powerful others: Distinctions within the concept of internal–external control. *Journal of Personality Assessment, 38,* 377–383.

3231

Test Name: LINDGREN EMBEDDED FIGURES TEST

Purpose: To measure field independence.

Number of Items: 20

Format: For each item, the subject finds a figure among lines in a rectangle.

Reliability: Test–retest reliability was .81.

Validity: Correlation with Group Embedded Figures Test was .61.

Author: Hicks, L. A., and Lindgren, H. C.

Article: Field dependence and ability to judge spatial coordinates.

Journal: *Perceptual and Motor Skills*, December 1985, *61*(3, Part 1), 984–986.

∎ ∎ ∎

3232

Test Name: LIPSITT SELF-CONCEPT SCALE

Purpose: To measure positive and negative evaluations of self.

Number of Items: 22

Format: Subjects rate themselves on a 5-point scale on traits such as friendly, obedient, and lazy.

Reliability: Internal reliability ranged from .84 to .85 in three separate administrations.

Validity: Significant negative relationships to Children's Manifest Anxiety and positive relationships to academic motivation.

Author: Peterson, G. W., et al.

Article: Children's self-esteem and maternal behavior in three low-income samples.

Journal: *Psychological Reports*, 1983, *52*(1), 79–86.

3233

Test Name: LOCUS OF CONTROL INVENTORY FOR THREE ACHIEVEMENT DOMAINS (LOCITAD)

Purpose: To measure locus of control perceived for intellectual, physical, and social activities.

Number of Items: 47

Reliability: Minimum item-total correlation was .30. Kuder-Richardson formula 20 ranged between .52 and .53 (.75 total scale).

Validity: Correlated .78 with Intellectual Achievement Responsibility Scale.

Author: Williams, R. E., et al.

Article: Effects of STEP on parental attitudes and locus of control of their learning disabled children.

Journal: *The School Counselor*, November 1984, *32*(2), 126–133.

Related Research: Bradley, R., et al. (1977). A new scale to assess locus of control in three achievement domains. *Psychological Reports, 41*, 656–661.

∎ ∎ ∎

3234

Test Name: LOCUS OF CONTROL MEASURE

Purpose: To measure locus of control of college students.

Number of Items: 4

Format: Responses to each item are made on a 5-point scale ranging from 1 (*strongly agree*) to 5 (*strongly disagree*).

Reliability: Coefficient alphas ranged from .49 to .57.

Author: Behuniak, P., Jr., and Gable, R. K.

Article: A longitudinal study of

self-concept and locus of control for persisters in six college majors.

Journal: *Educational Research Quarterly,* Spring 1981, *6*(1), 3–12.

Related Research: Conger, A. S., et al. (1977). *National longitudinal study of high school seniors: Group profiles on self-esteem, locus of control and life goals* (NCES 77-260). Washington, DC: U.S. Department of Health, Education and Welfare.

∎ ∎ ∎

3235

Test Name: LOCUS OF CONTROL SCALE

Purpose: To measure locus of control.

Number of Items: 12

Format: Likert scale.

Reliability: Test–retest reliability coefficient was .75 (1-week interval).

Validity: Correlation with the Marlowe-Crowne Social Desirability Scale was .09.

Author: Harris, R. M., and Salomone, P. R.

Article: Toward an abbreviated internal-external locus of control scale.

Journal: *Measurement and Evaluation in Guidance,* January 1981, *13*(4), 229–234.

Related Research: MacDonald, A. R., & Tseng, M. S. (1976). Dimensions of internal versus external control revisited. In R. K. Gable & D. L. Thompson (Eds.), Perception of personal control and conformity of vocational choice as correlates of vocational development. *Journal of Vocational Behavior, 8*, 259–267.

3236

Test Name: LOCUS OF CONTROL SCALE

Purpose: To assess locus of control.

Number of Items: 24

Format: Includes three scales: internal, powerful others, and chance.

Reliability: Kuder-Richardson reliabilities ranged from .67 to .82. Test–retest reliabilities ranged from .08 to .78.

Author: Harris, R. M., and Salomone, P. R.

Article: Toward an abbreviated internal–external locus of control.

Journal: *Measurement and Evaluation in Guidance,* January 1981, *13*(4), 229–234.

Related Research: Levenson, H. (1972). *Distinctions within the concept of internal–external control: Development of a new scale.* Proceedings of the 80th Annual Convention of the American Psychological Association, *7,* 259–260.

■ ■ ■

3237

Test Name: LOCUS OF CONTROL SCALE

Purpose: To measure locus of control.

Number of Items: 88

Format: Likert scale for 46 items.

Reliability: Test–retest reliability coefficients for the 46 items ranged from .18 to .75 (*N* = 300).

Validity: Correlation of the 46 items with the Rotter I-E Scale was .82.

Author: Harris, R. M., and Salomone, P. R.

Article: Toward an abbreviated internal–external locus of control.

Journal: *Measurement and Evaluation in Guidance,* January 1981, *13*(4), 229–234.

Related Research: Collins, B. E. (1974). Form components of the Rotter Internal–External Scale. *Journal of Personality and Social Psychology, 29,* 381–391.

■ ■ ■

3238

Test Name: LOCUS OF CONTROL SCALE

Purpose: To assess locus of control.

Number of Items: 40

Format: High scores indicate externality.

Reliability: Alpha was .72 (American children) and .61 (Venezuelans).

Author: Prawat, R. S., et al.

Article: Attitude development in American and Venezuelan schoolchildren.

Journal: *Journal of Social Psychology,* December 1981, *115*(second half), 149–158.

Related Research: Nowicki, S., & Strickland, B. (1973). A locus of control scale for children. *Journal of Consulting and Clinical Psychology, 40,* 148–154.

■ ■ ■

3239

Test Name: LOCUS OF CONTROL SCALE

Purpose: To measure locus of control.

Number of Items: 11

Format: For each item subjects select either the internal or the external locus of control statement, whichever they more strongly believe is true. Examples are presented.

Reliability: Cronbach's alpha was .60.

Validity: Correlations with loneliness scores ranged from –.02 to –.46.

Author: Schmitt, J. P., and Kurdek, L. A.

Article: Age and gender differences in and personality correlates of loneliness in different relationships.

Journal: *Journal of Personality Assessment,* October 1985, *49*(5), 485–496.

Related Research: Valecha, G. K., & Ostrum, T. M. (1974). An abbreviated measure of internal–external locus of control. *Journal of Personality Assessment, 38,* 369–376.

■ ■ ■

3240

Test Name: LOCUS OF CONTROL SCALE

Purpose: To measure internal locus of control.

Number of Items: 29

Format: Subjects choose two statements for each item: One statement reflects an external frame of reference, the other an internal frame of reference.

Reliability: Cronbach's alpha was .78.

Validity: Correlations with social anxiety were –.38 (college students) and –.31 (homosexuals).

Author: Schmitt, J. P., and Kurdek, L. A.

Article: Correlates of social anxiety in college students and homosexuals.

Journal: *Journal of Personality Assessment,* August 1984, *48*(4), 403–409.

Related Research: Rotter, J. B.

(1966). Generalized expectancies for internal versus external control of reinforcement. *Psychological Monographs, 80,* 1–28.

Martin, J. D., & Coley, L. A. (1984). *Educational and Psychological Measurement, 44*(2), 517–521.

■ ■ ■

3241

Test Name: LOCUS OF CONTROL SCALE FOR CHILDREN

Purpose: To measure generalized expectancy for the locus of control of reinforcement in children.

Number of Items: 21

Format: Yes–no.

Reliability: Test–retest reliability was .83. Internal consistency was .72.

Author: Lokan, J. J., et al.

Article: A study of vocational maturity during adolescence and locus of control.

Journal: *Journal of Vocational Behavior,* June 1982, *20*(3), 331–342.

Related Research: Nowicki, S., Jr., & Strickland, B. R. (1973). A locus of control scale for children. *Journal of Consulting and Clinical Psychology, 40,* 148–154.

■ ■ ■

3242

Test Name: LOCUS OF CONTROL SCALE FOR CHILDREN'S PERCEPTIONS OF SOCIAL INTERACTIONS

Purpose: To measure children's perceptions of social interactions.

Number of Items: 48

Format: Includes three scores:

number of items answered in the internal direction, number of positive content items answered in the internal direction, and number of negative content items answered in the internal direction. A social desirability scale is included.

Reliability: Coefficients of internal consistency ranged from .75 to .81. Test–retest correlations (10 days) ranged from .65 to .70.

Validity: Correlations with other measures ranged from .30 to .44.

Author: Dahlquist, L. M., and Ottinger, D. R.

Article: Locus of control and peer status: A scale for children's perceptions of social interactions.

Journal: *Journal of Personality Assessment,* June 1983, *47*(3), 278–287.

■ ■ ■

3243

Test Name: MANAGERIAL COMPETENCE SCALE

Purpose: To measure perceptions of the competence of female managers.

Number of Items: 17

Format: Likert format.

Reliability: Alphas ranged from .69 to .82 across subscales.

Author: Ezell, H. F., et al.

Article: The effects of having been supervised by a woman on perceptions of female managerial competence.

Journal: *Personnel Psychology,* Summer 1981, *34*(2), 291–299.

Related Research: Snyder, R. A., & Morris, J. H. (1978). Reliability of the factor structure of the Wagner and Morse Competence Index. *Psychological Reports, 43,* 419–425.

Wagner, F. R., & Morse, J. J.

(1975). A measure of individual sense of competence. *Psychological Reports, 36,* 451–459.

■ ■ ■

3244

Test Name: MATHEMATICS ACHIEVEMENT QUESTIONNAIRE

Purpose: To assess locus of control.

Number of Items: 20

Format: Includes obtaining students' views of mathematics, problem-solving, their mathematics teachers, their fellow mathematics students. Students responded to each item by choosing either an internal or an external point of view.

Reliability: Kuder-Richardson formula 20 reliability coefficients ranged from .5 to .6. Also reliability coefficients ranged from .6 to .8.

Validity: Correlation with SAT was .07.

Author: McLeod, D. B., and Adams, V. M.

Article: Locus of control and mathematics instruction: Three exploratory studies.

Journal: *Journal of Experimental Education,* Winter 1980/81, *49*(2), 94–99.

■ ■ ■

3245

Test Name: MATHEMATICS AS A MALE DOMAIN SCALE

Purpose: To measure the extent to which subjects stereotype mathematics as being a male domain.

Number of Items: 12

Format: Likert items. Higher scores indicate weaker stereotyping by the subjects.

Reliability: Split-half reliability coefficient was .87.

Validity: Correlation with other variables ranged from −.23 to .34.

Author: Llabre, M. M., and Suarez, E.

Article: Predicting math anxiety and course performance in college women and men.

Journal: *Journal of Counseling Psychology*, April 1985, *32*(2), 283–287.

Related Research: Fennema, E., & Sherman, J. (1976). Fennema-Sherman Mathematics Attitude Scales: Instruments designed to measure attitudes toward the learning of mathematics by females and males. *JSAS Catalog of Selected Documents in Psychology*, *6*, 31.

■ ■ ■

3246

Test Name: MATHEMATICS ATTRIBUTION SCALE

Purpose: To assess high school students' attributions of achievement in algebra or geometry.

Number of Items: 32

Format: Consists of eight 4-item subscales.

Validity: Correlations with the Multidimensional-Multi-attributional Causality Scale ranged from −.31 to .52.

Author: Powers, S., et al.

Article: Convergent validity of the Multidimensional-Multi-attributional Causality Scale with the Mathematics Attribution Scale.

Journal: *Educational and Psychological Measurement*, Autumn 1985, *45*(3), 689–692.

Related Research: Fennema, E., et al. (1979). Mathematics Attribution Scale: An instrument

designed to measure students' attributions of the causes of their successes and failures in mathematics. *Journal Abstract Service of the American Psychological Association: Catalog of Selected Documents in Psychology*, *9*(2), 26.

Douglas, P., et al. (1985). Achievement motivation and attributions for success and failure. *Psychological Reports*, *57*(3), 751–754.

■ ■ ■

3247

Test Name: MATHEMATICAL SELF-CONCEPT QUESTIONNAIRE

Purpose: To measure pupils' self-concept of mathematical achievement, ability, and affect.

Number of Items: 21

Format: Items rated on a 3-point Likert scale. One sample item presented.

Reliability: Alpha was .83.

Validity: Construct validity tested with factor analysis of items. Two achievement factors, two affective factors, and one ability factor were extracted.

Author: Mevarech, Z. R., and Rich, Y.

Article: Effects of computer-assisted mathematics instruction on disadvantaged pupils' cognitive and affective development.

Journal: *Journal of Educational Research*, September/October 1985, *79*(1), 5–11.

■ ■ ■

3248

Test Name: MATHEMATICS SELF-CONCEPT SCALE

Purpose: To measure student mathematics self-concept.

Number of Items: 24

Format: Double-Q sort of mathematics student behavior and attitude descriptors, one sort for ideal student and one sort for themselves. Sample items presented.

Reliability: Test–retest reliability was .92.

Author: Peterson, K., et al.

Article: Geometry students' role-specific self-concept: Success, teacher, and sex differences.

Journal: *Journal of Educational Research*, November/December 1983, *77*(2), 122–126.

Related Research: Peterson, K., et al. (1980). Science students' role-specific self-concept: Course, success and gender. *Science Education*, *64*, 169–174.

■ ■ ■

3249

Test Name: MATHEMATICS SELF-EFFICACY SCALE

Purpose: To measure math-related self-efficacy.

Number of Items: 52

Format: Includes three subscales: Math tasks, math courses, and math problems.

Validity: Correlations with other variables ranged from −.25 to .66.

Author: Hackett, G.

Article: Role of mathematics self-efficacy in the choice of math-related majors of college women and men: A path analysis.

Journal: *Journal of Counseling Psychology*, January 1985, *32*(1), 47–56.

Related Research: Betz, N. E., & Hackett, G. (1983). The relationship of mathematics self-efficacy expectations to the selection of science-based college majors. *Journal of Vocational Behavior, 23,* 329–345.

■ ■ ■

3250

Test Name: ME SCALE

Purpose: To measure self-concept of gifted children.

Number of Items: 40

Format: Students respond to each item by agreeing or disagreeing. All items are presented.

Reliability: Kuder-Richardson formula 20 was .80.

Validity: Correlation with the Piers-Harris Self-Concept Scale was .65.

Author: Feldhusen, J. F., and Kolloff, M. B.

Article: Me: A self-concept scale for gifted children.

Journal: *Perceptual and Motor Skills,* August 1981, *53*(1), 319–323.

■ ■ ■

3251

Test Name: MULTIDIMENSIONAL HEALTH LOCUS OF CONTROL SCALE

Purpose: To assess locus of control as a multidimensional health construct.

Number of Items: 18

Format: Includes three subscales: internal, powerful others, and chance.

Reliability: Cronbach's alpha reliabilities ranged from .59 (internal) to .76 (powerful others).

Author: Desmond, S., et al.

Article: Health locus of control and voluntary use of seat belts among high school students.

Journal: *Perceptual and Motor Skills,* August 1985, *61*(1), 315–319.

Related Research: Wallston, K. A., et al. (1978). Development of the Multidimensional Health Locus of Control (MHLC) scales. *Health, Education Monographs, 6,* 160–170.

Slenker, S. E., et al. (1985). Health locus of control of joggers and nonexercisers. *Perceptual and Motor Skills, 61,* 323–328.

Winefield, H. R. (1982). Reliability and validity of the Health Locus of Control Scale. *Journal of Personality Assessment, 46*(6), 614–619.

Adler, D., & Price, J. H. (1985). Relation of agoraphobics: Health locus of control orientation to severity of agoraphobia. *Psychological Reports, 56*(2), 619–625.

■ ■ ■

3252

Test Name: MULTIDIMENSIONAL MEASURE OF CHILDREN'S PERCEPTIONS OF CONTROL

Purpose: To measure children's perceived control.

Number of Items: 48

Format: Represented by the items are: each source of control, within each domain, for each outcome. Responses to each item are made on a 4-point Likert format. All items are presented.

Reliability: Subscale coefficient alphas ranged from .39 to .70. Test–retest reliabilities ranged from .30 to .48 (9 months); and from .25 to .50 (17 months).

Author: Connell, J. P.

Article: A new multidimensional measure of children's perceptions of control.

Journal: *Child Development,* August 1985, *56*(4), 1018–1041.

Related Research: Harter, S., &

Connell, J. P. (1984). A model of the relationships among children's academic achievement and their self-perceptions of competence, control and motivational orientation. In J. Nichols (Ed.), *The development of achievement motivation* (pp. 219–250). Greenwich, CT: JAI.

■ ■ ■

3253

Test Name: MULTIDIMENSIONAL-MULTIATTRIBUTIONAL CAUSALITY SCALE

Purpose: To measure attributions of general school achievement to four causal factors.

Number of Items: 24

Format: Includes eight 3-item subscales.

Validity: Correlations with the Mathematics Attribution Scale ranged from –.31 to .52.

Author: Powers, S., et al.

Article: Convergent validity of the Multidimensional–Multiattributional Causality Scale with the Mathematics Attribution Scale.

Journal: *Educational and Psychological Measurement,* Autumn 1985, *45*(3), 689–692.

Related Research: Lefcourt, H. M., et al. (1979). The Multidimensional-Multiattributional Causality Scale: The Development of a Goal-Specific Locus of Control Scale. *Canadian Journal of Behavioral Science, 11,* 286–304.

Powers, S., et al. (1985). Applicability and validity investigation of the Multidimensional-Multiattributional Causality Scale. *Educational and Psychological Measurement, 45*(4), 897–901.

3254

Test Name: NONSEXIST PERSONAL ATTRIBUTE INVENTORY FOR CHILDREN

Purpose: To measure self-concept.

Number of Items: 32

Format: Subjects indicate which 10 words on a list best describe them. All items are presented.

Reliability: Test–retest correlations ranged from .35 to .74 (Ns = 29 to 272).

Validity: Correlations with Piers-Harris Children's Self-Concept scale ranged from .29 to .72 (Ns = 31 to 297).

Author: Parish, T. S., and Rankin, C. I.

Article: The Nonsexist Personal Attribute Inventory for Children: A report on its validity and reliability as a self-concept scale.

Journal: *Educational and Psychological Measurement*, Spring 1982, *42*(1), 339–343.

■ ■ ■

3255

Test Name: NOWICKI-STRICKLAND INTERNAL–EXTERNAL CONTROL SCALE FOR ADULTS

Purpose: To measure locus of control with simpler language than Rotter's scale.

Number of Items: 40

Format: Yes–no.

Reliability: Alpha was .69.

Validity: Correlated from .48 to .68 with Rotter's scale among college students.

Author: Tiggemann, M., and Winefield, A. H.

Article: The effects of unemployment on the mood, self-esteem, locus of control and depressive affect of school-leavers.

Journal: *Journal of Occupational Psychology*, March 1984, *57*(1), 33–42.

Related Research: Nowicki, S., & Duke, M. P. (1974). A locus of control scale for non-college as well as college adults. *Journal of Personality Assessment, 38*, 136–137.

■ ■ ■

3256

Test Name: OCCUPATIONAL SELF-EFFICACY SCALE

Purpose: To measure occupational self-efficacy.

Number of Items: 68 (4 items each for 17 different occupations).

Format: Items rated on 7-point Likert response categories. All items are presented.

Reliability: Test–retest ranged from .73 to .77.

Author: Wheeler, K. G.

Article: Comparisons of self-efficacy and expectancy models of occupational preferences for college males and females.

Journal: *Journal of Occupational Psychology*, March 1983, *56*(1), 73–78.

Related Research: Hackett, G., & Betz, N. E. (1981). A self-efficacy approach to the career development of women. *Journal of Vocational Behavior, 18*, 326–339.

■ ■ ■

3257

Test Name: ORIENTATION TO LITERACY TEST

Purpose: To measure the child's understanding of the purpose of literacy.

Number of Items: 10 sets of four drawings.

Format: Child instructed to point to correct response in drawings.

Reliability: Cronbach internal consistency was .717.

Author: Mayfield, M.

Article: Code systems instruction and kindergarten children's perception of the nature and purpose of reading.

Journal: *Journal of Educational Research*, January/February 1983, *76*(3), 161–168.

Related Research: Evanechko, P., et al. (1973). An investigation of the reading readiness domain. *Research in the Teaching of English, 7*, 61–78.

■ ■ ■

3258

Test Name: PAY EXPECTATION SCALE

Purpose: To measure pay expectation in other employment situations.

Number of Items: 5

Format: High scores reflect stronger expectations of earning higher pay by taking other employment.

Reliability: Cronbach's alpha was .78.

Validity: Correlations with other variables ranged from –.39 to .02.

Author: Motowidlo, S. J.

Article: Predicting sales turnover from pay satisfaction and expectation.

Journal: *Journal of Applied Psychology*, August 1983, *68*(3), 484–489.

■ ■ ■

3259

Test Name: PEER ROLE-TAKING QUESTIONNAIRE

Purpose: To serve as a measure of role-taking.

Number of Items: 10

Format: The subject names one person from the group who is most like each of the 10 presented descriptions. All items are presented.

Reliability: Intraclass correlations representing reliability ratings ranged from .85 to .99.

Validity: Spearman correlation with the Role-Taking Task was .22.

Author: Moser, R. S.

Article: The measurement of role taking in young adults.

Journal: *Journal of Personality Assessment*, August 1984, *48*(4), 380–387.

• • •

3260

Test Name: PERCEIVED COMPETENCE SCALE FOR CHILDREN

Purpose: To measure children's self-perception of competence.

Number of Items: 28

Format: Includes three domains of perceived competence: cognitive, social, and physical as well as children's general self-esteem.

Reliability: Coefficient alphas ranged from .54 to .78.

Author: Stigler, J. W., et al.

Article: The self-perception of competence by Chinese children.

Journal: *Child Development*, October 1985, *56*(5), 1259–1270.

Related Research: Harter, S. (1982). The Perceived Competence Scale for Children. *Child Development*, *53*, 87–97.

Horn, T. S. Coaches' feedback and changes in children's perceptions of their physical competence. *Journal of Educational Psychology*, *77*(2), 174–186.

3261

Test Name: PERCEIVED CONFIRMATION SCALE

Purpose: To determine the degree to which the respondent perceives the partner to have confirmed and supported the respondent's identity in the interaction.

Number of Items: 6

Format: The items are global judgment items.

Reliability: Coefficient alpha was .82 and .69.

Validity: Correlation with rating of altercompetence was .71.

Author: Spitzberg, B. H., and Cupach, W. R.

Article: Conversational skill and locus of perception.

Journal: *Journal of Psychopathology and Behavioral Assessment*, September 1985, *7*(3), 207–220.

Related Research: Cissna, K. N. (1976). *Interpersonal confirmation: A review of current theory, measurement and research* (ED 126 544). Paper presented at the Central States Speech Association Convention, Chicago.

• • •

3262

Test Name: PERCEIVED PARTICIPATION SCALE

Purpose: To measure perceptions faculty have of decision-making at their colleges.

Number of Items: 3

Format: Multiple-choice. All items are presented.

Reliability: Alpha was .76.

Validity: Correlated .68 (*p* < .05) with distribution of control in colleges.

Author: Peterson, M. F., and Cook, R. A.

Article: Attitudinal and contextual variables explaining teachers' leadership behavior.

Journal: *Journal of Educational Psychology*, February 1983, *71*(1), 50–62.

• • •

3263

Test Name: PERCEIVED SOMATATYPE SCALE

Purpose: To measure perceived somatatype.

Number of Items: 7 male figures, 2 questions per figure.

Format: Subject selects which figure best resembles his own body-build and the figure that best appears to be what he would like to be.

Reliability: Test–retest ranged from .94 to .96 over 2 weeks.

Validity: Significant associations between somatatype and Body Cathexis Scale (Secord & Jourard).

Author: Tucker, L. A.

Article: Relationship between perceived somatatype and body cathexis of college males.

Journal: *Psychological Reports*, 1982, *50*(3, Part 1), 983–989.

Related Research: Secord, P. F., & Jourard, S. M. (1953). The appraisal of body-cathexis: Body-cathexis and the self. *Journal of Consulting Psychology*, *17*, 343–347.

• • •

3264

Test Name: PERCEIVED UNDERSTANDING SCALE

Purpose: To measure perception of being understood or misunderstood.

Number of Items: 16

Format: Items rated on a 5-point scale.

Reliability: Test–retest reliability was .90. Cronbach's alpha was .89.

Author: Cahn, D. D.

Article: Relative importance of perceived understanding in initial interaction and development of interpersonal relationships.

Journal: *Psychological Reports,* June 1983, *52*(3), 923–929.

Related Research: Cahn, D. D., & Shulman, G. M. (1982). *Measurement of the perception of being understood/misunderstood: Development and assessment.* Paper presented at the annual meeting of the Central States Speech Association, Milwaukee, WI.

• • •

3265

Test Name: PERCEPTION OF CHILD PSYCHOLOGIST QUESTIONNAIRE

Purpose: To measure perception of child psychologists held by parents.

Number of Items: 7

Format: Seven problem situations are presented to respondents who then choose one of nine professional occupations that might help. Child psychology is one of the nine. All problems are presented.

Reliability: Test–retest yielded 85% agreement (over 8 weeks, $N = 18$).

Author: Murphy, G. C., et al.

Article: Perceptions of child psychologists held by parents of Australian school children.

Journal: *Psychological Reports,* 1982, *51*(1), 47–51.

Related Research: Murphy, G. C., et al. (1978). Client perceptions of professional helpers. *Australian Journal of Social Issues, 13,* 207–215.

• • •

3266

Test Name: PERCEPTUAL ABERRATION SCALE

Purpose: To measure transient aberrations in perception.

Number of Items: 35

Format: True–false. Sample items presented.

Reliability: Alpha ranged from .88 to .90.

Validity: Correlated .70 to Perceptual Aberration (Chapman et al., 1981).

Author: Chapman, L. J., et al.

Article: Reliabilities and intercorrelations of eight measures of proneness to psychosis.

Journal: *Journal of Consulting and Clinical Psychology,* April 1982, *50*(2), 187–195.

Related Research: Chapman, L. J., et al. (1978). Body-image aberration in schizophrenia. *Journal of Abnormal Psychology, 87,* 399–407.

• • •

3267

Test Name: PERFORMANCE EXPECTANCY SCALE

Purpose: To measure perceptions of performance and expectancy on the job.

Number of Items: 8

Format: Likert format. All items presented.

Reliability: Alpha was .86.

Author: Lee, C., and Schuler, R. S.

Article: A constructive replication and extension of a role and expectancy perception model of participation decision making.

Journal: *Journal of Occupational Psychology,* June 1982, *55*(2), 109–118.

Related Research: House, R. J., & Dessler, J. (1974). The path-goal theory of leadership: Some post hoc and a priori tests. In J. G. Hunt & L. L. Larson (Eds.), *Contingency approaches to leadership.* Carbondale: Southern Illinois Press.

• • •

3268

Test Name: PERFORMANCE SELF-ATTRIBUTION SCALE

Purpose: To measure attributions a child makes about his or her task performance.

Number of Items: 20

Format: Number of statements circled as descriptive of child's own behavior are summed to yield a total score on each of four subscales. All statements are presented.

Validity: Three independent judges classified states into four categories with 90% agreement.

Author: Ames, C.

Article: Achievement attributions and self-instructions under competitive and individualistic goal structures.

Journal: *Journal of Educational Psychology,* June 1984, *76*(3), 478–487.

Related Research: Diener, C., & Dweck, C. (1978). An analysis of learned helplessness: Continuous changes in performance, strategy and achievement cognitions following failure. *Journal of Personality and Social Psychology, 36,* 451–462.

3269

Test Name: PERSONAL ATTRIBUTE INVENTORY

Purpose: To identify 30 adjectives that subjects believe are most descriptive of a target group.

Number of Items: 100 adjectives.

Format: Half of the adjectives are positive and half are negative.

Reliability: Test–retest reliabilities ranged from .90 to .95.

Author: Eberly, C., et al.

Article: Mental health professionals' attitudes toward physically handicapped groups in attributionally ambiguous and non-ambiguous situations.

Journal: *Journal of Counseling Psychology*, May 1981, *28*(3), 276–278.

Related Research: Parish, T. S., et al. (1976). The personal attribute inventory. *Perceptual and Motor Skills, 42,* 715–720.

■ ■ ■

3270

Test Name: PERSONAL ATTRIBUTE INVENTORY FOR CHILDREN

Purpose: To measure children's perceptions of self.

Number of Items: 48

Format: Contains positive and negative descriptors from which the children choose 15 that best describe themselves.

Validity: Correlations with: Behavior Rating Profile, Student Scales ranged from .28 to .48 (Ns = 276 to 628); State-Trait Anxiety Inventory for Children ranged from –.44 to –.56 (Ns = 279 to 631).

Author: Nunn, G. D., et al.

Article: Concurrent validity of the Personal Attribute Inventory for Children with the State-Trait Anxiety Inventory for Children

and the Behavior Rating Profile Student Scales.

Journal: *Educational and Psychological Measurement,* Summer 1983, *43*(2), 639–641.

Related Research: Parish, T., & Taylor, J. (1978). The Personal Attribute Inventory for Children: A report on its reliability and validity as a self-concept scale. *Educational and Psychological Measurement,* 1978, *38,* 565–569.

■ ■ ■

3271

Test Name: PERSONAL ATTRIBUTES QUESTIONNAIRE

Purpose: To measure sexual identity.

Number of Items: 24

Format: Items rated on a 5-point continuum bounded by extreme adjective pairs. Sample items presented.

Reliability: Alpha was .79 (masculinity) and .84 (femininity).

Author: Hirschman, E. C.

Article: Sexual identity and the acquisition of rational, absorbing, escapist and modeling experiences.

Journal: *Journal of Social Psychology,* February 1985, *125*(1), 63–73.

Related Research: Spence, J. T., et al. (1975). Ratings of self and peers on sex-role attributes. *Journal of Personality and Social Psychology, 32,* 19–39.

Arnold, S. T. (1981). Attitudes of counselors-in-training toward career goals of a male client. *Vocational Guidance Quarterly, 29*(3), 221–228.

■ ■ ■

3272

Test Name: PERSONAL CONTROL SCALE

Purpose: To measure extent to which respondents believe luck or personal control shapes events.

Number of Items: 5

Format: Forced-choice paired statements.

Reliability: .52.

Author: Begley, T. M., and Alker, H.

Article: Anti-busing protest: Attitudes and actions.

Journal: *Social Psychology Quarterly,* December 1983, *45*(4), 187–197.

Related Research: Forward, J. P., & Williams, J. R. (1970). Internal–external control and Black militancy. *Journal of Social Issues, 26,* 75–93.

■ ■ ■

3273

Test Name: PERSONAL DYNAMICS PROFILES

Purpose: To measure major aspects of self-perception.

Number of Items: 60

Format: Subjects respond to each adjective on a 5-point Likert scale.

Reliability: Ranged from .704 to .938.

Validity: Predictive validity ranged from .498 to .627.

Author: Mann, J., and Houston, S.

Article: Profile of women managers.

Journal: *Colorado Journal of Educational Research,* Spring 1981, *20*(3), 5–6.

Related Research: Houston, S. R., & Solomon, D. (1978). *Personal Dynamics Profiles Occupational Survey* (Research Methodology Monographs No. 4), University of Northern Colorado.

3274

Test Name: PERSONAL REACTION SCALE

Purpose: To measure locus of control perceptions of college and non-college adults.

Number of Items: 41

Format: Includes six factors: fate, social self, personal self, self-determination, luck, and powerlessness. All items are presented.

Reliability: Spearman-Brown reliability estimates for each factor ranged from .39 to .84.

Author: Galejs, I., et al.

Article: Personal reaction scale for college and non-college adults: Its development and factorial validity.

Journal: *Educational and Psychological Measurement,* Summer 1984, *44*(2), 383–393.

Related Research: Nowicki, S., & Duke, M. P. (1974). A locus of control scale for non-college as well as college adults. *Journal of Personality Assessment, 36,* 136–137.

■ ■ ■

3275

Test Name: PHYSICAL ATTRACTIVENESS SCALE

Purpose: To measure peoples' perception of their own attractiveness.

Number of Items: 24

Format: Items rated on 5-point Likert response categories.

Reliability: Internal consistency ratings were .88 and .90.

Author: Starr, P.

Article: Physical attractiveness and self-esteem ratings of young adults with cleft lip and/or palate.

Journal: *Psychological Reports,* 1982, *50*(2), 467–470.

Related Research: Lerner R. M., et al. (1973). Relations among Physical attractiveness, body attitudes and self-conception in male and female college students. *Journal of Psychology, 85,* 119–129.

■ ■ ■

3276

Test Name: PIERS-HARRIS SELF-CONCEPT SCALE

Purpose: To measure pupil self-esteem.

Number of Items: 80

Time Required: 15–20 minutes.

Format: True–false self-descriptive statements.

Reliability: Internal consistency was .93. Test–retest reliability was .71.

Author: Fox, R., et al.

Article: Student evaluation of teacher as a measure of teacher behavior and teacher impact on students.

Journal: *Journal of Educational Research,* September/October 1983, *77*(1), 16–21.

Related Research: Piers, E. V., & Harris, D. B. (1964). Age and other correlates of self-concept in children. *Journal of Educational Psychology, 55,* 91–95.

■ ■ ■

3277

Test Name: PORTER NEEDS SATISFACTION QUESTIONNAIRE—REVISED

Purpose: To assess the level of need deficiencies perceived by educators in five need categories.

Number of Items: 13

Format: Includes five subscales:

security, social interaction, esteem, autonomy, and self-actualization. A 7-point rating scale is used ranging from 1 (*minimum*) to 7 (*maximum*). All items are presented.

Reliability: Cronbach's alpha reliability coefficients were .89 (Factor I) and .46 (Factor II).

Author: Pierson, D., et al.

Article: A cross validation of the Porter Needs Satisfaction Questionnaire for Educators.

Journal: *Educational and Psychological Measurement,* Autumn 1985, *45*(3), 683–688.

Related Research: Trusty, F., & Sergiovanni, T. (1966). Perceived need deficiencies of teachers and administrators: A proposal for restructuring teacher roles. *Educational Administration Quarterly, 2,* 168–180.

■ ■ ■

3278

Test Name: PRIMARY PICTORIAL SELF-ESTEEM TEST

Purpose: To measure general or global academic self-esteem.

Number of Items: 26

Format: Each item consists of a statement read to the examinee who selects one of three pictures of faces perceived as reflecting the respondent's feeling relative to the statement read.

Reliability: Test–retest reliability ranged from .58 to .64

Validity: Correlations with CIRCUS ranged from .00 to .24 (*N* ranged from 69 to 74).

Author: Snyder, S. C., and Michael, W. B.

Article: The relationship of performance on standardized tests in mathematics and reading to two measures of social intelligence and one of academic self-esteem for two samples of primary school children.

Journal: *Educational and Psychological Measurement,* Winter 1983, *43*(4), 1141–1148.

Related Research: Kirkwood, W. J. (1978). *The development and validation of the Primary Pictorial Self-Esteem Test: Intellectual development.* Unpublished manual. Downey, CA: Downey Unified School District.

■ ■ ■

3279

Test Name: PRIMARY SELF-CONCEPT INVENTORY

Purpose: To measure self-concept.

Number of Items: 18

Format: Child is told a story about a picture and is asked to circle the person in the picture most like himself or herself.

Reliability: Test–retest ranged from .51 to .91.

Author: Summerlin, M. L., et al.

Article: The effect of magic circle participation on a child's self-concept.

Journal: *The School Counselor,* September 1983, *31*(1), 49–52.

Related Research: Muller, D. G., & Leonetti, R. (1974). *Primary self-concept inventory test manual.* Austin, TX: Learning Concepts.

■ ■ ■

3280

Test Name: PROBLEM-SOLVING INVENTORY

Purpose: To assess people's perceptions of their personal problem-solving behaviors and attitudes.

Number of Items: 32

Format: Employs a 6-point Likert scale. Low scores reflect effective problem-solving.

Reliability: Internal consistency ranged from .72 to .90 (*N* = 140). Test–retest (2 weeks) ranged from .83 to .89 (*N* = 31).

Validity: Correlations with vocational identity ranged from –.18 to –.40.

Author: Heppner, P. P., and Krieschok, T. S.

Article: An applied investigation of problem-solving appraisal, vocational identity, and career service requests, utilization, and subsequent evaluations.

Journal: *Vocational Guidance Quarterly,* June 1983, *31*(4), 240–249.

Related Research: Heppner, P. P., & Petersen, C. H. (1982). The development and implications of a personal problem-solving inventory. *Journal of Counseling Psychology, 29,* 66–75.

■ ■ ■

3281

Test Name: PROCRASTINATION INVENTORY

Purpose: To measure beliefs regarding the causes of procrastination and the likelihood of changing those causes.

Number of Items: 40

Format: Includes 4 scales: controllability, justification, motivation to change, and expectation to change. Responses to each item are made on a 7-point scale ranging from *true* to *false*.

Reliability: Test–retest reliabilities ranged from .73 to .83. Internal consistency reliabilities ranged from .37 to .84.

Author: Claiborn, C. D., et al.

Article: Effects of congruence

between counselor interpretations and client beliefs.

Journal: *Journal of Counseling Psychology,* March 1981, 28(2), 101–109.

Related Research: Strong, S. R., et al. (1979). Motivational and equipping functions of interpretation in counseling. *Journal of Counseling Psychology, 26,* 98–107.

■ ■ ■

3282

Test Name: PUPIL CONTROL IDEOLOGY SCALE

Purpose: To measure a respondent's pupil control orientation on a humanistic-custodial continuum.

Number of Items: 20

Format: Employs a Likert scale from 5 (*strongly agree*) to 1 (*strongly disagree*).

Reliability: Split-half Spearman-Brown corrected coefficients were .95 (*N* = 170) and .91 (*N* = 55).

Author: Graham, S., et al.

Article: A factor analysis of the pupil control ideology scale.

Journal: *Journal of Experimental Education,* Summer 1985, *53*(4), 202–206.

Related Research: Willower, D. J., et al. (1967/1973). *The school and pupil control ideology* (The Pennsylvania State University Studies, No. 24). University Park: The Pennsylvania State University.

Halpin, G., et al. (1982). Personality characteristics and self-concept of preservice teachers related to their pupil control orientation. *Journal of Experimental Education, 50*(4), 195–199.

3283

Test Name: PUPIL CONTROL IDEOLOGY SCALE—REVISED

Purpose: To measure a respondent's pupil control orientation on a humanistic-custodial continuum.

Number of Items: 10

Format: Responses are made on a 5-point Likert scale ranging from 5 (*strongly agree*) to 1 (*strongly disagree*). All items are presented.

Reliability: Coefficient alpha was .71.

Author: Graham, S., et al.

Article: An analysis of the dimensionality of the Pupil Control Ideology Scale.

Journal: *Educational and Psychological Measurement,* Winter 1985, *45*(4), 889–896.

Related Research: Graham, S., et al. (1985). A factor analysis of the Pupil Control Ideology Scale. *Journal of Experimental Education, 53,* 202–206.

■ ■ ■

3284

Test Name: RATIONAL BEHAVIOR INVENTORY

Purpose: To assess irrational beliefs.

Number of Items: 37

Format: Items rated on a 5-point scale (*agree–disagree*).

Reliability: Test–retest ranged from .71 to .82 (3 and 10-day intervals). Split-half reliability was .73.

Author: Ray, J. B., and Friedlander, R. B.

Article: Changes in rational beliefs among treated alcoholics.

Journal: *Psychological Reports,* December 1984, *55*(3), 883–886.

Related Research: Sharkey, C. T., & Sutton-Simon, K. (1983). Reliability and validity of the rational behavior inventory with a clinical population. *Journal of Clinical Psychology, 39,* 34–38.

■ ■ ■

3285

Test Name: REFLECTIONS OF SELF AND ENVIRONMENT

Purpose: To measure self-actualization.

Number of Items: 80

Format: Responses are recorded on a 5-point rating scale from 1 (*no*) to 5 (*definitely*). Some items are presented.

Reliability: Hoyt internal consistency coefficient was .90 ($N = $ 31 men) and .94 ($N = 85$ women).

Validity: Correlations with other variables ranged from .14 to .73.

Author: Buckmaster, L. R., and Davis, G. A.

Article: ROSE: A measure of self-actualization and its relationship to creativity.

Journal: *Journal of Creative Behavior,* 1985, *19*(1), 30–37.

■ ■ ■

3286

Test Name: REFLECTIONS OF SELF BY YOUTH

Purpose: To measure self-actualizing growth in preadolescents.

Number of Items: 62

Format: Includes two factors: feelings and perceptions of self. All items are presented.

Reliability: Test–retest Pearson product–moment correlation was .84.

Author: Schatz, E. M., and Buckmaster, L. R.

Article: Development of an instrument to measure self-actualizing growth in preadolescents.

Journal: *Journal of Creative Behavior,* 1984, *18*(4), 263–272.

Related Research: Buckmaster, L. R. (1980). *Development of an instrument to measure self-actualization and an investigation into the relationship between self-actualization and creativity.* Unpublished master's thesis, University of Wisconsin.

■ ■ ■

3287

Test Name: RELATIONSHIP BELIEF INVENTORY

Purpose: To assess irrational beliefs about self.

Number of Items: 40

Format: Items rated on a 6-point *strongly true* to *strongly false* scale. Sample items are presented.

Reliability: Alpha ranged from .72 to .81 across 5 subscales.

Validity: All subscales correlated positively with the Irrational Beliefs Test ($rs = .11$ to .31, $N = 200$, $p < .05$). All subscales correlated negatively with Locke-Wallace Marital Adjustment Scale ($rs = -.18$ to $-.38$, $N = 200$, $p < .05$).

Author: Eidelson, R. J., and Epstein, N.

Article: Cognition and relationship maladjustment: Development of a measure of dysfunctional relationship beliefs.

Journal: *Journal of Consulting and Clinical Psychology,* October 1982, *50*(5), 715–720.

■ ■ ■

3288

Test Name: ROLE AMBIGUITY SCALE

Purpose: To measure clarity of responsibilities, authority, and expectations of supervisor for jobs.

Number of Items: 6

Format: Items rated in 5-point Likert format.

Reliability: Alpha was .79.

Author: Ashford, S. J., and Cummings, L. L.

Article: Proactive feedback seeking: The instrumental use of the information environment.

Journal: *Journal of Occupational Psychology*, March 1985, *58*(1), 67–79.

Related Research: Rizzo, J. R., et al. (1970). Role conflict and ambiguity in complex organizations. *Administrative Science Quarterly, 15,* 150–163.

Bedeian, A. G., et al. (1981). The relationship between role stress and job-related, interpersonal, and organizational climate factors. *Journal of Social Psychology, 113*(second half), 247–260.

■ ■ ■

3289

Test Name: ROLE CONFLICT SCALE

Purpose: To measure role conflict of nursing staff.

Number of Items: 8

Format: A 5-point response scale from *very false* to *very true* was used.

Reliability: Alpha was .89.

Validity: Zero-order correlations with variables ranged from –.48 to .69.

Author: Bedeian, A. G., et al.

Article: The relationship between role stress and job-related interpersonal and organizational climate factors.

Journal: *Journal of Social Psychology,* April 1981, *113*(second half), 247–260.

Related Research: Rizzo, J. R., et al. (1970). Role conflict and ambiguity in complex organizations. *Administrative Science Quarterly, 15,* 150–163.

■ ■ ■

3290

Test Name: ROLE CONFLICT AND AMBIGUITY SCALE

Purpose: To measure role conflict and role ambiguity.

Number of Items: 14

Format: Includes 8 conflict items and 6 ambiguity items. Responses are made on a 5-point scale ranging from *always* to *never.* Examples are given.

Reliability: Reliabilities ranged from .78 to .82.

Validity: Correlations with other variables ranged from –.07 to .45.

Author: Eisenhauer, J. E., et al.

Article: Role conflict, role ambiguity and school principals' job robustness.

Journal: *Journal of Experimental Education,* Winter 1984/1985, *53*(2), 86–90.

Related Research: Rizzo, J. R., et al. (1970). Role conflict and ambiguity in complex organizations. *Administrative Science Quarterly, 15,* 150–163.

House, R. J., et al. (1983). Role conflict and ambiguity scales: Reality or artifacts? *Journal of Applied Psychology, 68*(2), 334–337.

Rosenkrantz, S. A., et al. (1983). Role conflict and ambiguity scales: An evaluation of psychometric properties and the role of social desirability response bias. *Educational and Psychological Measurement, 43*(4), 957–970.

3291

Test Name: ROLE EXPECTATIONS SCALE

Purpose: To measure managers' business view, management style, relationships to subordinates, and technical orientation.

Number of Items: 15

Format: Items rated on 5-point importance scales. All items are presented.

Reliability: Alphas ranged from .74 to .84 across subgroups.

Validity: Four factors can be extracted from the 15 items but median reliability of the resulting subscales is only .58.

Author: Berger-Gross, V., and Kraut, A. I.

Article: Great expectations: A no-conflict explanation of role conflict.

Journal: *Journal of Applied Psychology,* May 1984, *69*(2), 261–271.

■ ■ ■

3292

Test Name: ROLE QUESTIONNAIRE

Purpose: To assess one's perceived level of role conflict and role ambiguity.

Number of Items: 14

Format: Includes two factors: role conflict and role ambiguity. All items are presented.

Reliability: Reliability coefficients ranged from .78 to .86.

Author: Schwab, R. L., et al.

Article: Assessing role conflict and role ambiguity: A cross validation study.

Journal: *Educational and Psychological Measurement,* Summer 1983, *43*(2), 587–593.

Related Research: Rizzo, J. R., et al. (1970). Role conflict and ambiguity in complex organizations. *Administrative Science Quarterly, 15,* 150–163.

■ ■ ■

3293

Test Name: ROSENBERG SELF-ESTEEM SCALE

Purpose: To provide a global measure of self-esteem.

Number of Items: 10

Format: Each item is rated on a 4-point Likert scale ranging from *strongly agree* (1) to *strongly disagree* (4).

Reliability: Test–retest (2 weeks) reliability was .85. Coefficient alpha was .75.

Author: Robbins, S. B.

Article: Validity estimates for the Career Decision-Making Self-Efficacy Scale.

Journal: *Measurement and Evaluation in Counseling and Development,* July 1985, *18*(2), 64–71.

Related Research: Rosenberg, M. (1979). *Conceiving the self.* New York: Basic Books.

Stafford, I. P. (1984). Relation of attitudes toward women's roles and occupational behavior to women's self-esteem. *Journal of Counseling Psychology, 31*(3), 332–338.

■ ■ ■

3294

Test Name: RRF ANDRO SCALES

Purpose: To measure sex-role identity and self-esteem.

Number of Items: 85

Format: Includes scales measuring: masculinity, femininity, and self-esteem.

Reliability: Coefficient alphas ranged from .65 to .79.

Validity: Correlations with Scales for Investigation of the Dual-Career Family—Revised ranged from −.38 to .43.

Author: Gaddy, C. D., et al.

Article: A study of the Scales for Investigation of the Dual-Career Family.

Journal: *Measurement and Evaluation in Counseling and Development,* October 1985, *18*(3), 120–127.

Related Research: Berzins, J. I., et al. (1978). A new measure of psychological androgyny based on the Personality Research Form. *Journal of Consulting and Clinical Psychology, 46,* 126–138.

■ ■ ■

3295

Test Name: SCALE OF SELF-ESTEEM

Purpose: To measure self-esteem.

Format: Responses were made on a 5-point scale from *strongly agree* (1) to *strongly disagree* (5).

Reliability: Alpha reliability was .81.

Validity: Correlations with other variables ranged from .20 to .43.

Author: Keith, P. M.

Article: Sex-role attitudes, family plans, and career orientations: Implications for counseling.

Journal: *Vocational Guidance Quarterly,* March 1981, *29*(3) 244–252.

Related Research: Rosenberg, M. (1965). *Society and the adolescent self-image.* Princeton, NJ: Princeton University Press.

■ ■ ■

3296

Test Name: SELF-ACCEPTANCE SCALE

Purpose: To measure self-esteem.

Number of Items: 36

Format: Responses were made on a 5-point continuum.

Reliability: Alpha reliability estimate was .89.

Validity: Correlations with Interpersonal Jealousy Scale ranged from −.34 to −.40.

Author: Stewart, R. A., and Beatty, M. J.

Article: Jealousy and self-esteem.

Journal: *Perceptual and Motor Skills,* February 1985, *60*(1), 153–154.

Related Research: Berger, E. M. (1952). The relation between expressed acceptance of self and expressed acceptance of others. *Journal of Abnormal and Social Psychology, 47,* 778–782.

■ ■ ■

3297

Test Name: SELF-CONCEPT AND MOTIVATION INVENTORY (SCAMIN)

Purpose: To measure motivation and self-concept.

Number of Items: 24

Format: Items read to children who then circle their choice of a face pictured on an answer sheet.

Reliability: Test–retest reliability was .77 (elementary form).

Author: Soule, J. C., et al.

Article: Dimensions of self-concept for children in kindergarten and grades 1 and 2.

Journal: *Psychological Reports,* February 1981, *48*(1), 83–88.

Related Research: Farrah, G. A., et al. (1968). *Self-concept and motivation inventory: What face you wear.* Dearborn Heights, MI: Person-O-Metrics.

3298

Test Name: SELF-CONCEPT APPRAISAL SCALES

Purpose: To measure self-concept, appraisal of spouses' self-concept and perceived appraisal by spouse.

Number of Items: 21

Format: Semantic differential. All adjective-pairs presented.

Reliability: Alpha ranged between .78 and .82.

Author: Schafer, R. B.

Article: Equity/inequity and self-concept: An interactionist analysis.

Journal: *Social Psychology Quarterly,* March 1984, *47*(1), 42–49.

Related Research: Sherwood, J. J. (1962). *Self-identity and self-actualization: A theory and research.* Unpublished doctoral dissertation, University of Michigan.

■ ■ ■

3299

Test Name: SELF-CONCEPT AS A LEARNER SCALE

Purpose: To measure one's self-concept as a learner in the school context.

Number of Items: 50

Format: Includes four subscales: motivation, task orientation, problem-solving or intellectual ability, and class membership.

Reliability: Test–retest reliability for the total score ranged from .79 to .90 (time between testing ranged from 7 days to 3 months). Coefficient alphas ranged from .88 to .91.

Author: Baldauf, R. B., Jr., et al.

Article: The reliability and factorial validity of the Self Concept as a Learner (SCAL) measure for year seven students in Australia.

Journal: *Educational and Psychological Measurement,* Autumn 1985, *45*(3), 655–659.

Related Research: Waetjen, W. (1972). *Procedure for the analysis of the self-concept as a learner scale* (mimeo, 5 pages).

Lunenburg, F. C. (1983). Pupil control ideology and self-concept as a learner. *Educational Research Quarterly, 8*(3), 33–39.

■ ■ ■

3300

Test Name: SELF-CONCEPT MEASURE

Purpose: To measure self-concept of college students.

Number of Items: 4

Format: Responses to each item are made on a 5-point scale ranging from 1 (*strongly agree*) to 5 (*strongly disagree*).

Reliability: Coefficient alphas ranged from .66 to .79.

Author: Behuniak, P., Jr., and Gable, R. K.

Article: A longitudinal study of self-concept and locus of control for persisters in six college majors.

Journal: *Educational Research Quarterly,* Spring 1981, *6*(1), 3–12.

Related Research: Conger, A. S., et al. (1977). *National longitudinal study of high school seniors: Group profiles on self-esteem, locus of control, and life goals* (NCES 77-260). Washington, DC: U.S. Department of Health, Education and Welfare.

■ ■ ■

3301

Test Name: SELF-CONCEPT OF ABILITY SCALE

Purpose: To measure academic self-concept.

Number of Items: 8

Format: Employs a 5-point Likert scale. Students rate present school ability on five items and they rate their future academic ability on three items.

Reliability: Test–retest reliability coefficients (1 year) ranged from .69 to .77.

Author: Byrne, B. M.

Article: Investigating measures of self-concept.

Journal: *Measurement and Evaluation in Guidance,* October 1983, *16*(3), 115–126.

Related Research: Brookover, W. B., et al. (Eds). (1967). *Self-concept of ability and school achievement III: Relationship of self-concept to achievement in high school* (Educational Research series No. 36). East Lansing, MI: Educational Publication Services.

■ ■ ■

3302

Test Name: SELF-CONSCIOUSNESS SCALE

Purpose: To measure self-consciousness.

Number of Items: 23

Format: Subjects respond to each item on a 5-point scale from 0 (*extremely uncharacteristic*) to 4 (*extremely characteristic*) as to how well each item describes them. Includes three scales: private self-consciousness, public self-consciousness, and social anxiety. Examples are presented.

Reliability: Cronbach's alphas ranged from .56 to .84.

Validity: Correlations with loneliness scores ranged from −.18 to .38.

Author: Schmitt, J. P., and Kurdek, L. A.

Article: Age and gender differences in and personality correlates of loneliness in different relationships.

Journal: *Journal of Personality Assessment,* October 1985, *49*(5), 485–496.

Related Research: Fenigstein, A., et al. (1975). Public and private self-consciousness: Assessment and theory. *Journal of Consulting and Clinical Psychology, 43,* 522–527.

Vleeming, R. G., & Engelse, J. A. (Assessment of private and public self-consciousness: A Dutch replication). *Journal of Personality Assessment, 45*(4), 385–389.

■ ■ ■

3303

Test Name: SELF-DESCRIPTION QUESTIONNAIRE

Purpose: To measure academic and non-academic self-concept.

Number of Items: 72

Format: Items rated on a 5-point response scale from 1 (*true*) to 5 (*false*).

Reliability: Alpha ranged from .65 to .95 across subscales and grade level.

Author: Marsh, H. W., et al.

Article: Self-descriptive questionnaire: Age–sex effects in the structure and level of self-concept for preadolescent children.

Journal: *Journal of Educational Psychology,* October 1984, *76*(5), 940–956.

Related Research: Marsh, H. W., et al. (1983). Preadolescent self-concept: Its relation to self-concept as inferred by teachers and to academic ability. *British Journal of Educational Psychology, 53,* 60–78.

Marsh, H. W., et al. (1983). Self-

concept, reliability, stability, dimensionality, validity, and the measurement of change. *Journal of Educational Psychology, 75*(5), 772–790.

■ ■ ■

3304

Test Name: SELF-DESCRIPTION QUESTIONNAIRE

Purpose: To measure student self-concept (preadolescent).

Number of Items: 56

Format: Multiple-choice and rating scales. Sample item descriptions presented.

Reliability: Alpha ranged from .80s to .90s over subscales.

Author: Marsh, H. W., et al.

Article: The relationship between dimensions of self-attribution and dimensions of self-concept.

Journal: *Journal of Educational Psychology,* February 1984, *76*(1), 3–32.

Related Research: Marsh, H. W., et al. (1983). Preadolescent self-concept: Its relation to self-concept as inferred by teachers and to academic ability. *British Journal of Occupational Psychology, 53,* 60–78.

■ ■ ■

3305

Test Name: SELF-DESCRIPTION QUESTIONNAIRE III

Purpose: To measure university-aged respondents' self-concept.

Number of Items: 136

Format: Includes 13 factors: mathematics, verbal, academic, problem-solving/creativity, physical abilities/sports, physical appearance, relations with same-sex peers, relations with opposite-sex peers, relations with parents, religion/spirituality, honesty/reliability, emotional stability/

security, general self-concept. Students respond to each item on an 8-point scale from 1 (*definitely false*) to 8 (*definitely true*). All items are presented.

Reliability: Coefficient alphas ranged from .75 to .95.

Validity: Correlations with other criteria ranged from –.24 to .61.

Author: Marsh, H. W., and O'Neill, R.

Article: Self-Description Questionnaire III: The construct validity of multidimensional self-concept ratings by late adolescents.

Journal: *Journal of Educational Measurement,* Summer 1984, *21*(2), 153–174.

Related Research: Marsh, H. W., et al. (1983). Multitrait–multimethod analyses of the Self-Description Questionnaire: Student–teacher agreement on multidimensional ratings of student self-concept. *American Educational Research Journal, 20,* 333–357.

■ ■ ■

3306

Test Name: SELF-EFFICACY MEASURES

Purpose: To measure four aspects of self-efficacy with respect to science and engineering field achievement.

Number of Items: 15

Format: Subjects indicate whether they believe they could successfully complete the educational requirements of and job duties performed in 15 science and engineering fields. Subjects indicate their degree of confidence and their ability to complete the educational requirements and job duties. A 10-point scale was employed to indicate strength of confidence.

Reliability: Test–retest correlations for the four efficacy scales (8 week interval) ranged from .58 to .89. Coefficient alphas ranged from .79 to .89.

Validity: Correlation of level of educational requirements with PSAT was .41 and with high school rank was .38. Correlation with strength of educational requirement with PSAT was .53 and with high school rank was .37.

Author: Lent, R.W., et al.

Article: Relation of self-efficacy expectations to academic achievement and persistence.

Journal: *Journal of Counseling Psychology*, July 1984, *31*(3), 356–362.

Related Research: Betz, N. E., & Hackett, G. (1981). The relationship of career-related self-efficacy expectations to perceived career options in college women and men. *Journal of Counseling Psychology, 28*, 399–410.

■ ■ ■

3307

Test Name: SELF-EFFICACY SCALE

Purpose: To measure self-efficacy.

Format: 14-point Likert scale. All items presented.

Reliability: Alphas ranged from .71 to .86.

Validity: Correlated significantly with locus of control (Rotter), personal contact (Gurin et al.), social desirability (Crowne and Marlowe), ego strength (Barron), interpersonal competency (Holland and Baird), and self-esteem (Rosenberg).

Author: Sherer, M., et al.

Article: The self-efficacy scale: Construction and validation.

Journal: *Psychological Reports*, 1982, *51*(2), 663–671.

3308

Test Name: SELF-EFFICACY SCALE

Purpose: To measure perceived self-efficacy.

Number of Items: 6

Format: Items were based on an 11-point scale ranging from 0 to 100.

Reliability: Cronbach's alpha coefficient was .87.

Author: Valerio, H. P., and Stone, G. L.

Article: Effects of behavioral, cognitive, and combined treatments for assertion as a function of differential deficits.

Journal: *Journal of Counseling Psychology*, March 1982, *29*(2), 158–168.

Related Research: Bandura, A. (1977). Self-efficacy: Toward a unifying theory of behavior change. *Psychological Review, 84*, 191–215.

■ ■ ■

3309

Test Name: SELF-ESTEEM INVENTORY

Purpose: To measure self-concept.

Number of Items: 58

Format: Includes a lie scale and four subscales assessing perception of peers, parents, school, and self.

Reliability: Coefficient alpha was .86 for total test and for subscales coefficients ranged from .61 to .71.

Validity: Correlation with Children's Self-Concept Scale, $r = $ .63; Behavioral Academic Assessment Scale, $r = $ .47; Children's Social Desirability Scale, $r = $ .17.

Author: Johnson, B. W., et al.

Article: The Coopersmith Self-

Esteem Inventory: A construct validation study.

Journal: *Educational and Psychological Measurement*, Autumn 1983, *43*(3), 907–913.

Related Research: Coopersmith, S. (1967). *The antecedents of self-esteem*. San Francisco: Freeman.

■ ■ ■

3310

Test Name: SELF-ESTEEM INVENTORY—FORM B

Purpose: To enable teachers to evaluate students' self-esteem.

Number of Items: 25

Reliability: Test–retest (2 months) reliability coefficients ranged from .72 to .85.

Validity: Correlations with other variables ranged from .05 to .62.

Author: Chiu, L-H.

Article: The reliability and validity of the Coopersmith Self-Esteem Inventory—Form B.

Journal: *Educational and Psychological Measurement*, Winter 1985, *45*(4), 945–949.

Related Research: Coopersmith, S. (1967). *The antecedents of self-esteem*. San Francisco: Freeman.

■ ■ ■

3311

Test Name: SELF-ESTEEM INVENTORY—GENERAL SELF SUBSCALE

Purpose: To measure general self-concept.

Number of Items: 26

Format: Each item is answered either *like me* or *unlike me*.

Reliability: Test–retest coefficients ranged from .52 to .60 (6 months).

Author: Byrne, B. M.

Article: Investigating measures of self-concept.

Journal: *Measurement and Evaluation in Guidance*, October 1983, *16*(3), 115–126.

Related Research: Drummond, R. J., et al. (1977). Stability and sex differences on the Coopersmith Self-Esteem Inventory for students in grades two to twelve. *Psychological Reports, 40,* 943–946.

■ ■ ■

3312

Test Name: SELF-ESTEEM SCALE

Purpose: To assess a person's general feeling toward self.

Number of Items: 6

Format: Respondents asked if feelings are similar to those described on a 7-point favorableness scale.

Reliability: Coefficient of reproducibility was 90.2%.

Author: Starr, P., et al.

Article: Physical attractiveness and self-esteem ratings of young adults with cleft lip and/or palate.

Journal: *Psychological Reports,* 1982, *50*(2), 467–470.

Related Research: Simmons, R. G., et al. (1973). Disturbance in the self-image at adolescence. *American Sociological Review, 38,* 553–568.

■ ■ ■

3313

Test Name: SELF-ESTEEM SCALE

Purpose: To provide a unidimensional measure of general self-concept of high school students.

Number of Items: 10

Format: A Guttman scale with a 4-point Likert-scaling format ranging from *strongly agree* to *strongly disagree.*

Reliability: Test–retest coefficient was .85 for 28 college students over a 2-week interval.

Author: Byrne, B. M.

Article: Investigating measures of self-concept.

Journal: *Measurement and Evaluation in Guidance*, October 1983, *16*(3), 115–126.

Related Research: Silber, E., & Tippett, J. (1965). Self-esteem: Clinical assessment and measurement validation. *Psychological Reports, 16,* 1017–1071.

■ ■ ■

3314

Test Name: SELF-ESTEEM SCALE

Purpose: To measure self-esteem.

Number of Items: 10

Format: Respondents indicate degree of agreement to adjective list corresponding to how well each describes themselves on a 7-point response scale.

Reliability: Alpha was .79.

Author: Hansen, G.

Article: Perceived threats and marital jealousy.

Journal: *Social Psychology Quarterly,* September 1985, *48*(3), 262–268.

Related Research: Anderson, N. H. (1968). Likeableness ratings of 555 personality trait words. *Journal of Personality and Social Psychology, 9,* 272–279.

■ ■ ■

3315

Test Name: SELF-ESTEEM SCALE

Purpose: To measure self-esteem.

Number of Items: 10

Reliability: Coefficient alpha was .84.

Validity: Correlations with other variables ranged from –.22 to .27.

Author: Keller, R. T.

Article: Predicting absenteeism from prior absenteeism, attitudinal factors, and nonattitudinal factors.

Journal: *Journal of Applied Psychology,* August 1983, *68*(3), 536–540.

Related Research: Ellis, R. A., & Taylor, M. S. (1983). Role of self-esteem within the job search process. *Journal of Applied Psychology, 68,* 632–640.

Rosenberg, M. (1965). *Society and the adolescent self-image.* Princeton, NJ: Princeton University Press.

■ ■ ■

3316

Test Name: SELFISM SCALE

Purpose: To measure beliefs about how one should best construe problem situations involving a variety of needs.

Number of Items: 28

Format: Responses are made on a 5-point Likert scale from (1) *strongly agree* to (5) *strongly disagree.* Examples are presented. Also contains 12 filler items to disguise somewhat the purpose of the scale.

Reliability: Spearman-Brown split-half reliabilities were .84 (men) and .83 (women). Test–retest reliability for 7 weeks was .61 ($N=$ 92) and for 4 weeks was .91 ($N=$ 66).

Validity: Correlations with other measures ranged from –.37 to .43.

Author: Phares, E. J., and Erskine, N.

Article: The measurement of selfism.

Journal: *Educational and Psychological Measurement,* Autumn 1984, *44*(3), 597–608.

■ ■ ■

3317

Test Name: SENSE OF COMPETENCE MEASURE

Purpose: To measure an individual's sense of competence resulting from mastering the work setting.

Number of Items: 23

Format: A 5-point Likert scale is employed.

Reliability: Alpha coefficient was .94.

Validity: Correlations with other variables ranged from .11 to .52.

Author: Tharenou, P., and Harker, P.

Article: Moderating influence of self-esteem on relationships between job complexity, performance, and satisfaction.

Journal: *Journal of Applied Psychology,* November 1984, *69*(4), 623–632.

Related Research: Wagner, F. R., & Morse, J. J. (1975). A measure of individual sense of competence. *Psychological Reports, 36,* 451–459.

■ ■ ■

3318

Test Name: SEX STEREOTYPE MEASURE (KOREAN)

Purpose: To measure awareness of sex-trait stereotypes.

Number of Items: 32

Format: Subjects assign each of 32 traits to male or female silhouetted figures.

Reliability: Test–retest reliabilities were .69 and .70 for Korean girls and boys, respectively.

Author: Lee, J. Y., and Sugawara, A. I.

Article: Awareness of sex-trait stereotypes among Korean children.

Journal: *Journal of Social Psychology,* August 1982, *117*(second half), 161–170.

Related Research: Williams, J. E., et al. (1977). *Sex stereotype measure II* (Tech. Rep.). Winston-Salem, NC: Wake Forest University, Department of Psychology.

■ ■ ■

3319

Test Name: SEX STEREOTYPE QUESTIONNAIRE

Purpose: To assess attitudes toward gender role.

Number of Items: 122

Format: Employs a modified semantic differential format. Subjects respond to the statements by first identifying their ideal man, then their ideal woman, and then they identify the characteristics that reflect themselves.

Reliability: Reliability is reported to range from .56 to .70.

Author: Stevens, G., et al.

Article: Factor analyses of two "attitude toward gender role" questionnaires.

Journal: *Journal of Personality Assessment,* June 1984, *48*(3), 312–316.

Related Research: Rosenkrantz, P., et al. (1968). Sex-role stereotypes and self-concepts in college students. *Journal of Consulting and Clinical Psychology, 32*(3), 287–297.

3320

Test Name: SKILLS RATING INVENTORY

Purpose: To measure self-assessment of personal skills.

Number of Items: 44

Format: Two ratings were made on each item: frequency of activity and quality of performance. Each rating was made on a 5-point rating scale.

Reliability: Alphas were .93 (number of skills) and .93 (quality of skills).

Validity: Number and quality correlated at .38.

Author: Prager, K. J.

Article: Educational aspirations and self-esteem in returning and traditional community college students.

Journal: *Journal of College Student Personnel,* March 1983, *24*(2), 144–147.

■ ■ ■

3321

Test Name: STUDENT SELF-CONCEPT SCALE

Purpose: To measure intellectual and academic self-concept and interpersonal and social self-concept.

Number of Items: 11

Format: Rating scale from above to below average.

Reliability: Intellectual and academic (5 items) alpha was .68. Interpersonal and social (6 items) alpha was .63.

Author: Pascarella, E. T.

Article: The influence of on-campus living versus commuting to college on intellectual and interpersonal self-concept.

Journal: *Journal of College*

Student Personnel, July 1985, *26*(4), 292–299.

Related Research: Pascarella, E. T. (1984). Reassessing the effects of living on-campus versus commuting to college: A causal modelling approach. *Review of Higher Education, 7,* 247–260.

■ ■ ■

3322

Test Name: STUDENT PERCEPTION SCALES

Purpose: To measure perceptions of academic preparation, university demands, institutional climate, and personal adjustment.

Number of Items: 31

Format: Items rated on a 5-point scale.

Reliability: Cronbach's alpha ranged from .57 to .77.

Author: Holahan, C. K., et al.

Article: The formation of student performance expectancies: The relationship of student perceptions and social consequences.

Journal: *Journal of College Student Personnel,* November 1982, *23*(6), 497–502.

■ ■ ■

3323

Test Name: STUDENT PERFORMANCE ATTRIBUTION SCALE

Purpose: To assess how students attribute cause of performance on tests.

Number of Items: 22

Format: 7-point Likert format.

Reliability: Cronbach's alpha was .84; Spearman-Brown odd–even reliability was .88.

Validity: Does not significantly correlate with social desirability (r = .06) or self-esteem (r = .11).

Author: Ames, R., and Lau, S.

Article: An attributional analysis of student help-seeking in academic settings.

Journal: *Journal of Educational Psychology,* June 1982, *74*(3), 414–423.

■ ■ ■

3324

Test Name: SUBORDINATE PERCEPTIONS SCALE

Purpose: To measure subordinates' perception of psychological influence.

Number of Items: 6

Format: Likert format.

Reliability: Alpha was .82.

Author: James, L. R., et al.

Article: Perceptions of psychological influence: A cognitive information processing approach for explaining moderated relationships.

Journal: *Personnel Psychology,* Autumn 1981, *34*(3), 453–475.

Related Research: James, L. R., et al. (1979). Correlates of psychological influence: An illustration of the psychological climate approach to work environment perceptions. *Personnel Psychology, 32,* 563–588.

■ ■ ■

3325

Test Name: SUPERVISEE LEVELS QUESTIONNAIRE

Purpose: To identify counselor supervisees' perceptions of their counseling and supervision behavior.

Number of Items: 24

Format: Responses to each item were made on a 7-point Likert scale. Includes three subscales: self-awareness, dependency-autonomy, and theory/skills

acquisition. Sample items are presented.

Reliability: Cronbach's alpha ranged from .55 to .76.

Author: McNeill, B. W., et al.

Article: Supervisees' perceptions of their development: A test of the counselor complexity model.

Journal: *Journal of Counseling Psychology,* October 1985, *32*(4), 630–633.

Related Research: Stoltenberg, C. D. (1981). Approaching supervision from a developmental perspective: The counselor complexity model. *Journal of Counseling Psychology, 28,* 59–65.

■ ■ ■

3326

Test Name: SUPERVISOR'S APPLICATION OF DISCIPLINE SCALE

Purpose: To measure employees' perception of their boss and the manner they use in disciplinary actions.

Number of Items: 38

Format: Five-point agreement scale.

Reliability: Alpha ranged from .88 to .90 across two subscales. Interrater reliability ranged from .31 to .43.

Validity: Two factors extracted (style and consistency) that together explain 95% of variance.

Author: Arvey, R. D., et al.

Article: Use of discipline in an organization: A field study.

Journal: *Journal of Applied Psychology,* August 1984, *69*(3) 448–460.

■ ■ ■

3327

Test Name: SYDNEY ATTRIBUTION SCALE

Purpose: To measure students' perception of causes of academic success and failure.

Number of Items: 72

Format: Items rated on a 5-point response scale.

Reliability: Alphas ranged from .57 to .86 across subscales.

Author: Marsh, H. W.

Article: Relations among dimensions of self-attribution, dimensions of self-concept, and academic achievements.

Journal: *Journal of Educational Psychology*, December 1984, *76*(6), 1291–1308.

Related Research: Marsh, H. W., et al. (1984). The relationship between dimensions of self-attribution and dimensions of self-concept. *Journal of Educational Psychology*, *76*, 3–32.

. . .

3328

Test Name: TASK-SPECIFIC AND SOCIAL SELF-ESTEEM SCALES

Purpose: To measure self-evaluation of ability and performance on a particular task, and self-perception of how others view ability on a particular task.

Number of Items: 41

Format: Items rated in 5-point Likert format. Sample items are presented.

Reliability: Alphas were above .80.

Validity: Academic ability and satisfaction correlated significantly ($r = .81$, $p < .001$) as did athletic ability and satisfaction ($r = .84$, $p < .001$).

Author: McIntire, S. A., and Levine, E. L.

Article: An empirical investigation of self-esteem as a composite construct.

Journal: *Journal of Vocational Behavior*, December 1984, *25*(3), 290–303.

. . .

3329

Test Name: TASK-SPECIFIC SELF-ESTEEM SCALE

Purpose: To measure task-specific self-esteem in the job search context.

Number of Items: 10

Format: Items deal with individuals' confidence in general search ability and in specific job search knowledge and skills. Responses are made on a 5-point Likert scale. All items are presented.

Reliability: Coefficient alphas were .82 and .83.

Validity: Correlations with other variables ranged from –.40 to .54.

Author: Ellis, R. A., and Taylor M. S.

Article: Role of self-esteem within the job search process.

Journal: *Journal of Applied Psychology*, November 1983, *68*(4), 632–640.

. . .

3330

Test Name: TEACHING EFFECTIVENESS QUESTIONNAIRE

Purpose: To measure what teachers believe to be effective teaching.

Number of Items: 20

Format: Items rated on 5-point Likert scales. All items presented.

Reliability: Cronbach's alphas all above .84 (for pre- and posttests).

Author: Guskey, T.

Article: The effects of staff development on teachers' perceptions about effective teaching.

Journal: *Journal of Educational Research*, July/August 1985, *78*(6), 378–381.

Related Research: Guskey, T. R. (1984). The influence of change in instructional effectiveness upon the affective characteristics of teachers. *American Educational Research Journal*, *7*, 265–274.

. . .

3331

Test Name: TEACHER EFFICACY SCALE

Purpose: To measure the belief that teachers can help even the most difficult or unmotivated students.

Number of Items: 30

Format: Likert format. All items presented.

Validity: Convergent and discriminant validity assessed by multitrait–multimethod analysis supported use of the construct.

Author: Gibson, S., and Demba, M. H.

Article: Teacher efficacy: A construct validation.

Journal: *Journal of Educational Psychology*, August 1984, *76*(4), 569–582.

Related Research: Gibson, S., & Brown, R. (1982). *The development of teacher's personal responsibility/self-efficacy scale.* Paper presented at the annual meeting of the American Educational Research Association, New York.

. . .

3332

Test Name: TEACHER LOCUS OF CONTROL SCALE

Purpose: To measure teacher locus of control.

Number of Items: 24

Format: Likert scale including 4 response choices: *strongly agree, agree, disagree, strongly disagree.* One half of the items are oriented toward internal locus of control and one half toward external locus of control.

Reliability: Coefficient alphas were .85 (*N*= 111) and .78 (*N*= 130).

Author: Halpin, G., et al.

Article: Teacher stress as related to locus of control, sex, and age.

Journal: *Journal of Experimental Education,* Spring 1985, *53*(3), 136–139.

Related Research: Hall, B. W., et al. (1980). *Development and validation of a teacher locus of control scale.* Paper presented at the meeting of the National Council on Measurement in Education, Boston.

■ ■ ■

3333

Test Name: TEACHER LOCUS OF CONTROL

Purpose: To measure teacher expectancies for internal or external control of aspects of teacher role.

Number of Items: 32

Format: Each item is a contrast between an internal and external belief. Sample item is presented.

Reliability: Alpha was .86. Temporal stability coefficients were .75 (2 weeks) and .62 (3 weeks).

Validity: Factorial four factors were extracted (recognition, teaching/learning process, relations with teachers, attitudes of parents and society).

Author: Maes, W. R., and Anderson, D. E.

Article: A measure of teacher locus of control.

Journal: *Journal of Educational Research,* September/October 1985, *79*(1), 27–32.

■ ■ ■

3334

Test Name: TEACHER LOCUS OF CONTROL SCALE

Purpose: To measure perceptions of control in the classroom.

Number of Items: 28

Format: Forced-choice items.

Reliability: Kuder-Richardson formula 20 was .81 (I– subscale). Kuder-Richardson formula 20 was .71 (I + subscale).

Validity: TCL more predictive of teacher and student behavior than E-1 scale according to correlations presented.

Author: Rose, J. S., and Medway, F. J.

Article: Measurement of teachers' beliefs in their control over student outcome.

Journal: *Journal of Educational Research,* January/February 1981, *74*(3), 185–190.

Related Research: Rotter, J. B. (1966). Generalized expectancies for internal vs. external control of reinforcement. *Psychological Monographs, 80*(1, Whole No. 609).

■ ■ ■

3335

Test Name: TEMPORAL INTEGRATION SCALES

Purpose: To measure time perspective in terms of long-term personal direction and time utilization.

Number of Items: 40

Format: Items rated on 7-point Likert response scales. Sample items are presented.

Reliability: Alpha ranged from .80 to .83.

Author: Wolf, F. M., and Savickas, M. L.

Article: Time perspective and causal attributions for achievement.

Journal: *Journal of Educational Psychology,* August 1985, *77*(4), 471–488.

Related Research: Wessman, A. E. (1973). Personality and the subjective experience of time. *Journal of Personality Assessment, 37,* 103–114.

■ ■ ■

3336

Test Name: THERAPIST EXPECTANCY INVENTORY

Purpose: To measure therapists' pretreatment expectancies.

Number of Items: 29

Format: Likert scale (1 = *not at all expect*; 8 = *greatly expect*). All items are presented.

Reliability: Cronbach's alphas ranged from .67 to .87 on four subscales.

Validity: Four-factor solution accounted for 34% of the variance in the responses.

Author: Bernstein, B. L., et al.

Article: Therapist expectancy inventory: Development and preliminary validation.

Journal: *Psychological Reports,* April 1983, *52*(2), 479–487.

■ ■ ■

3337

Test Name: UNDERSTANDING LITERACY BEHAVIOR TEST

Purpose: To measure child's recognition of reading and writing activities.

Number of Items: 10 sets of four drawings.

Format: Child instructed to point to each person who is reading.

Reliability: Cronbach internal consistency was .758.

Author: Mayfield, M.

Article: Code systems instructions and kindergarten children's perception of the nature of and purpose of reading.

Journal: *Journal of Educational Research*, January/February 1983, *76*(3), 161–168.

Related Research: Evanechko, P., et al. (1973). An investigation of the reading readiness domain. *Research in the Teaching of English*, 7, 61–78.

■ ■ ■

3338

Test Name: WALLACE SELF-CONCEPT SCALE

Purpose: To estimate the perception one holds toward the concept *myself as a person.*

Number of Items: 15

Format: Items are bipolar.

Reliability: Test–retest coefficients ranged from .72 to .81. Coefficient alpha was .81.

Validity: Convergent validity correlations ranged from .45 to .64. Discriminant validity correlation with the Crowne-Marlowe Social Desirability Scale was .23.

Author: Wallace, G. R., et al.

Article: Factorial comparison of the Wallace Self-Concept Scale between special education teachers and regular classroom teachers.

Journal: *Educational and*

Psychological Measurement, Summer 1984, *44*(2), 199–207.

Related Research: White, G., & Chan, E. (1983). A comparison of self-concept scores of Chinese and White graduate students and professionals. *Journal of Non-White Concerns, 11*(4), 138–141.

■ ■ ■

3339

Test Name: WALLSTON HEALTH LOCUS OF CONTROL SCALE

Purpose: To measure sense of control of health.

Number of Items: 9

Format: Items rated on a 4-point agree–disagree scale. All items are presented.

Reliability: Alpha was .65.

Author: Seeman, M., et al.

Article: Social networks and health status: A longitudinal analysis.

Journal: *Social Psychology Quarterly,* September 1985, *48*(3), 237–248.

Related Research: Wallston, K. A., & Wallston, B. S. (1980). Health locus of control scales. In J. Lefcourt (Ed.), *Advances and innovation in locus of control research* (pp. 189–243). New York: Academic Press.

■ ■ ■

3340

Test Name: WEIGHT LOCUS OF CONTROL SCALE

Purpose: To measure locus of control with respect to weight.

Number of Items: 4

Format: Employs a 6-point Likert format ranging from 1 (*strongly disagree*) to 6 (*strongly agree*) for the two externally worded items and reverse scoring for the two internally worded items. All items are presented.

Reliability: Test–retest reliability was .67 (*N* = 110). Cronbach's alphas were .58 (*N* = 113) and .56 (*N* = 112).

Validity: Correlations with other scales ranged from –.30 to .35.

Author: Saltzer, E. B.

Article: The Weight Locus of Control (WLOC) Scale: A specific measure for obesity research.

Journal: *Journal of Personality Assessment,* December 1982, *46*(6), 620–628.

■ ■ ■

3341

Test Name: WORK–NONWORK CONFLICT SCALE

Purpose: To measure perceived conflict between work and nonwork.

Number of Items: 6

Format: Items rated on a 5-point response scale (*completely true* to *completely not true*). All items are presented.

Reliability: Alpha was .69.

Validity: Correlates significantly with "inclusiveness" among army personnel.

Author: Shamir, B.

Article: Some antecedents of work–nonwork conflict.

Journal: *Journal of Vocational Behavior,* August 1983, *23*(1), 98–111.

CHAPTER 17
Personality

3342

Test Name: ABBREVIATED TEMPERAMENT QUESTIONNAIRE

Purpose: To assess temperament.

Number of Items: 30

Format: For children 5 to 7 years. Includes 4 components and uses a 5-point rating scale.

Reliability: A total of 50% of item reliabilities (1 month) were greater than .80 (N= 15); 80% of item reliabilities were greater than .60.

Author: Hubert, N. C., et al.

Article: The study of early temperament: Measurement and conceptual issues.

Journal: *Child Development,* June 1982, *53*(3), 571–600.

Related Research: Garside, R. F., et al. (1975). Dimensions of temperament in infant school children. *Journal of Child Psychology and Psychiatry and Allied Disciplines, 16,* 219–231.

· · ·

3343

Test Name: ACT UNISEX INTEREST INVENTORY

Purpose: To measure Holland personality types.

Number of Items: 90 (6 subscales of 15 items each).

Format: Item responses are *like, indifferent,* and *dislike.*

Reliability: Alpha ranged from .85 to .92 across subscales.

Author: Wolfe, L. K., and Betz, N.

Article: Traditionality of choice and sex-role identification as moderators of the congruence of occupational choice in college women.

Journal: *Journal of Vocational Behavior,* February 1981, *18*(1), 43–55.

Related Research: Hanson, G. R. (1974). *Assessing the interest of college youth: Summary of research and applications* (ACT Research Report No. 67). Iowa City, Iowa: American College Testing Program.

Hanson, G. R., et al. (1977). *Development and validation of sex-balanced interest inventory scales* (ACT Research Report No. 78). Iowa City, Iowa: American College Testing Program.

· · ·

3344

Test Name: AGREEMENT RESPONSE SCALE—REVISED

Purpose: To measure the agreeing response tendency.

Number of Items: 15

Format: Each item reflects value or belief-oriented statements about oneself. Subjects respond on a 7-point scale from 1 (*strongly disagree*) to 7 (*strongly agree*).

Reliability: Internal consistency was .71.

Validity: Correlation with satisfaction was .21.

Author: Blau, G., and Katerberg, R.

Article: Agreeing response set: Statistical nuisance or meaningful personality concept?

Journal: *Perceptual and Motor Skills,* June 1982, *54*(3-I), 851–857.

Related Research: Couch, A., & Keniston, K. (1961). Agreeing response set and social desirability. *Journal of Abnormal and Social Psychology, 62,* 175–179.

· · ·

3345

Test Name: BABY BEHAVIOR QUESTIONNAIRE

Purpose: To assess temperament.

Number of Items: 54

Format: Includes 7 factors: intensity/activity, regularity, approach/withdrawal, sensory sensitivity, attentiveness, manageability, sensitivity to new foods.

Reliability: Test–retest correlation coefficients ranged from .63 to .93 (N= 26). Alphas ranged from .51 to .72.

Author: Hubert, N. C., et al.

Article: The study of early temperament: Measurement and conceptual issues.

Journal: *Child Development,* June 1982, *53*(3), 571–600.

Related Research: Bohlin, G., et al. (1981). Dimensions of infant behavior. *Infant Behavior and Development, 4,* 83–96.

3346

Test Name: BASIC PERSONALITY INVENTORY

Purpose: To measure independent components of psychopathology.

Number of Items: 220

Format: True–false.

Reliability: Kuder-Richardson formula 20 ranged from .47 to .83 across subscales. Item-total correlations ranged from .29 to .44.

Validity: Validity coefficients averaged .21.

Author: Holden, R. R., and Jackson, D. N.

Article: Disguise and the structured self-report assessment of psychopathology: I. An analogue investigation.

Journal: *Journal of Consulting and Clinical Psychology*, April 1985, *53*(2), 211–222.

Related Research: Jackson, D. H. (1976). *The basic personality inventory*. London, Ontario, Canada: Author.

■ ■ ■

3347

Test Name: BEHAVIOR CHECKLIST

Purpose: To assess temperament.

Number of Items: 25

Format: For children 4–14 years. Includes 5 temperament types: easy, difficult, slow warmer, environmentalist, emotionally fragile.

Reliability: Test–retest correlation coefficients (8 weeks) ranged from .44 to .82 (*N* = 50).

Validity: Correlation with parent ratings of behavior description items ranged from .27 to .70.

Author: Hubert, N. C., et al.

Article: The study of early

temperament: Measurement and conceptual issues.

Journal: *Child Development*, June 1982, *53*(3), 571–600.

■ ■ ■

3348

Test Name: BEHAVIORAL STYLES QUESTIONNAIRE

Purpose: To assess temperament.

Number of Items: 100

Format: For children 3–7 years. Includes 9 categories: activity level, rhythmicity, approach/ withdrawal, adaptability, intensity, sensory threshold, mood, distractibility, attention span/persistence.

Reliability: Test–retest reliability coefficients (1 month) ranged from .67 to .94 (*N* = 53). Alphas ranged from .47 to .80 (*N* = 350).

Validity: Correlations with other measures ranged from .29 to .35.

Author: Hubert, N. C., et al.

Article: The study of early temperament: Measurement and conceptual issues.

Journal: *Child Development*, June 1982, *53*(3), 571–600.

Related Research: McDevitt, S. C., & Carey, W. B. (1978). Measurement of temperament in 3- to 7-year-old children. *Journal of Child Psychology and Psychiatry and Allied Disciplines, 19*, 245–253.

■ ■ ■

3349

Test Name: BIOGRAPHICAL QUESTIONNAIRE

Purpose: To identify a variety of biographical information.

Number of Items: 118

Format: Includes 15 factors for women and 13 factors for men.

Reliability: Coefficient alphas for women's data ranged from .70 to .89 and coefficient alphas for men's data ranged from .67 to .89.

Author: Eberhardt, B. J., and Muchinsky, P. M.

Article: Biodata determinants of vocational typology: An integration of two paradigms.

Journal: *Journal of Applied Psychology*, December 1982, *67*(6), 714–727.

Related Research: Owens, W. A., & Schoenfeldt, L. F. (1979). Toward a classification of persons. *Journal of Applied Psychology, 64*, 569–607.

■ ■ ■

3350

Test Name: CHILD ABUSE POTENTIAL INVENTORY

Purpose: A screening device to differentiate abusers from nonabusers.

Number of Items: 160

Format: Agree–disagree format.

Reliability: Kuder-Richardson formula 20 ranged from .92 to .96.

Validity: Classification rate for abusers is 94%. Eight subscales correlate between .19 and .34 with abuse (all significant, *p* < .05 or .01); .15 to .26 with neglect (7 of 8 significant, *p* < .05 or .01); and .10 to .29 with failure to thrive (3 of 8 significant *p* < .01).

Author: Milner, J. S., et al.

Article: Predictive validity of the child abuse potential inventory.

Journal: *Journal of Consulting and Clinical Psychology,* October 1984, *52*(5), 879–884.

Related Research: Milner, J. S. (1980). *The Child Abuse Potential Inventory Manual*. Webster, NC: Psytec.

3351

Test Name: CHILD STIMULUS SCREENING SCALE

Purpose: To assess temperament.

Number of Items: 46

Format: For children 3 months to 7 years. Employs a 9-point rating scale.

Reliability: Kuder-Richardson formula coefficient was .82 ($N=$ 157).

Validity: Correlations with other measures ranged from –.42 to .54.

Author: Hubert, N. C., et al.

Article: The study of early temperament: Measurement and conceptual issues.

Journal: *Child Development*, June 1982, *53*(3), 571–600.

Related Research: Mehrabian, A., & Falander, C. (1978). A questionnaire measure of individual differences in child stimulus screening. *Educational and Psychological Measurement, 38*, 1119–1127.

• • •

3352

Test Name: COLORADO CHILDHOOD TEMPERAMENT INVENTORY

Purpose: To assess temperament.

Number of Items: 30

Format: Includes the following content: sociability, emotionality, activity, attention span-persistence, reaction to food, soothability.

Reliability: Test–retest (1 week) correlation coefficients ranged from .43 to .80 ($N=$ 31 twins). Alphas ranged from .73 to .88.

Author: Hubert, N. C., et al.

Article: The study of early temperament: Measurement and conceptual issues.

Journal: *Child Development*, June 1982, *53*(3), 571–600.

Related Research: Rowe, D. C., & Plomin, R. (1977). Temperament in early childhood. *Journal of Personality Assessment, 41*, 150–156.

• • •

3353

Test Name: COUNSELOR RATING FORM

Purpose: To measure the interviewer's perception of the student's persuasiveness.

Number of Items: 12

Format: Includes the dimensions expertness, attractiveness, and trustworthiness. The format is semantic differential with 7-point items.

Reliability: Split-half reliabilities ranged from .84 to .90.

Author: Wild, B. K., and Kerr, B. A.

Article: Training adolescent job-seekers in persuasion skills.

Journal: *Vocational Guidance Quarterly*, September 1984, *33*(1), 63–69.

Related Research: Barak, A., & LaCrosse, M. B. (1977). Comparative perception of practicum counselor behavior: A process and methodological investigation. *Counselor Education and Supervision, 16*, 202–208.

• • •

3354

Test Name: DAYDREAM ASSESSMENT QUESTIONNAIRE

Purpose: To rate daydreams.

Number of Items: 7

Format: All items except two are in Likert-scale form. All items are presented.

Reliability: Interjudge reliability for each item ranged from .36 to .91.

Author: Ireland, M. S., and Kernan-Schloss, L.

Article: Pattern analysis of recorded daydreams, memories and personality types.

Journal: *Perceptual and Motor Skills*, February 1983, *56*(1), 119–125.

Related Research: Starker, S. (1973). Aspects of inner experience: Autokinesis, daydreaming, dream recall and cognitive style. *Perceptual and Motor Skills, 36*, 663–673.

• • •

3355

Test Name: DEFENSE MECHANISMS INVENTORY

Purpose: To determine characteristic coping mechanisms employed by individuals when faced with a series of conflict situations.

Number of Items: 40

Format: Scores are derived for the relative usage of five major groups of defenses. Subjects indicate how they would respond if faced with each of the 10 conflicts.

Validity: Correlations with the percent of menstrual complaints ranged from –.350 to .487. Correlations with the sum of menstrual complaints ranged from –.220 to .168.

Author: Greenberg, R. P., and Fisher, S.

Article: Menstrual discomfort, psychological defenses and feminine identification.

Journal: *Journal of Personality Assessment*, December 1984, *48*(6), 643–648.

Related Research: Gleser, G. C., & Ihilevich, D. (1969). An objective instrument for measuring defense mechanisms. *Journal of Consulting and Clinical Psychology, 33,* 51–60.

■ ■ ■

3356

Test Name: DIMENSIONS OF TEMPERAMENT SURVEY

Purpose: To assess the dimensions of temperamental individuality across the life span.

Number of Items: 34

Format: Includes five factors: activity level, attention span/distractibility, adaptability/approach-withdrawal, rhythmicity, and reactivity.

Reliability: Test–retest reliability ranged from .60 to .93.

Author: Lerner, R. M., et al.

Article: Assessing the dimensions of temperamental individuality across the life span: The Dimensions of Temperament Survey (DOTS).

Journal: *Child Development,* February 1982, *53*(1), 149–159.

Related Research: Thomas, A., & Chess, S. (1981). The role of temperament in the contributions of individuals to their development. In R. M. Lerner & N. A. Busch-Rossnagel (Eds.), *Individuals as producers of their development: A life-span perspective.* New York: Academic Press.

■ ■ ■

3357

Test Name: EASI-I TEMPERAMENT SURVEY

Purpose: To assess temperament.

Number of Items: 20

Format: For children 1–9 years. Includes the following categories: emotionality, activity, sociability, impulsivity.

Reliability: Test–retest (21 days) correlation coefficients ranged from .75 to .92 ($N = 20$) and from .59 to .68 ($N = 27$). Alphas ranged from .69 to .76 ($N = 66$).

Author: Hubert, N. C., et al.

Article: The study of early temperament: Measurement and conceptual issues.

Journal: *Child Development,* June 1982, *53*(3), 571–600.

Related Research: Buss, A. H., et al. (1973). The inheritance of temperament. *Journal of Personality, 4,* 513–524.

■ ■ ■

3358

Test Name: EASI-III TEST

Purpose: To measure temperament.

Number of Items: 57

Format: Includes the following scales: emotionality, activity, sociability, and impulsivity. This latter scale was further divided into a planning scale.

Reliability: Alpha reliabilities for the scales ranged from .65 to .81.

Author: Harburg, E., et al.

Article: Handedness and temperament.

Journal: *Perceptual and Motor Skills,* February 1981, *52*(1), 283–290.

Related Research: Buss, A. H., & Plomin, R. (1974). *A temperament theory of personality development.* New York: Wiley.

■ ■ ■

3359

Test Name: EGO INVOLVEMENT SCALE

Purpose: To measure subjective relevance regarding the areas of achievement and interpersonal contact.

Number of Items: 25

Format: Items rated in 6-point Likert format. All items are presented.

Reliability: Alpha ranged from .76 to .86 in two subscales (interpersonal contact and achievement).

Validity: Men and women did not differ, $F(1, 102) = .63, p < .80$, and both sexes assigned greater relevance to interpersonal contact than to achievement ($p < .01$).

Author: Krahé, B.

Article: Self-serving biases in perceived similarity and causal attributions of other people's performance.

Journal: *Social Psychology Quarterly,* December 1983, *46*(4), 318–329.

■ ■ ■

3360

Test Name: EGO PERMISSIVENESS QUESTIONNAIRE

Purpose: To measure the relative amount of ego energy.

Number of Items: 50

Format: Includes five subscales: peak experience, dissociated experiences, openness to experience, belief in the supernatural, and intrinsic arousal. Range of scores is from 0 to 200.

Reliability: Test–retest reliability ranged from .20 to .50. Coefficient alpha was .87 ($N = 120$).

Validity: Correlation with TAT Expression scores was .40.

Author: Daly, E. B.

Article: Relationship of stress and ego energy to field-dependent perception in older adults.

Journal: *Perceptual and Motor*

Skills, December 1984, *59*(3), 919–926.

Related Research: Taft, R. (1970). Measurement of the dimension of ego permissiveness. *Personality: An International Journal, 1,* 163–184.

■ ■ ■

3361

Test Name: EXPRESSION OF EMOTION SCALE

Purpose: To measure the extent to which each of four different types of emotions are expressed.

Number of Items: 16

Format: Includes emotions of: love, hate, happiness, and sadness. Responses are made on Likert scale from 1 (*never*) to 4 (*very often*).

Reliability: Test–retest reliabilities were .83 (1 week, *N* = 34) and .72 (6 weeks, *N* = 33).

Author: Dosser, D. A. (Jr)., et al.

Article: Situational context of emotional expressiveness.

Journal: *Journal of Counseling Psychology,* July 1983, *30*(3), 375–387.

Related Research: Davidson, B., et al. (1983). Affective self-disclosure and marital adjustment: A test of equity theory. *Journal of Marriage and the Family, 45,* 93–102.

■ ■ ■

3362

Test Name: INFANT BEHAVIOR QUESTIONNAIRE

Purpose: To assess temperament.

Number of Items: 87

Format: For infants 3 to 12 months. Includes 6 scales: activity level, smiling and laughing distress to limitations, fear, soothability, duration of orienting.

Reliability: Test–retest correlation

coefficients ranged from –.02 to .74 (3–12 months, *N* = 36–105) and –.14 to .81 (3–12 months, *N* = 36). Alphas ranged from .63 to .88 (*N* = 464).

Author: Hubert, N. C., et al.

Article: The study of early temperament: Measurement and conceptual issues.

Journal: *Child Development,* June 1982, *53*(3), 571–600.

Related Research: Rothbart, M. (1981). Measure of temperament in infancy. *Child Development, 52,* 569–578.

■ ■ ■

3363

Test Name: INFANT CHARACTERISTICS QUESTIONNAIRE

Purpose: To assess temperament.

Number of Items: 24

Format: For infants 4–6 months. Includes the following categories: activity level, rhythmicity, approach/withdrawal, adaptability, intensity, sensory threshold, mood, distractibility, attention span/persistence, fussiness, sociability, changeability, and soothability.

Reliability: Test–retest correlation coefficients ranged from .47 to .70 (1 month, *N* = 112). Alphas ranged from .39 to .79 (*N* = 196).

Validity: Correlations with other measures ranged from –.25 to .40.

Author: Hubert, N. C., et al.

Article: The study of early temperament: Measurement and conceptual issues.

Journal: *Child Development,* June 1982, *53*(3), 571–600.

Related Research: Bates, J., et al. (1979). Measurement of infant difficultness. *Child Development, 50,* 794–803.

3364

Test Name: INFANT TEMPERAMENT QUESTIONNAIRE

Purpose: To assess temperament.

Number of Items: 70

Format: For infants 3.5 to 8.5 months. Includes 9 categories: activity level, rhythmicity, approach/withdrawal, adaptability, intensity, sensory threshold, mood, distractibility, attention span/persistence.

Reliability: Test–retest reliability coefficients (2 weeks to 5 months) ranged from .27 to .93 (*N* ranged from 20 to 151).

Validity: Correlations with Infant Characteristics Questionnaire ranged from –.06 to .22; with Bayley mental series, *r* = .58 (*N* = 12); with teacher-rated adjustment scores, *r* = .42; and with mother's mood, *r* = .28 (*N* = 132).

Author: Hubert, N. C., et al.

Article: The study of early temperament: Measurement and conceptual issues.

Journal: *Child Development,* June 1982, *53*(3), 571–600.

Related Research: Carey, W. B. (1970). A simplified method for measuring infant temperament. *Journal of Pediatrics, 77,* 188–194.

■ ■ ■

3365

Test Name: INFANT TEMPERAMENT QUESTIONNAIRE

Purpose: To provide infant temperament ratings.

Number of Items: 70

Time Required: Approximately 20 minutes.

Format: Includes the following scales: activity, rhythmicity, adaptability, approach, threshold, intensity, mood, distractibility, and persistence.

Reliability: Cronbach's alphas ranged from .20 to .67.

Validity: Correlations with observed behavior ranged from −.26 to .17.

Author: Sameroff, A. J., et al.

Article: Sociocultural variability in infant temperament ratings.

Journal: *Child Development,* February 1982, *53*(1), 164–173.

Related Research: Carey, W. B. (1972). Measuring infant temperament. *Journal of Pediatrics, 81,* 414.

■ ■ ■

3366

Test Name: MANAGING PEOPLE INVENTORY

Purpose: To assess trust and respect.

Number of Items: 26

Format: Responses to each item were either *usually true* or *not usually true.* All items are presented.

Reliability: Kuder-Richardson formula 20 estimates were .937 and .927.

Validity: Correlations with a criterion item were .796 and .783.

Author: Drehmer, D. E., and Grossman, J. H.

Article: Scaling managerial respect: A developmental perspective.

Journal: *Educational and Psychological Measurement,* Autumn 1984, *44*(3), 763–767.

■ ■ ■

3367

Test Name: NEED FOR COGNITION SCALE

Purpose: To assess individual differences in need for cognition.

Number of Items: 18

Format: All items are presented.

Reliability: Theta coefficient was .90 (*N* = 527).

Author: Cacioppo, J. T., et al.

Article: The efficient assessment of need for cognition.

Journal: *Journal of Personality Assessment,* June 1984, *48*(3), 306–307.

Related Research: Cacioppo, J. T., & Petty, R. E. (1982). The need for cognition. *Journal of Personality and Social Psychology, 42,* 116–131.

■ ■ ■

3368

Test Name: OFFICE ATTITUDE QUESTIONNAIRE

Purpose: To assess tendencies to be a "power seeker" or "politician" in the office.

Number of Items: 50

Format: *Mostly true* to *mostly false* format.

Reliability: Alpha was .90. Split-half reliability was .88.

Author: Biberman, G.

Article: Personality and characteristic work attitudes of persons with high, moderate, and low political tendencies.

Journal: *Psychological Reports,* December 1985, *57*(3-II), 1303–1310.

Related Research: Dubrin, A. J. (1981). Winning at office politics: 50 questions to help you play like a pro. *Success, 46,* 26–28.

■ ■ ■

3369

Test Name: OPEN PROCESSING STYLE SCALE

Purpose: To measure the "open processing" cognitive style.

Number of Items: 24

Format: Items rated on 5-point descriptive verbal anchors for each of 12 "open" and 12 "cautious" styles.

Reliability: Kuder-Richardson formula 8 was .82. Test–retest reliability was .72.

Author: Joseph, W. B.

Article: Receivers' open processing style as a moderator of communications persuasiveness.

Journal: *Psychological Reports,* June 1983, *52*(3), 963–967.

Related Research: Walton, J., et al. (1978). Validation of the consumer creativity scale. *Proceedings of the 86th annual convention of the American Psychological Association, Division 23* (pp. 47–48). Washington, DC: American Psychological Association.

■ ■ ■

3370

Test Name: PARENT TEMPERAMENT QUESTIONNAIRE

Purpose: To assess temperament.

Number of Items: 72

Format: For children 3 to 7 years. Includes 9 categories: activity level, rhythmicity, approach/withdrawal, adaptability, intensity, sensory threshold, mood, distractibility, attention span/persistence.

Reliability: Estimated correlations ranged from .15 to .74 (*N* = 126).

Validity: Correlations between mother and teacher ranged from −.08 to .31; between father and teacher ranged from −.02 to .34.

Author: Hubert, N. C., et al.

Article: The study of early temperament: Measurement and conceptual issues.

Journal: *Child Development,* June 1982, *53*(3), 571–600.

Related Research: Thomas, A., & Chess, S. (1971). *Temperament and development.* New York: Brunner/Mazel.

. . .

3371

Test Name: PERSONAL STYLE INVENTORY

Purpose: To measure Jungian personality types.

Number of Items: 32

Format: Bipolar items.

Reliability: Values of –1.00 take the opposite side of each scale (multitrait–multimethod).

Validity: Validity coefficients ranged from .52 to .70.

Author: Ware, R., et al.

Article: A preliminary study to assess validity of the personal style inventory.

Journal: *Psychological Reports,* June 1985, *56*(3), 903–910.

. . .

3372

Test Name: PSYCHOLOGICAL INVENTORY OF PERSONALITY AND SYMPTOMS

Purpose: To assess personality and symptoms of individuals.

Number of Items: 346

Format: Built from descriptors and criteria of the DSM-III.

Reliability: Test–retest (1 week) ranged from .62 to .93.

Validity: No significant differences

between ratings of 3 attending clinicians.

Author: Vincent, K. R.

Article: Rated clinical utility of the Psychological Inventory of Personality and Symptoms.

Journal: *Psychological Reports,* June 1985, *56*(3), 847–850.

Related Research: McMurrey, A. D., & Vincent, K. R. (1985). Reliability of the Psychological Inventory of Personality and Symptoms. *Psychological Reports, 56,* 902.

. . .

3373

Test Name: POST COLLEGE EXPERIENCE INVENTORY

Purpose: To measure individual life experiences 3–4 years after college graduation.

Number of Items: 97

Reliability: Kuder-Richardson formula 20 ranged from .50 to .85 over 12 factors (*mdn* = .64).

Validity: Four factors differentiated men ($p < .01$), three factors differentiated women ($p < .05$).

Author: Davis, K. R., Jr.

Article: A longitudinal analysis of biographical subgroups using Owens' developmental–integrative model.

Journal: *Personnel Behavior,* Spring 1984, *37*(1), 1–14

Related Research: Davis, K. R. (1978). Biographical correlates of post-college experience (Doctoral dissertation, University of Georgia). *Dissertation Abstracts International, 38,* 3940B.

. . .

3374

Test Name: PUPIL EVALUATION INVENTORY

Purpose: To provide an instrument for peer assessment.

Number of Items: 35

Format: Includes 3 factors: likeability, aggression, and withdrawal.

Reliability: Test–retest (8 weeks) reliability coefficients ranged from .70 to .93.

Validity: Correlations with other variables ranged from –.74 to .83.

Author: Vogel, J., et al.

Article: Comparability of peer-assessment measures: A multitrait–multimethod and selection analytic approach.

Journal: *Journal of Psychopathology and Behavioral Assessment,* December 1985, *7*(4), 385–396.

Related Research: Pekarik, E. G., et al. (1976). The pupil evaluation inventory. *Journal of Child Psychology, 4,* 93–97.

. . .

3375

Test Name: REVISED INFANT TEMPERAMENT QUESTIONNAIRE

Purpose: To assess temperament.

Number of Items: 95

Format: For infants 4 to 8 months. Includes 9 categories: activity level, rhythmicity, approach/ withdrawal, adaptability, intensity, sensory threshold, mood distractibility, attention span/ persistence.

Reliability: Test–retest reliability coefficients (25.1 days) ranged from $r = .66$ to $r = .81$ ($N = 41$).

Validity: Correlations with: Piagetian sensorimotor development $r = .58$ ($N = 100$); a variety of factors' rs ranged from .66 to .46 ($N = 29$).

Author: Hubert, N. C., et al.

Article: The study of early temperament: Measurement and conceptual issues.

Journal: *Child Development,* June 1982, *53*(3), 571–600.

Related Research: Carey, W. B., & McDevitt, S. C. (1978). Revision of the Infant Temperament Questionnaire. *Pediatrics, 61,* 735–739.

Field, T., & Greenberg, R. (1982). Temperament ratings by parents and teachers of infants, toddlers, and preschool children. *Child Development, 53*(1), 160–163.

■ ■ ■

3376

Test Name: SELF-CONSCIOUSNESS SCALE

Purpose: To measure self-consciousness.

Number of Items: 23

Format: Includes four factors: social anxiety, public self-consciousness, self-reflectiveness, internal state awareness. Responses to each item are made on a 5-point scale from *extremely characteristic* (0) to *extremely uncharacteristic* (4). All items are presented.

Reliability: Cronbach's alphas ranged from .71 to .79.

Author: Burnkrant, R. E., and Page, T. J., Jr.

Article: A modification of the Fenigstein, Scheier, and Buss self-consciousness scales.

Journal: *Journal of Personality Assessment,* December 1984, *48*(6), 629–637.

Related Research: Fenigstein, A., et al. (1975). Public and private self-consciousness: Assessment and theory. *Journal of Consulting and Clinical Psychology, 43,* 522–527.

3377

Test Name: SERVICE ORIENTATION INDEX FOR NURSES AIDES

Purpose: To measure the disposition to be helpful, thoughtful, considerate, and cooperative.

Number of Items: 92

Reliability: Internal consistency = .81.

Validity: Correlated .42 with overall job performance; .22 with communications skills; .20 with relational skills; .23 with working under pressure.

Author: Hogan, J., et al.

Article: How to measure service orientation.

Journal: *Journal of Applied Psychology,* February 1984, *69*(1), 167–173.

Related Research: Hogan, R. A. (1983). Socioanalytic Theory of Personality. In M. Page (Ed.), *Nebraska Symposium on Motivation.* Lincoln: University of Nebraska Press.

■ ■ ■

3378

Test Name: SWEDISH SIX-MONTH TEMPERAMENT QUESTIONNAIRE

Purpose: To assess temperament.

Number of Items: 41

Format: For children 5–8 months. Includes 9 categories: activity level, rhythmicity, approach/withdrawal, adaptability, intensity, sensory threshold, mood, distractibility, attention span/persistence.

Reliability: Test–retest reliability coefficients (2 to 3 weeks) ranged from .40 to .86 (*N*= 14).

Author: Hubert, N. C., et al.

Article: The study of early temperament: Measurement and conceptual issues.

Journal: *Child Development,* June 1982, *53*(3), 571–600.

Related Research: Persson-Blennow, I., & McNeil, T. (1979). A questionnaire for measurement of temperament in six-month-old infants: Development and standardization. *Journal of Child Psychology and Psychiatry and Allied Disciplines, 20,* 1–13.

■ ■ ■

3379

Test Name: SWEDISH TEMPERAMENT QUESTIONNAIRE

Purpose: To assess temperament.

Number of Items: 55 at 12 months, 50 at 24 months.

Format: For infants 12 and 24 months old. Includes 9 categories: activity level, rhythmicity, approach/withdrawal, adaptability, intensity, sensory threshold, mood, distractibility, attention span/persistence.

Reliability: For 12-month-olds, test–retest correlation coefficients ranged from .05 to .84 (3–6 weeks, *N*= 11). For 24-month-olds, coefficients ranged from .00 to .95 (2–4 weeks, *N*= 11).

Author: Hubert, N. C., et al.

Article: The study of early temperament: Measurement and conceptual issues.

Journal: *Child Development,* June 1982, *53*(3), 571–600.

Related Research: Persson-Blennow, I., & McNeil, T. (1980). Questionnaire for measurement of temperament in one and two year old children. *Journal of Child Psychology and Psychiatry, 21,* 37–46.

3380

Test Name: TEACHER TEMPERAMENT QUESTIONNAIRE

Purpose: To assess temperament.

Number of Items: 64

Format: For children 3 to 7 years. Includes eight categories: activity level, approach/withdrawal, adaptability, intensity, sensory threshold, mood, distractibility, attention span/persistence.

Reliability: Correlations ranged from .69 to .87 ($N = 10$).

Validity: Correlations with Behavioral Styles Questionnaire ranged from .18 to .46 ($N = 78$).

Author: Hubert, N. C., et al.

Article: The study of early temperament: Measurement and conceptual issues.

Journal: *Child Development,* June 1982, *53*(3), 571–600.

Related Research: Thomas, A., & Chess, S. (1977). *Temperament and development.* New York: Brunner/Mazel.

■ ■ ■

3381

Test Name: TEACHER TEMPERAMENT QUESTIONNAIRE—SHORT FORM

Purpose: To assess teacher's perceptions of children's temperament.

Number of Items: 23

Format: Includes three factors: task orientation, personal-social flexibility, and reactivity.

Reliability: Alpha coefficients for the three factors were .94, .88, and .62, respectively.

Author: Keogh, B. K., et al.

Article: A short form of the Teacher Temperament Questionnaire.

Journal: *Journal of Educational Measurement,* Winter 1982, *19*(4), 323–329.

Related Research: Pullis, M. E. (1982). *An investigation of the relationship between children, temperament and school adjustment.* Unpublished doctoral dissertation, University of California, Los Angeles.

■ ■ ■

3382

Test Name: THEMATIC APPERCEPTION TEST FOR URBAN HISPANIC CHILDREN

Purpose: To measure thematic apperception.

Number of Items: 23 pictures.

Format: Sample pictures presented. Stories told to bilingual interns in either English or Spanish.

Reliability: Interrater agreement achieved .80 after training.

Validity: Multiple correlations were .32 to .51 with measures of ego development, trait anxiety, and adaptive behavior.

Author: Malgady, R. G., et al.

Article: Development of a thematic apperception test (TEMAS) for urban Hispanic children.

Journal: *Journal of Consulting and Clinical Psychology,* December 1984, *52*(6), 986–996.

Related Research: Constantino, G., & Malgady, R. (1983). Verbal fluency of Hispanic, Black, and White children on TAT and TEMAS. *Hispanic Journal of Behavioral Sciences, 5,* 291–300.

■ ■ ■

3383

Test Name: THERAPEUTIC TALENT INDEX

Purpose: To measure acceptingness, understanding, and openness.

Format: Items rated on 6-point Likert categories. Sample items presented.

Reliability: Cronbach's alpha was .76.

Validity: Correlated significantly with love (.25), dominance (.28), aggressive–sadistic (−.24), and distrust (−.30, $ps < .05$).

Author: Jackson, E.

Article: Interpersonal traits and facilitative helping characteristics.

Journal: *Psychological Reports,* December 1985, *57*(3-I), 995–999.

Related Research: Goodman, G., 1972. *Companionship therapy.* San Francisco, CA: Jossey-Bass.

■ ■ ■

3384

Test Name: TODDLER BEHAVIOR QUESTIONNAIRE

Purpose: To measure temperament.

Number of Items: 60

Format: Includes 8 factors: intensity/activity, regularity, approach/withdrawal, sensory sensitivity, attentiveness, manageability, sensitivity to new foods, adaptability.

Reliability: Test–retest reliability coefficients ranged from .64 to .87 ($N = 26$). Alphas ranged from .59 to .77 ($N = 357$).

Author: Hubert, N. C., et al.

Article: The study of early temperament: Measurement and conceptual issues.

Journal: *Child Development,* June 1982, *53*(3), 571–600.

Related Research: Hagekull, B., et al. (1980). Behavioral dimensions in one year olds and dimensional stability in infancy. *International Journal of Behavioral Development, 3,* 351–364.

■ ■ ■

3385

Test Name: TODDLER TEMPERAMENT SCALE

Purpose: To measure toddler temperament.

Number of Items: 97

Format: Each item was rated on a 6-point scale. All items were combined into nine temperament categories: activity level, rhythmicity, approach/withdrawal, adaptability, intensity of reaction, quality of mood, attention span and persistence, distractibility, threshold of responsiveness.

Reliability: Median test–retest correlation for the nine scales was .81.

Author: Matheny, A. P., Jr., et al.

Article: Toddler temperament: Stability across settings and over ages.

Journal: *Child Development,* August 1984, *55*(4), 1200–1211.

Related Research: Rullard, W., et al. (1984). Assessing temperament in one to three year old children.

Journal of Pediatric Psychology.

Field, T., & Greenberg, R. (1982). Temperament ratings by parents and teachers of infants, toddlers and preschool children. *Child Development, 53*(1), 160–163.

Hubert, N. C., et al. (1982). The study of early temperament: Measurement and conceptual issues. *Child Development, 53*(3), 571–600.

■ ■ ■

3386

Test Name: WHAT ABOUT YOU

Purpose: To evaluate personality and biographical traits of creative people.

Number of Items: 87

Format: Responses are recorded on a 5-point rating scale from *no* to *definitely.*

Reliability: Hoyt internal reliability was .95.

Validity: Correlations with other variables ranged from .15 to .73.

Author: Buckmaster, L. R., and Davis, G. A.

Article: ROSE: A measure of self-actualization and its relationship to creativity.

Journal: *Journal of Creative*

Behavior, 1985, *19*(1), 30–37.

Related Research: Davis, G. A., & Bull, K. S. (1978). Strengthening affective components of creativity in a college course. *Journal of Educational Psychology, 70,* 833–836.

■ ■ ■

3387

Test Name: WIGGINS PERSONALITY INVENTORY

Purpose: To assess self-rated personality.

Number of Items: 128

Format: Items rated on 8-point self-applicability scales.

Reliability: Reliabilities of eight subscales all greater than .80.

Author: Gifford, R.

Article: Projected interpersonal distance and orientation choices: Personality, sex, and social situations.

Journal: *Social Psychology Quarterly,* September 1982, *44*(3), 145–152.

Related Research: Wiggins, J. S. (1979). A psychological taxonomy of trait-descriptive terms: The interpersonal domain. *Journal of Personality and Social Psychology, 37,* 395–412.

CHAPTER 18
Preference

3388

Test Name: ACTIVITY PREFERENCE SCALE

Purpose: To identify activity preference.

Number of Items: 170

Format: Items consist of randomly ordered pairs of skilled and chance activities.

Reliability: Uncorrected split-half reliabilities ranged from .85 to .89.

Validity: Correlation with the Rotter I-E Scale was .19.

Author: Harris, R. M., Jr., and Salomone, P. R.

Article: Toward an abbreviated internal-external locus of control scale.

Journal: *Measurement and Evaluation in Guidance,* January 1981, *13*(4), 229–234.

Related Research: Schneider, J. H. (1968). Skill versus chance activity preference and locus of control. *Journal of Consulting and Clinical Psychology, 32,* 333–337.

■ ■ ■

3389

Test Name: BEM SEX-ROLE INVENTORY

Purpose: To measure sex-role orientation.

Number of Items: 54

Reliability: Coefficient alphas ranged from .80 to .86.

Validity: Correlations with the Intellectual Achievement Responsibility Questionnaire

ranged from −.41 to .56 (Ns = 12 to 404); with Fear of Success Scale ranged from −.37 to .33 (Ns = 12 to 404); with sex ranged from .30 to .56 (Ns = 26 to 404).

Author: Ireland-Galman, M. M., and Michael, W. B.

Article: The relationship of a measure of the fear of success construct to scales representing the locus of control and sex-role orientation constructs for a community college sample.

Journal: *Educational and Psychological Measurement,* Winter 1983, *43*(4), 1217–1225.

Related Research: Bem, S. L. (1974). The measurement of psychological androgyny. *Journal of Consulting and Clinical Psychology, 42,* 155–162.

■ ■ ■

3390

Test Name: CHOICE-MONITOR SCALE

Purpose: To measure intrinsic and extrinsic reasons for making choices.

Number of Items: 20

Format: Subjects select one of two choices (vocational or activity and check a reason for making it from among 10 alternatives, half extrinsic and half intrinsic).

Reliability: Cronbach's alpha was .65.

Author: Tzuriel, D., and Haywood, H. C.

Article: Locus of control and child-rearing practices in intrinsically

motivated and extrinsically motivated children.

Journal: *Psychological Reports,* December 1985, *57*(3-I), 887–894.

Related Research: Hamlin, R. M, & Nemo, R. S. (1962). Self-actualization in choice scores of improved schizophrenics. *Journal of Clinical Psychology, 18,* 51–54.

■ ■ ■

3391

Test Name: COGNITIVE PREFERENCE READING INSTRUMENT

Purpose: To measure degree of preference for four cognitive modes.

Number of Items: 15 paragraphs.

Format: Students indicate the most and least interesting sentences in paragraphs. Sentences written to be easily classified into four cognitive modes.

Reliability: Split-half reliability ranged from .60 to .71.

Validity: Correlations with an alternative cognitive preference measure ranged from .04 to .43.

Author: van den Berg, E., et al.

Article: Index of distinctness: A measure of the intensity of cognitive preferences.

Journal: *Journal of Educational Research,* March/April 1982, *75*(4), 197–203.

Related Research: van den Berg, E., et al. (1982). The convergent validity of the cognitive preference construct. *Journal of Research in Science Teaching, 19*(5), 337–350.

3392

Test Name: COUNSELOR PREFERENCE QUESTIONNAIRE

Purpose: To assess Black students' preferences for counselors of their own race.

Number of Items: 19

Format: Items rated on Likert scales.

Reliability: Kuder-Richardson formula 20 was .85.

Validity: A total of 13 of 17 expert judges had to approve items.

Author: Abott, K., et al.

Article: Counselor race as a factor in counselor preference.

Journal: *Journal of College Student Personnel,* January 1982, *23*(1), 36–40.

■ ■ ■

3393

Test Name: EDUCATIONAL ORIENTATION QUESTIONNAIRE

Purpose: To measure and rate characteristics of educational orientation in working with adults.

Number of Items: 60

Format: Agreement scale.

Reliability: Test–retest (2 weeks) reliability was .89. Alpha was .94. Item-total correlations ranged from .27 to .40 across subscales.

Author: Hyman, R. B., and Top, D.

Article: Effects of andragogical educational experience on andragogical orientation of nurses.

Journal: *Psychological Reports,* December 1984, *55*(3), 829–830.

Related Research: Hadley, H. N. (1975). Development of an instrument to determine adult educators' orientation: Andragogical or pedagogical. Doctoral dissertation, Boston University. *Dissertation Abstracts International, 35,* 75955. (University Microfilms No. 75–12, 228)

■ ■ ■

3394

Test Name: ENDEMIC IMAGERY QUESTIONNAIRE

Purpose: To measure the appeal of relaxing images and scenes.

Number of Items: 10

Format: Items rated on 5-point Likert response categories. All items are presented.

Reliability: Test–retest reliability was .79 (2-week interval).

Author: Saigh, P. A., and Antoun, F. T.

Article: Endemic images and the desensitization process.

Journal: *Journal of School Psychology,* 1984, *22*(2), 177–184.

Related Research: Saigh, P. A. (1980). The use of endemic images as a means of inducing relaxation and desensitization. *Mediterranean Journal of Social Psychiatry, 1,* 11–16.

■ ■ ■

3395

Test Name: EQUITY SENSITIVITY INSTRUMENT

Purpose: To tap an individual's preference for outcomes versus inputs in a general work situation.

Number of Items: 5

Format: Respondents address each item by distributing 10 points between an entitled response and a benevolent response.

Reliability: Coefficient alpha was .83.

Validity: Correlations with other variables ranged from –.10 to .20.

Author: Huseman, R. C., et al.

Article: Test for individual perception of job equity: Some preliminary findings.

Journal: *Perceptual and Motor Skills,* December 1985, *61*(3-II), 1055–1064.

■ ■ ■

3396

Test Name: FOOD PREFERENCE SURVEY

Purpose: To measure attitudes toward trying new foods.

Number of Items: 13

Format: Items rated on 5-point Likert response categories. Sample items are presented.

Reliability: Alpha was .86.

Validity: Correlated .62 ($p < .001$) with willingness to try unfamiliar food.

Author: Otis, L. P.

Article: Factors influencing the willingness to taste unusual foods.

Journal: *Psychological Reports,* June 1984, *54*(3), 739–745.

■ ■ ■

3397

Test Name: IMAGERY DIFFERENCE QUESTIONNAIRE

Purpose: To determine students' preference for visual or verbal imagery.

Number of Items: 54

Format: Items are forced-choice statements.

Reliability: Alpha coefficients were .74 and .72.

Author: Sheckles, M. P., and Eliot, J.

Article: Preference and solution patterns in mathematics performance.

Journal: *Perceptual and Motor Skills,* December 1983, *57*(3-I), 811–816.

Related Research: Paivio, A. (1971). *Imagery and verbal processes.* New York: Holt, Rinehart & Winston.

■ ■ ■

3398

Test Name: INSTITUTIONAL/ GOAL COMMITMENT

Purpose: To measure importance of college to freshmen.

Number of Items: 6

Format: Likert items.

Reliability: Alpha was .71.

Author: Pascarella, E. T., and Terenzini, P. T.

Article: Contextual analysis as a method for assessing resident group effects.

Journal: *Journal of College Student Personnel,* March 1982, *23*(2), 108–114.

Related Research: Pascarella, E. T., & Terenzini, P. T. (1980). Predicting persistence and voluntary dropout decisions from a theoretical model. *Journal of Higher Education, 51,* 60–75.

■ ■ ■

3399

Test Name: INTENTION TO SUPPORT UNION SCALE

Purpose: To measure favorable intentions to faculty union membership.

Number of Items: 28

Format: Items rated on 5-point agreement scales (7 items), 7-point bipolar evaluative scales (2 items), 3-point bipolar scales, and 5-point change scale (19 items).

Reliability: Internal consistency ranged from .87 to .88 across two subscales (one reliability not reported).

Author: Zalesny, M. D.

Article: Comparison of economic and noneconomic factors in predicting faculty veto preference in a union representation election.

Journal: *Journal of Applied Psychology,* May 1985, *70*(2), 243–256.

Related Research: Terborg, J. R. (1982, August). *University faculty dispositions toward unionization: A test of Triandis' model.* Paper presented at the meeting of the American Psychological Association, Washington, DC.

■ ■ ■

3400

Test Name: INTERVENTION RATING PROFILE

Purpose: To assess acceptability of interventions.

Number of Items: 20

Format: Items rated on 6-point Likert categories ranging from *strongly agree* to *strongly disagree.*

Reliability: Cronbach's alpha was .91 (from previous study, see related research).

Author: Elliott, S. N., et al.

Article: Acceptability of positive and reductive behavioral interventions: Factors that influence teachers' decisions.

Journal: *Journal of School Psychology,* 1984, *22*(4), 353–360.

Related Research: Witt, J. C., et al. (1983). Assessing the acceptability of behavioral interventions. *Psychology in the Schools, 20,* 510–517.

■ ■ ■

3401

Test Name: LEAST PREFERRED CO-WORKER SCALE

Purpose: To measure perception of least preferred co-workers.

Number of Items: 8

Format: Bipolar adjective pairs. Sample items presented.

Reliability: Alpha was .85.

Author: Hoffman, E., and Roman, P. M.

Article: Criterion-related validity of the least preferred co-worker measure.

Journal: *Journal of Social Psychology,* February 1984, *122*(first half), 79–84.

Related Research: Fiedler, F. E. (1981). Leadership effectiveness. *American Behavior Science, 24,* 619–632.

Hoffman, E. (1984). An internal dimensional analysis of the least preferred co-worker measure. *Journal of Social Psychology, 123,* 35–42.

■ ■ ■

3402

Test Name: LOGO SCALE

Purpose: To assess whether students are primarily oriented to learning (LO) or grades (GO).

Number of Items: 12

Format: Two-point agree–disagree format. All items are presented.

Reliability: Test–retest reliability was .71 (6 weeks). Median item total was .48.

Validity: 34 of 36 students known to be one or the other of the two orientations could be placed in their correct group by LOGO scores.

Author: Eison, J. A.

Article: A new instrument for assessing students' orientations towards grades or learning.

Journal: *Psychological Reports,* June 1983, *48*(3), 919–924.

■ ■ ■

3403

Test Name: MASCULINE GENDER IDENTITY SCALE

Purpose: To measure feminine identity.

Number of Items: 20

Format: Multiple-choice. All items presented. Adapted from Feminine Gender Identity Scale.

Reliability: Alpha was .89.

Validity: Discriminates transsexual, homosexual, and heterosexual subjects (69% of subjects classified correctly).

Author: Blanchard, R., and Freund, K.

Article: Measuring masculine gender identity in females.

Journal: *Journal of Consulting and Clinical Psychology,* April 1983, *51*(2), 205–214.

Related Research: Freund, K., et al. (1974). Extension of the Gender Identity Scale for Males. *Archives of Sexual Behavior, 3,* 249–260.

■ ■ ■

3404

Test Name: MIRENDA LEISURE INTEREST FINDER

Purpose: To identify leisure interests.

Number of Items: 90

Format: Includes a mixture of activities: games, sports, nature, and so forth. Employs a 5-point scale from like very much (5) to dislike very much (1).

Reliability: Internal reliability of .87.

Author: McDowell, C. F., and Clark, P.

Article: Assessing the leisure needs of older persons.

Journal: *Measurement and Evaluation in Guidance,* October 1982, *15*(3), 228–239.

Related Research: Wilson, G. T., & Mirenda, J. J. (1975). The Milwaukee leisure counseling model. *Counseling and Values, 20,* 42–46.

3405

Test Name: PREFERENCE FOR JOB ENRICHMENT SCALE

Purpose: To measure willingness to have jobs changed and enriched.

Number of Items: 6

Format: Items rated in 6-point Likert format. Sample items presented.

Reliability: Alpha was .85.

Author: Holley, W. H., et al.

Article: Negotiating quality of worklife, productivity and traditional issues: Union members' preferred roles of their union.

Journal: *Personnel Psychology,* Summer 1981, *34*(2), 309–328.

Related Research: Hackman, J. R., & Lawler, E. E. (1971). Employee reactions to job characteristics. *Journal of Applied Psychology, 16,* 259–286.

■ ■ ■

3406

Test Name: PREFERRED INSTRUCTOR CHARACTERISTICS SCALE

Purpose: To disclose the level of personal–social or cognitive–intellectual preference students have for teacher behaviors.

Number of Items: 36

Format: For each item students select one of two statements expressing a personal–social teacher behavior or a cognitive–intellectual teacher behavior. An example is presented.

Reliability: Test–retest reliability (4 weeks) was .88. Internal consistency reliability coefficient was .90.

Author: Dorhout, A.

Article: Student and teacher perceptions of preferred teacher behaviors among the academically gifted.

Journal: *Gifted Child Quarterly,* Summer 1983, *27*(3), 122–125.

Related Research: Krumholtz, J. D., & Faquhar, W. W. (1957). The effect of three teaching methods on achievement and motivation outcomes in a how-to-study course. *Psychological Monographs, 71*(14), 1–26.

■ ■ ■

3407

Test Name: RECREATION EXPERIENCE PREFERENCE SCALES

Purpose: To measure the need-satisfying properties of leisure activities.

Number of Items: 82

Format: Includes 41 two-item scales grouped into 18 preference domains. Items are rated on a Likert format with 6 response options from *not important* (1) to *extremely important* (6).

Reliability: Cronbach's alpha internal consistency reliability coefficient for 34 of the two-item scales ranged from .46 to .80.

Author: Tinsley, H. E. A., et al.

Article: Reliability and concurrent validity of the Recreation Experience Preference Scales.

Journal: *Educational and Psychological Measurement,* Autumn 1982, *41*(3), 897–907.

Related Research: Driver, B. L., & Cooksey, R. (1977). Preferred psychological outcomes of recreational fishing. *Proceedings of the Catch-and-Release Fishing as a Management Tool, National Sport Fishing Symposium.* Arcata, CA: Humboldt State University.

■ ■ ■

3408

Test Name: ROLE CATEGORY QUESTIONNAIRE

Purpose: To measure cognitive complexity.

Number of Items: 2

Format: Respondent writes a 5-minute essay describing a "liked" peer and a "disliked" peer. Descriptive constructs are counted and totalled from each essay.

Reliability: Interrater reliability exceeds .90.

Author: Capurso, R. J., and Blocher, D. H.

Article: The effects of sex-role consistent and inconsistent information on the social perceptions of complex, noncomplex, androgynous and sex-typed women.

Journal: *Journal of Vocational Behavior*, February 1985, *26*(1), 79–91.

Related Research: O'Keefe, D. J., & Sypher, H. E. 1980. *Cognitive complexity and communication: A critical review of alternative measures.* Unpublished manuscript, Department of Speech Communication, Pennsylvania State University.

■ ■ ■

3409

Test Name: SCALE OF COUNSELING DIMENSION PREFERENCES

Purpose: To assess preferences of bereaved parents for counseling during difficult phases of grieving.

Number of Items: 24

Format: Includes items dealing with: action orientation, insight orientation, cognition, conation, structure, and ambiguity.

Reliability: Interrater agreement for the 6 dimensions ranged from .83 to .94.

Author: Alexy, W. D.

Article: Dimensions of psychological counseling that

facilitate the grieving process of bereaved parents.

Journal: *Journal of Counseling Psychology*, September 1982, *29*(5), 498–507.

Related Research: Bowlby, J. (1980). *Loss: Sadness and depression.* New York: Basic Books.

■ ■ ■

3410

Test Name: SCIENCE COGNITIVE PREFERENCE INVENTORY

Purpose: To measure degree of preference for four cognitive modes.

Number of Items: 30

Format: Four correct response statements to items are ranked and rated according to preference.

Reliability: Cronbach's alpha ranged from .26 to .90.

Validity: Correlations with an alternative measure of cognitive preference ranged from .04 to .43.

Author: van den Berg, E., et al.

Article: Index of distinctiveness: A measure of the intensity of cognitive preferences.

Journal: *Journal of Educational Research*, March/April 1982, *75*(4), 197–203.

Related Research: van den Berg, E., et al. (1982). The convergent validity of the cognitive preference construct. *Journal of Research in Science Teaching, 19*(5), 337–350.

■ ■ ■

3411

Test Name: SEX-ROLE IDEOLOGY SCALE

Purpose: To measure prescriptive beliefs about appropriate behavior to men and women.

Number of Items: 30

Format: Items rated on a 7-point

Likert agreement–disagreement scale.

Reliability: Interitem Cronbach's alpha (total scale) was .82. Cronbach's alphas across subscales ranged from .28 to .82.

Author: Milo, T., et al.

Article: Conceptual analysis of the Sex-Role Ideology Scale.

Journal: *Psychological Reports*, August 1983, *53*(1), 139–146.

Related Research: Kalin, R., & Tilby, P. (1978). Development and validation of a Sex-Role Ideology Scale. *Psychological Reports, 42,* 731–738.

■ ■ ■

3412

Test Name: SOCIAL BEHAVIOR INVENTORY—REVISED

Purpose: To measure preference for cooperation and competition by self-report.

Number of Items: 25

Format: Items rated on 5-point Likert type agree–disagree response categories. All items are presented.

Reliability: Spearman-Brown reliability ranged from .77 to .78 over two factors.

Validity: Low but significant correlations found with mothers', fathers', and teachers' ratings of behavior and children's ratings.

Author: Stockdale, D. F., et al.

Article: Cooperative-competitive preferences and behavioral correlates as a function of sex and age of school-age children.

Journal: *Psychological Reports,* December 1983, *53*(3-I), 739–750.

Related Research: Galejs, I., & Stockdale, D. F. (1980). Cooperative preferences and locus of control of school-age children. *Home Economics Research Journal, 8,* 386–393.

3413

Test Name: STUDENT-ATHLETE RECRUITMENT DECISION-MAKING SURVEY

Purpose: To measure importance student athletes attach to coach, campus, athletics, friends, and academics.

Number of Items: 59

Format: Items rated on 5-point Likert scales.

Reliability: Alphas were coach, .95; campus, .93; athletics, .83; friends, .75; academics, .83.

Author: Mathes, S., and Gurney, G.

Article: Factors in student athletes' choices of colleges.

Journal: *Journal of College Student Personnel,* July 1985, *26*(4), 327–333.

Related Research: Swaim, N. M. (1983). *Factors influencing college basketball players to attend selected NCAA Division I colleges, NCAA Division II colleges or NAIA colleges or NCAA Division III colleges.* Unpublished master's thesis, Iowa State University.

■ ■ ■

3414

Test Name: TOY PREFERENCE TEST

Purpose: To measure children's sex-role preference.

Format: Consists of a booklet of pictures of toys and the child selects those with which the child would most like to play.

Reliability: Test–retest reliabilities ranged from .011 to .818.

Validity: Correlations with mother's preference was .204 (daughter) and –.087 (son); father's preference was –.089

(daughter) and –.046 (son).

Author: Newman, R. C., and Carney, R. E.

Article: Cross-validation of sex-role measures for children with correlation of sex-role measures for children and parents.

Journal: *Perceptual and Motor Skills,* June 1981, *52*(3), 883–890.

Related Research: DeLucia, L. A. (1963). The toy preference test: A measure of sex-role identification. *Child Development, 34,* 107–117.

■ ■ ■

3415

Test Name: UNIONISM SCALE

Purpose: To measure the value of union representation.

Number of Items: 6

Format: Items rated on 6-point agreement scales. All items are presented.

Reliability: Internal consistency was .80.

Validity: Correlated .56 and .42 ($p < .001$) with direct questions about instrumentality of union as a mechanism for change.

Author: Hammer, T. H.

Article: Absenteeism when workers have a voice: The case of employee ownership.

Journal: *Journal of Applied Psychology,* October 1981, *66*(5), 561–573.

■ ■ ■

3416

Test Name: VALANCE OF OUTCOMES SCALE

Purpose: To measure importance of instrumental outcomes.

Number of Items: 13

Format: Items rated on a 5-point desirability scale.

Reliability: Alphas ranged from .79 to .87 for extrinsic and intrinsic items.

Validity: Did not correlate with pro-strike attitude or locus of control. Did correlate significantly with intention to join a union ($r = .27$).

Author: Beutell, N. J., and Biggs, D. L.

Article: Behavioral intentions to join a union: Instrumentality x valence, locus of control and strike attitudes.

Journal: *Psychological Reports,* August 1984, *55*(1), 215–222.

■ ■ ■

3417

Test Name: WOLOWITZ FOOD PREFERENCE INQUIRY

Purpose: To measure food preferences.

Number of Items: 103

Format: Items contrast food preferences (spicy vs. bland, sweet vs. sour, soft vs. hard).

Reliability: Kuder-Richardson formula 20 was .62 for men ($N = 73$) and .74 for women ($N = 122$).

Validity: Correlates with orality (.27 for men, –.18 for women), but not with sadism (.10 for men, .13 for women).

Author: Juni, S.

Article: Food preference and orality.

Journal: *Psychological Reports,* June 1983, *52*(3), 842.

Related Research: Wolowitz, H. M. (1964). Food preference as an index of orality. *Journal of Abnormal Social Psychology, 69,* 650–654.

CHAPTER 19
Problem Solving and Reasoning

3418

Test Name: ANALOGICAL REASONING TEST

Purpose: To measure analogical reasoning of kindergarten and first-grade children.

Number of Items: 10

Format: Students supplied the missing word in each analogy. Each response was scored *pass* (1) or *fail* (0). Examples are presented.

Reliability: Coefficient alpha was .74.

Validity: Correlation with English proficiency ranged from .01 to .15.

Author: Diaz, R. M.

Article: Bilingual cognitive development: Addressing three gaps in current research.

Journal: *Child Development,* December 1985, *56*(6), 1376–1388.

■ ■ ■

3419

Test Name: ARLIN TEST OF FORMAL REASONING

Purpose: To measure formal reasoning.

Number of Items: 42

Format: Consists of 4-response multiple-choice items and includes 9 classical types of thinking operations and schemata.

Reliability: Interrater reliabilities ranged from .52 to .97.

Validity: Construct validity coefficients ranged from .55 to .74. Correlations with predictor and criterion variables ranged from

−.32 to .45 (*N* = 218) and −.32 to .47 (*N* = 259).

Author: Bloland, R. M., and Michael, W. B.

Article: A comparison of the relative validity of a measure of Piagetian cognitive development and a set of conventional prognostic measures in the prediction of the future success of ninth- and tenth-grade students in algebra.

Journal: *Educational and Psychological Measurement,* Winter 1984, *44*(4), 925–943.

■ ■ ■

3420

Test Name: BALANCE BEAM TEST

Purpose: To measure proportional reasoning.

Number of Items: 16

Format: Multiple-choice.

Reliability: .75

Author: Linn, M. C., and Swiney, J. F.

Article: Individual differences in formal thought: Role of expectations and aptitudes.

Journal: *Journal of Educational Psychology,* April 1981, *73*(2), 274–286.

Related Research: Linn, M. C., & Pulos, S. (1980). *Proportional reasoning during adolescence: The balance puzzle* (Adolescent Reasoning Project, Rep. No. 25). Berkeley: The University of California, Lawrence Hall of Science.

3421

Test Name: BIERI GRID

Purpose: To measure cognitive complexity.

Number of Items: 10

Format: Semantic differential.

Reliability: Test–retest reliability was .86.

Author: Wexley, K. N., and Youtz, M. A.

Article: Rater beliefs about others: Their effects on rating errors and rater accuracy.

Journal: *Journal of Occupational Psychology,* December 1985, *58*(4), 265–275.

Related Research: Tripodi, T., & Bieri, J. (1963). Cognitive complexity as a function of own and provided constructs. *Psychological Reports, 13,* 26.

■ ■ ■

3422

Test Name: COGNITIVE LATERALITY QUESTIONNAIRE

Purpose: To measure hemispheric dominance.

Number of Items: 3 left and 3 right hemisphere tests.

Format: Varies by test—all tests are described.

Reliability: Cronbach's alphas were .80 or more.

Validity: Correctly classifies 95% of brain-damaged patients.

Author: Harpaz, I.

Article: Asymmetry of cognitive

functioning as a possible predictor for vocational counseling and personnel classification.

Journal: *Journal of Vocational Behavior,* December 1983, *23*(3), 305–317.

Related Research: Benton, S., & Gordon, H. W. (1979). Assessment of cognitive asymmetries in brain-damaged and normal subjects: Validation of a test battery. *Journal of Neurology, Neurosurgery and Psychiatry, 42,* 715–723.

■ ■ ■

3423

Test Name: COGNITIVE PROCESS QUESTIONNAIRE

Purpose: To measure students' thought processes during periods of teaching-learning.

Number of Items: 23

Format: Items rated on 5-point response categories (*usually* to *almost never*, plus *don't know*). Sample items presented.

Reliability: Alpha –.71 (alphas vary from .22 to .65 on subscales).

Author: Peterson, P. L., et al.

Article: Students' aptitudes and their reports of cognitive processes during direct instruction.

Journal: *Journal of Educational Psychology,* August 1972, *74*(4), 535–547.

■ ■ ■

3424

Test Name: CONCEPTUAL LEVEL ANALOGY TEST

Purpose: To measure abstract reasoning predictive of morbidity and mortality following cardiac surgery.

Number of Items: 41

Format: Multiple-choice.

Reliability: Point-biserial correlations between correct item

response and total score were all significant (*p* < .05).

Validity: Significant differences by age, education, and occupation.

Author: Kelleher, W. J., and Townes, B. D.

Article: The conceptual level analogy test: Internal consistency and relationship to demographic variables.

Journal: *Psychological Reports,* June 1984, *54*(3), 971–976.

■ ■ ■

3425

Test Name: DECISION-MAKING STYLE SCALE (subscale of the ACDM)

Purpose: To measure how respondents make important decisions. Respondents choose between rational, intuitive, and dependent styles.

Number of Items: 30

Format: Dichotomous agree–disagree. Sample items presented.

Reliability: Test–retest ranged from .76 to .85. Internal consistency ranged from .60 to .72.

Author: Phillips, S. D., et al.

Article: A factor analytic investigation of career decision-making styles.

Journal: *Journal of Vocational Behavior,* February 1985, *26*(1), 106–115.

Related Research: Harren, V. A. (1978). *Assessment of career decision-making (ACDM): Counselor/Instructor Guide.* Unpublished manuscript, Southern Illinois University.

■ ■ ■

3426

Test Name: DEDUCTIVE/INDUCTIVE REASONING TESTS

Purpose: To measure deductive and inductive reasoning ability.

Number of Items: 14 (7 deductive, 7 inductive).

Format: Multiple-choice. Sample items are presented.

Reliability: Kuder-Richardson formula 20 coefficients were .45 (deductive) and .42 (inductive).

Validity: Correlations between each test with 11 other tests (reading, inference, tabular completion, letter series, figure analogies, judgment, logical order, computation, arithmetic reasoning) ranged from .23 to .62.

Author: Colberg, M., et al.

Article: Convergence of the inductive and deductive models in the measuring of reasoning abilities.

Journal: *Journal of Applied Psychology,* November 1985, *70*(4), 681–694.

■ ■ ■

3427

Test Name: FORMAL OPERATIONS ASSESSMENT BATTERY

Purpose: To measure logical reasoning skills.

Time Required: 45 minutes.

Reliability: Cronbach's alpha was .83.

Validity: Correlates with Wechsler Intelligence Scale for children (.57 with full scale, .48 with verbal scale, and .24 with performance scale). Correlates .56 with Raven's Progressive Matrices.

Author: Lonky, E.

Article: Logical concept prerequisites to political development in adolescence.

Journal: *Psychological Reports,* December 1983, *53*(3-I), 947–954.

Related Research: Arnold, D., et

al. (1980). *The relationship of two measures of formal operations to psychometric intelligence.* Paper presented at the annual meeting of the Eastern Psychological Association, Hartford, CT.

■ ■ ■

3428

Test Name: FORMAL OPERATIONAL REASONING TEST

Purpose: To assess a subject's comprehension of second-order operations that are used as barometers of formal thought.

Number of Items: 25

Time Required: 45 minutes.

Format: One sorting problem, 16 proportional logic items, and 8 proportionality items. Sample items are presented.

Reliability: Test–retest (sorting problem) reliability ranged from .80 to .81. Kuder-Richardson formula 20 (proportional and proportionality) ranged from .52 to .75.

Validity: Subscales factored with other scales in an interpretable manner.

Author: Roberge, J. J., and Flexer, B. K.

Article: The formal operational reasoning test.

Journal: *Journal of General Psychology,* January 1982, *106*(first half), 61–67.

■ ■ ■

3429

Test Name: INTERPERSONALLY BASED PROBLEM-SOLVING SCALE (IBPS)

Purpose: To assess how consultants facilitate problem-solving.

Number of Items: 42

Reliability: Cronbach's alpha was .96.

Validity: Correlates with behavior change (.37); with teacher satisfaction (.71); with problem resolution (.74); and with professional growth (.67). All $ps <$ .01.

Author: Maitland, R. E., et al.

Article: The effects of an interpersonally based problem-solving process on consultation outcomes.

Journal: *Journal of School Psychology,* Winter 1985, *23*(4), 337–345.

Related Research: Maitland, R. E., et al. (1981). *The interpersonally-based problem-solving scale field test instrument.* Lawrence: University of Kansas.

■ ■ ■

3430

Test Name: INTUITIVE ABILITY TEST

Purpose: To measure ability to reach a successful conclusion based upon insufficient information.

Number of Items: 20

Format: Includes verbal–serial, verbal analogy, numerical–serial, and numerical analogy items.

Reliability: Split-half reliabilities ranged from .36 to .91 ($Ns = 28$ to 38). Internal consistency ranged from .27 to .51. Test–retest reliability (3 years) ranged from .50 to .66 ($N = 95$).

Author: Fallik, B., and Eliot, J.

Article: Intuition, cognitive style and hemispheric processing.

Journal: *Perceptual and Motor Skills,* June 1985, *60*(3), 683–697.

Related Research: Westcott, M. R. (1968). *Psychology of intuition.* New York: Holt, Rinehart & Winston.

3431

Test Name: INVENTORY OF LEARNING PROCESSES

Purpose: To measure learning processes.

Number of Items: 62 (four subscales).

Format: True–false questions. Sample items presented.

Reliability: Ranged from .79 to .88 across subscales.

Author: Alesandrini, K. L., et al.

Article: Visual-verbal and analytic-holistic strategies, abilities, and styles.

Journal: *Journal of Educational Research,* January/February 1984, *77*(3), 150–157.

Related Research: Schmeck, R. R., et al. (1977). Development of a self-report inventory for assessing individual differences in learning process. *Applied Psychological Measurement, 1,* 413–431.

■ ■ ■

3432

Test Name: KIRTON ADAPTATION INVENTORY

Purpose: To measure adaptation of innovative styles of problem-solving.

Number of Items: 32

Reliability: Internal reliability (alpha) ranged from .85 to .88. Test–retest ranged from .82 to .85.

Validity: Correlates .40 with ratings of innovativeness ($p <$ .001).

Author: Kirton, M. J., and McCarthy, R. M.

Article: Personal and group estimates of the Kirton inventory scores.

Journal: *Psychological Reports,* December 1985, *57*(3-II), 1067–1070.

Related Research: Kirton, M. J. (1976). Adaptors and innovators: A description and measure. *Journal of Applied Psychology, 61,* 622–629.

• • •

3433

Test Name: MEANS-ENDS PROBLEM-SOLVING TEST

Purpose: To measure means-ends problem-solving ability.

Number of Items: 6

Format: The child is presented the beginning and the outcome of each of six stories. The child is asked to fill in the middle part or to explain how the ending occurred.

Reliability: Interrater reliabilities ranged from .86 to .98. Cronbach's alphas ranged from .62 to .88.

Validity: Correlations with other variables ranged from −.02 to .56.

Author: Pellegrini, D. S.

Article: Social cognition and competence in middle childhood.

Journal: *Child Development,* February 1985, *56*(1), 253–264.

Related Research: Shure, M. B., & Spivack, G. (1972). Means–ends thinking, adjustment and social class among elementary school-aged children. *Journal of Consulting and Clinical Psychology, 38,* 348–353.

• • •

3434

Test Name: PREACTIVE DECISION EXERCISES

Purpose: To measure teachers' ability to make teaching decisions.

Number of Items: 131

Format: Problem situation described and followed by several courses of action that teachers may choose or may not choose.

Sample problem and items are presented.

Reliability: Kuder-Richardson formula 20 was .72.

Author: McNergney, R. F., et al.

Article: Assessing teachers' planning abilities.

Journal: *Journal of Educational Research,* November/December 1983, *77*(2), 108–111.

Related Research: Frederiksen, N., et al. (1957). The in-basket test. *Psychological Monographs: General and Applied, 71*(9), 1–28.

• • •

3435

Test Name: PREDICTING DISPLACED VOLUME TEST

Purpose: To assess predictions made about displacement of water.

Number of Items: 8

Format: Multiple-choice. Sample items presented.

Reliability: Alpha ranged from .82 (7th grade) to .88 (11th grade).

Validity: Correlates .68 with test using real water and real blocks to displace it.

Author: Linn, M. C., and Pulos, S.

Article: Male-female differences in predicting displaced volume: Strategy, usage, aptitude relationships and experience influences.

Journal: *Journal of Educational Psychology,* February 1983, *75*(1), 86–96.

• • •

3436

Test Name: PROBLEM-SOLVING INVENTORY

Purpose: To measure problem-solving strategies in children.

Number of Items: 25

Format: Items rated on a 5-point

rating scale for importance of each item.

Reliability: Alphas ranged from .61 to .75 across subscales.

Author: Fry, P. S., and Addington, J.

Article: Comparison of social problem-solving of children from open and traditional classrooms: A two-year longitudinal study.

Journal: *Journal of Educational Psychology,* April 1984, *76*(2), 318–329.

Related Research: Heppner, P. P., & Petersen, C. H. (1977). *The development, factor analysis, and validation of a problem-solving instrument.* Unpublished manuscript. Lincoln, NE: University of Nebraska.

• • •

3437

Test Name: PROBLEM-SOLVING INVENTORY

Purpose: To provide an estimate of self-appraised problem-solving behaviors and attitudes.

Number of Items: 32

Format: Includes three dimensions: problem-solving confidence, approach-avoidance, and personal control.

Reliability: Reliability ranged from .72 to .90.

Validity: Correlations with decision-making scales ranged from −.55 to .38.

Author: Phillips, S. D., et al.

Article: Decision-making styles and problem-solving appraisal.

Journal: *Journal of Counseling Psychology,* October 1984, *31*(4), 497–502.

Related Research: Heppner, P. P., & Petersen, C. H. (1982). The development and implications of a personal problem-solving inventory. *Journal of Counseling Psychology, 29*, 66–75.

■ ■ ■

3438

Test Name: PROBLEM-SOLVING INVENTORY

Purpose: To measure beliefs about problem-solving skills and behavior patterns.

Number of Items: 35

Format: Items rated in 6-point Likert format.

Reliability: Internal consistency ranged from .72 to .90. Test–retest ranged from .83 to .89 across three subscales.

Validity: Significant correlations between subscales and dimensions of coping ranged from .04 to .54 in absolute value.

Author: Ritchey, K. M., et al.

Article: Problem-solving appraisal versus hypothetical problem-solving.

Journal: *Psychological Reports,* December 1984, *55*(3), 815–818.

■ ■ ■

3439

Test Name: PROBLEM-SOLVING INVENTORY

Purpose: To assess attitudes and behaviors associated with effective problem-solving.

Number of Items: 35

Format: True–false format.

Validity: Correlates significantly (.47) with rational beliefs. Mothers low in intensity of punishment score high on problem-solving.

Author: Shorkey, C. T., and McRoy, R. G.

Article: Intensity of parental punishments and problem-solving attitudes and behaviors.

Journal: *Psychological Reports,*

February 1985, *56*(1), 283–286.

Related Research: Heppner, P. P., & Petersen, C. H. (1983). The development and implications of a personal problem-solving inventory. *Journal of Counseling Psychology, 30*, 537–545.

■ ■ ■

3440

Test Name: REVISED INDIVIDUAL DIFFERENCES QUESTIONNAIRE

Purpose: To assess the extent to which an individual typically uses imagery and verbal processes in thinking, studying, and problem-solving.

Number of Items: 54

Format: Includes two factors: verbal and imaginal.

Reliability: Coefficient alphas were .72 (verbal) and .74 (imagery).

Author: Fallik, B., and Eliot, J.

Article: Intuition, cognitive style and hemispheric processing.

Journal: *Perceptual and Motor Skills,* June 1985, *60*(3), 683–697.

Related Research: Perunko, M. (1982). *Relationships among mental imagery, spatial ability, analytic and synthetic processing and performance on mathematical problems.* Unpublished doctoral dissertation, University of Maryland.

Paivio, A., & Harshman, R. A. (1983). Factor analysis of a questionnaire in imagery and verbal habits and skills. *Canadian Journal of Psychology, 37*, 461–483.

■ ■ ■

3441

Test Name: SHIGAKI-WOLF LOGIC TEST

Purpose: To measure children's

class and conditional logic abilities.

Number of Items: 33

Format: Includes three or four items to measure each of 10 principles of logic. Subjects are required to generate the appropriate missing element for each syllogism.

Reliability: Test–retest (1 week) reliabilities ranged from .87 to .94 (*N* = 36).

Author: Shigaki, I. S., and Wolf, W.

Article: Comparison of class and conditional logic abilities of gifted and normal children.

Journal: *Child Study Journal,* 1982, *12*(3), 161–170.

Related Research: Shigaki, I. S., & Wolf, W. (1980). Hierarchies of formal syllogistic reasoning of young gifted children. *Child Study Journal, 10*, 87–106.

■ ■ ■

3442

Test Name: TEST OF FORMAL REASONING

Purpose: To assess levels of reasoning.

Number of Items: 48

Format: Multiple-choice organized into nine subtests: classification, volume, combinations, isolation of variables, proportions, probability, correlation, mechanical equilibrium, coordination of two frames of reference. A few examples are presented.

Reliability: Coefficients ranged from .52 to .85.

Validity: Kendall's tau ranged from .55 to .74.

Author: Arlin, P. K.

Article: A multitrait–multimethod

validity study of a test of formal reasoning.

Journal: *Educational and Psychological Measurement,* Winter 1982, *42*(4), 1077–1088.

■ ■ ■

3443

Test Name: TEST OF TEST-WISENESS—REVISED

Purpose: To measure test-wiseness of college students.

Number of Items: 41

Format: Includes measures of two test-wiseness elements: deductive reasoning strategies and cue-using strategies.

Reliability: Coefficient alpha was .844.

Validity: Correlations with other variables ranged from −.40 to .70.

Author: Borrello, G. M., and Thompson, B.

Article: Correlates of selected test-wiseness skills.

Journal: *Journal of Experimental Education,* Spring 1985, *53*(3), 124–128.

Related Research: Ferrell, G. M. (1972). The relationship of scores on a measure of test-wiseness to performance on teacher-made objective achievement examinations and on standardized ability and achievement tests, to grade-point average, and to sex for each of five high school samples. Doctoral dissertation, University of Southern California. *Dissertation Abstracts International, 33,* 1510-A. (University Microfilms No. 72-26,013)

CHAPTER 20
Status

3444

Test Name: HOME INDEX

Purpose: To measure SES by asking children about parent's home and activities.

Number of Items: 22

Format: Factual question format.

Validity: Thirteen items were validated against known father's occupation.

Author: Hailer, E. J., and Davis, S. A.

Article: Teacher perceptions, parental social status and grouping for reading instruction.

Journal: *Sociology of Education,* July 1981, *54*(3), 162–174.

Related Research: Gough, H. (1949). A short social status inventory. *Journal of Educational Psychology, 40,* 42–56.

Robinson, J., et al. (1969). *Measures of occupational attitudes and occupational characteristics.* Ann Arbor, MI: Institute for Social Research.

• • •

3445

Test Name: INDEX OF EVALUATED INEQUALITY

Purpose: To measure perceptions of the fairness of social inequalities.

Number of Items: 5

Format: Items rated in 4-point agree–disagree format. Sample item presented.

Reliability: Cronbach's alpha was .51.

Author: Smith, K. B., and Green, D. N.

Article: Individual correlates of the belief in a just world.

Journal: *Psychological Reports,* April 1984, *54*(2), 435–438.

Related Research: Robinson, R., & Bell, W. (1978). Equality, success, and social justice. *American Sociological Review, 43,* 65–89.

• • •

3446

Test Name: INDEX OF PERCEIVED INEQUALITY

Purpose: To measure perceptions of the extensiveness of social inequalities.

Number of Items: 20

Format: Agree–disagree response categories. Sample item presented.

Reliability: Cronbach's alpha was .71.

Author: Smith, K. B., and Green, D. N.

Article: Individual correlates of the belief in a just world.

Journal: *Psychological Reports,* April 1984, *54*(2), 435–438.

Related Research: Bell, W., & Robinson, R. (1980). Cognitive maps of class and racial inequalities in England and the United States. *American Journal of Sociology, 43,* 320–349.

• • •

3447

Test Name: OCCUPATIONAL ASPIRATION SCALE

Purpose: To measure the level of occupational prestige.

Number of Items: 8

Format: Includes four specific domains and four goal levels. The score for each question ranged from 0 to 9.

Reliability: Test–retest reliability coefficients were .78 (2 weeks) and .88 (5 weeks).

Author: Moracco, J., et al.

Article: A comparison of the occupational aspirations of a select group of military men and women.

Journal: *Vocational Guidance Quarterly,* December 1981, *30*(2), 149–156.

Related Research: Hailer, A. O., & Miller, I. W. (1963). *The Occupational Aspiration Scale: Theory, structure and correlates* (Technical Bulletin No. 288). East Lansing: Michigan State University.

• • •

3448

Test Name: RACIAL SEMANTIC DIFFERENTIAL

Purpose: To assess racial evaluation.

Number of Items: 60

Format: Includes five color-person concepts each rated on 12 bipolar scales.

Validity: Correlation with Tennessee Self-Concept Scale was .02; with Index of Adjustment and Values (self-ideal) was –.02; with Index of Adjustment and Values (self-acceptance) was .05.

Author: Hines, P., and Berg-Cross, L.

Article: Racial differences and global self-esteem.

Journal: *Journal of Social Psychology*, April 1981, *113*(second half), 271–281.

Related Research: Williams, J. (1964). Connotations of color names among Negros and Caucasians. *Perceptual and Motor Skills, 18,* 721–731.

■ ■ ■

3449

Test Name: SOCIOMETRIC PEER-RATING SCALE

Purpose: To provide a measure of social status for first- and second-graders.

Number of Items: 28

Format: Each child rates every classmate by marking a happy face (likes to play with), neutral face (sometimes likes to play with), or sad face (do not like to play with).

Reliability: Test–retest (7 months) Spearman rho was .69. Split-half corrected Spearman rho was .83.

Validity: Correlations with other variables ranged from –.46 to .88.

Author: Riley, W. T.

Article: Reliability and validity of a cost-efficient sociometric measure.

Journal: *Journal of Psychopathology and Behavioral Assessment,* September 1985, *7*(3), 235–241.

Related Research: Asher, S. R., et al. (1979). A reliable sociometric measure for preschool children. *Developmental Psychology, 15,* 443–444.

CHAPTER 21
Trait Measurement

3450

Test Name: A–B RATING SCALE

Purpose: To measure type A behavior pattern in children.

Number of Items: 24

Format: Each item is answered on a 7-point scale arranged as a ladder. All items are presented.

Reliability: Spearman-Brown odd–even correlation coefficient was .59 ($N = 336$).

Author: Wolf, T. M., et al.

Article: Validation of a measure of type A behavior pattern in children: Bogalusa heart study.

Journal: *Child Development,* February 1982, *53*(1), 126–135.

Related Research: Bortner, R. (1969). A short ruling scale as a potential measure of pattern A behavior. *Journal of Chronic Diseases, 22,* 87–91.

■ ■ ■

3451

Test Name: ADULT SELF-EXPRESSION SCALE

Purpose: To measure assertive behavior.

Number of Items: 48

Format: Includes 25 positively worded and 23 negatively worded items. Responses to each item are recorded on a 5-point Likert format (0–4).

Reliability: Test–retest reliability estimate was .89.

Author: Lafromboise, T. D.

Article: The factorial validity of the adult self-expression scale with American Indians.

Journal: *Educational and Psychological Measurement,* Summer 1983, *43*(2), 547–555.

Related Research: Gay, M. L, et al. (1975). An assertiveness inventory for adults. *Journal of Counseling Psychology, 22,* 340–344.

■ ■ ■

3452

Test Name: AGGRESSION WORD ASSOCIATION TEST

Purpose: To measure aggressive associations.

Number of Items: 5 stimulus words denoting aggression embedded in a total of 11 words.

Format: Subjects given 30 seconds to produce 5 associations to each of 11 stimulus words. Primary associations are scored.

Reliability: .72 to .83.

Author: Russell, G. W.

Article: A comparison of hostility measures.

Journal: *Journal of Social Psychology,* February 1981, *113*(first half), 45–55.

Related Research: Gellerman, S. (1956). The *effects of experimentally induced aggression and inhibition on word-association sequences.* Unpublished dissertation, University of Pennsylvania.

3453

Test Name: AGGRESSIVE BEHAVIOR SCALE

Purpose: To measure aggressive behavior in children.

Number of Items: 10

Format: 0 to 3 severity rating. Sample item presented.

Reliability: Alphas ranged from .78 to .92 across subscales.

Author: Margalit, M.

Article: Perception of parents' behavior, familial satisfaction, and sense of coherence in hyperactive children.

Journal: *Journal of School Psychology,* Winter 1985, *23*(4), 355–364.

Related Research: Prinz, R. J., et al. (1981). Hyperactive and aggressive behaviors in childhood: Intertwined dimensions. *Journal of Abnormal Child Psychology, 9,* 191–202.

Stewart, M. A., et al. (1980). Aggressive conduct disorders of children. *Journal of Nervous and Mental Disease, 168,* 605–610.

■ ■ ■

3454

Test Name: ANGER INVENTORY

Purpose: To provide an index of anger reactions to a wide range of provocations.

Number of Items: 80

Format: Each item consists of an anger provoking incident to which the subject responds on a 5-point scale according to the perceived degree of provocation if the incident actually happened.

Reliability: Test–retest reliability coefficient was .17.

Author: Biaggio, M. K., et al.

Article: Reliability and validity of four anger scales.

Journal: *Journal of Personality Assessment*, December 1981, *45*(6), 639–648.

Related Research: Biaggio, M. K. (1980). Assessment of anger arousal. *Journal of Personality Assessment, 44*, 289–298.

■ ■ ■

3455

Test Name: ANGER SELF-REPORT

Purpose: To differentiate between the awareness and expression of anger/aggression.

Number of Items: 64

Format: Likert questionnaire yielding scores for awareness of anger, expression of anger (including subscales for general, physical, and verbal expression), guilt, condemnation of anger, and mistrust.

Reliability: Test–retest reliability coefficients ranged from .28 to .76 for subscales and .54 for total.

Author: Biaggio, M. K., et al.

Article: Reliability and validity of four anger scales.

Journal: *Journal of Personality Assessment,* December 1981, *45*(6), 639–648.

Related Research: Zelin, M. L., et al. (1972). Anger and self-report: An objective questionnaire for the measurement of aggression. *Journal of Consulting and Clinical Psychology, 39*, 340.

3456

Test Name: ARGUMENTATIVENESS SCALE

Purpose: To measure the individual's general trait to be argumentative.

Number of Items: 20

Format: A self-report scale on which the subject indicates for each item whether it is *almost never true* (1), *rarely true* (2), *occasionally true* (3), *often true* (4), or *almost always true* (5). All items are presented.

Reliability: Cronbach's coefficient alphas were .91 and .86 (*N* = 692). Test–retest (1 week) reliabilities were .87 and .86 (*N* = 35).

Validity: Correlations with communication predispositions ranged from –.45 to .47. Correlations with behavioral choices ranged from –.39 to .35.

Author: Infante, D. A., and Rancer, A. S.

Article: A conceptualization and measure of argumentativeness.

Journal: *Journal of Personality Assessment,* February 1982, *46*(1), 72–80.

■ ■ ■

3457

Test Name: ASSERTION INVENTORY

Purpose: To measure assertion.

Number of Items: 40

Format: Responses to each item are first made on a 5-point scale from 1 (*none*) to 5 (*very much*), indicating degree of discomfort in various situations. Responses are then made on another 5-point scale from 1 (*always*) to 5 (*never*), indicating the probability of engaging in those behaviors.

Reliability: Test–retest (5 weeks)

reliability was .87 and .81 (*N* = 49).

Author: Ramanaiah, N. V., et al.

Article: Personality and self-actualizing profiles of assertive people.

Journal: *Journal of Personality Assessment,* August 1985, *49*(4), 440–443.

Related Research: Gambrill, E., & Ritchey, C. (1975). An assertion inventory for use in assessment and research. *Behavior Therapy, 6*, 550–561.

■ ■ ■

3458

Test Name: ASSERTIVE JOB-HUNTING SURVEY

Purpose: To assess self-reported job-hunting assertiveness.

Number of Items: 25

Format: Subjects respond on a 1 to 6 point scale as to how likely they would be to respond in the described manner, where 1 is *very unlikely* and 6 is *very likely*.

Reliability: Cronbach's measure of internal consistency was .82. Test–retest (2 months) correlation was .77.

Validity: Point-biserial correlations with sex, *r* = .13 and with previous job-hunting experience, *r* = .19.

Author: Becker, H. A.

Article: The assertive job-hunting survey.

Journal: *Measurement and Evaluation in Guidance,* April 1980, *13*(1), 43–48.

■ ■ ■

3459

Test Name: ASSERTIVENESS SELF-REPORT INVENTORY

Purpose: To provide a self-report measure of assertiveness.

Number of Items: 25

Format: Subjects respond by answering *true* or *false* to each item. All items are presented.

Reliability: Test–retest reliability (5 weeks) was .81; for women, r = .80 and for men, r = .96.

Validity: Correlations with the Rathus Assertiveness Schedule were .70 and .63; for women correlations were .69 and .60 and for men correlations were .74 and .77.

Author: Herzberger, S. D., et al.

Article: The development of an assertiveness self-report inventory.

Journal: *Journal of Personality Assessment,* June 1984, *48*(3), 317–323.

• • •

3460

Test Name: BALANCED F SCALE (SHORT FORM)

Purpose: To measure authoritarianism.

Number of Items: 14

Format: Likert format. All items presented for this scale and several others that measure authoritarianism.

Reliability: Alpha was .87.

Author: Ray, J. J.

Article: The workers are not authoritarian: Attitude and personality data from six countries.

Journal: *Sociology and Social Research,* January 1983, *67*(2), 166–189.

Related Research: Ray, J. J. (1979). A short balanced F scale. *Journal of Social Psychology, 109,* 309–310.

3461

Test Name: BEHAVIORAL ASSERTIVENESS TEST

Purpose: To measure assertiveness.

Number of Items: 7

Format: Seven interpersonal situations requiring assertive responses played to subjects on videotape.

Reliability: Interrater reliability was .71.

Author: Nesbitt, E.

Article: Use of assertive training in teaching the expression of positively assertive behavior.

Journal: *Psychological Reports,* 1981, *49*(1), 155–161.

Related Research: Nesbitt, E. B. (1977). *Comparison of two measures of assertiveness and the modification of non-assertive behaviors.* Unpublished doctoral dissertation, University of Tennessee.

• • •

3462

Test Name: BELIEFS AND FEARS SCALE

Purpose: To measure pattern of beliefs and fears associated with type A behavior.

Number of Items: 48

Format: Items rated on 7-point Likert response categories.

Reliability: Ranged from .42 to .70 over seven constructs.

Validity: Modest correlations with type A behavior; 9 of 28 correlations significant, but none above .30.

Author: Burke, R. J.

Article: Beliefs and fears underlying type A behavior.

Journal: *Psychological Reports,* April 1984, *54*(2), 655–662.

3463

Test Name: BUSS-DURKEE HOSTILITY INVENTORY

Purpose: To assess different forms of aggression and hostility

Number of Items: 66

Format: Includes seven subscales: assault, indirect aggression, irritability, negativism, resentment, suspicion, verbal aggression.

Reliability: Test–retest correlations ranged from .64 to .82.

Validity: Correlations with other variables ranged from −.53 to .67.

Author: Selby, M. J.

Article: Assessment of violence potential using measures of anger, hostility and social desirability.

Journal: *Journal of Personality Assessment,* October 1984, *48*(5), 531–544.

Related Research: Buss, A. H., & Durkee, A. (1957). An inventory for assessing different kinds of hostility. *Journal of Consulting Psychology, 21,* 343–349.

Biaggio, M. K., et al. (1981). Reliability and validity of four anger scales. *Journal of Personality Assessment, 45*(6), 639–648.

• • •

3464

Test Name: CHILDREN'S ACTION TENDENCY SCALE

Purpose: To measure aggressiveness, assertiveness, and submissiveness in children.

Number of Items: 39

Format: Consists of 13 situations, each of which is followed by three pairs of responses. The child selects one response in each pair. An example is presented.

Validity: Correlations with observed behaviors ranged from

−.60 to .53 for boys ($N = 21$) and −.54 to .46 for girls ($N = 24$).

Author: Deluty, R. H.

Article: Behavioral validation of the Children's Action Tendency Scale.

Journal: *Journal of Behavioral Assessment*, June 1984, *6*(2), 115–130.

Related Research: Deluty, R. H. (1979). Children's Action Tendency Scale: A self-report measure of aggressiveness, assertiveness and submissiveness in children. *Journal of Consulting and Clinical Psychology, 47*, 1061–1071.

■ ■ ■

3465

Test Name: CHILDREN'S ASSERTIVE BEHAVIOR SCALE

Purpose: To measure children's assertive behavior.

Number of Items: 27

Format: Subjects respond to each item by selecting one of five responses, which represent very passive, passive, assertive, aggressive, and very aggressive behavior. All items are presented.

Reliability: Test–retest (4 weeks) reliabilities were .86 and .66. Kuder-Richardson formula 20 internal consistency was .78 and .80.

Validity: Correlation with behavioral observations was .38.

Author: Michelson, L., and Wood, R.

Article: Development and psychometric properties of the Children's Assertive Behavior Scale.

Journal: *Journal of Behavioral Assessment*, March 1982, *4*(1), 3–13.

Related Research: Michelson, L., & Wood, R. (1980). A group

assertive training program for elementary school children. *Child Behavior Therapy, 2*, 1–9.

■ ■ ■

3466

Test Name: CHILDREN'S AUTHORITARIAN PERSONALITY SCALE

Purpose: To measure authoritarian personality among children in grades 7–11.

Number of Items: 20

Format: Yes–?–No format. All items are presented.

Reliability: Alpha was .84.

Validity: Correlates .65 with attitude toward authority.

Author: Ray, J. J., and Jones, J. M.

Article: Attitude to authority and authoritarianism among school children.

Journal: *Journal of Social Psychology*, April 1983, *119*(second half), 199–203.

Related Research: Jones, J. M., & Ray, J. J. (1984). Validating the school children's attitude toward authority and authoritarianism scales. *Journal of Social Psychology, 122*(first half), 141–142.

■ ■ ■

3467

Test Name: COLLEGE SELF-EXPRESSION SCALE

Purpose: To measure assertiveness.

Format: Items rated on a 5-point rating scale (*always* to *never*).

Reliability: Test–retest ranged from .80 to .90.

Validity: Correlated .28 with response latency and .80 with eye contact.

Author: Williams, J. M.

Article: Assertiveness as a mediating variable in conformity to confederates of high and low status.

Journal: *Psychological Reports*, October 1984, *55*(2), 415–418.

Related Research: Galassi, J. P., et al. (1975). The college self-expression scale: A measure of assertiveness. *Behavior Therapy, 6*, 217–221.

Gorecki, P. R., et al. (1981). Convergent and concurrent validation for four measures of assertion. *Journal of Behavioral Assessment, 3*(2), 85–91.

■ ■ ■

3468

Test Name: COLLEGE WOMEN'S ASSERTION SAMPLE

Purpose: To provide a controlled observational measure of assertion.

Number of Items: 52

Format: Items are audiotaped and present a brief description of a realistic interpersonal encounter. Subjects respond to each item exactly as they would if actually experiencing it as they hear it.

Reliability: Average coefficient of agreement across all items was .91.

Validity: Correlations with other variables ranged from −.31 to .42.

Author: MacDonald, M. L., and Tyson, P.

Article: The College Women's Assertion Sample (CWAS): A cross-validation.

Journal: *Educational and Psychological Measurement*, Summer 1984, *44*(2), 405–412.

Related Research: MacDonald, M. L. (1978). Measuring assertion: A model and method. *Behavior Therapy, 9*, 889–899.

3469

Test Name: DEL GRECO ASSERTIVE BEHAVIOR INVENTORY

Purpose: To measure assertive, aggressive, nonassertive, and passive aggressive behavior in the college dormitory population.

Number of Items: 86

Format: Subjects respond to each item on a 5-point Likert scale from *almost never* to *almost always.* All items are presented.

Reliability: Coefficient alphas ranged from .83 to .91.

Validity: Correlations with other scales ranged from −.65 to .58.

Author: Del Greco, L.

Article: The Del Greco Assertive Behavior Inventory.

Journal: *Journal of Behavioral Assessment,* March 1983, *5*(1), 49–63.

Related Research: DeGiovanni, I. S. (1978). Development and validation of an assertiveness scale for couples. Doctoral dissertation, State University of New York at Buffalo. *Dissertation Abstracts International, 39*(9-B), 4573.

● ● ●

3470

Test Name: DIRECTIVENESS SCALE

Purpose: To measure domineering, aggressive behavior.

Number of Items: 8

Format: Yes–No–Undecided format. All items presented.

Reliability: Alpha was .63.

Author: Ray, J. J.

Article: Achievement motivation as a source of racism, conservativism and authoritarianism.

Journal: *Journal of Social*

Psychology, June 1984, *123*(first half), 21–28.

Related Research: Ray, J. J. (1976). Do authoritarians hold authoritarian attitudes? *Human Relations, 29,* 307–325.

● ● ●

3471

Test Name: DIRECTIVENESS SCALE

Purpose: To measure directiveness.

Number of Items: 14

Reliability: Coefficient alphas ranged from .74 to .79.

Validity: Correlations with dominance was .429; with submissiveness was -.322; with aggressiveness was .241.

Author: Ray, J. J.

Article: Authoritarianism, dominance and assertiveness.

Journal: *Journal of Personality Assessment,* August 1981, *45*(4), 390–397.

Related Research: Ray, J. J. (1980). Authoritarianism in California 30 years later—With some cross-cultural comparisons. *Journal of Social Psychology, 111,* 9–17.

● ● ●

3472

Test Name: DOMINANCE SCALE

Purpose: To measure dominance.

Number of Items: 30

Format: All items are presented.

Reliability: Coefficient alpha was .89.

Validity: Correlation with rated dominance was .54; with rated submissiveness was −.39.

Author: Ray, J. J.

Article: Authoritarianism, dominance and assertiveness.

Journal: *Journal of Personality Assessment,* August 1981, *45*(4), 390–397.

● ● ●

3473

Test Name: EMOTIONAL EMPATHY SCALE

Purpose: To measure empathy.

Number of Items: 33

Format: Modified for children to 3 response categories (*completely disagree, disagree to some extent, completely agree*).

Reliability: Alpha was .68 (children). Split-half reliability was .84 (adults).

Validity: Correlates slightly (.11) with social desirability (Crandall et al., 1965).

Author: Kalliopuska, M.

Article: Relationship between moral judgement and empathy.

Journal: *Psychological Reports,* October 1983, *53*(2), 575–578.

Related Research: Mehrabian, A., & Epstein, N. (1972). A measure of emotional empathy. *Journal of Personality, 40,* 525–543.

● ● ●

3474

Test Name: EMPATHIC RESPONSE INSTRUMENT

Purpose: To measure empathic response of teachers.

Number of Items: 15 vignettes (one example given).

Format: Raters judge students' written responses to vignettes on a 5-point scale of empathy.

Reliability: Interrater reliability was .90.

Author: Higgins, E., et al.

Article: Effects of human relations training on education students.

Journal: *Journal of Educational Research*, September/October 1981, *75*(1), 22–25.

Related Research: Egan, G. (1974). *The skilled helper.* Monterey, CA: Brooks/Cole.

■ ■ ■

3475

Test Name: EMPATHIC UNDERSTANDING SUBSCALE OF THE BARRETT-LENNARD RELATIONSHIP INVENTORY FORM OS–64

Purpose: To measure empathy between counselor and client.

Number of Items: 16

Format: The client indicates one of three degrees of agreement or disagreement with no neutral ground for each item. A sample item is presented.

Reliability: Test–retest correlation is .89. Spearman-Brown split-half correlations ranged from .82 to .93.

Validity: Correlations with other variables ranged from .033 to .617.

Author: Robinson, J. W., et al.

Article: Autonomic responses correlate with counselor–client empathy.

Journal: *Journal of Counseling Psychology*, March 1982, *29*(2), 195–198.

Related Research: Barrett-Lennard, G. T. (1972). *Resource bibliography of reported studies using the relationship inventory.* Unpublished manuscript, University of Waterloo, Waterloo, Canada.

■ ■ ■

3476

Test Name: EMPATHY TEST

Purpose: To measure emotional empathy.

Number of Items: 33

Format: Includes six subscales. Subjects respond on a scale from –4 (*completely disagree*) to +4 (*completely agree*).

Reliability: Split-half reliability was .84 (*N* = 202). Alpha-coefficient was .79.

Validity: Correlation with Marlowe and Crowne's social desirability scale was .06.

Author: Kalliopuska, M.

Article: Verbal components of emotional empathy.

Journal: *Perceptual and Motor Skills*, April 1983, *56*(2), 487–496.

Related Research: Mehrabian, A., & Epstein, N. (1972). A measure of emotional empathy. *Journal of Personality, 40,* 525–543.

■ ■ ■

3477

Test Name: FASTE

Purpose: To measure children's empathy.

Format: Subjects are asked how they feel after being shown slides of children experiencing emotions of happiness, sadness, anger, or fear.

Reliability: Test–retest (1 week) reliability was .84.

Validity: Correlations with other variables ranged from –.35 to .83 (entire group); from –.16 to .48 (girls); from –.08 to .85 (boys).

Author: Marcus, R. F., et al.

Article: Verbal and non-verbal empathy and prediction of social behavior of young children.

Journal: *Perceptual and Motor Skills*, February 1985, *60*(1), 299–309.

Related Research: Feshbach, N. D.

(1975). Empathy in children: Some theoretical and empirical considerations. *Counseling Psychology, 5,* 25–30.

■ ■ ■

3478

Test Name: FEAR OF NEGATIVE EVALUATION SCALE

Purpose: To measure situation-specific trait anxiety.

Number of Items: 30

Format: Contains true–false items.

Validity: Correlations with other variables ranged from .29 to .67.

Author: Smith, T. W., et al.

Article: Irrational beliefs and the arousal of emotional distress.

Journal: *Journal of Counseling Psychology*, April 1984, *31*(2), 190–201.

Related Research: Watson, S. R., & Friend, R. (1969). Measurement of social-evaluative anxiety. *Journal of Consulting and Clinical Psychology, 83,* 448–457.

■ ■ ■

3479

Test Name: FRAMINGHAM TYPE A SCALE

Purpose: To assess type A behavior.

Number of Items: 10

Format: Respondents indicate extent to which items are self-descriptive. Sample items presented.

Reliability: Alpha was .71.

Author: Matteson, M. T.

Article: Relation of type A behavior to performance and satisfaction among sales personnel.

Journal: *Journal of Vocational Behavior*, October 1984, *25*(2), 203–214.

Related Research: Haynes, S. G.,

et al. The relationship of psychosocial factors to coronary heart disease in the Framingham Study. *American Journal of Epidemiology, 107,* 362–383.

■ ■ ■

3480

Test Name: GENERAL POPULATION ASSERTIVENESS CONTINGENCY SCHEDULE

Purpose: To measure assertiveness.

Number of Items: 20

Format: Statements are followed by four response categories ranging from *very much like me* to *very much unlike me.* All items are presented.

Reliability: Cronbach's alpha was .70. Item-total correlations ranged from –.06 to .36.

Validity: Assertiveness correlated –.08 with anxiety and –.13 with mood state (*p* < .05 or better).

Author: Sundel, M., and Lobb, M. L.

Article: Reinforcement contingencies and role relationships in assertiveness within a general population.

Journal: *Psychological Reports,* December 1982, *51*(3-I), 1007–1015.

■ ■ ■

3481

Test Name: HYPOTHETICAL, ROLE-PLAYING TEST

Purpose: To provide a behavioral measure of assertion.

Number of Items: 12

Format: Includes six refusal items and six general items. A 5-point scale is used. Subjects are instructed to respond as a highly assertive person would.

Reliability: Interrater reliability was .88.

Author: Valerio, H. P., and Stone, G. L.

Article: Effects of behavioral, cognitive, and combined treatments for assertion as a function of differential deficits.

Journal: *Journal of Counseling Psychology,* March 1982, *29*(2), 158–168.

Related Research: Schwartz, R., & Gottman, J. (1976). Toward a task analysis of assertive behavior. *Journal of Consulting and Clinical Psychology, 44,* 910–920.

■ ■ ■

3482

Test Name: IMPULSIVENESS SCALE

Purpose: To measure workplace impulsiveness.

Number of Items: 13

Format: Likert.

Reliability: Alpha was .77.

Author: James, L. R., et al.

Article: Perceptions of psychological influence: A cognitive information processing approach for explaining moderated relationships.

Journal: *Personnel Psychology,* Autumn 1981, *34*(3), 453–475.

Related Research: Barratt, E. S. (1959). Anxiety and impulsiveness related to psychomotor efficiency. *Perceptual and Motor Skills, 9,* 191–198.

■ ■ ■

3483

Test Name: INDEX OF EMPATHY FOR CHILDREN AND ADOLESCENTS

Purpose: To measure empathy for

children and adolescents.

Number of Items: 22

Format: Half the items require an affirmative response and half require a negative response to indicate au empathic tendency. All items are presented.

Reliability: Cronbach's alpha coefficients ranged from .54 for first graders, to .68 for fourth graders, to .79 for seventh graders. Test–retest reliability coefficients were .74 (1st graders) and .83 (7th graders).

Validity: Correlations with other measures ranged from –.57 to .77.

Author: Bryant, B. K.

Article: An index of empathy for children and adolescents.

Journal: *Child Development,* April 1982, *53*(2), 413–425.

Related Research: Feshbach, N. D., & Roe, K. (1968). Empathy in six- and seven-year-olds. *Child Development, 39,* 133–145.

■ ■ ■

3484

Test Name: INNOVATIVENESS SCALE

Purpose: To measure innovativeness.

Number of Items: 20

Format: Likert format.

Reliability: Split-half reliability was .94. Alpha was .82.

Author: Evans, R. H.

Article: Innovativeness and information processing confidence.

Journal: *Psychological Reports,* April 1985, *56*(2), 557–558.

Related Research: Hurt, H. T., et al. (1977). Scales for the measurement of innovativeness. *Human Communication Research, 4,* 58–65.

3485

Test Name: INTERPERSONAL JEALOUSY SCALE

Purpose: To measure jealousy.

Number of Items: 28

Format: Items rated on 9-point *agree–disagree* response categories. Sample items are presented.

Reliability: Alpha was .92.

Validity: Significant correlations between jealousy and romantic love were .47 (men) and .41 (women), nonsignificant correlations between liking and jealousy were .05 (men) and .15 (women).

Author: Mathes, E. W., and Severa, N.

Article: Jealousy, romantic love and liking: Theoretical considerations and preliminary scale development.

Journal: *Psychological Reports,* 1981, *49*(1), 23–31.

● ● ●

3486

Test Name: MACH IV SCALE

Purpose: To measure Machiavellianism.

Number of Items: 20

Reliability: Nunnally (Equation 6–18) was .73.

Validity: Correlated .34 with role ambiguity (Rizzo et al., 1970); –.26 with perceived participation in decision-making (Vroom, 1960); –.35 with job satisfaction (Vroom, 1960); –.28 with job involvement (Lodahl & Kejner, 1965); –.28 with job tension (Kahn et al., 1965); .13 with perceived job performance (Porter & Lander, 1968).

Author: Hallon, C. J.

Article: Machiavellianism and

managerial work attitudes and perceptions.

Journal: *Psychological Reports,* April 1983, *52*(2), 432–434.

Related Research: Christie, R., & Geis, F. (1970). *Studies in Machiavellianism.* New York: Academic Press.

● ● ●

3487

Test Name: MACH V SCALE

Purpose: To measure a respondent's Machiavellian orientation.

Number of Items: 20 triads.

Format: Each triad contains: A statement tapping Machiavellianism, a statement unrelated to the Mach item but matched in social desirability, and a statement of different social desirability. Respondents indicate which of the three statements they most agree with and which they least agree with.

Reliability: Spearman-Brown adjusted split-half reliability coefficients were .45 and .53. Alphas were .44 and .55

Author: Shea, M. T., and Beatty, J. R.

Article: Measuring Machiavellianism with Mach V: A psychometric investigation.

Journal: *Journal of Personality Assessment,* October 1983, *47*(5), 509–513.

Related Research: Christie, R. (1970). Scale construction. In R. Christie & F. L. Geis (Eds.), *Studies in Machiavellianism.* New York: Academic Press.

● ● ●

3488

Test Name: MANIFEST ANXIETY DEFENSIVENESS SCALE

Purpose: To differentiate the highly trait anxious from those lower in anxiety.

Number of Items: 63 (men) and 59 (women).

Format: A self-report questionnaire.

Reliability: Test–retest (2 months) reliability coefficient was .95. Kuder-Richardson formula 20 coefficient was .91. Split-half (Spearman-Brown correction) reliability was .90.

Validity: Correlations with the Byrne R-S scale were .97 (men) and .94 (women); with the Taylor Manifest Anxiety Scale was .92 (both men and women).

Author: Gard, K. A., et al.

Article: Accuracy in nonverbal communication as affected by trait and state anxiety.

Journal: *Perceptual and Motor Skills,* December 1982, *55*(3-I), 747–753.

● ● ●

3489

Test Name: MATTHEWS YOUTH TEST FOR HEALTH

Purpose: To assess children's type A behaviors.

Number of Items: 17

Format: Items are statements descriptive of type A adults and include competitive achievement striving, impatience, aggressiveness, and easily arousal hostility. The teacher rates the child on a 5-point scale as to how characteristic each statement is of the child.

Reliability: Pearson correlation coefficients over a 1-year period ranged from .47 to .59 (*N*s ranged from 121 to 208). Pearson correlation coefficients over a 3-week period ranged from .84 to .87 (*N*s ranged from 121 to 127).

Author: Matthews, K. A., and Avis, NE.

Article: Stability of overt Type A behaviors in children: Results from a one-year longitudinal study.

Journal: *Child Development,* December 1983, *54*(6), 1507–1512.

Related Research: Matthews, K. A., & Angulo, J. (1980). Measurement of the Type A behavior pattern in children: Assessment of children's competitiveness, impatience-anger and aggression. *Child Development, 51,* 466–475.

∎ ∎ ∎

3490

Test Name: MEHRABIAN AND EPSTEIN EMOTIONAL EMPATHY SCALE

Purpose: To measure emotional empathy.

Number of Items: 33

Format: Items rated on an 8-point agreement scale.

Reliability: Split-half reliability was .84.

Validity: High-scorers have higher rates of helping behavior than low scorers.

Author: Bohlmeyer, E. M., et al.

Article: Differences between education and business students in cooperative and competitive attitudes, emotional empathy and self-esteem.

Journal: *Psychological Reports,* February 1985, *56*(1), 247–253.

Related Research: Mehrabian, A., & Epstein, A. (1972). A measure of emotional empathy. *Journal of Personality, 40,* 523–543.

∎ ∎ ∎

3491

Test Name: NARCISSISTIC PERSONALITY INVENTORY

Purpose: To identify narcissistic personality.

Number of Items: 54

Format: A forced-choice test.

Reliability: Coefficient alpha was .86. Correlation between alternate forms (8-week interval) was .72.

Validity: Correlation with the Millon Clinical Multiofial Inventory Narcissistic Scale was .55. Correlation with the Marlowe-Crowne Social Desirability Scale was −.01.

Author: Auerbach, J. S.

Article: Validation of two scales for narcissistic personality disorder.

Journal: *Journal of Personality Assessment,* December 1984, *48*(6), 649–653.

Related Research: Raskin, R. N., & Hall, C. S. (1981). The Narcissistic Personality Inventory: Alternate form reliability and further evidence of construct validity. *Journal of Personality Assessment, 45,* 159–162.

Emmons, R. A. (1984). Factor analysis and construct validity of the Narcissistic Personality Inventory. *Journal of Personality Assessment, 48*(3), 291–300.

∎ ∎ ∎

3492

Test Name: NEGATIVE ASSERTION QUESTIONNAIRE

Purpose: To measure assertiveness by self-report.

Number of Items: 17

Format: Yes–no format. Sample items presented.

Reliability: Alpha was .70.

Validity: Correlated −.50 with Fear of Negative Evaluation Scale. Correlated .31 with the Provocative Situation Questionnaire.

Author: Quinsey, V. L., et al.

Article: Assertion and overcontrolled hostility among mentally disordered murderers.

Journal: *Journal of Consulting and Clinical Psychology,* August 1983, *51*(4), 550–556.

∎ ∎ ∎

3493

Test Name: NONPATHOLOGICAL COMPULSIVENESS SCALE

Purpose: To measure compulsiveness.

Number of Items: 11

Format: Yes–no.

Reliability: Alpha was .80.

Validity: Three factors extracted indecision and double-checking, order and regularity, and detail and perfectionism.

Author: Kagan, D., and Squires, R. L.

Article: Measuring nonpathological compulsiveness.

Journal: *Psychological Reports,* October 1985, *57*(2), 559–563.

Related Research: Cooper, J. (1970). The Leyton Obsessional Inventory. *Psychological Medicine, 1,* 48–64.

∎ ∎ ∎

3494

Test Name: NOVACO ANGER INVENTORY—REVISED

Purpose: To measure the potential for becoming angry when provoked.

Number of Items: 80

Format: Subjects respond to each item on a 5-point scale indicating the degree to which the situation makes them angry. Some items are presented.

Reliability: Pre–posttest correlation was .74. Internal consistency was .90.

Validity: Correlations with other variables ranged from .08 to .82.

Author: Selby, M. J.

Article: Assessment of violence potential using measures of anger, hostility, and social desirability.

Journal: *Journal of Personality Assessment,* October 1984, *48*(5), 531–544.

Related Research: Novaco, R. (1975). *Anger control: The development and evaluation of an experimental treatment.* Lexington, MA: D. C. Heath.

■ ■ ■

3495

Test Name: OVEREXCITABILITY QUESTIONNAIRE

Purpose: To assess five forms of overexcitability.

Number of Items: 21

Format: A free response instrument including five forms of overexcitability: psychomotor, sensual, intellectual, imaginational, and emotional. All items are presented.

Reliability: Interrater correlations ranged from .56 to .80.

Author: Piechowski, M. M., and Cunningham, K.

Article: Patterson of overexcitability in a group of artists.

Journal: *Journal of Creative Behavior,* 1985, *19*(2), 153–172.

Related Research: Piechowski, M. M. (1979). Developmental potential. In N. Colangelo & R. T. Zaffrann (Eds.), *New voices in counseling the gifted.* Dubuque, IA: Kendall/Hunt.

■ ■ ■

3496

Test Name: NEO INVENTORY

Purpose: To measure personality

traits by means of three broad domains.

Number of Items: 144

Format: Includes three broad domains of neuroticism, extroversion, and openness. Within each domain are six specific traits and 8-item scales for each specific trait.

Reliability: Internal consistency ranged from .61 to .81 for specific traits. Test–retest reliability (6 months) ranged from .66 to .92. Internal consistency and test–retest for the three domains ranged from .85 to .93.

Validity: Correlation of the three domains with the Self-Directed Search ranged from –.22 to .65 for men ($N = 217$) and from –.26 to .53 for women ($N = 144$).

Author: Costa, P. T., et al.

Article: Personality and vocational interests in an adult sample.

Journal: *Journal of Applied Psychology,* August 1984, *69*(3), 390–400.

Related Research: McCrae, R. R., and Costs, P. T., Jr. (1983). Joint factors in self-reports and ratings: Neuroticism, extroversion, and openness to experience. *Personality and Individual Differences, 4,* 245–255.

■ ■ ■

3497

Test Name: OBSESSIVE–COMPULSIVE SCALE

Purpose: To measure the degree of obsessive–compulsive traits.

Number of Items: 22

Format: Subjects respond to each item as being either true or false. Two items are validity check-items. All items are presented.

Reliability: Test–retest reliability coefficient was .82.

Validity: Correlations with

clinicians' evaluations were .79; with roommate evaluations were .45; with other measures ranged from –.57 to .83 (Ns ranged from 34 to 114).

Author: Gibb, G. D., et al.

Article: The measurement of the obsessive–compulsive personality.

Journal: *Educational and Psychological Measurement,* Winter 1983, *43*(4), 1233–1238.

■ ■ ■

3498

Test Name: PEER RATING INDEX OF AGGRESSION

Purpose: To identify aggressive and nonaggressive children.

Number of Items: 9

Format: Children rate all other classmates on a series of aggressive items. An example is presented.

Reliability: Coefficient alpha was .95. Test–retest reliability (over 1 month) was .91.

Author: Graybill, D., et al.

Article: Effects of playing violent versus nonviolent video games on the aggressive ideation of aggressive and nonaggressive children.

Journal: *Child Study Journal,* 1985, *15*(3), 199–205.

Related Research: Walder, L. O., et al. (1961). Development of a peer-rating measure of aggression. *Psychological Reports, 9,* 497–556.

■ ■ ■

3499

Test Name: PEER RATING OF PERSONALITY TRAITS SCALE

Purpose: To measure and rate college faculty members.

Number of Items: 29

Format: Nine-point scales followed each of 29 adjectives.

Reliability: Interrater reliability ranged from .61 to .94.

Validity: Items factor into two dimensions: achievement orientation and interpersonal orientation.

Author: Erdle, S., et al.

Article: Personality, classroom behaviors and student ratings of college teaching effectiveness: A path analysis.

Journal: *Journal of Educational Psychology,* August 1985, *77*(4), 394–407.

■ ■ ■

3500

Test Name: Q-TAGS TEST OF PERSONALITY

Purpose: To measure hostility.

Number of Items: 54

Format: Subject indicates which items are descriptive of self. Items are selected primarily from the Minnesota Multiphasic Personality Inventory. The score for an item ranges from 1 to 11.

Reliability: Test–retest reliability was .69.

Author: Roberts, A., and Jenkins, P. A.

Article: Teachers' perceptions of assertive and aggressive behavior at school: A discriminant analysis.

Journal: *Psychological Reports,* 1982, *50*(3-I), 827–832.

Related Research: Storey, A. G., & Mason, L. I. (1967). *The Q-Tags Test of Personality.* Montreal: Institute of Psychological Research.

■ ■ ■

3501

Test Name: RATHUS ASSERTIVENESS SCHEDULE— MODIFIED

Purpose: To measure early

adolescent assertiveness.

Number of Items: 30

Format: Responses to each item are made on a 6-point scale from *very like me* to *very unlike me.* All items are presented.

Reliability: Odd–even, split-half Spearman-Brown adjusted coefficients ranged from .69 to .81 (*N*s = 25 to 28).

Validity: Correlations with peer rating scores ranged from .25 to .52 (*N*s ranging from 25 to 28).

Author: Del Greco, L., et al.

Article: The Rathus Assertiveness Schedule modified for early adolescents.

Journal: *Journal of Behavioral Assessment,* December 1981, *3*(4), 321–328.

Related Research: Rathus, S. A. (1973). A 30-item schedule for assessing assertive behavior. *Behavior Therapy, 4,* 398–406.

■ ■ ■

3502

Test Name: REDUCED BEHAVIORAL REHEARSAL ASSERTION TEST

Purpose: To assess the quality of assertive responses under conditions that simulated reality.

Number of Items: 12

Format: Items consist of taped situations half of which were specific refusal tasks and half of a general assertive nature. Oral responses were rated on a 5-point scale, ranging from 1 (*unqualified nonassertive response*) to 5 (*unqualified assertive response*).

Reliability: Interrater reliability was .94.

Author: Valerio, H. P., and Stone, G. L.

Article: Effects of behavioral, cognitive, and combined

treatments for assertion as a function of differential deficits.

Journal: *Journal of Counseling Psychology,* March 1982, *29*(2), 158–168.

Related Research: Schwartz, R., & Gottman, J. (1976). Toward a task analysis of assertive behavior. *Journal of Consulting and Clinical Psychology, 44,* 910–920.

■ ■ ■

3503

Test Name: REPRESSION– SENSITIZATION SCALE

Purpose: To measure repression– sensitization.

Number of Items: 127

Reliability: Test–retest reliability was .82 (3 months). Internal consistency was .94.

Validity: Correlations with internal–external locus of control were .35 (*N* = 73) and .85 (*N* = 16).

Author: Valliant, P. M., et al.

Article: Variations in locus of control and repression– sensitization in acute schizophrenics, schizophrenic criminals and criminal psychiatric offenders.

Journal: *Perceptual and Motor Skills,* December 1982, *55*(3-I), 919–924.

Related Research: Byrne, D., et al. (1963). Relation of the Revised Repression–Sensitization Scale to measures of self-description. *Psychological Reports, 13,* 323– 334.

■ ■ ■

3504

Test Name: REPRESSION– SENSITIZATION SCALE— SHORT VERSION

Purpose: To measure sensitization.

Number of Items: 90

Format: Subjects indicate whether

each item is true or false of them.

Reliability: Cronbach's alpha was .92.

Validity: Correlations with social anxiety were .63 (college students) and .48 (homosexuals).

Author: Schmitt, J. P., and Kurdek, L. A.

Article: Correlates of social anxiety in college students and homosexuals.

Journal: *Journal of Personality Assessment*, August 1984, *48*(4), 403–409.

Related Research: Byrne, D., et al. (1963). Relation of the Revised Repression–Sensitization Scale to measure of self-description. *Psychological Reports, 13*, 323–334.

■ ■ ■

3505

Test Name: RESPONSE EMPATHY RATING SCALE

Purpose: To measure the empathic quality of counselor behavior.

Format: Includes nine components: intention to enter client's frame of reference, perceptual inference and clarification, accuracy–plausibility, here and now, topic centrality, choice of words, voice quality, exploratory manner, impact. Ratings were made on 5-point behaviorally anchored rating scale.

Reliability: Interrater reliability for total empathy was .91. Interitem reliability (alpha) for total empathy was .82.

Validity: Correlations between empathy components and response modes ranged from −.71 to .61.

Author: Elliott, R., et al.

Article: Measuring response empathy: Development of a multicomponent rating scale.

Journal: *Journal of Counseling*

Psychology, July 1982, *29*(4), 379–387.

Related Research: Hargrove, D. S. (1974). Verbal interaction analysis of empathic and nonempathic responses of therapists. *Journal of Consulting and Clinical Psychology, 42*, 305.

■ ■ ■

3506

Test Name: REVISED EMPATHY SCALE

Purpose: To measure perceived empathy.

Number of Items: 13

Format: Includes a 6-point response scale.

Reliability: Cronbach's alpha was .79.

Author: Hammer, A. L.

Article: Matching perceptual predicates: Effect on perceived empathy in a counseling analogue.

Journal: *Journal of Counseling Psychology*, April 1983, *30*(2), 172–179.

Related Research: Barrett-Lennard, G. T. (1981). The empathy cycle: Refinement of a nuclear concept. *Journal of Counseling Psychology, 28*, 91–100.

■ ■ ■

3507

Test Name: REVISED F SCALE

Purpose: To measure authoritarianism.

Number of Items: 20

Format: Includes 4 factors: leadership/dominance, achievement motivation, interpersonal conflict, and verbal hostility. All items are presented.

Reliability: Ranged from .70 to .79.

Author: Heaven, P. C. L.

Article: Construction and validation of a measure of authoritarian personality.

Journal: *Journal of Personality Assessment,* October 1985, *49*(5), 545–551.

Related Research: Heaven, P. C. L. (1984). Predicting authoritarian behavior: Analysis of three measures. *Personality and Individual Differences, 5*, 251–253.

■ ■ ■

3508

Test Name: SALES TYPE A PERSONALITY INDEX— SHORT FORM

Purpose: To tap Type A characteristics.

Number of Items: 9

Format: Attempts to measure Type A characteristics including sense of time urgency, challenge of responsibilities, job involvement, speed and impatience, involved striving, and competitiveness.

Reliability: Internal reliability coefficients ranged from .75 to .80. Cronbach's alpha was .76.

Author: Abush, R., and Burkhead, E. J.

Article: Job stress in midlife working women: Relationships among personality type, job characteristics, and job tension.

Journal: *Journal of Counseling Psychology,* January 1984, *31*(1), 36–44.

Related Research: Jolly, J. A. (1979). Job change: Its relationship to role stresses and stress symptoms according to personality and environment. *Dissertation Abstracts International, 32*, 4518B. (University Microfilms No. 79-25475)

3509

Test Name: SCALE OF TOLERANCE–INTOLERANCE OF AMBIGUITY

Purpose: To measure authoritarianism.

Number of Items: 16

Format: Items rated in 7-point Likert format. Sample items are presented.

Validity: Mean correlation with other measures of tolerance of ambiguity is .46.

Author: Tom, D. Y. H., et al.

Article: Influences of student background and teacher authoritarianism on teacher expectations.

Journal: *Journal of Educational Psychology,* April 1984, *76*(2), 259–265.

Related Research: Budner, S. (1962). Tolerance of ambiguity as a personality variable. *Journal of Personality, 30,* 29–50.

Robinson, J. P., & Shaver, P. R. (1973). *Measures of Social Psychological Attitudes* (Rev. ed.). Ann Arbor: University of Michigan.

■ ■ ■

3510

Test Name: SELF-DECEPTION QUESTIONNAIRE

Purpose: To measure denial.

Number of Items: 20

Format: Subjects respond as to the extent to which they can answer each item in the affirmative. A 7-point Likert scale is employed.

Reliability: Correlations with lateral eye-movements ranged from .15 to .28 (*N*s = 43 to 16).

Author: Pierro, R. A., and Goldberger, L.

Article: Lateral eye-movement,

field dependence and denial.

Journal: *Perceptual and Motor Skills,* October 1982, *55*(2), 371–378.

Related Research: Gur, R. C., & Sackeim, H. A. (1979). Self-deception: A concept in search of a phenomenon. *Journal of Personality and Social Psychology, 37,* 147–169.

■ ■ ■

3511

Test Name: SELF-REPORT PSYCHOPATHY SCALE

Purpose: To assess personality traits and anti-social behaviors.

Number of Items: 22

Format: 1–5 scale.

Reliability: Alpha was .80.

Validity: Correlated .26 with MMPI Psychopathic Deviate Scale (*ns*); .36 with MMPI Hypomania Scale (*p* < .05); and −.53 with Socialization Scale of CPI.

Author: Hare, R. D.

Article: Comparison of procedures for the assessment of psychopathy.

Journal: *Journal of Consulting and Clinical Psychology,* February 1985, *53*(1), 7–16.

Related Research: Hare, R. D. (1980). A research scale for the assessment of psychopathy in criminal populations. *Personality and Individual Differences, 1,* 111–117.

■ ■ ■

3512

Test Name: SELF-RIGHTEOUSNESS SCALE

Purpose: To measure self-righteousness.

Number of Items: 4

Format: Responses to each item are made on a 5-point rating scale

from *strongly agree* to *strongly disagree.* All items are presented.

Reliability: Cronbach's alpha was .60. Test–retest correlation coefficient was .53.

Validity: Correlations with age were −.26 and −.21. Correlations with other variables ranged from .05 to .48.

Author: Falbo, T., and Belk, S. S.

Article: A short scale to measure self-righteousness.

Journal: *Journal of Personality Assessment,* April 1985, *49*(2), 172–177.

■ ■ ■

3513

Test Name: SOCIAL RETICENCE SCALE

Purpose: To measure shyness.

Number of Items: 22

Format: A self-report instrument.

Reliability: Coefficient alpha was .91. Test–retest reliability was .88 (8 weeks) and .78 (12 weeks).

Author: Jones, W. H., and Russell, D.

Article: The Social Reticence Scale: An objective instrument to measure shyness.

Journal: *Journal of Personality Assessment,* December 1982, *46*(6), 629–631.

Related Research: Zimbardo, P. G. (1977). *Shyness.* Reading, MA: Addison-Wesley.

■ ■ ■

3514

Test Name: S-R INVENTORY OF MACHIAVELLIANISM

Purpose: To measure Machiavellianism.

Number of Items: 9

Format: Nine situations are

followed by six modes of response, each of which was rated on a 5-point scale of how much respondents would be inclined to use it. All items are presented.

Reliability: Alpha ranged from .45 to .84 for situations and .72 to .92 for modes of response.

Author: Vleeming, R. G.

Article: Some sources of behavioral variance as measured by an S-R Inventory of Machiavellianism.

Journal: *Psychological Reports,* April 1981, *48*(2), 359–368.

Related Research: Endler, N. S., & Hunt, J. M. (1976). S-R inventories of hostility and comparisons of the proportions of variance from persons, responses and situations for hostility and anxiousness. In N. S. Endler & D. Magnusson (Eds.), *International psychology and personality* (pp. 288–298). New York: Hemisphere.

■ ■ ■

3515

Test Name: THRESHOLD TRAITS ANALOGY

Purpose: To provide a reliable, comprehensive system for defining and establishing the human attributes required to perform a wide variety of jobs.

Number of Items: 33

Format: Checklist. All items presented.

Reliability: Spearman-Brown Prophecy Formula was .86 (33 traits, 100 jobs). Interform reliability ranged from .42 to .67.

Validity: Validity coefficients were all significant ($p < .01$) for criterion variables, including overall job performance.

Author: Lopez, F. M., et al.

Article: An empirical test of a trait-oriented job analysis technique.

Journal: *Personnel Psychology,* Autumn 1981, *34*(3), 479–502.

■ ■ ■

3516

Test Name: TOLERANCE FOR AMBIGUITY SCALE

Purpose: To measure ambiguity in members of organizations.

Number of Items: 6

Format: Items rated in 5-point Likert format.

Reliability: Alpha was .69.

Author: Ashford, S. J., and Cummings, L. L.

Article: Proactive feedback seeking: The instrumental use of the information environment.

Journal: *Journal of Occupational Psychology,* March 1986, *58*(1), 67–79.

Related Research: Norton, R. W. (1975). Measure of ambiguity tolerance. *Journal of Personality Assessment, 39,* 607–619.

■ ■ ■

3517

Test Name: TRAIT FRUSTRATION SCALE

Purpose: To measure trait frustration.

Number of Items: 8

Format: An 8-point response scale is used with each of the 8 items, which describe frustrating situations.

Reliability: Test–retest reliability was .79.

Validity: Frustration scores were related positively but not significantly to aggression.

Author: Bergandi, T. A., et al.

Article: Trait frustration and aggression in adult humans.

Journal: *Psychological Reports,* December 1982, *51*(3-I), 815–819.

■ ■ ■

3518

Test Name: TYPE A BEHAVIOR SCALE

Purpose: To measure type A behavior.

Number of Items: 14

Format: Items rated on a 7-point bipolar scale.

Reliability: Internal consistency was .49.

Author: Burke, R. J.

Article: Career orientations and type A behavior in police officers.

Journal: *Psychological Reports,* December 1985, *57*(3-II), 1239–1246.

Related Research: Bortner, R. W., & Rosenman, R. H. (1967). The measurement of pattern A behavior. *Journal of Chronic Diseases, 20,* 525–533.

CHAPTER 22
Values

3519

Test Name: ACCULTURATION SCALE FOR MEXICAN-AMERICAN CHILDREN

Purpose: To assess acculturation of Mexican-American children by responses of teachers and counselors who can report about particular children.

Number of Items: 10

Format: Likert format. All items presented.

Reliability: Test–retest (5 week interval) reliability was .97. Alpha was .77. Interrater agreement was .93.

Validity: Correlates .76 with the Acculturation Rating Scale for Mexican-Americans. Mean difference between Anglo-Americans and Mexican-Americans was in correct direction and significant ($t = 12.62$, $p < .001$).

Author: Franco, J. N.

Article: An acculturation scale for Mexican-American children.

Journal: *Journal of General Psychology*, April 1983, *108*(second half), 175–181.

Related Research: Cuellar, I., et al. (1980). An acculturation scale for Mexican-American normal and clinical populations. *Hispanic Journal of Behavioral Science, 2,* 199–217.

• • •

3520

Test Name: AFFECTIVE WORK COMPETENCIES INVENTORY

Purpose: To measure work attitudes, values, and habits desired by industry and educators.

Number of Items: 45

Format: Includes five factors: ambition, self-control, organization, enthusiasm, and conscientiousness.

Reliability: Kuder-Richardson formula 20 reliability estimates ranged from .64 to .89.

Author: Brauchle, P. E., et al.

Article: The factorial validity of the affective work competencies inventory.

Journal: *Educational and Psychological Measurement,* Summer 1983, *43*(2), 603–609.

Related Research: Kazanas, H. C. (1978). *Affective work competencies for vocational education.* Columbus, OH: ERIC Clearinghouse for Vocational and Technical Education, The Ohio State University. (ERIC Document Reproduction Service No. ED 166420)

• • •

3521

Test Name: ANTI-INDUSTRIAL VALUES SCALE

Purpose: To measure perceived faults of society and to measure perceptions of ideal society.

Number of Items: 14

Format: Semantic differential format. All items presented.

Reliability: Cronbach's alpha was .78.

Author: Duff, A., and Cotgrove, S.

Article: Social values and the choice of careers in industry.

Journal: *Journal of Occupational Psychology,* June 1982, *55*(2), 97–107.

Related Research: Cotgrove, S., & Duff, A. (1980). Environmentalism, middle-class radicalism and politics. *Sociological Review, 28,* 333–351.

• • •

3522

Test Name: BELIEF IN A JUST WORLD

Purpose: To measure the extent a person believes that people experience the fates that they deserve.

Number of Items: 16

Format: Respondents indicate agreement or disagreement with each item on a 6-point scale.

Reliability: Coefficient alpha was .62.

Validity: Correlations with other variables ranged from −.16 to .17.

Author: Smith, C. A.

Article: Organizational citizenship behavior: Its nature and antecedents.

Journal: *Journal of Applied Psychology,* November 1983, *68*(4), 653–663.

Related Research: Miller, D. T. (1977). Altruism and threat to a belief in a just world. *Journal of Experimental Social Psychology, 13,* 113–124.

3523

Test Name: BILLS JUNIOR HIGH SCHOOL INDEX OF ADJUSTMENT AND VALUES

Purpose: To measure self-described values, how subject feels about them, and how subject would like to be.

Number of Items: 35

Format: 35 trait words are rated: self, self-acceptance, and ideal self.

Reliability: Test–retest (6 weeks) reliability was .53 to .89 across three types of ratings.

Author: Hines, P., and Berg-Cross, L.

Article: Racial differences in global self-esteem.

Journal: *Journal of Social Psychology*, April 1981, *113*(second half), 271–281.

Related Research: Bills, R. E. (No date). *Index Adjustment Values—Forms: Elementary, Junior High School and High School Manual* (mimeo). University of Alabama.

■ ■ ■

3524

Test Name: BIOPHILIA SCALE

Purpose: To measure the meaning of life.

Number of Items: 22

Format: Yes–Undecided–No format. All items are presented.

Reliability: Alpha was .77.

Author: Ray, J. J.

Article: Attitude to abortion, attitude to life and conservatism in Australia.

Journal: *Sociology and Social Research*, January 1984, *68*(2), 236–246.

Related Research: Ray, J. J., & Lovejoy, F. H. (1982). Conservatism, attitude toward abortion and Maccoby's Biophilia. *Journal of Social Psychology, 118*, 143–144.

■ ■ ■

3525

Test Name: CREEDAL ASSENT INDEX

Purpose: To measure general adherence to traditional Christian creeds.

Number of Items: 7

Format: Responses to each item are made on a 5-point Likert scale ranging from 5 (*strongly agree*) to 1 (*strongly disagree*). An example is presented.

Reliability: Cronbach's alphas ranged from .85 to .94.

Author: Hoge, D. R., et al.

Article: Transmission of religious and social values from parents to teenage children.

Journal: *Journal of Marriage and the Family*, August 1982, *44*(3), 569–580.

Related Research: King, M. B., & Hunt, R. A. (1975). Measuring the religious variable: National replication. *Journal for the Scientific Study of Religion, 14,* 13–22.

■ ■ ■

3526

Test Name: DEVOTIONALISM INDEX

Purpose: To measure religious devotionalism.

Number of Items: 5

Format: Responses to each item are made on a 5-point Likert scale ranging from 5 (*strongly agree*) to 1 (*strongly disagree*). An example is given.

Reliability: Cronbach's alphas ranged from .84 to .90.

Author: Hoge, D. R., et al.

Article: Transmission of religious and social values from parents to teenage children.

Journal: *Journal of Marriage and the Family,* August 1982, *44*(3), 569–580.

Related Research: King, M. B., & Hunt, R. A. (1975). Measuring the religious variable: National replication. *Journal for the Scientific Study of Religion, 14,* 13–22.

■ ■ ■

3527

Test Name: DUALISM SCALE

Purpose: To measure dualism–relativism.

Number of Items: 7

Format: Uses a 5-point Likert format for rating how often respondents experience a feeling. All items are presented.

Reliability: Test–retest reliability was .80.

Author: Ryan, M. P.

Article: Monitoring text comprehension: Individual differences in epistemological standards.

Journal: *Journal of Educational Psychology,* April 1984, *76*(2), 248–258.

Related Research: Perry, W. G., Jr. (1968). *Patterns of development in thought and values of students in a liberal arts college: A validation of a scheme.* Cambridge, MA: Harvard University. (ERIC Document Reproduction Service No. ED 024315)

■ ■ ■

3528

Test Name: ECLECTIC PROTESTANT ETHIC SCALE

Purpose: To measure traditional Protestant beliefs.

Number of Items: 18

Format: Items rated in 5-point Likert format. All items are presented.

Reliability: Alpha was .82.

Validity: Correlates with Mirels and Garrett Scale (.36), and Ray Scale (.59).

Author: Ray, J. J.

Article: The Protestant ethic in Australia.

Journal: *Journal of Social Psychology*, February 1982, *116*(first half), 127–138.

▪ ▪ ▪

3529

Test Name: ETHICAL BEHAVIOR RATING SCALE

Purpose: To identify and quantify moral behavior.

Number of Items: 15

Format: Includes two factors: personal moral character and verbal moral assertiveness. Teachers rate students on a 5-point rating scale from 1 (*never*) to 5 (*always*). All items are presented.

Reliability: Test–retest reliability coefficient was .54. Coefficient alpha was .96.

Validity: Correlations with the Ethical Reasoning Inventory ranged from –.10 to .37.

Author: Hill, G., and Swanson, H. L.

Article: Construct validity and reliability of the Ethical Behavior Rating Scale.

Journal: *Educational and Psychological Measurement*, Summer 1985, *45*(2), 285–292.

Related Research: Blasi, A. (1980). Bridging moral cognition and moral action: A critical review of literature. *Psychological Bulletin*, *88*, 1–45.

3530

Test Name: ETHICAL CONFLICT QUESTIONNAIRE

Purpose: To measure degree of perceived ethical conflict.

Number of Items: 20

Format: Items rated on a 7-point scale. All items are presented.

Reliability: Test–retest reliability was .84. Interval was not reported.

Author: Morrison, J. K., et al.

Article: Ethical conflict among clinical psychologists and other mental health workers.

Journal: *Psychological Reports*, December 1982, *51*(3-I), 703–714.

▪ ▪ ▪

3531

Test Name: ETHICAL REASONING INVENTORY

Purpose: To measure moral reasoning.

Number of Items: 26

Format: Multiple-choice format. Stories include six of Kohlberg's moral dilemmas.

Validity: Correlations with the Ethical Behavior Rating Scale ranged from –.10 to .37.

Author: Hill, G., and Swanson, H. L.

Article: Construct validity and reliability of the Ethical Behavior Rating Scale.

Journal: *Educational and Psychological Measurement*, Summer 1985, *45*(2), 285–292.

Related Research: Page, R., & Bode, J. (1980). Comparison of measures of moral reasoning and development of a new objective measure. *Educational and Psychological Measurement*, *40*, 317–329.

3532

Test Name: FREE WILL– DETERMINISM SCALE

Purpose: To measure beliefs in free will and determinism.

Number of Items: 7

Format: Semantic-differential format.

Reliability: Alpha ranged from .62 to .79.

Validity: Student essays that successfully defend a position on the free will-determinism issue correlated with scores on the scale. Correlations ranged from .54 to .59.

Author: Viney, W., et al.

Article: Validity of a scale designed to measure beliefs in free will and determinism.

Journal: *Psychological Reports*, June 1984, *54*(3), 867–872.

Related Research: Viney, W., et al. (1982). Attitudes toward punishment in relation to belief in free will and determinism. *Human Relations*, *35*, 939–949.

▪ ▪ ▪

3533

Test Name: FRIEDMAN'S SCALE

Purpose: To measure degree of agreement with economic-ideological structure of M. and R. Friedman's book, *Free to Choose*.

Number of Items: 30

Format: All items presented. Response categories not presented.

Reliability: Item-test correlations ranged from .13 to .65. Kuder-Richardson formula 20 was .80.

Validity: Loads highly (.58) on a factor that measures Western modes of thought and loads only slightly on a factor measuring Eastern modes of thought (.16).

Author: Krus, D. J., and Kennedy, P. H.

Article: Some characteristics of Apollonian and Dionysian dimensions of economic theories.

Journal: *Psychological Reports,* 1982, *50*(3-I), 967–974.

■ ■ ■

3534

Test Name: IDEOLOGICAL SCALE

Purpose: To measure traditional religious values.

Number of Items: 5

Format: Multiple-choice format.

Reliability: Alpha was .79.

Author: Frost, T. F., and Rogers, B. G.

Article: Attitudes toward technology and religion among collegiate undergraduates.

Journal: *Psychological Reports,* June 1985, *56*(3), 943–946.

Related Research: Faulkner, J. E., & DeJong, F. (1966). Religiosity in 5-D: An empirical analysis. *Social Forces, 45,* 246–254.

■ ■ ■

3535

Test Name: INDEX OF ADJUSTMENT AND VALUES

Purpose: To measure adjustment and values.

Number of Items: 35

Format: Includes 35 trait words for which the subject indicates how descriptive it is, how the subject feels about it, and how the subject would like it to be. Provides self-acceptance and self-ideal scores.

Reliability: Test–retest for self-acceptance ranged from .74 to .89 (6 weeks); for self-ideal ranged from .53 to .81 (6 weeks).

Validity: Correlation with Tennessee Self-Concept Scale was .31 (self-acceptance) and –.17 (self-ideal); with racial evaluation scale was –.01 (self-ideal) and .05 (self-acceptance).

Author: Hines, P., and Berg-Cross, L.

Article: Racial differences in global self-esteem.

Journal: *Journal of Social Psychology,* April 1981, *113*(second half), 271–281.

Related Research: Bills, R. E. (No date). *Index of adjustment and values–Forms: Elementary, junior high school and high school manual.* Mimeographed manuscript, University of Alabama.

■ ■ ■

3536

Test Name: INDIVIDUAL TRADITION–MODERNITY SCALE—REVISED

Purpose: To measure modern attitudes in Chinese adults.

Number of Items: 40

Format: Items rated in 6-point Likert format. Sample items are presented.

Validity: Correlates with Kahl's Modernism Scale at .38 for men and .32 for women.

Author: Yang, K-S.

Article: Social orientation and individual modernity among Chinese students in Taiwan.

Journal: *Journal of Social Psychology,* April 1981, *113*(second half), 159–170.

Related Research: Yang, K-S., & Hchu, H-Y. (1974). Determinants, correlates, and consequents of Chinese individual modernity. *Bull. Inst. Ethnol. Academic Sinica, 37,* 1–28. (In Chinese with English summary.)

3537

Test Name: JUST WORLD SCALE

Purpose: To measure perception of justice.

Number of Items: 20

Format: Paper-and-pencil test. All items are presented.

Reliability: Split-half reliability was .81.

Validity: Correlations with other scales ranged from –.60 to .61.

Author: Ahmed, S. M. S., and Stewart, R. A. C.

Article: Factor analytical and correlational study of Just World Scale.

Journal: *Perceptual and Motor Skills,* February 1985, *60*(1), 135–140.

Related Research: Rubin, Z., & Peplau, L. A. (1975). Who believes in just world? *Journal of Social Issues, 31,* 65–89.

■ ■ ■

3538

Test Name: JUST WORLD SCALE—CHINESE VERSION

Purpose: To measure adherence to the belief in a just world.

Number of Items: 20

Format: Items rated in 6-point Likert format.

Reliability: Alpha was .78.

Validity: Correlated with alienation (rs = .33 to .54, $p < .01$) and with support for work ethic (.33, $p < .01$).

Author: Ma, L.-C., and Smith, K. B.

Article: Individual and social correlates of the Just World Belief: A study of Taiwanese college students.

Journal: *Psychological Reports,*

August 1985 *57*(1), 35–38.

Related Research: Rubin, Z., & Peplau, L. A. (1975). Who believes in just world? *Journal of Social Issues, 31*, 65–89.

■ ■ ■

3539

Test Name: MAGICAL IDEATION SCALE

Purpose: To measure belief in forms of causation that are invalid by conventional standards.

Number of Items: 30

Format: True–false format. All items are presented.

Reliability: Alpha was .82 (men) and .85 (women).

Validity: Correlation with Eysenck Psychoticism was .32 (men); with perceptual aberration, .68 (men); with physical anhedonia, –.29 (men).

Author: Eckbad, M., and Chapman, L. J.

Article: Magical ideation as an indicator of schizotypy.

Journal: *Journal of Consulting and Clinical Psychology,* April 1983, *51*(2), 215–225.

Related Research: Chapman, L. J., et al. (1982). Reliabilities and intercorrelations of eight measures of proneness to psychosis. *Journal of Consulting and Clinical Psychology, 50*(2), 187–195.

■ ■ ■

3540

Test Name: MAGNITUDE ESTIMATION SCALE FOR HUMAN VALUES

Purpose: To assess human values at a ratio level of measurement. Terminal and instrumental goals are assessed.

Number of Items: 18

Format: Subjects rank 18 values,

the first of which then receives the value of 100. Respondents enter numbers for subsequent values that are equal to or less than the number given to the prior value in the ranked list.

Reliability: Test–retest (rho) values were .73 (terminal) and .72 (instrumental). Rank-value correlations were .78 (terminal) and .78 (instrumental).

Author: Cooper, D. R., and Clare, D. A.

Article: A magnitude estimation scale for human values.

Journal: *Psychological Reports,* 1981, *49*(2), 431–438.

Related Research: Rokeach, M. (1967). *Value summary.* Sunnyvale, CA: Halgren Press.

■ ■ ■

3541

Test Name: MORAL COMMITMENT SCALE

Purpose: To measure organizational commitment.

Number of Items: 4

Format: Responses are made on a 5-point scale.

Reliability: Coefficient alpha was .85.

Validity: Correlations with other variables ranged from –.18 to .16.

Author: Werbel, J. D., and Gould, S.

Article: A comparison of the relationship of commitment to turnover in recent hires and tenured employees.

Journal: *Journal of Applied Psychology,* November 1984, *69*(4), 687–690.

Related Research: Gould, S., & Penley, L. (1982). *Organizational commitment: A test of the model Working Paper Series.* San

Antonio: The University of Texas at San Antonio.

■ ■ ■

3542

Test Name: MORAL CONTENT COMPONENTS TEST

Purpose: To measure the content of moral thought.

Number of Items: 50

Format: The subject reads a series of moral dilemmas or stories and then after each the subject ranks statements reflecting possible moral considerations. Includes three factors.

Reliability: Average reliability coefficients were .69 and .75.

Author: Jensen, L., et al.

Article: A factorial study of the Moral Content Components Test.

Journal: *Educational and Psychological Measurement,* Autumn 1981, *41*(3), 613–624.

Related Research: Boyce, D., & Jensen, L. (1978). *Moral reasoning: Psychological philosophical perspectives.* Lincoln: The University of Nebraska Press.

■ ■ ■

3543

Test Name: MORAL JUDGEMENT SCALE

Purpose: To measure moral judgment.

Number of Items: 43

Format: Subjects evaluate each item as to its "rightness" or "wrongness" on a scale from 1 to 5. All items are presented.

Validity: Correlation of each item with locus of control scores ranged from –.26 to .09.

Author: Frost, T. F., and Wilmesmeier, J. M.

Article: Relationship between locus of control and moral judgements among college students.

Journal: *Perceptual and Motor Skills,* December 1983, *57*(3-I), 931–939.

Related Research: Rettig, S., & Pasamanick, B. (1959). Changes in moral values among college students: A factorial study. *American Sociological Review, 10,* 856–863.

. . .

3544

Test Name: MYSTICISM SCALE

Purpose: To measure mystical experience.

Number of Items: 32

Format: Includes two factors: general mysticism, religious interpretation.

Reliability: Internal consistency reliability correlations included item to total scale .29 to .52 ($N = 300$); subscale to total scale .39 to .62 ($N = 300$).

Validity: Correlation with the Religious Experience Episodes Measure was .47 ($N = 52$).

Author: Cowling, W. R., III.

Article: Relationship of mystical experience, differentiation, and creativity.

Journal: *Perceptual and Motor Skills,* October 1985, *61*(2), 451–456.

Related Research: Hood, R. W., Jr. (1975). The construction and preliminary validation of a measure of reported mystical experience. *Journal of the Scientific Study of Religion, 14,* 29–41.

. . .

3545

Test Name: NATIVE AMERICAN VALUE–ATTITUDE SCALE

Purpose: To assess attitude-value orientations of elementary age American Indian children on four dimensions.

Number of Items: 64

Format: Auditory dialogues followed by a typical Indian and typical Anglo response. Sample item presented.

Reliability: Alpha was .65 (school goals), .74 (sense of community), .50 (indirectness), .50 (noninterference).

Validity: Anglo responses increased as grade level increases for school goals and noninterference. Increased Indian responses occurred as grade level increases for sense of community and indirectness.

Author: Plas, J. M., and Bellet, W.

Article: Assessment of the value–attitude orientations of American Indian children.

Journal: *Journal of School Research,* 1983, *21*(1), 57–64.

. . .

3546

Test Name: NATURE OF EPISTEMOLOGICAL BELIEFS SCALE

Purpose: To classify students as dualists or relativists.

Number of Items: 7

Format: Items rated on a 5-point Likert scale.

Reliability: Test–retest reliability was .84.

Author: Ryan, M. P.

Article: Conceptions of prose coherence: Individual differences in epistemological standards.

Journal: *Journal of Educational Psychology,* December 1984, *76*(6), 1226–1238.

Related Research: Perry, W. G., Jr. (1968). *Patterns of*

development in thought and values of students in a liberal arts college: A validation of a scheme. Cambridge, MA: Harvard University. (ERIC Document Reproduction Service No. ED 024315)

. . .

3547

Test Name: ORIENTATION TO LEARNING SCALE

Purpose: To measure student orientation to humanistic instructional values.

Number of Items: 135

Format: Two equivalent forms, A and B. Responses to each item are made on a 5-point scale from *strongly agree* to *strongly disagree.*

Reliability: Odd–even and split-half reliabilities ($N = 20$) ranged from .93 to .95.

Validity: Correlations with other variables ranged from .119 to .513 ($N = 31$).

Author: Shapiro, S. B.

Article: The development and validation of an instrument to measure student orientation to humanistic instructional values.

Journal: *Educational and Psychological Measurement,* Winter 1985, *45*(4), 869–880.

Related Research: Shapiro, S. B. (1983). *An empirical value analysis of humanistic approaches to educational psychology.* Paper presented at the Western Psychological Association annual meeting, San Francisco.

. . .

3548

Test Name: PERSONAL SPHERE MODEL

Purpose: To measure people, ideas, and things that are or have been important.

Time Required: 10–15 minutes.

Format: The respondent draws symbols of people, ideas, or things important to him or her and indicates level of importance by connecting them with one, two, or three lines to a symbol for himself or herself. Respondents also cross out connecting lines for interrupted relationships.

Validity: Six factors account for 86% of the common variance. Concurrent validity: Beck Depression Scale correlated significantly with some subscales (sometimes opposite to expected direction). No correlations with fear of success, age, or class in school. Correlation between some subscales and locus of control.

Author: Sollod, R. N.

Article: The personal sphere model: Psychometric properties and concurrent validity in a college population.

Journal: *Psychological Reports,* December 1984, *55*(3), 727–736.

Related Research: Schmiedeck, R. (1978). *The personal sphere model.* New York: Grune & Stratton.

■ ■ ■

3549

Test Name: POLYPHASIC VALUES INVENTORY

Purpose: To reflect the existence of a broad range of values.

Number of Items: 20

Format: Subjects respond to a value-laden situation by selecting a philosophically defensible response ranging between conservative and liberal alternatives. Examples are presented.

Reliability: Average item reliability was .63.

Author: Kayne, J. B., and Houston, S. R.

Article: Values of American college students.

Journal: *Journal of Experimental Education,* Summer 1981, *49*(4), 199–206.

Related Research: Roscoe, J. T. (1965). Report of first research with the Polyphasic Values Inventory. *Journal of Research Services, 5,* 3–12.

■ ■ ■

3550

Test Name: PROTESTANT SCALE

Purpose: To measure orientation to work that conforms to the Protestant work ethic.

Number of Items: 19

Format: Forced-choice 9-point agreement scale.

Reliability: Alpha was .75.

Author: Ganster, D. C.

Article: Protestant ethic and performance: A re-examination.

Journal: *Psychological Reports,* February 1981, *48*(1), 335–338.

Related Research: Mirels, J. L., & Garrett, J. B. (1971). The Protestant ethic as a personality variable. *Journal of Consulting and Clinical Psychology, 36,* 40–44.

■ ■ ■

3551

Test Name: PROTESTANT ETHIC SCALE

Purpose: To measure attitudes toward work.

Number of Items: 19

Format: Forced-choice, 9-point response scale ranging from *very strong disagreement* to *very strong agreement.*

Reliability: Internal consistency reliability of .75.

Author: Ganster, D. C.

Article: Protestant ethic and performance: A re-examination.

Journal: *Psychological Reports,* February 1981, *48*(1), 335–338.

Related Research: Mirels, J. L., & Garrett, J. B. (1971). The Protestant ethic as a personality variable. *Journal of Consulting and Clinical Psychology, 36,* 40–44.

■ ■ ■

3552

Test Name: RAM SCALE— REVISED

Purpose: To measure student philosophical orientation in terms of relative, absolute, or mixed biases or preferences toward issues of knowledge, methods, and values.

Number of Items: 36

Format: Includes three scales of knowledge, methods, and values, employing a Likert format.

Reliability: Internal consistency (alpha) estimate for total-scale was .79 and .38, .71, and .76 for subscales of knowledge, methods, and values, respectively.

Author: Wright, C. R., et al.

Article: The RAM Scale: Development and validation of the revised scale in Likert format.

Journal: *Educational and Psychological Measurement,* Winter 1983, *43*(4), 1089–1102.

Related Research: Brown, G. F., et al. (1977). The relationship of scores of community college students on a measure of philosophical orientation to the nature of reality to their standing in selected school-related variables. *Educational and Psychological Measurement, 37,* 939–947.

3553

Test Name: RELIGIOSITY INDEX

Purpose: To measure religiosity among Jews.

Number of Items: 7

Format: Guttmann. All items presented.

Reliability: Coefficient of reproducibility was .91.

Validity: Correlates with age and marriage, ideal number of births, mean number of births, and work experience ($p < .05$).

Author: Hartman, M.

Article: Pronatalist tendencies and religiosity in Israel.

Journal: *Sociology and Social Research,* January 1984, *68*(2), 247–258.

■ ■ ■

3554

Test Name: RELIGIOSITY SCALE

Purpose: To measure religiosity.

Number of Items: 37

Format: Orthodox-liberal response continuum. Sample item presented.

Reliability: Alphas were .81 and .83 for husbands and wives, respectively.

Author: Filsinger, E. E., and Wilson, M. R.

Article: Religiosity, socioeconomic rewards, and family development: Predictors of marital adjustment.

Journal: *Journal of Marriage and the Family,* August 1984, *46*(3), 663–670.

Related Research: DeJong, G. F., et al. (1976). Dimensions of religiosity reconsidered: Evidence from a cross-cultural study. *Social Focus, 54,* 866–889.

3555

Test Name: RELIGIOUS RELATIVISM INDEX

Purpose: To measure belief that all religions are equally true vs. belief that only followers of Jesus Christ can be saved.

Number of Items: 5

Format: Responses to each item are made on a 5-point Likert scale ranging from 5 (*strongly agree*) to 1 (*strongly disagree*). An example is given.

Reliability: Cronbach's alphas ranged from .73 to .76.

Author: Hoge, D. R., et al.

Article: Transmission of religious and social values from parents to teenage children.

Journal: *Journal of Marriage and the Family,* August 1982, *44*(3), 569–580.

Related Research: Hoge, D. R., & Petrillo, G. H. (1978). Determinants of church participation and attitudes among high school youth. *Journal for the Scientific Study of Religion, 17,* 359–379.

■ ■ ■

3556

Test Name: REST'S TEST OF MORAL COMPREHENSION

Purpose: To measure moral comprehension.

Number of Items: 11-item version.

Format: Multiple-choice.

Validity: Reproducibility was .93. Scalability was .84.

Author: Tsujimoto, R. N.

Article: Guttmann scaling of moral comprehension stages.

Journal: *Psychological Reports,* 1982, *51*(2), 550.

Related Research: Rest, J. R.

(1979). *Development of judging moral issues.* Minneapolis: University of Minnesota Press.

■ ■ ■

3557

Test Name: SOCIAL ORDER SCALE

Purpose: To measure acceptance of feminist ideology.

Number of Items: 14

Format: Items rated in 6-point Likert format.

Reliability: Item-total correlations were .40 or higher. Average interitem correlation was .59. Test–retest (2 weeks) reliability was .86.

Author: Koupman-Boydan, P. G., and Abbott, M.

Article: Expectations for household task allocation and actual task allocation: A New Zealand study.

Journal: *Journal of Marriage and the Family,* February 1985, *47*(1), 211–219.

Related Research: Worell, J., & Worell, L. (1977). Support and opposition to the women's liberation movement: Some personality and parental correlates. *Journal of Research in Personality, 11,* 10–20.

■ ■ ■

3558

Test Name: SOCIOMORAL REFLECTION MEASURE

Purpose: To assess nonnative values and how they guide reason and reflective sociomoral thought.

Number of Items: 15

Format: Paper-and-pencil test in which respondents justify norms by responding to dilemmas.

Reliability: Interrater, test–retest, parallel forms, and internal consistency generally were in the .70s.

Validity: Correlated .85 with Moral Judgement Interview (Colby et al.).

Author: Gibbs, J. C.

Article: Facilitation of sociomoral reasoning in delinquents.

Journal: *Journal of Consulting and Clinical Psychology*, February 1984, *52*(1), 37–45.

Related Research: Gibbs, J. C., et al. (1982). Construction and validation of a simplified, group-administered equivalent to the Moral Judgement Interview. *Child Development, 53,* 875–910.

3559

Test Name: SURVEY OF WORK VALUES—MODIFIED

Purpose: To identify intrinsic and extrinsic work values.

Number of Items: 54

Format: Includes intrinsic and extrinsic work values. A 7-point Likert format was used. A sample item is presented.

Reliability: Coefficient alpha reliability estimates were .77 (intrinsic work values) and .69 (extrinsic work values).

Author: Phillips, J. S., and Freedman, S. M.

Article: Contingent pay and intrinsic task interest: Moderating effects of work values.

Journal: *Journal of Applied Psychology*, May 1985, *70*(2), 306–313.

Related Research: Wollack, S., et al. (1971). Development of the Survey of Work Values. *Journal of Applied Psychology, 55,* 331–338.

Hazer, J. T., & Alvarez, K. M. (1981). Police work values during organizational entry and assimilation. *Journal of Applied Psychology, 66*(1), 12–18.

CHAPTER 23
Vocational Evaluation

3560

Test Name: BEHAVIORAL OBSERVATION SCALES

Purpose: To measure the behavior of managers on the dimensions of support, interaction facilitation, goal emphasis, work facilitation.

Number of Items: 75

Format: Items rated on 5-point Likert response categories. Sample items presented.

Reliability: Alpha ranged from .85 to .92 across subscales.

Author: Wexley, K. N., and Pulakos, E. D.

Article: Sex effects on performance ratings in manager–subordinate dyads: A field study.

Journal: *Journal of Applied Psychology*, August 1982, *67*(4), 433–439.

Related Research: Stogdill, R. M., et al. (1962). New leader behavior description scales. *Journal of Psychology, 54,* 259–269.

Taylor, J. C., & Bowers, D. G. (1972). *Survey of organizations: A machine-scored standardized questionnaire instrument.* Ann Arbor: University of Michigan, IRSS.

●●●

3561

Test Name: BOREDOM IN DRIVING SCALE

Purpose: To measure boredom among truck drivers while driving on the job.

Number of Items: 6

Format: Items rated on 5-point scales, each point representing the percent of time the driver feels bored. All items are presented.

Reliability: Alpha was .86.

Validity: Boredom scores do not differ between "monotonous" and "more stimulating" routes. Scores were significantly and positively related to age ($p < .04$), length of residency ($p < .04$), tenure ($p < .03$), and health ($p < .05$).

Author: Drory, A.

Article: Individual differences in boredom proneness and test effectiveness at work.

Journal: *Personnel Psychology,* Spring 1982, *35*(1), 141–151.

●●●

3562

Test Name: CLINTON ASSESSMENT OF PROBLEM IDENTIFICATION SKILLS

Purpose: To assess problem identification skills of instructional supervisors.

Number of Items: 3

Format: Includes three scenarios, each of which contains a description of a situation or dilemma with explicit or implied problems to be solved. An example is provided. Two forms are included.

Reliability: Equivalence reliability estimate was .76. Score–rescore coefficients were .71 and .67 for forms A and B, respectively.

Validity: Correlations of forms A and B with the Merrifield-Guilford Seeing Problems test were .42 and .54, respectively.

Author: Clinton, B. J., et al.

Article: The development and validation of an instrument to assess problem identification skills of instructional supervisors.

Journal: *Educational and Psychological Measurement,* Summer 1983, *43*(2), 581–586.

●●●

3563

Test Name: COGNITIVE CONTRIBUTION TEST

Purpose: To measure cognitive contribution of teaching.

Number of Items: 8

Format: Likert items.

Reliability: .81 to .91.

Author: Neumann, L., and Neumann, Y.

Article: Determinants of students' instructional evaluation: A comparison of four levels of academic areas.

Journal: *Journal of Educational Research,* January/February 1985, *73*(3), 152–158.

Related Research: Bloom, B. S. (1956). *Taxonomy of Educational Objectives: Handbook I–Cognitive Domain.* New York: David McKay.

●●●

3564

Test Name: COUNSELING EVALUATION INVENTORY

Purpose: To assess client satisfaction with counseling.

Number of Items: 21

Format: Three satisfaction components identified through factor analysis include counseling climate, counselor comfort, and client satisfaction.

Reliability: Test–retest (14 days) reliability ($N = 163$) ranged from .63 to .78.

Author: Heesacker, M., and Heppner, P. P.

Article: Using real-client perceptions to examine psychometric properties of the Counselor Rating Form.

Journal: *Journal of Counseling Psychology*, April 1933, *30*(2), 180–187.

Related Research: Linden, J. D., et al. (1965). Development and evaluation of an inventory for rating counseling. *Personnel and Guidance Journal, 44,* 267–276.

■ ■ ■

3565

Test Name: COUNSELOR BEHAVIOR EVALUATION FORM

Purpose: To assess whether or not trainees observed in counseling interviews performed specific behaviors in the decision-making counseling paradigm.

Number of Items: 10

Format: Ratings on each of 10 behaviors are made on a 3-point scale from *clearly displays the behavior* (3) to *completely fails to display the behavior* (1). Scores ranged from 10 to 30.

Reliability: Internal consistency reliability coefficient equivalent to a Kuder-Richardson formula 20 estimate was .85 ($N = 216$).

Author: Baker, S. B., et al.

Article: Microskills practice versus

mental practice training for competence in decision-making counseling.

Journal: *Journal of Counseling Psychology*, January 1984, *31*(1), 104–107.

Related Research: Herr, E. L., et al. (1973). Clarifying the counseling mystique. *American Vocational Journal, 48*(4), 66–72.

■ ■ ■

3566

Test Name: COUNSELOR EFFECTIVENESS SCALE

Purpose: To measure client attitudes toward the counselor.

Number of Items: 25

Format: Items consist of 7-point semantic differentials. A parallel form was prepared.

Reliability: Coefficient of equivalence was .98.

Author: Ponterotto, J. G., and Furlong, M. J.

Article: Evaluating counselor effectiveness: A critical review of rating scale instruments.

Journal: *Journal of Counseling Psychology*, October 1985, *32*(4), 597–616.

Related Research: Ivey, A. E., & Authier, J. (1978). *Microcounseling: Innovations in interviewing, counseling, psychotherapy, and psychoeducation* (2nd ed.). Springfield, IL: Charles C Thomas.

■ ■ ■

3567

Test Name: COUNSELOR EFFECTIVENESS RATING SCALE

Purpose: To measure client perception of counselor credibility.

Number of Items: 10

Format: Items are rated on a 7-point semantic differential scale.

Reliability: Cronbach's alphas ranged from .75 to .90.

Validity: Concurrent validity with the Counselor Rating Form, $r = .80$.

Author: Ponterotto, J. G., and Furlong, M. J.

Article: Evaluating counselor effectiveness: A critical review of rating scale instruments.

Journal: *Journal of Counseling Psychology*, October 1985, *32*(4), 597–616.

Related Research: Furlong, M. J., et al. (1979). Effects of counselor ethnicity and attitudinal similarity on Chicano students' perceptions of counselor credibility and attractiveness. *Hispanic Journal of Behavorial Sciences, 1,* 41–53.

■ ■ ■

3568

Test Name: COUNSELOR DEVELOPMENT QUESTIONNAIRE

Purpose: To provide a trainee self-report instrument.

Number of Items: 157

Format: Includes two subscales: trainee and supervisory needs. Employs a 5-point Likert scale from *strongly agree* to *strongly disagree*.

Reliability: Cronbach's alpha ranged from .82 to .88.

Author: Reising, G. N., and Daniels, M. H.

Article: A student of Hogan's model of counselor development and supervision.

Journal: *Journal of Counseling Psychology*, April 1983, *30*(2), 235–244.

Related Research: Worthington, E. L., Jr., & Roehlke, H. J.

(1979). Effective supervision as perceived by beginning counselors-in-training. *Journal of Counseling Psychology, 26,* 64–73.

■ ■ ■

3569

Test Name: COUNSELOR EVALUATION INVENTORY

Purpose: To measure counselor effectiveness.

Number of Items: 21

Format: Includes three factors: counseling climate, counselor comfort, client satisfaction. A 5-point Likert scale is used. Examples are presented.

Reliability: Test–retest (14 days) reliability ranged from .63 to .83.

Author: Ponterotto, J. G., and Furlong, M. J.

Article: Evaluating counselor effectiveness: A critical review of rating scale instruments.

Journal: *Journal of Counseling Psychology,* October 1985, *32*(4), 597–616.

Related Research: Linden, J. D., et al. (1965). Development and evaluation of an inventory for rating counseling. *Personnel and Guidance Journal, 44,* 267–276.

Heppner, P. P., & Heesacker, M. (1983). Perceived counselor characteristics, client expectation and client satisfaction with counseling. *Journal of Counseling Psychology, 30*(1), 31–39.

■ ■ ■

3570

Test Name: COUNSELOR EVALUATION AND RATING SCALE

Purpose: To provide a measure of practicum student competence.

Number of Items: 27

Format: Responses are recorded on a Likert scale of 6 values

ranging from 3 (*I strongly agree*) to –3 (*I strongly disagree*).

Reliability: Split-half reliability was .95 (*N* = 45). Test–retest reliability was .94.

Author: Handley, P.

Article: Relationship between supervisors' and trainees' cognitive styles and the supervision process.

Journal: *Journal of Counseling Psychology,* September 1982, *29*(5), 508–515.

Related Research: Myrick, R. D., & Kelly, D. F., Jr. (1971). A scale for evaluating practicum students in counseling and supervision. *Counselor Education and Supervision, 10,* 330–336.

■ ■ ■

3571

Test Name: COUNSELOR INTERVIEW COMPETENCE SCALE

Purpose: To evaluate counselors' interpersonal competence in client interviews.

Number of Items: 5

Format: Ratings are made on a 7-point continuum for each of five dimensions: empathy, attractiveness, trustworthiness, interpretation, and expertness.

Reliability: Hoyt coefficients were reported to be .96 and .896. Interrater agreement was reported to be .86.

Author: Baker, S. B., et al.

Article: Microskills practice versus mental practice training for competence in decision-making counseling.

Journal: *Journal of Counseling Psychology,* January 1984, *31*(1), 104–107.

Related Research: Jenkins, W. W., et al. (1982). *The development of behaviorally anchored rating*

scales to evaluate counselor interview competence. Unpublished manuscript, Pennsylvania State University.

■ ■ ■

3572

Test Name: COUNSELOR RATING FORM—SHORT VERSION

Purpose: To assess counselor characteristics of attractiveness, expertness, and trustworthiness.

Number of Items: 12

Format: Each item is rated on a 7-point scale from *not very* (1) to *very* (7).

Reliability: Coefficient alphas ranged from .63 to .89.

Author: Epperson, D. L., and Pecnik, J. A.

Article: Counselor Rating Form—Short Version: Further validation and comparison to the long form.

Journal: *Journal of Counseling Psychology,* January 1985, *32*(1), 143–146.

Related Research: Corrigan, J. D., & Schmidt, L. D. (1983). Development and validation of revisions in the Counselor Rating Form. *Journal of Counseling Psychology, 30,* 64–75.

Lee, D. Y., et al. (1985). Counselor verbal and nonverbal responses and perceived expertness, trustworthiness and attractiveness. *Journal of Counseling Psychology, 32,* 181–187.

Vandecreek, L., & Angstadt, L. (1985). Client preferences and anticipation about counselor self-discipline. *Journal of Counseling Psychology, 32,* 206–214.

Brooks, L., et al. (1982). The effects of nontraditional role modeling intervention on the sex typing of occupational preference and career salience in adolescent females. *Journal of Vocational Behavior, 26*(3), 264–275.

■ ■ ■

3573

Test Name: COUNSELOR RATING FORM

Purpose: To measure clients' perceptions of counselors' expertness, attractiveness, and trustworthiness.

Number of Items: 36

Format: Includes three scales containing 7-point bipolar items.

Reliability: Split-half reliability ranged from .75 to .92.

Validity: Correlation with congruence measures ranged from –.05 to .41.

Author: Hill, C. E., et al.

Article: Nonverbal communication and counseling outcome.

Journal: *Journal of Counseling Psychology,* May 1981, *28*(3), 203–212.

Related Research: Barak, A., & LaCrosse, M. B. (1975). Multidimensional perceptions of counselor behavior. *Journal of Counseling Psychology, 22,* 471–476.

Banikiotes, P. G., & Merluzzi, T. V. (1981). Impact of counselor gender and counselor sex role orientation on perceived counselor characteristics. *Journal of Counseling Psychology, 28,* 342–348.

McKitrick, D. (1981). Generalizing from counseling analogue research on subjects' perceptions of counselors. *Journal of Counseling Psychology, 28,* 357–360.

Heppner, P. P., & Handley, P. C. (1981). A study of the interpersonal influence process in supervision. *Journal of Counseling Psychology, 28,* 437–444.

Zamostny, K. P., et al. (1981).

Replication and extension of social influence processes in counseling: A field study. *Journal of Counseling Psychology, 28,* 481–489.

Atkinson, D. R., et al. (1981). Sexual preference similarity, attitude similarity, and perceived counselor credibility and attractiveness. *Journal of Counseling Psychology, 28,* 504–509.

Hubble, M. A., et al. (1981). The effect of counselor touch in an initial counseling session. *Journal of Counseling Psychology, 28,* 533–535.

Hardin, S. I., & Yanico, B. J. (1981). A comparison of modes of presentation in vicarious participation counseling analogues. *Journal of Counseling Psychology, 28,* 540–543.

Dowd, E. T., & Bororo, D. R. (1982). Differential effects of counselor self-disclosure, self-involving statements, and interpretation. *Journal of Counseling Psychology, 29,* 8–13.

McCarthy, P. R. (1982). Differential effects of counselor self-referent responses and counselor status. *Journal of Counseling Psychology, 29,* 125–131.

Porché, L. M., & Banikiotes, P. G. (1982). Racial and attitudinal factors affecting the perceptions of counselors by Black adolescents. *Journal of Counseling Psychology, 29,* 169–174.

Dowd, E. T., & Pety, J. (1982). Effect of counselor predicate matching on perceived social influence and client satisfaction. *Journal of Counseling Psychology, 29,* 206–209.

Heppner, P. P., & Heesacker, M. (1982). Interpersonal influence process in real-life counseling: Investigating client perceptions, counselor experience level, and

counselor power over time. *Journal of Counseling Psychology, 29,* 215–223.

Hackman, H. W., & Claiborn, C. D. (1982). An attributional approach to counselor attractiveness. *Journal of Counseling Psychology, 29,* 224–231.

Ruppel, G., & Kaul, T. J. (1982). Investigation of social influence theory's conception of client resistance. *Journal of Counseling Psychology, 29,* 232–239.

Paurohit, N., et al. (1982). The role of verbal and nonverbal cues in the formation of first impressions of Black and White counselors. *Journal of Counseling Psychology, 29,* 371–378.

Heppner, P. P., & Heesacker, M. (1983). Perceived counselor characteristics, client expectations, and client satisfaction with counseling. *Journal of Counseling Psychology, 30,* 31–39.

Corrigan, J. D., & Schmidt, L. D. (1983). Development and validation of revisions in the Counselor Rating Form. *Journal of Counseling Psychology, 30,* 64–75.

Remer, P., et al. (1983). Differential effects of positive versus negative self-involving counselor responses. *Journal of Counseling Psychology, 30,* 121–125.

Heesacker, M., & Heppner, P. P. (1983). Using real-client perceptions to examine psychometric properties of the counselor rating form. *Journal of Counseling Psychology, 30,* 180–187.

Strohmer, D. C., & Biggs, D. A. (1983). Effects of counselor disability status on disabled subjects, perceptions of counselor attractiveness and expertness. *Journal of Counseling Psychology, 30,* 202–208.

Merluzzi, T. V., & Brischetto, C. S. (1983). Breach of confidentiality and perceived trustworthiness of counselors. *Journal of Counseling Psychology, 30,* 245–251.

Lee, D. Y., et al. (1983). Effects of counselor race on perceived counselor effectiveness. *Journal of Counseling Psychology, 30,* 447–450.

Reynolds, C. L., & Fischer, C. H. (1983). Personal versus professional evaluations of self-disclosing and self-involving counselors. *Journal of Counseling Psychology, 30,* 451–454.

Milne, C. R., & Dowd, E. T. (1983). Effect of interpretation style on counselor social influence. *Journal of Counseling Psychology, 30,* 603–606.

Angle, S. S., & Goodyear, R. K. (1984). Perceptions of counselor qualities: Impact on subjects' self-concepts, counselor gender, and counselor introduction. *Journal of Counseling Psychology, 31,* 576–579.

Robbins, E. S., & Haase, R. F. (1985). Power of nonverbal cues in counseling interactions: Availability, vividness, or salience? *Journal of Counseling Psychology, 32,* 502–513.

Ponterotto, J. G., & Furlong, M. J. (1985). Evaluating counselor effectiveness: A critical review of rating scale instruments. *Journal of Counseling Psychology, 32,* 597–616.

Kraft, R. G., et al. (1985). Effects of positive refraining and paradoxical directives in counseling for negative emotions. *Journal of Counseling Psychology, 32,* 617–621.

Suiter, R. L., & Goodyear, R. K. (1985). Male and female counselor and client perceptions of four levels of counselor touch. *Journal*

of Counseling Psychology, 32, 645–648.

Corcoran, K. J. (1985). Unraveling subjects' perceptions of paraprofessionals and professionals: A pilot study. *Perceptual and Motor Skills, 60,* 111–114.

■ ■ ■

3574

Test Name: EMPLOYMENT INTERVIEW RATING SCALES

Purpose: To assess potential employees.

Number of Items: 7

Format: Items rated on 7-point rating scales. All items are presented.

Reliability: Interrater reliability ranged from .39 to .72 across items and age and sex categories. Overall reliability was .70 ($p <$ .001).

Validity: Comparable reliability ratings obtained for men and women and Blacks and Whites.

Author: Grove, D. A.

Article: A behavioral consistency approach to decision-making in employment selection.

Journal: *Personnel Psychology,* Spring 1981, *34*(1), 55–64.

■ ■ ■

3575

Test Name: EVALUATION RATING SCALE

Purpose: To evaluate job applicants (in an experimental setting where raters view taped simulated interviews).

Number of Items: 15

Format: Semantic differential. All adjective pairs presented.

Reliability: Alpha was .96.

Validity: Factor analysis showed

that the 15 items accounted for 68% of item variance.

Author: Mullins, T. W.

Article: Interviewer decisions as a function of applicant race, applicant quality and interviewer prejudice.

Journal: *Personnel Psychology,* Spring 1982, *35*(1), 163–174.

■ ■ ■

3576

Test Name: FACULTY PERFORMANCE CHECKLIST

Purpose: To measure college students' satisfaction with their course and instructor.

Number of Items: 64

Format: Students respond to each item with *Yes, No,* or *Does Not Apply.* Examples are presented.

Reliability: Coefficient alpha was .88.

Author: Strom, B., and Hocevar, D.

Article: Course structure and student satisfaction: An attribute–treatment interaction analysis.

Journal: *Educational Research Quarterly,* Spring 1982, *7*(1), 21–30.

Related Research: Schuler, G. (1974). *Report of the research team on faculty evaluation.* Unpublished manuscript, Ithaca College.

■ ■ ■

3577

Test Name: GLOBAL DIMENSION APPRAISAL FORM

Purpose: To rate performance of law enforcement personnel.

Number of Items: 40

Format: Includes nine dimensions.

Reliability: Interrater reliabilities

ranged from .53 to .71 (corrected by Spearman-Brown formula).

Validity: Correlations with age ranged from −.28 to .03. Correlations with tenure ranged from −.21 to .15.

Author: Lee, R., et al.

Article: Multitrait–multimethod–multirater analysis of performance ratings for law enforcement personnel.

Journal: *Journal of Applied Psychology*, October 1981, *66*(5), 625–632.

■ ■ ■

3578

Test Name: HELPING BELIEFS INVENTORY

Purpose: To measure basic counseling skills.

Number of Items: 10 (all nonhelpful response items).

Format: Items rated on 5-point response categories (*almost always helpful* to *almost never helpful*). All items presented.

Reliability: Alpha was .84.

Validity: Correlates .32 with authoritarianism, −.36 with flexibility, −.28 with psychological mindedness (all *p* < .01).

Author: McLennan, P. P.

Article: Helping beliefs inventory: Brief screening measure for training volunteer applicants in counseling.

Journal: *Psychological Reports*, June 1985, *56*(3), 843–846.

■ ■ ■

3579

Test Name: HIGHWAY PATROL PERFORMANCE ASSESSMENT FORM

Purpose: To measure job performance of highway patrol officers.

Number of Items: 78

Format: Statements appeared in 3-statement triads, each covering one aspect of the work of patrolmen. 26 triads were grouped into 9 performance areas. Sample items presented. Supervisors check the one statement out of three that best describes job performance of ratee.

Reliability: Triads all exceed the reproducibility of .80. Alpha (computed on triad scores) was .72. Interrater reliability was .90.

Validity: Correlations ranged between .62 and .78 with external indicator of job performance. Trooper of the year nominees rated higher than others (*p* < .001).

Author: Rosinger, G., et al.

Article: Development of behaviorally based performance appraisal system.

Journal: *Personnel Psychology*, Spring 1982, *35*(1), 75–88.

■ ■ ■

3580

Test Name: INDEX OF PERFORMANCE EVALUATION

Purpose: To measure performance of managers.

Number of Items: 5

Format: Items rated on 7-point response scales. All items are presented.

Reliability: Alpha was .89.

Author: Izraeli, D. N., and Izraeli, D.

Article: Sex effects in evaluating leaders: A replication study.

Journal: *Journal of Applied Psychology*, August 1985, *70*(3), 540–546.

Related Research: Bartol, K. M., & Butterfield, D. A. (1976). Sex effects in evaluating leaders.

Journal of Applied Psychology, 61, 446–454.

■ ■ ■

3581

Test Name: INSTRUCTOR RATING FORM

Purpose: To evaluate instructor performance using a longitudinal approach.

Number of Items: 33

Format: Items rated on 7-point bipolar adjective scales.

Validity: Seven first-order and two second-order factors were identified using the Chain-P technique.

Author: Hundleby, J. D., and Gluppe, M. R.

Article: Dimensions of change in instructor presentations.

Journal: *Journal of Educational Research*, January/February 1984, *74*(3), 133–138.

Related Research: Luborsky, L., & Mintz, J. (1972). The contributions of P-technique to personality, psychotherapy, and psychosomatic research. In R. M. Dreger (Ed.), *Multivariate personality research: Contributors to the understanding of personality in honor of Raymond B. Cattell*. Baton Rouge, LA: Claton Publishing Division.

■ ■ ■

3582

Test Name: ISRAELI ARMY QUESTIONNAIRE FOR PERSONALITY AND MOTIVATION MEASUREMENT

Purpose: To measure and predict success in military training.

Number of Items: 29

Format: Multiple-choice. "Choose the answer that best describes your behavior."

Reliability: Alpha was .88.

(Subscales ranged between .59 and .65.)

Validity: Questionnaire results correlated .34 with some criterion performance, compared to .36 for existing interview scores.

Author: Tubiana, J. H., and Ben-Shakhar, G.

Article: An objective group questionnaire as a substitute for a personal interview in the prediction of success in military training in Israel.

Journal: *Personnel Psychology,* Summer 1982, *35*(2), 349–357.

■ ■ ■

3583

Test Name: JOB INVOLVEMENT AND PSYCHOLOGICAL SUCCESS SCALES

Purpose: To measure to what extent a person "eats, sleeps, and lives" his or her job and feelings of competence and success.

Number of Items: 10

Format: Likert format.

Reliability: Alpha was .79 (involvement) and .78 (success).

Author: Slocum, J. W. (Jr)., and Cron, W. L.

Article: Job attitudes and performance during three career stages.

Journal: *Journal of Vocational Behavior,* April 1985, *26*(2), 126–145.

Related Research: Hall, T., et al. (1978). Effects of top-down departmental and job change upon perceived employee behavior and attitudes: A national field experiment. *Journal of Applied Psychology, 63,* 62–72.

■ ■ ■

3584

Test Name: JOB PERFORMANCE SCALES

Purpose: To provide self- and supervisor-ratings of performance.

Number of Items: 10

Format: Self-ratings consisted of 3 items, including measures of quantity, quality, and overall performance. Supervisory ratings consisted of 7 items including speed of performance, quality of performance, attitude to the job, initiative, cooperation, punctuality, and ability to learn. Five-point response scales were employed.

Reliability: Alpha coefficients were .93 (self-rating) and .97 (supervisor rating, $N = 166$).

Validity: Correlations with other variables ranged from .04 to .37.

Author: Tharenou, P., and Harker, P.

Article: Moderating influence of self-esteem on relationships between job complexity, performance, and satisfaction.

Journal: *Journal of Applied Psychology,* November 1984, *69*(4), 623–632.

■ ■ ■

3585

Test Name: MANAGERIAL PERFORMANCE SCALE

Purpose: To measure eight dimensions of managerial importance (know-how, administration, training, direction, feedback, motivating, innovation, and consideration).

Number of Items: 8

Format: Items rated on a 9-point rating scale. Items described.

Reliability: Split-half reliability was .87.

Validity: Convergent validity: superiors–subordinates, .24; self–subordinate, .19; superior–self, .16.

Author: Mount, M. K.

Article: Psychometric properties of subordinate ratings of managerial performance.

Journal: *Personnel Psychology,* Winter 1984, *37*(4), 687–702.

Related Research: Tornow, W. W., & Pinto, P. R. (1976). The development of a managerial taxonomy: A system for describing, clarifying, and evaluating executive positions. *Journal of Applied Psychology, 61,* 410–418.

■ ■ ■

3586

Test Name: MANAGERIAL POTENTIAL SCALE

Purpose: To measure managerial competence and managerial interest.

Number of Items: 34

Format: Items are from the California Psychological Inventory. Sample items are presented.

Reliability: Alpha was .75.

Validity: Correlates .88 (men) and .89 (women) with Goodstein and Schrader Scale.

Author: Gough, H. G.

Article: A managerial potential scale for the California Psychological Inventory.

Journal: *Journal of Applied Psychology,* May 1984, *69*(2), 233–240.

Related Research: Goodstein, L. D., & Schrader, W. J. (1963). An empirically-derived managerial key for the California Psychological Inventory. *Journal of Applied Psychology, 47,* 42–45.

■ ■ ■

3587

Test Name: MULTIPLE ITEM APPRAISAL FORM

Purpose: To rate performance of law enforcement personnel.

Number of Items: 40

Format: Includes nine dimensions.

Reliability: Coefficient alphas ranged from .73 to .95. Interrater reliabilities ranged from .61 to .80 (corrected by Spearman-Brown formula).

Validity: Correlations with age ranged from −.15 to .09. Correlations with tenure ranged from −.09 to .17.

Author: Lee, R., et al.

Article: Multitrait–multimethod–multirater analysis of performance ratings for law enforcement personnel.

Journal: *Journal of Applied Psychology,* October 1981, *66*(5), 625–632.

■ ■ ■

3588

Test Name: NONVERBAL APPLICANT RATING SCALE

Purpose: To rate applicants on poise, clothing, cleanliness, posture, articulation, voice, answering behavior, and eye contact.

Number of Items: 8

Format: Items rated on a 5-point multiple-choice format.

Reliability: Ranged from .62 to .88 across items. (Winer formula for interviewer reliability.)

Validity: Correlations among items ranged from .54 to .90. Mixed sex and race ratings were reported (men rated cleanliness, poise, clothing, posture, articulation, and eye contact lower than did women; Blacks rated lower than Whites on voice intensity and articulation).

Author: Parsons, C. K., and Liden, R. C.

Article: Interviewer perceptions of applicant qualifications: A multivariate field study of demographic characteristics and nonverbal cues.

Journal: *Journal of Applied Psychology,* December 1984, *69*(4), 557–568.

■ ■ ■

3589

Test Name: PERCEPTIONS OF CLASSROOM INSTRUCTOR SCALES

Purpose: To measure student perceptions of classroom teachers.

Number of Items: 40

Format: Semantic differential. All items presented.

Reliability: Cronbach's alpha ranged from .72 to .90 across subscales.

Validity: Identical factors (subscales) extracted for men and women.

Author: Bennett, S. K.

Article: Student perceptions and expectations for male and female instructors: Evidence relating to the question of gender bias in teaching evaluation.

Journal: *Journal of Educational Psychology,* April 1982, *74*(2), 170–179.

■ ■ ■

3590

Test Name: PERFORMANCE IMPROVEMENT GUIDE

Purpose: To evaluate student teachers on seven dimensions: Instruction, curriculum, relations to peers and principals, professional qualities, personal qualities.

Number of Items: 78 statements.

Format: Respondents rate student teachers on a 6-point scale from 1

(*strongly disagree*) to 6 (*strongly agree*).

Reliability: Cronbach's alpha ranged from .56 to .94 across dimensions.

Validity: Valid according to Fiske's multitrait–multimethod test for convergent, but not discriminant, validity.

Author: Wheeler, A. E., and Knoop, H. R.

Article: Self, teacher, and faculty assessments of student teaching performance.

Journal: *Journal of Educational Research,* January–February 1982, *75*(3), 178–181.

Related Research: Chiu, L. H. (1975). Influence of student teaching on perceived teaching competence. *Perceptual and Motor Skills, 40,* 872–874.

■ ■ ■

3591

Test Name: PRESENTER'S QUALITIES RATING FORM

Purpose: To measure subjects' perception of the presenter's competence.

Number of Items: 36

Format: Items are bipolar and rated from 1 to 7. Includes three dimensions: prepared–unprepared, likeable–unlikable, genuine–phony.

Reliability: Coefficient alpha was .87.

Author: Gilver, L. A., et al.

Article: Influence of presenter's gender on students' evaluations of presenters discussing sex fairness in counseling: An analogue study.

Journal: *Journal of Counseling Psychology,* May 1981, *28*(3), 258–264.

Related Research: LaCrosse, M. B. (1977). Comparative perceptions of counselor behavior: A replication and extension. *Journal of Counseling Psychology, 24,* 464–471.

■ ■ ■

3592

Test Name: RATING SCALE FOR ENTRY-LEVEL PSYCHIATRIC AIDS

Purpose: To assess potential psychiatric aid employees.

Number of Items: 78

Format: 1–5 rating scale format (1 = *seldom performs correctly;* 5 = *performs consistently above average*).

Reliability: Alpha ranged between .97 and .99 across rating categories. Test–retest reliability was .84 (10–14-day interval).

Validity: Correlated .26 with wide range vocabulary test; .24 with personnel tests for industry.

Author: Distefano, M. K., et al.

Article: Application of content validity methods to the development of a job-related performance rating criterion.

Journal: *Personnel Psychology,* Autumn 1983, *36*(3), 621–631.

■ ■ ■

3593

Test Name: RATING SCALE FOR JOB-RELATED WORK

Purpose: To measure performance of job-related work.

Number of Items: 50

Format: The 5-point rating format ranges from 1 (*seldom performs correctly*) to 5 (*performs consistently above acceptable level*).

Reliability: Alphas ranged from .91 to .98 across categories of work.

Validity: Correlated (mean

validity) .23 with verbal ability test.

Author: Distefano, M. K., and Pryer, M. W.

Article: Verbal selection test and work performance validity with aides from three psychiatric hospitals.

Journal: *Psychological Reports,* June 1985, *56*(3), 811–815.

Related Research: Distefano, M. K., et al. (1983). Application of content validity methods to the development of a job-related performance rating criterion. *Personnel Psychology, 36,* 621–631.

■ ■ ■

3594

Test Name: RELATIONSHIP INVENTORY

Purpose: To measure subjects' ratings of the interviewer.

Number of Items: 36

Format: Includes 5 subscales: empathic understanding, unconditional regard, level of regard, congruence, and resistance. Responses to each item were made on a 7-point scale from *mostly disagree* to *mostly agree.*

Reliability: Cronbach's alphas ranged from .54 to .85.

Author: Lopez, F. G., and Wambach, C. A.

Article: Effects of paradoxical and self-control directives in counseling.

Journal: *Journal of Counseling Psychology,* March 1982, *29*(2), 115–124.

Related Research: Strong, S., et al. (1979). Motivational and equipping functions of interpretation in counseling. *Journal of Counseling Psychology, 26,* 98–107.

3595

Test Name: RELATIONSHIP QUESTIONNAIRE

Purpose: To measure clients' ratings of counselors' performance.

Number of Items: 24

Format: Items rated on 7-point Likert response categories.

Reliability: Internal consistency ranged from .85 to .90 over two subscales.

Author: Loeb, R. G., and Curtis, J. M.

Article: Effects of counselors' self-references on subjects' first impressions in an experimental psychological interview.

Journal: *Psychological Reports,* December 1984, *55*(3), 803–810.

Related Research: Sorenson, A. G. (1967). *Toward an instructional model for counseling* (Occasional Report No. 6). Center for the Study of Instructional Programs, UCLA.

Curtis, J. M. (1981). Effect of therapist's self-disclosure on patients' impressions of empathy, competence, and trust in an analogue of psychotherapeutic interaction. *Psychological Reports, 48*(1), 127–136.

■ ■ ■

3596

Test Name: SALES PERFORMANCE CHART

Purpose: To evaluate salespeople on seven key dimensions: volume, new accounts, selling results, leadership, planning, initiative, resourcefulness.

Number of Items: 7

Format: Items rated on a 5-point Likert format.

Reliability: Alpha was .89.

Validity: Actual sales volume

correlates .41 with evaluation of sales volume.

Author: Slocum, J. W., Jr., and Cron, W. L.

Article: Job attitudes and performance during three career stages.

Journal: *Journal of Vocational Behavior*, April 1985, *26*(2), 126–145.

■ ■ ■

3597

Test Name: SLATER NURSING COMPETENCE RATING SCALE

Purpose: To measure performance of nurses on the job.

Number of Items: 84

Format: Supervisors rate observed behaviors. Six behavioral dimensions are scored.

Reliability: Split-half reliability was .98.

Author: Martin, T. N.

Article: Job performance and turnover.

Journal: *Journal of Applied Psychology*, February 1981, *66*(1), 116–119.

Related Research: Slater, D. (1967). *The Slater Nursing Competence Rating Scale.* Detroit, MI: Wayne State University College of Nursing.

■ ■ ■

3598

Test Name: SELF-EVALUATED SALES PERFORMANCE MEASURE

Purpose: To provide a self-evaluation of sales job activities.

Number of Items: 47

Format: Responses were made on a 5-point scale ranging from *much below average* to *much above average.*

Reliability: Cronbach's alpha was .88.

Validity: Correlations with other variables ranged from –.11 to .27.

Author: Motowidlo, S. J.

Article: Relationship between self-rated performance and pay satisfaction among sales representatives.

Journal: *Journal of Applied Psychology*, April 1982, *67*(2), 209–213.

■ ■ ■

3599

Test Name: SESSION EVALUATION QUESTIONNAIRE

Purpose: To measure novice counselors' and their clients' view of counseling session impact.

Number of Items: 19

Format: Includes four dimensions: depth, smoothness, positivity, and arousal. All items are bipolar adjectives with responses to each made on a 1–7 scale. All items presented.

Reliability: Coefficient alphas ranged from .78 to .93.

Author: Stiles, W. B., and Snow, J. S.

Article: Counseling session impact as viewed by novice counselors and their clients.

Journal: *Journal of Counseling Psychology*, January 1984, *31*(1), 3–12.

Related Research: Stiles, W. B., et al. (1982). Participants' perceptions of self-analytic group sessions. *Small Group Behavior, 13,* 237–254.

■ ■ ■

3600

Test Name: STUDENT EVALUATION OF TEACHING

Purpose: To measure student opinion of teacher behavior and its effect on the student.

Number of Items: 8

Format: Rating scales.

Reliability: Internal consistency was .76; Intraclass correlation was .89; Cross-year correlation was .68.

Author: Fox, R., et al.

Article: Student evaluation of teacher as a measure of teacher behavior and teacher impact on students.

Journal: *Journal of Educational Research,* September/October 1983, *77*(1), 16–21.

Related Research: Veldman, D. J., & Peck, R. F. (1979). Student teacher characteristics from the pupil's viewpoint. *Journal of Educational Psychology, 71,* 117–124.

■ ■ ■

3601

Test Name: STUDENT RATINGS OF TEACHERS SCALE

Purpose: To measure student evaluations of teachers.

Number of Items: 18

Format: Items rated on a 7-point agreement scale.

Validity: Factors emerged that were similar to Marsh and Ware's five-factor structure of teacher qualities.

Author: Basow, S. A., and Distenfeld, M. S.

Article: Teacher expressiveness: More important for male than female teachers.

Journal: *Journal of Educational Psychology*, February 1985, *77*(1), 45–52.

Related Research: Marsh, H. W., & Ware, J. E. (1982). Effects of expressiveness, content coverage, and incentive on multi-dimensional student rating scales: New interpretations of the Dr. Fox Effect. *Journal of Educational Psychology, 74,* 126–134.

■ ■ ■

3602

Test Name: STUDENT TEACHER RATING SCALE

Purpose: To measure level of professional development in student teachers.

Number of Items: 19

Format: Multiple-choice. Sample items presented.

Reliability: Alphas ranged from .87 to .90 across subgroups.

Author: Hattie, J., et al.

Article: Assessment of student teachers by supervising teachers.

Journal: *Journal of Educational Psychology,* October 1982, *74*(5), 778–785.

■ ■ ■

3603

Test Name: SUPERVISORY STYLES INVENTORY

Purpose: To study supervisors' self-perceptions and trainees' perceptions of their supervisors.

Number of Items: 25

Format: Includes three factors: attractive, interpersonally sensitive, and task-oriented. There are two versions: supervisor and trainee.

Reliability: Cronbach's alpha ranged from .70 to .84 for the SSI-S and from .84 to .89 for the SSI-T (Ns = 105 to 202). Test–retest reliabilities for the SSI-T ranged from .78 to .94 (N = 32).

Author: Friedlander, M. L., and Ward, L. G.

Article: Development and

validation of the Supervisory Styles Inventory.

Journal: *Journal of Counseling Psychology,* October 1984, *31*(4), 541–557.

Related Research: Stenack, R. J., & Dye, H. A. (1982). Behavioral descriptions of counseling supervision roles. *Counselor Education and Supervision, 21,* 295–304.

■ ■ ■

3604

Test Name: TEACHER SCORING KEYS

Purpose: To score teacher behaviors measured by existing teacher behavior instruments.

Number of Items: 42

Format: Varied with instrument used.

Reliability: Special measures of reliability varied from 0 to .62 with an average of .23. A total of 22 of the 42 were significant at the .05 level.

Validity: Problematic validity revealed by factor analysis.

Author: Medley, D. M., et al.

Article: Assessing teacher performance from observed competency indicators defined by classroom teachers.

Journal: *Journal of Educational Research,* March/April 1981, *74*(4), 197–216.

■ ■ ■

3605

Test Name: TEACHER BEHAVIORS INVENTORY

Purpose: To rate teacher classroom behavior.

Number of Items: 60

Format: Items rated on a 5-point

frequency scale (1 = *almost never* to 5 = *almost always*).

Reliability: SB ranged from .24 to .97 for individual items (*Mdn* = .76).

Author: Murray, H. G.

Article: Low-inference classroom teaching behaviors and student ratings of college teaching effectiveness.

Journal: *Journal of Educational Psychology,* February 1983, *75*(1), 138–149.

Related Research: Tom, F. K. T., & Cushman, H. R. (1975). The Cornell diagnostic observation and reporting system for student descriptions of college teaching. *Search, 5*(8), 1–27.

■ ■ ■

3606

Test Name: TEACHER RATING SCALES

Purpose: To measure teacher behavior.

Number of Items: 12 behavioral incidents plus 8 judgments.

Format: Judgments made on a 5-point Likert scale. Behavior scales on an 8-point frequency scale.

Validity: Convergent validity ranged from .57 to .70. Discriminant validity ranged from .21 to .47.

Author: Murphy, K. R., et al.

Article: Effects of the purpose of rating on accuracy in observing teacher behavior and evaluating teacher performance.

Journal: *Journal of Educational Psychology,* February 1984, *76*(1), 45–54.

Related Research: Murphy, K. (1982). Do behavioral observation scales measure observation? *Journal of Applied Behavior, 67,* 562–567.

3607

Test Name: TEACHING EFFECTIVENESS INSTRUMENT

Purpose: To measure students' perceptions of teaching practice that contribute to or detract from learning.

Number of Items: Varies by respondent.

Format: Students list "things" that contribute to or detract from teaching. Lists then are content analyzed to ascertain the number, variety, and nature of reasons of things cited.

Reliability: Lights coefficients: number (.93); variety (.80); nature of reason (.72).

Author: Cruickshank, D. R., et al.

Article: Evaluation of reflective teacher questionnaire.

Journal: *Journal of Educational Research*, September/October 1981, *75*(1), 26–32.

Related Research: Nott, D. L., & Williams, E. J. (1980). *Experimental effects of reflective teaching on preservice teachers' ability to identify a greater number and wider variety of variables present during the act of teaching.* Paper presented at the meeting of the American Educational Research Association, Boston.

■ ■ ■

3608

Test Name: WORK OPINION QUESTIONNAIRE

Purpose: To measure job-related values that predict performance of low income workers at entry-level jobs.

Number of Items: 35

Format: 5-point Likert agreement scales. All items presented.

Reliability: Alphas ranged from .66 to .87 across subscales.

Validity: All subscales correlate significantly ($p < .05$) with the Job Performance Index.

Author: Johnson, C. D., et al.

Article: Predicting job performance of low income workers: The Work Opinion Questionnaire.

Journal: *Personnel Psychology*, Summer 1984, *37*(2), 291–299.

CHAPTER 24
Vocational Interest

3609

Test Name: AFFECTIVE COMMITMENT SCALE

Purpose: To assess commitment characterized by positive feelings of identification with, attachment to, and involvement in, the work organization.

Number of Items: 8

Format: Responses are made on a 7-point Likert scale from *strongly disagree* to *strongly agree*. Examples are presented.

Reliability: Coefficient alphas were .88 and .84.

Validity: Correlations with other commitment measures ranged from –.01 to .86.

Author: Meyer, J. P., and Allen, N. J.

Article: Testing the "side-bet theory" of organizational commitment: Some methodological considerations.

Journal: *Journal of Applied Psychology*, August 1984, *69*(3), 372–378.

Related Research: Jackson, D. N. (1970). A sequential system for personality scale development. In C. D. Spielberger (Ed.), *Current topics in clinical and community psychology* (Vol. 2, pp. 61–96). New York: Academic Press.

. . .

3610

Test Name: ASSESSMENT OF CAREER DECISION-MAKING SCALE

Purpose: To measure progress in career decision making.

Format: Agree–disagree.

Reliability: Test–retest ranged from .67 to .82 across subscales. Alphas ranged from .67 to .82.

Validity: Subscale intercorrelations presented and resemble previous patterns.

Author: Kahn, M. W., and Weare, C. R.

Article: The role of anxiety in the career decision-making of liberal arts students.

Journal: *Journal of Vocational Behavior*, June 1983, *22*(3), 312–323.

Related Research: Harren, V. A., et al. (1978). Influence of sex role attitudes and cognitive styles on career decision making. *Journal of Counseling Psychology, 25,* 390–395.

. . .

3611

Test Name: CAREER COMMITMENT SCALE

Purpose: To measure commitment to job.

Number of Items: 8

Format: Items rated in 5-point Likert format.

Reliability: Test–retest reliability was .67.

Validity: Correlated significantly with career withdrawal cognitions (–.41) and role ambiguity (–.38).

Author: Blau, G.

Article: The measurement and prediction of career commitment.

Journal: *Journal of Occupational Psychology*, December 1985, *58*(4), 277–288.

Related Research: Downing, P., et al. (1978). *Work attitudes and performance questionnaire.* San Francisco School of Nursing, University of California.

. . .

3612

Test Name: CAREER COMMITMENT SCALE

Purpose: To assess interest in long-term career prospects and advancement.

Number of Items: 17

Format: Items are rated on a 5-point scale with scores ranging from 17 to 85.

Reliability: Coefficient alpha was .83.

Author: Koski, L. K., and Subich, L. M.

Article: Career and homemaking choices of college preparatory and vocational education students.

Journal: *Vocational Guidance Quarterly*, December 1985, *34*(2), 116–123.

Related Research: Farmer, H. (1983). Career and homemaking plans for high school youth. *Journal of Counseling Psychology, 30,* 40–45.

Super, D. E., et al. (1978). *The Work Salience Inventory* (mimeo).

New York: Columbia University, Teachers College.

• • •

3613

Test Name: CAREER DECISION-MAKING QUESTIONNAIRE

Purpose: To assess readiness for career decision making.

Number of Items: 14

Format: Item presented; response categories not presented.

Reliability: Test–retest reliability was .83.

Validity: Factor analysis confirmed the constructs on which the CDM was based. High scorers on CDM likely to be successful users of the SIGI.

Author: Dungy, G.

Article: Computer-assisted guidance: Determining who is ready.

Journal: *Journal of College Student Personnel*, November 1984, *25*(6), 539–545.

• • •

3614

Test Name: CAREER EXPLORATION SURVEY

Purpose: To measure the reactions and beliefs of people to the way they get information about careers.

Number of Items: 59

Format: Multiple formats. All items are presented.

Reliability: Alphas ranged from .67 to .89 across subscales.

Validity: Factor analysis of items in different populations yielded similar results. Social Desirability did not correlate with CES dimensions. Other validity studies are presented.

Author: Stumpf, S. A., et al.

Article: Development of the Career Exploration Survey.

Journal: *Journal of Vocational Behavior*, April 1983, *22*(2), 191–226.

• • •

3615

Test Name: CAREER INDECISION FACTORS SURVEY

Purpose: To measure underlying reasons for career indecision as a means of differential diagnosis and treatment of career problems.

Number of Items: 47

Format: Includes six subscales with Likert and semantic differential items, each scaled along 5 points.

Reliability: Coefficient alpha for self-esteem subscale was .83. Coefficient alpha for choice anxiety was .87.

Author: Robbins, S. B., et al.

Article: Attrition behavior before career development workshops.

Journal: *Journal of Counseling Psychology*, April 1985, *32*(2), 232–238.

Related Research: Robbins, S., et al. (1983). *Career indecision factor survey.* Unpublished manuscript, Virginia Commonwealth University, Richmond.

• • •

3616

Test Name: CAREER INFORMATION-SEEKING SCALE

Purpose: To measure participants' amount of career information-seeking.

Number of Items: 17

Format: Respondents rate their frequency of performance on a 6-point scale for each of the 17 information-seeking behaviors.

Reliability: Internal consistency was .88.

Author: Remer, P., et al.

Article: Multiple outcome evaluation of a life-career development course.

Journal: *Journal of Counseling Psychology*, October 1984, *31*(4), 532–546.

Related Research: O'Neill, C. D. (1982). *The differential effectiveness of two dimension-making treatments on college freshmen.* Unpublished doctoral dissertation, University of Kentucky.

Krumboltz, J. D., & Schroeder, W. W. (1965). Promoting career planning through reinforcement. *Personnel and Guidance Journal, 44*, 19–26.

• • •

3617

Test Name: CAREER ORIENTATION INVENTORY

Purpose: To measure degree of expectation and aspiration for a high-level occupation.

Number of Items: 17

Format: Semantic differential. All items are presented.

Reliability: Hoyt reliabilities ranged from .84 to .85 across sex. Item-total correlations rho was .86.

Validity: Men tended to have stronger career orientations than women.

Author: Cochran, L. R.

Article: Level of career aspirations and strength of career orientation.

Journal: *Journal of Vocational Behavior*, August 1983, *23*(1), 1–10.

3618

Test Name: CAREER ORIENTATION SCALE

Purpose: To measure depth and intensity of interest in a career.

Number of Items: 27

Format: Likert format.

Reliability: .81

Author: Pedro, J. D.

Article: Induction into the workplace: The impact of internships.

Journal: *Journal of Vocational Behavior,* August 1984, *25*(1), 80–95.

Related Research: Greenhaus, J. (1971). An investigation of the role of career salience in vocational behavior. *Journal of Vocational Behavior, 2,* 209–216.

■ ■ ■

3619

Test Name: CAREER PLANNING QUESTIONNAIRE

Purpose: To measure career maturity in 11th grade students.

Number of Items: 130

Format: Agree–disagree and multiple-choice. Sample items presented.

Reliability: Kuder-Richardson formula 20 values ranged from .71 to .91 across subscales (*Mdn* = .70).

Validity: Not related to aptitude. Not related to frequency of discussion of plans after high school. Selected subscales correlated with knowledge of duties in occupations and level of certainty about entering occupations.

Author: Westbrook, B. W., et al.

Article: Predictive and construct validity of six experimental measures of career maturity.

Journal: *Journal of Vocational Behavior,* December 1985, *27*(3), 338–355.

Related Research: Tittle, C. K. (1982). Career, marriage and family: Values in adult roles and guidance. *Personnel and Guidance Journal, 61,* 154–158.

■ ■ ■

3620

Test Name: CAREER SALIENCE QUESTIONNAIRE

Purpose: To measure the importance of work.

Number of Items: 28

Format: All but one item is a 5-point Likert scale. The remaining item is a 6-response ranking item.

Reliability: Coefficient alpha was .81. Stability reliability coefficient was .89.

Validity: Correlations with other variables ranged from −.09 to .45.

Author: Thomas, R. G., and Bruning, C. R.

Article: Validities and reliabilities of minor modifications of the Central Life Interests and Career Salience Questionnaires.

Journal: *Measurement and Evaluation in Guidance,* October 1981, *14*(3), 128–135.

Related Research: Greenhaus, J. (1971). An investigation of the role of career salience in vocational behavior. *Journal of Vocational Behavior, 1,* 209–216.

■ ■ ■

3621

Test Name: CAREER SALIENCE SCALE

Purpose: To measure extent to which a career is a vital part of people's lives.

Number of Items: 7

Format: Likert format.

Reliability: Alpha was .83.

Author: Sekaran, U.

Article: Factors influencing the quality of life in dual-career families.

Journal: *Journal of Occupational Psychology,* June 1983, *56*(2), 161–174.

Related Research: Sekaran, U. (1982). An investigation of the career salience of men and women in dual career families. *Journal of Vocational Behavior, 20,* 111–119.

■ ■ ■

3622

Test Name: CENTRAL LIFE INTERESTS QUESTIONNAIRE–MODIFIED

Purpose: To measure the importance of work.

Number of Items: 30

Format: Multiple-choice items with three choices. A sample is presented.

Reliability: Stability reliability coefficient was .75.

Validity: Correlations with other variables ranged from −.26 to .45.

Author: Thomas, R. G., and Bruning, C. R.

Article: Validities and reliabilities of minor modifications of the Central Life Interests and Career Salience Questionnaires.

Journal: *Measurement and Evaluation in Guidance,* October 1981, *14*(3), 128–135.

Related Research: Dubin, R. (1956). *Central life interests questionnaire.* Unpublished manuscript, Graduate School of Administration, University of California, Irvine.

3623

Test Name: CERTAINTY OF OCCUPATIONAL PREFERENCE SCALE

Purpose: To measure how firm occupational aspirations are among secondary school students.

Number of Items: 8

Format: Items rated on 5-point agreement scales. Sample items are presented.

Reliability: Internal reliability was .79. Test–retest reliability was .79.

Author: Kidd, J. M.

Article: The relationship of self and occupational concepts to the occupational preferences of adolescents.

Journal: *Journal of Vocational Behavior*, February 1984, *24*(1), 48–65.

Related Research: Kidd, J. M. (1982). *Self and occupational concepts in occupational preferences and the entry into work: An overlapping longitudinal study.* Unpublished doctoral dissertation, The Hatfield Polytechnic.

■ ■ ■

3624

Test Name: COMMITMENT SCALE

Purpose: To measure commitment to organization of employment/membership.

Number of Items: 15 (continuance); 8 (affective).

Format: Items rated in 7-point response format. Sample item presented.

Reliability: Alpha was .77 (continuance). Alpha was .87 (affective).

Validity: Continuance did not correlate with Organizational Commitment Questionnaire (*r* = –.06). Affective did correlate with OCQ (*r* = .78).

Author: Meyer, J. P., and Allen, N. J.

Article: Testing the "side-bet theory" of organizational commitment: Some methodological considerations.

Journal: *Journal of Applied Psychology*, August 1984, *69*(3), 372–378.

Related Research: Ritzer, G., & Trice, H. M. (1969). An empirical test of Howard Becker's side-bet theory. *Social Forces, 47,* 475–479.

Mowday, R. T., et al. (1979). The measurement of organizational commitment. *Journal of Vocational Behavior, 14,* 224–257.

Hrebiniak, L. G., & Alluto, J. A. (1972). Personal and role-related factors in the development of organizational commitment. *Administrative Science Quarterly, 17,* 555–573.

■ ■ ■

3625

Test Name: CONTINUANCE COMMITMENT SCALE

Purpose: To assess the extent to which employees feel committed to their organizations by virtue of the costs that they feel are associated with leaving.

Number of Items: 8

Format: Responses are made on a 7-point scale from *strongly disagree* to *strongly agree.*

Reliability: Coefficient alphas were .73 and .74.

Validity: Correlations with other commitment measures ranged from –.06 to .33.

Author: Meyer, J. P., and Allen, N. J.

Article: Testing the "side-bet theory" of organizational commitment: Some methodological considerations.

Journal: *Journal of Applied Psychology*, August 1984, *69*(3), 372–378.

■ ■ ■

3626

Test Name: EMPLOYMENT COMMITMENT SCALE

Purpose: To provide an index of employment commitment.

Number of Items: 6

Format: Responses are made on a 5-point scale from 5 (*agree a lot*) to 1 (*disagree a lot*). Separate scales for the employed and unemployed. All items are presented.

Reliability: Alpha coefficients ranged from .64 to .71.

Validity: Correlation with psychological distress ranged from –.22 to .34 (*N*s ranged from 81 to 636).

Author: Jackson, P. R., et al.

Article: Unemployment and psychological distress in young people: The moderating role of employment commitment.

Journal: *Journal of Applied Psychology*, August 1983, *68*(3), 525–535.

Related Research: Warr, P. B., et al. (1979). Scales for the measurement of some work attitudes and aspects of psychological well-being. *Journal of Occupational Psychology, 52,* 129–148.

■ ■ ■

3627

Test Name: EMPLOYMENT IMMOBILITY QUESTIONNAIRE

Purpose: To provide administrators' assessment of how

locked-in to their job they feel.

Number of Items: 8

Format: The items are combined into a single score.

Reliability: Coefficient alpha was .70.

Validity: Correlations with a variety of variables ranged from −.30 to .28.

Author: Burke, R. J., and Weir, T.

Article: Occupational locking-in: Some empirical findings.

Journal: *Journal of Social Psychology*, December 1982, *118*(second half), 177–185.

Related Research: Quinn, R. P. (1975). *Locking-in as a moderator of the relationship between job satisfaction and mental health.* Unpublished manuscript, Surrey Research Centre, University of Michigan, Ann Arbor.

■ ■ ■

3628

Test Name: EMPLOYMENT IMPORTANCE SCALE

Purpose: To measure employment importance and work involvement.

Number of Items: 3

Format: Multiple-choice. All items presented.

Reliability: Alpha ranged from .34 to .73.

Author: Feather, N. T., and Bond, M. J.

Article: Time structure and purposeful activity among employed and unemployed university graduates.

Journal: *Journal of Occupational Psychology*, September 1983, *56*(3), 241–254.

Related Research: Feather, N. T.,

& Davenport, P. R. (1981). Unemployment and depressive affect: A motivational and attributional analysis. *Journal of Personality and Social Psychology, 41*, 422–436.

■ ■ ■

3629

Test Name: ENGINEERING INTEREST INVENTORY

Purpose: To measure interest in a career in engineering.

Number of Items: 111

Format: Formats include a 3-point *Yes-Doubtful-No* scale, and a 20-point rating scale.

Reliability: Alphas ranged from .68 to .93.

Author: Meir, E. E.

Article: Fostering a career in engineering.

Journal: *Journal of Vocational Behavior*, February 1981, *18*(1), 115–120.

Related Research: Dunnette, M. D. (1964). Further research on vocational interest differences among several types of engineers. *Personnel and Guidance Journal, 42*, 484–493.

■ ■ ■

3630

Test Name: FEEDBACK SHEET

Purpose: To measure satisfaction with CHOICES and SDS career exploration experiences.

Number of Items: 9

Format: Likert response categories.

Reliability: $R = .83$.

Author: Reardon, R. C., et al.

Article: Self-directed career exploration: A comparison of CHOICES and the Self-Directed Search.

Journal: *Journal of Vocational Behavior*, February 1982, *20*(1), 22–30.

Related Research: Talbot, D. B., & Birk, J. M. (1979). Does the vocational exploration and insight kit equal the sum of its parts? A comparison study. *Journal of Counseling Psychology, 26*, 359–362.

■ ■ ■

3631

Test Name: HOME ECONOMICS ATTITUDES SCALE

Purpose: To measure competence and interest in home economics.

Number of Items: 66

Format: Multiple-choice.

Reliability: Alpha ranged from .84 to .96 across subscales.

Author: Schumm, W. R., and Kennedy, C. E.

Article: Dimensions of competence and interest in home economics.

Journal: *Psychological Reports*, December 1985, *57*(3-I), 698.

Related Research: Nichols, C. W., et al. (1983). What home economics programs do mothers want for sons and daughters? *Journal of Home Economics, 75*, 28–30.

■ ■ ■

3632

Test Name: JOB DECISION STYLE QUESTIONNAIRE

Purpose: To measure manner in which a person chooses a job.

Number of Items: 6

Format: Subjects rank six statements as most to least descriptive of themselves.

Reliability: Test–retest (2 weeks) reliability was .87.

Author: Hesketh, B.

Article: Decision-making style and career decision-making behaviors among school leavers.

Journal: *Journal of Vocational Behavior,* April 1982, *20*(2), 223–234.

Related Research: Arroba, T. (1977). Styles of decision-making and their use: An empirical study. *British Journal of Guidance and Counseling, 5*(2), 149–158.

■ ■ ■

3633

Test Name: JOB INVOLVEMENT AND SEMANTIC DIFFERENTIAL

Purpose: To measure job involvement.

Number of Items: 8

Format: Semantic differential. All items presented.

Reliability: Item-total correlations ranged from .64 to .82 (*Mdn =* .75). Alpha was .83. Test–retest reliability was .74.

Validity: Correlated .27 (*p* < .01) with job satisfaction.

Author: Kanungo, R. N.

Article: Measurement of job and work involvement.

Journal: *Journal of Applied Psychology,* June 1982, *67*(3), 341–349.

■ ■ ■

3634

Test Name: JOB INVOLVEMENT SCALE

Purpose: To measure job involvement.

Number of Items: 20

Format: Items rated on a 4-point Likert format. Sample items are presented.

Reliability: .83 (unspecified).

Author: Drory, A.

Article: Organizational stress and job attitudes: Moderating effects of organizational level and task characteristics.

Journal: *Psychological Reports,* 1981, *49*(1), 139–146.

Related Research: Lodahl, T., & Kejner, J. (1965). The definition and measurement of job involvement. *Journal of Applied Psychology, 65,* 24–33.

■ ■ ■

3635

Test Name: JOB INVOLVEMENT MEASURE

Purpose: To measure job involvement.

Format: Responses to each item are made on a 7-point scale from 1 (*strongly disagree*) to 7 (*strongly agree*).

Reliability: Coefficient alpha was .86.

Validity: Correlations with other variables ranged from –.06 to .20.

Author: Graddick, M. M., and Farr, J. L.

Article: Professionals in scientific disciplines: Sex-related differences in working life commitments.

Article: *Journal of Applied Psychology,* November 1983, *68*(4), 641–645.

Related Research: Lodahl, T., & Kejner, J. (1965). The definition and measurement of job involvement. *Journal of Applied Psychology, 65,* 24–33.

Dubin, R. (1956). Industrial workers' worlds: A study of the central life interests of industrial workers. *Social Problems, 3,* 131–142.

■ ■ ■

3636

Test Name: JOB INVOLVEMENT SCALE

Purpose: To measure job involvement.

Number of Items: 4

Format: Items rated on a 5-point Likert format.

Reliability: Alpha was .69.

Author: Ashford, S. J., and Cummings, L. L.

Article: Proactive feedback seeking: The instrumental use of the information environment.

Journal: *Journal of Occupational Behavior,* March 1985, *58*(1), 67–79.

Related Research: Lawler, E. E., & Hall, D. T. (1970). Relationships of job characteristics to job involvement. *Journal of Applied Psychology, 54,* 305–312.

■ ■ ■

3637

Test Name: JOB INVOLVEMENT SCALE

Purpose: To measure job involvement.

Number of Items: 5

Format: Items deal with dislike of the work, reward value of the work, pride and accomplishments from the work, and opportunities to perform well.

Reliability: Coefficient alpha was .82.

Validity: Correlations with other variables ranged from –.16 to .47.

Author: Hammer, T. H., et al.

Article: Absenteeism when workers have a voice: The case of employee ownership.

Journal: *Journal of Applied Psychology,* October 1981, *66*(5), 561–573.

Related Research: Miller, G. A. (1967). Professionals in bureaucracy: Alienation among industrial scientists and engineers. *American Sociological Review, 32,* 755–768.

• • •

3638

Test Name: LIFESTYLE INDEX

Purpose: To measure career salience.

Number of Items: 9

Format: Multiple-choice.

Reliability: Test–retest ranged from .74 to .81 across items.

Author: Brooks, L., et al.

Article: The effects of a nontraditional role-modeling intervention on sex typing of occupational preferences and career salience in adolescent females.

Journal: *Journal of Vocational Behavior,* June 1985, *26*(3), 264–276.

Related Research: Angrist, S. S. (1972). Changes in women's work aspirations during college (or work does not equal career). *International Journal of Sociology of the Family, 2,* 27–37.

• • •

3639

Test Name: LIST OF COURSES IN NURSING

Purpose: To measure attractiveness of nursing courses representing nine clinical areas.

Number of Items: 90

Format: *Yes-Doubtful-No* response scale.

Reliability: Split-half reliability was .89. Equivalent test = .82.

Author: Hener, T., and Meir, E. I.

Article: Congruency, consistency and differentiation as predictors of job satisfaction with the nursing profession.

Journal: *Journal of Vocational Behavior,* June 1981, *18*(3), 304–309.

Related Research: Peiser, C., & Meir, E. I. (1978). Congruency, consistency, and differentiation of vocational interests as predictors of vocational satisfaction and preference stability. *Journal of Vocational Behavior, 12,* 270–278.

• • •

3640

Test Name: MEDICAL CAREER DEVELOPMENT INVENTORY

Purpose: To measure degree of development and readiness to cope with the career of physician.

Number of Items: 25

Format: Multiple-choice. All items presented.

Reliability: Alpha was .93 (total). Alphas ranged from .73 to .91 across subscales.

Validity: Did not correlate significantly with sex. Correlated significantly ($r = .41$) with career planfulness.

Author: Savickas, M. L.

Article: Construction and validation of a physician career development inventory.

Journal: *Journal of Vocational Behavior,* August 1984, *25*(1), 106–123.

• • •

3641

Test Name: NURSING COURSE ATTRACTIVENESS SCALE

Purpose: To measure the attractiveness of nursing courses.

Number of Items: 90

Format: *Yes-Doubtful-No* format for each item. Sample item presented.

Reliability: Split-half reliability was .89.

Validity: Nurses in specific clinical areas scored higher on that area than mean scores of all nurses for that area (no quantitative measure provided).

Author: Hener, T., and Meir, E. I.

Article: Congruency, consistency and differentiation as predictors of job satisfaction with the nursing profession.

Journal: *Journal of Vocational Behavior,* June 1981, *18*(3), 304–309.

• • •

3642

Test Name: OCCUPATIONAL RATING SCALE

Purpose: To rate to what degree people believe occupations are "appropriate" for men or women.

Number of Items: 14 (occupational titles).

Format: Items rated on a 7-point bipolar rating scale with anchors *appropriate for men* and *appropriate for women*.

Reliability: Test–retest reliability was .90 (2 weeks).

Author: Yanico, B. J.

Article: Androgyny and occupational sex-stereotyping of college students.

Journal: *Psychological Reports,* 1982, *50*(3-I), 875–878.

Related Research: Shinar, E. H. (1979). Sexual stereotypes of occupations. *Journal of Vocational Behavior,* 317–328.

• • •

3643

Test Name: ORGANIZATIONAL COMMITMENT QUESTIONNAIRE

Purpose: To assess an affective orientation to the organization.

Number of Items: 15

Format: Organizational commitment includes: a strong belief in and acceptance of the organization's goals and values, a willingness to exert considerable effort on behalf of the organization, and a strong desire to maintain membership in the organization. Responses are made on a 7-point Likert scale from *strongly disagree* to *strongly agree*.

Reliability: Coefficient alphas were .93 and .89.

Validity: Correlations with other commitment measures ranged from –.06 to .86.

Author: Meyer, J. P., and Allen, N. J.

Article: Testing the "side-bet theory" of organizational commitment: Some methodological considerations.

Journal: *Journal of Applied Psychology*, August 1984, *69*(3), 372–378.

Mowday, R. T., et al. (1979). The measurement of organizational commitment. *Journal of Vocational Behavior*, *14*, 224–257.

Graddick, M. M., & Farr, J. L. (1983). Professionals in scientific disciplines: Sex-related differences in working life commitments. *Journal of Applied Psychology*, *68*(4), 641–645.

• • •

3644

Test Name: ORGANIZATIONAL AND PROFESSIONAL COMMITMENT SCALES

Purpose: To measure commitment to an organization's (or a profession's) goals and values.

Number of Items: 15 each for organization and profession.

Format: Items rated on 7-point Likert scales.

Reliability: Alpha for organization

was .91. Alpha for profession was .87.

Author: Aranya, N., and Barak, A.

Article: A test of Holland's theory in a population of accountants.

Journal: *Journal of Vocational Behavior*, August 1981, *19*(1), 15–24.

Related Research: Porter, L. W., et al. (1974). Organizational commitment, job satisfaction and turnover among psychiatric technicians. *Journal of Applied Psychology*, *59*, 603–609.

• • •

3645

Test Name: ORGANIZATIONAL COMMITMENT SCALE

Purpose: To measure organizational commitment.

Number of Items: 9

Reliability: Cronbach's coefficient alpha was .90.

Validity: Correlation with other variables ranged from –.30 to .52.

Author: Chacko, T. I.

Article: Women and equal employment opportunity: Some unintended effects.

Journal: *Journal of Applied Psychology*, February 1982, *67*(1), 119–123.

Related Research: Porter, L. W., et al. (1974). Organizational commitment, job satisfaction, and turnover among psychiatric technicians. *Journal of Applied Psychology*, *59*, 603–609.

• • •

3646

Test Name: ORGANIZATIONAL COMMITMENT SCALE

Purpose: To measure commitment to stay (or leave) employing organization.

Number of Items: 4

Format: Items rated in 5-point Likert format. All items are presented.

Reliability: Alpha was .88.

Validity: Correlated –.17 with turnover intentions and –.23 with actual turnover (both *p*s < .001).

Author: Ferris, K. R., and Aranya, N.

Article: A comparison of two organizational commitment scales.

Journal: *Personnel Psychology*, Spring 1983, *36*(1), 87–98.

Related Research: Hrebiniak, L. G., & Alluto, J. A. (1972). Personal and role-related factors in the development of organizational commitment. *Administrative Science Quarterly*, *17*, 555–573.

• • •

3647

Test Name: ORGANIZATIONAL COMMITMENT SCALE

Purpose: To measure commitment to employing organizations.

Number of Items: 15

Format: Items rated in 7-point Likert format. All items are presented.

Reliability: Alpha was .90.

Validity: Correlated –.37 with turnover intentions and –.22 with actual turnover.

Author: Ferris, K. R., and Aranya, N.

Article: A comparison of two organizational commitment scales.

Journal: *Personnel Psychology*, Spring 1983, *36*(1), 87–98.

Related Research: Porter, L. W., et al. (1974). Organizational commitment, job satisfaction, and turnover among psychiatric technicians. *Journal of Applied*

Psychology, 59, 603–609.

Arnold, H. J., & Feldman, D. C. (1982). A multivariate analysis of the determinants of job turnover. *Journal of Applied Psychology, 67*(3), 350–360.

Drasgow, F., & Miller, H. E. (1982). Psychometric and substantive issues in scale construction and validation. *Journal of Applied Psychology, 67*(3), 268–279.

■ ■ ■

3648

Test Name: ORGANIZATIONAL COMMITMENT SCALE

Purpose: To measure "moral" commitment to organizations.

Number of Items: 4

Format: Items rated on 5-point response scales.

Reliability: Alpha was .65.

Author: Werbel, J. D., and Gould, S.

Article: A comparison of the relationship of commitment to turnover in recent hires and tenured employees.

Journal: *Journal of Applied Psychology,* December 1984, *69*(4), 687–690.

Related Research: Gould, S., & Penley, L. (1982). *Organizational commitment: A test of a model.* Working Paper Series. San Antonio: The University of Texas.

■ ■ ■

3649

Test Name: ORGANIZATIONAL IDENTIFICATION SCALE

Purpose: To measure the extent to which individuals take pride in and have a positive attitude toward their organization.

Number of Items: 4

Format: A sample item is presented.

Reliability: Coefficient alpha was .81.

Validity: Correlation with other variables ranged from –.28 to .46.

Author: Gould, S., and Werbel, J. D.

Article: Work involvement: A comparison of dual wage earner and single wage earner families.

Journal: *Journal of Applied Psychology,* May 1983, *68*(2), 313–319.

Related Research: Patchen, M. (1970). *Participation, achievement, and involvement on the job.* Englewood Cliffs, NJ: Prentice-Hall.

■ ■ ■

3650

Test Name: PROPENSITY TO LEAVE INDEX

Purpose: To measure propensity to leave job.

Number of Items: 3

Format: Items rated on 5-point Likert response categories.

Reliability: Median item intercorrelation was .57.

Author: Wright, D., and Thomas, J.

Article: Role strain among psychologists in the midwest.

Journal: *Journal of School Psychology,* 1982, *20*(2), 96–102.

Related Research: Lyons, T. F. (1971). Role clarity, need for clarity, satisfaction, tension, and withdrawal. *Organizational Behavior and Human Performance, 6,* 99–110.

■ ■ ■

3651

Test Name: RAMAK INTEREST INVENTORY

Purpose: To measure attractiveness of occupational titles.

Number of Items: 72

Format: Yes–no.

Reliability: Equivalent test was .76.

Author: Gati, I., and Meir, E. I.

Article: Congruence and consistency derived from the circular and hierarchical models as predictors of occupational choice satisfaction.

Journal: *Journal of Vocational Behavior,* June 1982, *20*(3), 354–365.

Related Research: Meir, E. I., & Barak, A. (1974). A simple instrument for measuring vocational interests based on Roe's classification of occupations. *Journal of Vocational Behavior, 4,* 33–42.

■ ■ ■

3652

Test Name: REENLISTMENT DECISIONS QUESTIONNAIRE

Purpose: To measure U.S. Army personnel's perceptions, expectancies, satisfactions, preferences, and intentions in regard to reenlistment.

Number of Items: Form 1: 63, Form 2: 59.

Format: Includes four sections of: perception, expectancies, satisfaction, intention and reenlistment.

Reliability: Internal consistency estimates ranged from .70 to .84.

Author: Motowidlo, S. J., and Lawton, G. W.

Article: Affective and cognitive factors in soldiers' reenlistment decisions.

Journal: *Journal of Applied Psychology,* May 1984, *69*(2), 157–166.

Related Research: Motowidlo, S. J., et al. (1980). Reenlistment factors for first-term enlisted personnel. *Proceedings of the 22nd Annual Conference of the Military Testing Association* (pp. 681–690). Toronto: Military Testing Association.

■ ■ ■

3653

Test Name: SELF-ASSESSMENT QUESTIONNAIRE

Purpose: To assist college students in identifying occupations consistent with a major field of study.

Number of Items: 107

Format: Includes six scales: appeal, practical, clues, aptitude, skills, and preferences. There are 4 forms.

Reliability: Coefficient alphas for the 4 forms ranged from .81 to .98.

Author: Turner, C. J.

Article: The reliability and factorial validity of the self-assessment questionnaire for liberal arts majors.

Journal: *Educational and Psychological Measurement,* Summer 1983, *43*(2), 509–516.

Related Research: Malnig, L. R., & Morrow, S. L. (1975). *What can I do with a major in...?* Jersey City, NJ: St. Peter's College Press.

■ ■ ■

3654

Test Name: SELF-CONCEPT/OCCUPATIONAL CONCEPT DISTANCE SCALE

Purpose: To assess similarity between actual and ideal self-concept and perceived occupational concepts.

Number of Items: 183 (three 61-item rating scales).

Format: 7-point response scale.

Reliability: Alpha ranged from .70 to .88.

Author: Kidd, J. M.

Article: The relationship of self and occupational concepts to the occupational preferences of adolescents.

Journal: *Journal of Vocational Behavior,* February 1984, *24*(1), 48–65.

Related Research: Kidd, J. M. (1982). *Self and occupational concepts in occupational preferences and the entry into work: An overlapping longitudinal study.* Unpublished doctoral dissertation, The Hatfield Polytechnic.

■ ■ ■

3655

Test Name: SPECIALITY INDECISION SCALE

Purpose: To measure indecision about specialities in professions.

Number of Items: 16

Format: Items rated in 4-point Likert format. All items are presented.

Reliability: Alpha was .82.

Validity: One general factor left residual correlations to produce three additional factors.

Author: Savickas, M. L., et al.

Article: Measuring specialty indecision among career-decided students.

Journal: *Journal of Vocational Behavior,* December 1985, *27*(3), 356–367.

■ ■ ■

3656

Test Name: VOCATIONAL COMMITMENT QUESTIONNAIRE

Purpose: To measure

organizational commitment and correlates of commitment.

Number of Items: 56

Format: Items rated on 5-point Likert agreement scales and multiple-choice. Sample items presented for all scales.

Reliability: Alpha ranged from .64 to .91 across subscales.

Author: Martin, T. N., and O'Laughlin, M. S.

Article: Predictors of organizational commitment: The study of part-time army reservists.

Journal: *Journal of Vocational Behavior,* December 1984, *25*(3), 270–283.

Related Research: Price, J. L., & Mueller, C. W. (1981). A causal model of turnover for nurses. *Academy of Management Journal, 24,* 543–565.

Ivancevich, J. W., & Matteson, M. T. (1980). *Stress and work: A managerial perspective.* Glenview, IL: Scott, Foresman.

Brayfield, A. H., & Rothe, H. F. (1951). An index of job satisfaction. *Journal of Applied Psychology, 63,* 677–688.

Martin, T. N. (1979). A contextual model of employee turnover intentions. *Academy of Management Journal, 22,* 313–324.

Mowday, R. T., et al. (1979). *Employee-organization linkages: The psychology of commitment, absenteeism, and turnover.* New York: Academic Press.

■ ■ ■

3657

Test Name: VOCATIONAL DECISION-MAKING DIFFICULTY SCALE

Purpose: To assess the number of reasons given by subjects for vocational indecision.

Number of Items: 13

Format: Each item is answered either *true* or *false*. *True* responses are summed to provide a total score.

Reliability: Kuder-Richardson formula 20 values ranged from .63 to .86.

Author: Slaney, R. B.

Article: Relation of career indecision to changes in expressed vocational interests.

Journal: *Journal of Counseling Psychology,* July 1984, *31*(3), 349–355.

Related Research: Holland, J. L., & Holland, J. E. (1977). Vocational indecision: More evidence and speculation. *Journal of Counseling Psychology, 24,* 404–414.

■ ■ ■

3658

Test Name: VOCATIONAL DECISION SCALE

Purpose: To measure degree of decidedness, comfort, and reasons for being decided or undecided about a career decision.

Number of Items: 38

Format: Items rated in a 5-point Likert format.

Reliability: Test-retest ranged from .36 to .64.

Author: Larson, L. M., and Heppner, P. P.

Article: The relationship of problem-solving appraisal to career decision and indecision.

Journal: *Journal of Vocational Behavior,* February 1985, *26*(1), 55–65.

Related Research: Jones, L. K., & Chenery, M. F. (1980). Multiple subtypes among vocationally undecided college students: A model and assessment instrument.

Journal of Counseling Psychology, 27, 469–477.

■ ■ ■

3659

Test Name: VOCATIONAL DECISION SCALE— DECIDEDNESS AND COMFORT DIMENSIONS

Purpose: To measure vocational decidedness, comfort, and reasons for undecidedness.

Number of Items: 14

Format: Items are rated on a 5-point Likert agree–disagree scale.

Reliability: Test–retest (2 weeks) reliabilities ranged from .61 to .77

Author: Jones, L. K., and Brooks, N.

Article: Outreach: A career exploration kit in the university library.

Journal: *Vocational Guidance Quarterly,* June 1985, *33*(4), 324–330.

Related Research: Jones, L. K., & Chenery, M. F. (1980). Multiple subtypes among vocationally undecided college students: A model and assessment instrument. *Journal of Counseling Psychology, 27,* 469–477.

■ ■ ■

3660

Test Name: VOCATIONAL ROLE PREFERENCE SCALE

Purpose: To measure stereotypical vocational role orientations.

Number of Items: 13

Format: Paired occupations, one "female" and one "male," one of which children are to choose as a future job.

Reliability: Test–retest reliability was .81.

Author: Weeks, M. O.

Article: A second look at the impact of nontraditional vocational role models and curriculum on the vocational role preferences of kindergarten children.

Journal: *Journal of Vocational Behavior,* August 1983, *23*(1), 64–71.

Related Research: Weeks, M. O., et al. (1977). The impact of exposure to nontraditional vocational role models on the vocational role preferences of five-year-old children. *Journal of Vocational Behavior, 10,* 139–145.

■ ■ ■

3661

Test Name: WORK INVOLVEMENT SEMANTIC DIFFERENTIAL

Purpose: To measure work involvement.

Number of Items: 8

Format: Semantic differential. All items are presented.

Reliability: Item-total correlations ranged from .71 to .82 (median .74). Alpha was .83. Test–retest reliability was .78.

Validity: Detailed convergent, discriminate criterion, and concurrent validity data reported.

Author: Kanungo, R. N.

Article: Measurement of job and work involvement.

Journal: *Journal of Applied Psychology,* June 1982, *67*(3), 341–349.

■ ■ ■

3662

Test Name: WORK INVOLVEMENT SCALE

Purpose: To measure psychological involvement in work.

Number of Items: 9

Format: 5- and 6-point rating scales.

Reliability: Alpha was .87.

Author: Pistrang, N.

Article: Women's work involvement and experience of new motherhood.

Journal: *Journal of Marriage and the Family*, May 1984, *46*(2), 433–447.

Related Research: Lodahl, T., & Kejner, M. (1965). The definition and measurement of job involvement. *Journal of Applied Psychology, 44*, 24–33.

Jiminez, M. H. (1977). *Relationships between job orientation in women and adjustment to the first pregnancy and postpartum period.* Doctoral dissertation, Northwestern University.

Thornton, A., & Camburn, D. (1979). Fertility, sex role attitudes, and labor force participation. *Psychology of Women Quarterly, 4*, 61–80.

■ ■ ■

3663

Test Name: WORK ORIENTATION SCALE

Purpose: To measure discipline and dedication to work as envisaged by Weber's concept of the Protestant ethic.

Number of Items: 40 (from California Personality Inventory).

Format: True–false format.

Reliability: Alpha was .75. Test–retest reliability was .70.

Validity: Correlated with CPI scales: well-being (.84); responsibility (.65); self-control (.67); socialization (.65); tolerance (.64); good impression (.66); achievement via conformance (.71); managerial potential (.74). Group norms presented for both males and females, by occupation.

Author: Gough, H. G.

Article: A Work Organization Scale for the California Personality Inventory.

Journal: *Journal of Applied Psychology*, August 1985, *70*(3), 505–513.

■ ■ ■

3664

Test Name: WORK PREFERENCE QUESTIONNAIRE

Purpose: To measure job attribute preferences in an ideal job.

Number of Items: 26

Format: Multiple-choice. All items presented.

Reliability: Alpha ranged from .43 to .95 across seven factors extracted by factor analysis.

Author: Sterns, L., et al.

Article: The relationship of extroversion and neuroticism with job preferences and job satisfaction for clerical employees.

Journal: *Journal of Occupational Psychology*, June 1983, *56*(2), 145–153.

Related Research: Barrett, G. V., et al. (1975). *Relationship among job structural attributes, retention, aptitude and work values* (Tech. Rep. No. 3). The University of Akron, Department of Psychology. Contract No. N00014-74-A-0202-0001, NR 151-351. Office of Naval Research (NTIS No. AD-A014466).

■ ■ ■

3665

Test Name: WORK-ROLE SALIENCE SCALE

Purpose: To measure importance of work and career in a person's life.

Number of Items: 27

Format: Items rated in a 5-point Likert format. Sample items are presented.

Reliability: Alpha ranged from .83 to .90.

Author: Beutell, N. J., and Greenhaus, J. H.

Article: Interrole conflict among married women: The influence of husband and wife characteristics on conflict and coping behavior.

Journal: *Journal of Vocational Behavior*, August 1982, *21*(1), 99–110.

Related Research: Greenhaus, J. (1971). An investigation of the role of career salience in vocational behavior. *Journal of Vocational Behavior, 1*, 209–216.

Author Index

All numbers refer to test numbers for the current volume.

Belsky, J., 2978, 3025
Bem, S. L., 3389
Ben-Shakhar, G., 3582
Bengston, V., 3028
Benner, E. H., 3213, 3222
Bennett, S. K., 3589
Benton, S., 3422
Berg-Cross, L., 3448, 3523, 3535
Bergandi, T. A., 3517
Berger, E. M., 3296
Berger-Gross, V., 3291
Berman, W. H., 2457, 2974
Bernal, H. H., 3068
Berndt, D. J., 2498, 2534
Bernstein, B., 3109
Bernstein, B. L., 3336
Bernstein, D. M., 2596
Berry, G. L., 2790
Berryman, J. D., 2694
Berscheid, E., 3177
Berzins, J. I., 3294
Betz, N., 3343
Betz, N. E., 2418, 3249, 3256, 3306
Betz, N. M., 3180
Beutell, N. J., 2669, 2703, 2796, 3416, 3664
Beyard-Tyler, K. C., 2700
Bhagat, R. S., 2466, 2488, 2504, 2543
Biaggio, M. K., 3106, 3454, 3455, 3463
Biberman, G., 3368
Bienvenu, M. J., 2897, 2905
Bieri, J., 3421
Bierman, K. L., 2794
Biggs, D. A., 3573
Biggs, D. L., 2669, 3416
Biggs, P., 2760
Bilderback, E. W., 2786
Bills, R. E., 3523, 3535
Birchler, G. R., 2966
Birk, J. M., 3630
Birleson, A. T., 2465
Bizzell, R. P., 3197
Blanchard, R., 3403
Blank, J. R., 2379, 3079
Blasi, A., 3529
Blatt, S. J., 2461
Blau, G., 3344, 3611
Blau, G. J., 3136, 3179
Bledsoe, J. C., 2389, 3151
Blocher, D. H., 3408
Bloland, R. M., 3419
Bloom, B. S., 3563
Blotcky, A. D., 2860
Blumenfield, P. C., 3187

Blyton, P., 2645, 2656
Bobo, J. K., 2803
Bode, J., 3531
Bohlin, G., 3345
Bohlmeyer, E. M., 3490
Bohra, K. A., 2841
Bohrnstedt, G. W., 3177
Bond, M. J., 3628
Bonge, D., 3226
Booth, A., 3023
Booth, R., 2615
Booth, R. Z., 3129
Borg, W. F., 2888
Borg, W. R., 2888
Borko, H., 2739
Bororo, D. R., 3573
Borrello, G. M., 3443
Bortner, R., 3450
Bortner, R. W., 3518
Bovermon, I. K., 3214
Bowen, D. E., 3054, 3066, 3077
Bowen, G. L., 3026
Bowers, D. G., 2889, 3560
Bowlby, J., 2977, 3409
Boyar, J. I., 2447
Boyce, D., 3542
Bradburn, N., 2436
Bradburn, N. M., 2466
Brader, P. K., 2778
Bradley, R., 2553, 3233
Bradley, R. H., 2997, 2998, 3182
Brauchle, P. E., 3520
Bray, D. W., 3145
Brayfield, A. H., 2625, 2634, 3656
Brenner, O. C., 2470
Bretell, D., 2462
Brett, J., 2986
Briggs, L. J., 2387
Brink, T. L., 2475
Brinkerhoff, M. B., 2759
Brischetto, C. S., 3573
Brogan, D., 2746, 2783
Brookover, W. B., 3301
Brooks, G. C., 2784
Brooks, G. C., Jr., 2684
Brooks, L., 3572, 3638
Brooks, N., 3659
Brophy, J., 2911
Brophy, J. E., 2804, 2821
Brown, D., 2415
Brown, D. R., 3199
Brown, D. S., 2574
Brown, G. F., 3552
Brown, R., 3331
Brown, R. A., 2452
Brown, R. D., 2917

Brown, S. A., 3159, 3160
Brown, S. D., 2403, 2977
Browning, D. L., 2959
Brozo, W. G., 2881
Bruch, M. A., 3201
Bruning, C. R., 2716, 3620, 3622
Bryant, B. K., 3483
Bryant, N. D., 2398
Bryne, D., 3504
Buckmaster, L. R., 3285, 3286, 3386
Budner, S., 3509
Buhrmester, D., 3044
Bull, K. S., 3386
Bunting, C. E., 2738
Burke, C., 2391
Burke, P., 3202
Burke, R. J., 2591, 3102, 3462, 3518, 3627
Burkhead, E. J., 2638, 3080, 3508
Burnkrant, R. E., 3376
Burr, R. G., 2641
Burton, R. L., 3229
Busch-Rossnagel, N. C., 3356
Bush, A. J., 2930
Buss, A. H, 3357, 3358, 3463
Butler, M. C., 2641
Butterfield, D. A., 3580
Byrne, B. M., 3301, 3311, 3313
Byrne, D., 3503
Byrnes, D. A., 2424

■ ■ ■

Cacioppo, J. T., 3367
Cadwell, J., 2739, 2817
Cahn, D. D., 3264
Caillet, K. C., 2585, 2949, 2951, 2955
Caldwell, B. M., 2997, 2998
Caldwell, D. F., 2569, 2636
Callero, P., 3174
Caltabiano, N. J., 3228
Camburn, D., 3662
Campbell, D. J., 2895
Campion, M. A., 3092
Cantwell, D. P., 2502
Caplan, R. D., 2516, 2537
Caplovitz, D., 2436
Capurso, R. J., 3408
Carey, W. B., 2811, 3348, 3364, 3365, 3375
Carlson, G. A., 2465, 2502
Carney, R. E., 3414
Carpenter, P. A., 2392
Carpenter, T. P., 2939

Diener, C., 3268

Diener, E., 2529

DiNola, A. J., 2381

Dishion, T. J., 2818

Distefano, M. K., 3059, 3592, 3593

Distenfeld, M. S., 3601

DiVesta, F. J., 2716

Dixon, D. N., 2900

Dixon, J. C., 2385, 2834

Dodge, K. A., 2613

Doherty, W. J., 3011, 3012, 3045

Dohrenwend, B. P., 3111

Dohrenwend, B. S., 2488, 2543, 3111

Dolan, L., 2994

Dolan, L. J., 2994

Dole, J. A., 2688

Dollinger, S. J., 2490

Domino, G., 2877, 3070

Dorhout, A., 3406

Dornbusch, S. M., 3166

Dosser, D. A., Jr., 3361

Douglas, P., 3246

Dourninck, W. J. van, 2969

Doverspike, D., 3061

Dowd, E. T., 3165, 3573

Dowd, J. J., 2496

Downey, A. M., 2447

Downey, R. G., 2407

Downing, P., 3611

Downs, C., 2904

Doyle, A., 2606

Drasgow, F., 2672, 3647

Dreger, R. M., 3581

Drehmer, D. E., 3366

Dressler, G., 2884

Driscoll, J. M., 2800, 2858

Driver, B. L., 3407

Drory, A., 3561, 3634

Drummond, R. J., 3311

Dubin, R., 2672, 3622, 3635

Dubrin, A. J., 3368

Duff, A., 3521

Duke, M. P., 3255, 3274

Dulaney, E., 2920

Duncan, R. B., 3072

Dungy, G., 3613

Dunham, F. Y., 3183

Dunnam, M., 2810

Dunnette, M. D., 3629

Dupuy, H. J., 2493

Durkee, A., 3463

Durlak, J. A., 2469

Duttweiler, P. C., 3223

Dweck, C., 3268

Dye, H. A., 3603

Dyer, L., 2719

■ ■ ■

Eagly, A. H., 3212, 3229

Eberhardt, B. J., 3349

Eberly, C., 3269

Eckbad, M., 3539

Edelbrock, C., 2816

Edelbrock, C. S., 2799

Edie, C. A., 2441

Edmonds, V. H., 2980, 3019

Edwards, J. N., 3023

Egan, G., 3474

Eggeman, K, 3021

Eidelson, R. J., 3287

Eisenhauer, J. E., 3107, 3290

Eison, J. A., 2757, 3402

Elardo, R., 2969

Eliot, J., 3397, 3430, 3440

Elliott, G. C., 2510

Elliott, R., 3505

Elliott, S. N., 2822, 3400

Ellis, R. A., 3315, 3329

Ellis, R. H., 2815

Ellithorpe, E., 2495

Emmons, R. A., 3491

Endicott, J., 2514

Endler, N. S., 3514

England, G. W., 2686

Englese, J. A., 3302

Epperson, D. L., 3572

Epstein, A., 3490

Epstein, N., 2952, 3287, 3473, 3476

Erdle, S., 3499

Erlenbacher, A., 2375

Erskine, N., 3316

Erwin, T. D., 2958

Estes, T. H., 2741

Etzion, D., 2619

Evanechko, P., 3257, 3337

Evans, D. R., 3106

Evans, R. H., 2907, 3484

Even, B., 2699

Eyberg, S. M., 2979

Ezell, H. F., 3243

■ ■ ■

Faguhar, W. W., 3406

Faigley, L., 2431

Fairbank, J. A., 2454

Falander, C., 3351

Falbo, T., 3512

Fallik, B., 3430, 3440

Farber, B. A., 2664

Farmer, H., 2996, 3612

Farr, J. L., 3085, 3635, 3643

Farrah, G. A., 3297

Farrell, J., 3028

Fasold, R., 2756

Faulkner, J. E., 3534

Favero, J., 2555, 2564

Fayne, H. R., 2398, 2821

Fazio, A. F., 2474

Feather, N. T., 3628

Feingold, A., 2378, 2680

Feldhusen, J. F., 3250

Feldman, D. C., 3647

Feletti, G. I., 3089

Felton, B. J., 2432

Fenigstein, A., 2605, 3302, 3376

Fenigstein, A. M., 2510

Fennema, E., 3245, 3246

Fergusson, D. M., 2987

Ferrell, G. M., 3443

Ferris, G. R., 2915

Ferris, K. R., 3646, 3647

Feshbach, N. D., 3477, 3483

Feuerstein, M., 2854

Fiebert, M. S., 2760

Fiedler, F. E., 2568, 3074, 3401

Field, T., 2811, 3375, 3385

Fielding, M., 3108

Figley, C. R., 2833

Filsinger, E. E., 2582, 2978, 3554

Fimian, M. J., 2666

Fine, M. A., 3034

Finnerty-Fried, P., 2697, 2755

Fischer, C. H., 3573

Fischer, E. H., 2698, 2743

Fischer, J. L., 2580

Fishbein, M., 2730

Fisher, D. L., 3093

Fisher, S., 3355

Fisher-Beckfield, D., 2409

Flanders, N. A., 2863

Fleishman, E. A., 2682

Flexer, B. K., 3428

Floyd, F. J., 2972

Foa, E. G., 2598, 3144

Foa, U. G., 2598, 3144

Fogarty, R., 2596

Fogerson, L., 3052

Fogl, A., 2877

Foley, T. S., 3120

Fonosch, G. G., 2717

Ford, D. L., Jr., 2628

Ford, M. R., 2848

Forehand, R., 2831

Forfar, C. S., 2453, 2458-, 2460, 2469, 2497

Hagan, J., 2874
Hage, G., 3088
Hagekull, B., 3384
Hagerty, B. K., 3112
Hahlweg, K., 2913
Hale, W. D., 2448
Hall, B. W., 3332
Hall, C. S., 3491
Hall, D., 3136
Hall, D. T., 3636
Hall, L. E., 2743
Hall, R. H., 2919
Hall, T., 3583
Hall, W. S., 2772
Haller, A. O., 3447
Haller, E. J., 3444
Halliday, M. A., 2370
Hallon, C. J., 3486
Halote, B., 3153
Halpin, G., 2665, 3197, 3222, 3282, 3332
Halsey, A. H., 3109
Hamerlynck, L. A., 3013
Hamilton, M., 2479
Hamilton, V., 2489, 2543
Hamlin, R. M., 3390
Hammer, A. L., 3506
Hammer, T. H., 3118, 3415, 3637
Handal, P. J., 2801
Handley, P., 3570
Handley, P. C., 3573
Hansell, S., 2948
Hansen, G., 2562, 2746, 3006, 3014, 3016, 3041, 3314
Hansen, G. L., 2749, 2750, 3019
Hanson, G. R., 3343
Hanson, R. A., 2952
Hanson, S. L., 2436
Harburg, E., 3358
Hardin, S. I., 3209, 3573
Hare, R. D., 2518, 3511
Hargrove, D. S., 3505
Haring, M. J., 2700
Harker, P., 2631, 3091, 3317, 3584
Harnisch, D. L., 2428
Harpaz, I., 3422
Harrell, T. H., 2442
Harren, V. A., 3425, 3610
Harris, D. B., 3276
Harris, K., 2665
Harris, K. R., 2771, 2917
Harris, R. M., 3225, 3235, 3236, 3237
Harris, R. M., Jr., 3388
Harshman, R. A., 3440
Harter, S., 2593, 3252, 3260

Hartman, B., 3199
Hartman, B. W., 2809
Hartman, M., 3553
Hartup, W. W., 2893
Harvey, D., 2694
Harvey, O. J., 2934
Hasan, R., 2370
Hatfield, J. D., 2633
Hattie, J., 3602
Hawk, J. W., 2763
Hawley, P., 2699
Haynes, S. G., 3479
Haywood, H. C., 3033, 3222, 3390
Hazen, M., 2904
Hazer, J. T., 3559
Hchu, H-Y., 3536
Heavan, P. C. L., 2732, 3507
Heeder, R., 2519
Heesacker, M., 3208, 3210, 3564, 3569, 3573
Heilbrun, A. B., Jr., 2489, 2932, 3135
Heimberg, L., 3156
Heller, R. M., 3050
Helmreich, R., 2614, 3206
Helmreich, R. L., 2704, 3036
Helms, B. J., 3195
Helms, J. E., 2772, 2773
Helwig, J., 2376
Henderson, R. W., 2993, 3076
Hendrix, W. H., 2535
Hener, T., 3639, 3641
Henry, R. M., 2437
Heppner, P. P., 3208, 3210, 3280, 3436, 3437, 3439, 3564, 3569, 3573, 3658
Hereford, C. F., 3032
Herman, M. W., 2696
Herold, D. M., 3083
Herr, E. L., 3565
Herrick, V. E., 2375
Herzberger, S. D., 3459
Hesketh, B., 3632
Heslin, R., 2908
Hicks, L. A., 3231
Higgins, E., 3474
Hill, C. E., 2899, 3063, 3573
Hill, G., 3529, 3531
Himmelfarb, S., 2474
Hines, P., 3448, 3523, 3535
Hirschfield, R. M. A., 2574
Hirschi, T., 2874
Hirschman, E., 3133
Hirschman, E. C., 2512, 2687, 2829, 3271
Hite, L. M., 2426

Ho, R., 2455
Hocevar, D., 2940, 3576
Hock, E., 2513, 2967
Hodapp, V., 2649
Hodges, W. F., 2856
Hoelter, J., 2497
Hoffman, E., 2919, 3401
Hoffman, J. A., 3040
Hoffman, L. W., 3009
Hofman, J. E., 3218
Hogan, H. W., 3189
Hogan, J., 3377
Hogan, R., 3377
Hoge, D. R., 2832, 3525, 3526, 3555
Hoge, R. D., 2606
Hojat, M., 2696
Holahan, C. K., 3322
Holcomb, H., 2823
Holcomb, W. R., 2539
Holden, R. R., 3346
Holland, J. E., 3657
Holland, J. L., 3657
Holley, W. H., 2719, 3405
Hollon, S. D., 2442
Holmes, T. H., 2423, 2481, 2531, 2533
Holt, M. L., 2837
Hong, S-M, 3167, 3230
Hong, S., 2455
Hood, A. B., 2588
Hood, J., 3224
Hood, R. W., Jr., 3544
Hopper, S., 2801
Hoppock, R., 2624
Hops, H., 3024
Horan, J., 2440
Horan, J. J., 2433, 2508
Horn, T. S., 3215, 3260
Hornung, C. A., 2973
Horowitz, J. E., 2921
Horowitz, M. J., 2484
Hosek, J., 2797
Hoskins, R., 2887
House, R. J., 2884, 3267, 3290
Houseknecht, S. K., 2978
Houston, S. R., 3273, 3549
Howard, A., 3145
Howard, K., 3191, 3200
Howard, K. I., 2847
Howe, A. C., 2880
Howell, F. M., 2416, 3005
Hrebiniak, L. G., 3624, 3646
Huba, M. E., 2390
Hubbard, F. O. A., 2742
Hubble, M. A., 3573
Huber, V. L., 3115, 3149

Kitson, G. C., 2963
Klaus, D., 2570
Klein, M. F., 3103
Klimoski, R. J., 2686
Knight, R. G., 2386
Knoop, H. R., 3590
Koch, H. L., 2806
Koch, J. L., 2617
Kochenour, E., 2883
Kogan, N. A., 2755
Kolko, D. J., 2570, 2603, 2885
Kolloff, M. B., 3250
Kontos, S., 2390
Korner, A. F., 2811
Kornhauser, A., 2504
Koski, L. K., 2996, 3612
Koss, M. P., 2875
Koupman-Boydan, P. G., 3557
Kourilsky, M., 2396
Kovacs, M., 2450
Kraft, R. G., 2445, 3573
Krahe, B., 3359
Kraut, A. I., 2918, 3291
Krefting, L. A., 2651
Krieschok, T. S., 3280
Krumboltz, J. D., 3406, 3616
Krus, D. J., 3533
Kuh, G. D., 2943
Kukulka, G., 2826, 2928
Kunce, J. T., 2983
Kundert, D. K., 2677
Kunkle, D., 3161
Kurdek, L. A., 2449, 2561, 2605, 2835, 3239, 3240, 3302, 3504,
Kurtines, W., 2957
Kurtzman, C., 2725
Kutner, N., 2783
Kutner, N. G., 2746

■ ■ ■

LaBaron, S., 2867
LaCrosse, M. B., 3353, 3591, 3753
Lafromboise, T. D., 3451
Lamb, C. W., Jr., 2798
Lamke, L. K., 2978
Lamont, D. J., 3069
Lange, A. J., 2573
LaRossa, R., 2496
Larsen, K. S., 2586, 2695, 2748
Larson, L. L., 2884, 3267
Larson, L. M., 3658
Larzelere, R. E., 2562
Latack, J. C., 2660
Lau, S., 3323
Lauton, G. W., 3652

Lawe, C. F., 2899
Lawler, E., 3136
Lawler, E. E., 2653, 3405, 3636
Lawson, J. S., 2681
Lawton, M. P, 2496, 2506
Leary, M. R., 2551, 2572
Lee, C., 3267
Lee, D. Y., 3572, 3573
Lee, G. R., 2495
Lee, J. Y., 3318
Lee, P. C., 3055
Lee, R., 2668, 3577, 3587
Lefcourt, H. M., 2587, 3157, 3253
Lefcourt, J., 3339
Lefebvre, M. F., 3192
Lefkowitz, J., 2671, 3143
Lefkowitz, M. M., 2502
Leighton, D. C., 2480
Lenihan, M., 3179
Lennox, R. D., 2558
Lent, R. W., 3306
Leonetti, R., 3279
Lerner, R. M., 3275, 3356
Lesser, G. S., 2437
Lessing, E. E., 2838
Lester, D., 2453, 2468
Levenson, H., 3230, 3236
Levine, E. L., 2614, 3328
Levine, J., 2594
Levinger, G., 2968
Levinson, D., 3047
Levy, D. A., 2487
Levy-Shiff, R., 2422
Lewinsohn, P. M., 3101
Lewis, J. M., 2765
Licata, J. W., 3107
Licht, B. G., 3205
Liden, R., 2916
Liden, R. C. 3588
Liebert, R. M, 2523
Lief, H. I., 2781
Likert, R., 2872, 3099
Lin, T., 2899
Lincoln, J. R., 2571
Linden, J. D., 3063, 3564, 3569
Lindgren, H. C., 3142, 3231
Linehan, M. M., 2521
Linkowski, D. S., 2432
Linn, B. S., 2425
Linn, M. C, 3420, 3435
Liska, A. E., 2706, 2714
Litt, M. D., 2499, 2635
Little, L. F., 3010
Litwin, G. H., 3097, 3098
Livch, H., 2468
Llabre, M. M., 2473, 3245

Lloyd, S. A., 2598
Lobb, M. L., 3480
Locke, H. J., 3011, 3015, 3027, 3035
Lodahl, T., 3634, 3635, 3662
Lodahl, T. M., 2986
Loeb, R. G., 3595
Loeber, R., 2818
Loesch, L. C., 2380
Loevinger, J., 2948, 2959
Lohr, J. M., 3226
Lokan, J. J., 3241
Loney, J., 2878
Long, T. J., 2522, 2532
Lonky, E., 3427
Lopez, F. G., 2769, 3594
Lopez, F. M., 3515
Lorge, I., 2697
Lorion, R. P., 2406, 2820, 2945
Louis, M. R., 2636
Lovejoy, F. H., 3524
Lovell-Troy, L. A., 2612
Low, B. P., 3056
Lowe, D. R., 2573
Lowe, M. R., 2608—2610
Lowry, N., 2733
Loyd, B. H., 2727
Loyd, D. E., 2727
Luborsky, L., 3581
Ludeke, R. J., 2893
Luenburg, F. C., 3299
Lumby, M. E., 2750
Lumpkin, J. R., 3178
Lunenburg, F. C., 3105
Lyons, T. F., 2542, 2640, 2647, 2657, 3650
Lysy, K. Z., 2852

■ ■ ■

Ma, L-C., 3538
MacDonald, A. P., Jr., 2713
MacDonald, A. R., 3235
MacDonald, M. L., 3468
Macke, A. S., 2978
Mackey, J., 2549
Mackle, M., 2759
Macklin, M. C., 2722
MacMillan, D. L., 2890
MacPhillamy, D. J., 3101
Madden, M. E., 3027
Madrid, D., 2933
Madsen, C. H., 2822
Maes, W. R., 3333
Magaro, P. A., 2491
Magnusson, D., 3514

Murphy, C. J., 2628
Murphy, G. C., 3265
Murphy, K. C., 2900
Murphy, K. R., 3606
Murphy, V. M., 2481
Murray, H. G., 3605
Myers, A. E., 3125
Myrick, R. D., 3570

■ ■ ■

Nagy, S., 2676, 3108
Naismith, D. C., 2650
Najman, J., 2458
Nall, R. L., 2872
Nambayan, A., 2767
Napoletano, M. A., 2736
Narayanan, S., 3099
Narikawa, D., 2779
Navran, L., 2921
Neal, W. R., 2694
Nelson, T. L., 2403
Nemo, R. S., 3390
Nesbitt, E., 3461
Nettler, G., 2734
Neumann, L., 3563
Neumann, Y., 3563
Nevid, J. S., 2748
Newfield, J., 3103
Newman, J. E., 2910
Newman, L. F., 3009
Newman, R. C., 3414
Newton, T. J., 2527
Nice, D. S., 2978
Nichols, C. W., 3631
Nichols, J., 3252
Noles, S. W., 3177
Norem-Hebeisen, A., 2785
Norton, R., 2978
Norton, R. W., 3516
Nott, D. L., 3607
Novaco, R., 3494
Nowack, K. M., 3075
Nowicki, S., 3238, 3255, 3274
Nowicki, S., Jr., 3183, 3241
Nowinski, J. K., 2576
Nunn, G. D., 3270
Nye, E. I., 2832

■ ■ ■

O'Brien, E. J., 3212
O'Connell, J. K., 3219
O'Conner, E. J., 2472, 2623
O'Dell, S. L., 2382
O'Donnell, J. P., 2490

O'Keefe, D. J., 3408
O'Laughlin, M. S., 3656
O'Leary, K. D., 2973
O'Leary, S., 2878
O'Malley, S. S., 2616
O'Neill, C. D., 3616
O'Neill, R., 3305
O'Reilly, C., 2636
O'Reilly, C. A., 2569
Oelke, M. C., 3199
Oetting, E. R., 2819
Okenek, K., 2516, 2517, 2627, 2642, 3071
Oldham, G. R., 2631, 2635, 3091
Olson, D. H., 2592, 2982, 2983
Omizo, M. M., 2897
Oppenheimer, B. T., 2604
Orbach, I., 2538
Oren, D. L., 3166
Ormrod, J. E., 2960
Oros, C. J., 2875
Orthner, D. K., 3026
Osterhouse, R. A., 2429
Ostrum, T. M., 3239
Otis, L. P., 3211, 3396
Ottinger, D. R, 3242
Owens, W. A., 3349
Ozawa, J. P., 2853

■ ■ ■

Page, R., 3531
Page, R. C., 3104
Page, T. J., Jr., 3376
Paivio, A., 3397, 3440
Palenzuela, D. L., 3196
Palmon, N., 2873
Pandey, J., 2841
Pappo, M., 2411, 2500
Paradise, L. V., 2590
Parham, T. A., 2772, 2773
Parish, T., 3270
Parish, T. S., 3186, 3254, 3269
Parkerson, J. A., 3114
Parrish, T. S., 3038
Parry, G., 3002
Parsons, C. K., 3083, 3588
Parten, M. B., 2861
Pasamanick, B., 3543
Pascarella, E. T., 2399, 2953, 2954, 3049, 3321, 3398
Patchen, M., 3649
Patrick, J., 3084
Pattengill, S. M., 3031
Patterson, J. M., 2975
Paurohit, N., 3573

Payne, B. D., 2428
Pearce, J. L., 3138
Pearlin, L., 2463
Pearlin, L. I., 2457
Pearlman, C., 3150
Pearson, J. E., 2522, 2532
Pearson, P., 3133
Peck, R. F., 3600
Pecnik, J. A., 3572
Pedhazur, E. J., 2739
Pedro, J. D., 3618
Peiser, C., 3639
Pekarik, E. G., 3374
Pellegrini, D. S., 3433
Pendleton, B. F., 3043
Penley, L., 3541, 3648
Peplau, L. A., 3537, 3538
Perry, J. D., 2601
Perry, W. G., Jr., 2958, 3527, 3546
Persson-Blennow, I., 3378, 3379
Perunko, M., 3440
Peters, K., 2546
Peters, L. H., 2472, 2623, 2796
Petersen, C. H., 3280, 3436, 3437, 3439
Peterson, C., 3165
Peterson, D. R., 2807
Peterson, G. W., 3232
Peterson, K., 3248
Peterson, L., 2607
Peterson, M. F., 2577, 2889, 3116, 3262
Peterson, P. L., 3423
Petrie, K., 2485, 2649
Petrillo, G. H., 3555
Pettegrew, L. S., 2839, 3220
Petty, R. E., 3367
Pety, J., 3573
Pfeiffer, E., 2544
Pfeiffer, J. W., 2896
Phares, E. J., 3316
Phelps, J., 2373
Phifer, S. J., 2720
Phillips, J. S., 2663, 3137, 3140, 3559
Phillips, S. D., 3425, 3437
Pichot, P., 2446
Piechowski, M. M., 2852, 3495
Pierro, R. A., 3510
Piers, E. V., 3276
Pierson, D., 3277 Pike, R., 2593
Pines, A., 2619, 2674
Pines, A. M., 2540, 2643
Pinkney, J. W., 2753
Pinsof, W., 2559
Pinto, P. R., 3585

Rullard, W., 3385
Runco, M. A., 2940, 2942
Rundquist, E. A., 3030
Runion, K. B., 3186
Ruppel, G., 3573
Rush, J. C., 3102
Russell, D., 2615, 3181, 3513
Russell, G. M., 3171, 3452
Ryan, M. P., 3527, 3546
Ryan, N. B., 2442
Ryder, R. G., 3012, 3045

■ ■ ■

Sabatelli, R. M., 2968, 3018
Sachs, J. S., 3119
Sackeim, H. A., 3510
Sackett, P. R., 3073
Sadock, B. J., 2520
Sadowski, C. J., 3100
Safran, J. S., 2865
Safran, S. P., 2865
Saigh, P. A., 3394
Saleh, S. D., 2797
Salomone, P. R., 3225, 3235—3237, 3388
Saltzer, E. B., 3340
Sameroff, A. J., 3365
Sampson, D. L., 2798
Sampson, J. P., 2380
Sanchez, A. R., 2698
Sarason, B., 2578
Sarason, I. G., 2402, 2473, 2489, 2508, 2543, 2578
Sarason, S. B., 2430
Saski, J., 2774
Saver, W., 2990
Savickas, M. L., 2483, 2950, 3156, 3157, 3335, 3640
Saxe, J. E., 2371, 2372, 2721
Saylor, C. F., 2450
Scandura, T. A., 2624, 2916
Schaefer, M. T., 2592
Schafer, R. B., 2463, 3298
Schatz, E. M., 3286
Schell, B. H., 2541
Schibeci, R. A., 2793
Schiemann, W., 2918
Schippman, J. S., 3131
Schludermann, E., 2971
Schludermann, S., 2971
Schmeck, R. R., 2420, 3431
Schmelzer, R. V., 2881
Schmidt, J. P., 2605
Schmidt, L. D., 3572, 3573
Schmidt, N., 2561
Schmiedeck, R., 3548

Schmitt, J. P., 2449, 2561, 2835, 3239, 3240, 3302, 3504
Schnake, M. E., 3097
Schneider, B., 3050, 3054, 3066, 3077
Schneider, J. H., 3388
Schoenfeldt, L. F., 3349
Schofield, H. L., 2715
Schon. I., 2758, 2768, 2775
Schooler, C., 2457
Schotte, D. E., 2530
Schrader, W. J., 3586
Schriesheim, C., 2842
Schroeder, M. L., 2518
Schroeder, W. W., 3616
Schuler, G., 3576
Schuler, R. S., 3267
Schumm, W. R., 2980, 3007, 3017, 3631
Schwab, L. O., 2717
Schwab, R. L., 3292
Schwartz, G. E., 2566
Schwartz, J. C., 3003
Schwartz, R., 3481, 3502
Schwartzbach, H., 2492, 3198
Schwarz, J. C., 2971
Schwarzwald, J., 3139
Scott, C., 2908
Scott, J. P., 2531
Scott, K. D., 2842
Scott, K. J., 2883
Scott, N. A., 2446
Scott, W. E., 3115, 3149
Scott, W. E., Jr., 2637
Scruggs, T. E. 2791, 2792
Seagoe, M. V., 2862
Seashore, S., 2569
Sebes, J. M., 2964, 2989
Secord, P. F., 3175, 3263
Sedlacek, W. E., 2684, 2784
Seelbach, W., 2990
Seelbach, W. C., 2991, 2992
Seeman, M., 3339
Segal, S. A., 2833
Seifert, E. H., 2882
Sekaran, V., 3621
Selby, M. J., 3463, 3494
Sells, S., 2601
Semmer, N., 2517, 2642, 3071
Senay, E. C., 2531
Sergiovanni, T., 3277
Sermat, V., 2561
Severa, N., 2575, 3485
Seyfarth, L. H., 2711
Shaha, S. H., 2429
Shamir, B., 3341

Shannon, M., 2690
Shanor, K., 2876
Shapiro, S. B., 3547
Sharkey, C. T., 3284
Sharpley, C. F., 2962, 3014
Shaver, P. R., 3509
Shaw, G. A., 2397, 2941
Shea, M. T., 3487
Sheckles, M. P., 3397
Shephatia, L., 2422
Sherer, M., 3307
Sherman, A. W., 3040
Sherman, J., 3245
Sherman, R. E., 2898
Sherman, T. M., 2766
Shermis, M. D., 2536
Sherwood, J. J., 3298
Shigaki, I. S., 3441
Shinar, E. H., 3642
Shinn, J. M., 3001
Shoham, M., 3139
Shorkey, C., 2871
Shorkey, C. T., 2505, 2774, 3439
Short, J. F., 2832
Shover, P. R., 2563
Shulman, G. M., 3264
Shumate, G. F., 3199
Shure, M. B., 3433
Shuy, R., 2756
Shwebel, A. I., 3034
Sid, A. K. W., 3142
Siegal, L. S., 2969
Siegelman, M., 3033
Siegfried, W. D., Jr., 2906
Sigman, M., 2935
Silber, E., 3313
Silverman, W. H., 3062
Silverstein, A. B., 2847, 3076, 3152
Simard, L. C., 2535
Simmons, R. G., 3312
Sims, E. V., Jr., 2376
Sims, H. P., Jr., 3080
Singer, S., 2961
Sinha, J. B. P., 2845
Siryk, B., 2400, 2401, 2611, 3123
Sjoberg, L., 2494
Slade, P., 2742
Slaney, R. B., 3657
Slater, D., 3597
Slaughter, H. B., 2395
Sleet, D. A., 2862
Slenker, S. E., 3251
Sletto, R. F., 3030
Sloan, V. J., 2779
Slocum, J. W., Jr., 3583, 3596
Smilanski, S., 2422

Thornton, A., 3662
Thumin, F. J., 2689
Thurlow, M., 2824
Thyer, B. A., 2871
Tiggemann, M., 3255
Tilby, P., 3411
Tinsley, H. E. A., 3209, 3210, 3407,
Tinto, V., 2399
Tippett, J., 3313
Tipton, T. M., 3216
Tisher, R. P., 2880
Tittle, C. K., 3619
Tobacyk, J., 2385, 2834
Tobin, D. L., 2830
Tolchinsky, P. D., 2752
Tolfa, D., 2792
Tolor, A., 2481
Tolsdorf, C., 2589
Tolstedt, B. E., 2965, 2976, 3035, 3039
Tom, D. Y. H., 3509
Tom, F. K. T., 3605
Tomkiewicz, J., 2470
Toobert, D. J., 2818
Top, D., 3393
Topf, M., 2850, 3110
Topkin, W. E., 3123
Topping, C., 2413
Tornow, W. W., 3585
Touhey, J. C., 2759
Townes, B. D., 3424
Tracey, T. S., 2684
Treadwell, T. W., 2579
Triandis, H. C., 3169
Trice, A. D., 3194
Trice, H. M., 3624
Tripodi, T., 3421
Trites, R. L., 2827
Trost, J., 2975
Trusty, F., 3277
Tsai, S-L., 2762
Tseng, M. S., 3235
Tsujimoto, R. N., 3556
Tubiana, J. H., 3582
Tuck, J. P., 2439
Tucker, C. M., 2743, 2921
Tucker, L. A., 3175, 3263
Tuckman, J., 2697
Tully, J., 3202
Tung, W. K., 2546
Turk, D. C., 2457, 2499, 2635, 2974
Turkat, I. D., 2839, 3220
Turner, C. J., 2492, 3198, 3653
Turner, J. L., 2698, 2743
Twentyman, C. T., 2885
Tybout, A., 2908

Tych, A. M., 2947
Tyson, P., 3468
Tzuriel, D., 3033, 3222, 3390

■ ■ ■

Udry, J. R., 3016
Ungerer, J. A., 2935

■ ■ ■

Valecha, G. K., 3239
Valencia, R. R., 2993
Valerio, H. P., 3308, 3481, 3502
Valliant, P. M., 3503
Van Bart, D., 2632, 2670, 3002
Van Ijzendoorn, M. H., 3037
Van Til, J., 3138
Vandecreek, L., 3572
VandenBerg, E., 3391, 3410
Vapava, J. R., 2692
Vaughn, E. S., III, 3068
Vaux, A., 2589
Vecchio, R. P., 2568, 2843, 3074
Veit, C. T., 2493
Veldman, D. J., 3600
Velluntino, F. R., 2377
Venkatachalam, R., 3099
Ventura, J. N., 2984
Vera, W., 2760
Verna, G. B., 3186
Vestre, N. D., 2931
Villemez, W. J., 2579
Vincent, J., 2982
Vincent, K. R., 2802, 3372
Viney, L. L., 2947
Viney, W., 3532
Vitale, M., 3154
Vizeltir, V., 3134
Vleeming, R. G., 3302, 3514
Vogel, J., 3374
Vojtisek, J. E., 2491
Volkin, J. I., 3015
Vroom, V. H., 2626

■ ■ ■

Waddell, F. T., 3141
Waetjen, W., 3299
Wagner, B., 2956
Wagner, F. R., 3243, 3317
Wakabayashi, M., 2926
Walberg, H. J., 3094, 3113
Walder, L. O., 3498
Walker, A. J., 3004
Walker, D. K., 2381

Walker, W. J., 3057
Walkey, F. H., 3230
Wall, S. M., 2590
Wallace, G. R., 3338
Wallace, K. M., 3011, 3015, 3035
Wallston, B. S., 3217, 3339
Wallston, K. A., 3251, 3339
Walsh, J. J., 2700
Walster, E., 2965
Walton, J., 3369
Wambach, C. A., 2769, 3594
Wampold, B. E., 3024
Warburton, D. M., 2489, 2543
Ward, L. G., 3603
Ware, E. E., 3224
Ware, J. E., 3601
Ware, J. E., Jr., 2493
Ware, R., 3371
Warehime, R. G., 2573
Warman, R., 2909
Warr, P., 2632, 2670, 3002, 3130
Warr, P. B., 3626
Wass, H., 2453, 2458—2460, 2469, 2497
Watson, D., 2604
Watson, J. M., 2740, 2795
Watson, S. R., 3478
Watt, N. F., 2870
Weare, C. R., 3610
Weaver, J. R., 2675
Webster-Stratton, C., 2799
Weeks, M. O., 3660
Wegener, C., 2913
Weinberg, J., 2520
Weiner, B., 2859
Weinstein, N., 2850, 3110
Weinstein, R. S., 2892
Weir, T., 3627
Weisberg, P., 2376
Weiss, D. J., 2995
Weiss, D. S., 2685
Weiss, H. M., 2533, 2650
Weiss, R. L., 2966, 3013
Weissberg, R. P., 2414, 2820
Wells, G. R., 3151
Werbel, J. D., 3541, 3648, 3649
Wessberg, H. W., 2610
Wessler, R., 2948
Wessman, A. E., 3335
West, D. J., Jr., 2639
Westbrook, B. W., 3619
Westbrook, M. T., 2981
Westcott, M. R., 3430
Westman, A. S., 2467
Wexley, K. N., 3421, 3560
Weyer, G., 2649

■ ■ ■

Subject Index

All numbers refer to test numbers. Numbers 1 through 3. 39 refer to entries in Volume 1, numbers 340 through 1034 refer to entries in Volume 2, numbers 1035 through 1595 refer to entries in Volume 3, numbers 1596 through 2369 refer to entries in Volume 4, and numbers 2370 through 3665 refer to entries in Volume 5.

tivity toward, 1784; opinions, 529; orientation, 3393; preference, 200; psychology, 684; quality, 663; research, 1752, 2710; set, 1068, 1350; vocational, 305—339

Effectiveness: advisor, 2329; college course, 2338; college instructor, 2338; college teacher(s), 1541, 1542, 2334; college students' perception of instructors, 2358; communication, 99, 148; counselor, 307, 312, 316, 325, 1001, 1002, 1559, 2335, 3566, 3567, 3569; counselor trainee's, 2337; elementary guidance, 316; instructor, 329; judgment by child, 243; organizational practices, 1972; peer counseling, 1973; perceptual, 214; personal, 214; practice teaching, 690; psychological, 1449; speakers, 1765; teacher, 335, 1026, 1030, 3607; teaching, 2333, 2347

Efficacy, 976, 3204, 3331

Effort, 575

Ego: -centrism, 579, 1109, 1480, 1484, 1485; closeness-distance, 913; cognitive, 1491; development, 135, 136, 629, 1944, 2948, 2959; functioning, 1417; identity, 949, 2241, 2949, 2950; identity development, 628, 2951; identity status, 628; involvement, 3359; organization, 749; permissiveness, 3360; role-taking, 1503; strength, 2164, 3206; sufficiency, 1929

Egotism, 417

Elaboration, 861

Elderly: attitudes toward, 2697, 2755; care, 2990; mental competence, 2385; morale, 2506; stress, 2531

Elementary: anaphora comprehension, 2370; children, attitudes, 1136; children, client centered approach, 249; children, creativity, 1927, 1932; children, interracial attitudes, 1168; children, teacher-pupil relations, 256; first grade adjustment, 2413; grades, 3—6, 696; grades, anthropology, 1044; guidance, 31; reading, 1455, 1460; school, 388, 389, 540, 595, 622, 688, 701, 1723, 1756,

1770; school, academic self-concept, 2147; school boys, 389; school child anxiety, 933; school children, 21, 101, 456, 491, 626, 1043; school climate, 1323; school counseling, 70, 315, 316, 671; school, English second language, 1598; school environment, 1316; school, inner city, 990; school openness, 1963; school perceptual abilities, 2098; school principals, 1680; school reading attitude, 1822; students academically talented, 1606; student teachers, 495, 701; teachers, 341, 488; teacher evaluation, 1036; visual discrimination, 2394

Embed(ded)(ness), 1417: figures, 770, 1386

Emotion(al)(s), 404, 593: arousal, 1231; control, peer counseling, 1973; dependence, 931, 1638; development, 637; distance, 1103; factors, 138; maturity, 621, 2952; reliance, 1715; self assessment, 2165; social climate, 583; -social state, 578; state, immediate, 416; support, university residence, 704; types, 3361; withdrawal, 405

Emotionality, 403, 944, 1641

Emotive imaging, 2063

Empath(ic)(y), 220, 227, 235, 328, 429, 757, 771, 1100, 1385, 1387, 1438, 2243, 2268, 3476, 3490: children, 3473, 3477, 3483; counselors, 309, 3475, 3505, 3506; police, 781; teachers, 3474; understanding, 431, 1370, 1538, 2344, 2353

Emphasis, 688

Empiricism, 301, 976

Employability, 310, 320: attitude(s), 188, 193, 1007, 1156, 2622; behavior, 2851; commitment, 1996; evaluation, 1007, 1016, 3574, 3575; motivation, 205; perceptions, 3326; rating, 327, 692; satisfaction, 164; self-evaluation, 1008; work relations, 1116; work values, 1532

Employee: appearance, 1007; aptitude, 1007

Employment: commitment, 3626; desire for, 3130; immobility, 3627; success, 241

Encoding, associative verbal, 1035

Encopresis, 846

Encounter groups, psychological state, 841

Encouragement, parental, 713

Engaged couples, 597

Engineer(ing)(s): career interests, 3629; correlates with success, 212; creative potential, 1933; motivation, 1366; performance, 1557; self perception, 829; students, 42, 95

English: black non-standard, 1046; invitation/comprehension, 1046; pressures for, 647, 673; proficiency, 1732; sound-symbol relations, 366

Enhancement, self, 1994

Enthusiasm, 679: toward learning, 540; toward school, 540

Enuresis, 846

Environment(al): assessment, 672; campus, 662; classroom, 1324, 1539, 3057, 3058, 3078, 3093, 3094; college, 165, 172, 184, 187, 212; community, 1060; control, 1997; coping, 1095; effects upon, 3069; forces, 673; geographic, 3070; issues, attitudes, 1152; learning, 473, 673, 686, 3076, 3109, 3114; living, 3087; medical school stress, 2419; orientation, 302; perception, 179; preserving the natural, 1776; press of, 704; psychosocial, 1960; satisfaction, 1965; school, 1316; stress, 3071; treatment, 1310; uncertainty, 3072; university, 1440

Envy, interpersonal, 439

Equalitarianism, 537, 1123, 1177

Equality, 301: ethnic, 976

Erikson(ian): ego epigenesis, 628; stages of development, 245, 632; theory, 628, 629, 949

Eroticism, 1157

Esprit, 688

Esteem: co-worker, 1458; father, 788; self, see Self-Esteem; self, adult male, 826; self, children, 458; self, college student, 816; self, high school students, 827; self, pre-adolescent, 825; self, student, 792

Estrangement: cultural, 1700, 1701; political, 1977; self, 430, 457

Ethic(al)(s), 1815, 3529: behavior, violations, 971; conflict, 3530;

cal development, 631; temperament, see: Temperament, child and infant

Inference(s), 2217: social, 114

Inferential reading comprehension, 1605

Inferiority, feelings, 515

Inflectional performance, 17

Influence, hierarchical, 2236: in counseling, 258; leader, 1554; psychological, 3324; work, 2626, 2653

Information, 575: acquisition, 1; amount, 2223; biographical, 703; community life, 1060; institutional, 150—193, 657—706, 1307—1336, 1959—1983; job training, 709, 3079; processing, 605, 2907; processing style, 443; seeking, adolescents, 868; seeking, careers, 3616; seeking strategies, 2223, 2814; sex, 2393; symbolic, 107; transformation abilities, 106—108

Ingratiating behavior, 2841

Inhibition(s), 1720, 1870: impulse, 386; motor, 59; reciprocal, 389

Initiative, 949, 2265, 2842, 3131: supervisors, 1023

Inmates, prison, 91

Inner-outer directedness, 789

Innocence-guilt, 381

Innovati(on)(veness), 3484: behaviors, 432, 621; educational, 1784; university residence, 704

Inpatient behavior, mood, 1862

Inquisitiveness, creative, 578

Insecurity, 515

Inservice evaluation, 1319

Insight, 1385

Institution(al)(s): attitudes, 82; authority, attitudes, 2747; helplessness, 1670; information, 150—193, 657—706, 1307—1336, 1959—1983; political, 1806; procedures, 682

Instruction(al): attitude toward, 2712; behavior, 322; programmed, 153; television, problems, 488; threat of, 488; values, 3547

Instructor, 527, 667: behavior, 2863; effectiveness, 329; evaluation, 698, 997, 1009, 1014, 1022, 1027—1029, 1032, 3581; quality, 667; university, 680

Integrat(ed)(ion), 517: attitude, 79; classrooms, 2189

Integrative complexity, 1910, 2214, 2934

Integrity: of man, 915; of social agents, 2288

Intellectual(ity), 624, 986: ability, children, 888; achievement responsibility, 786; development, 637, 2953, 2954, 2958; efficiency, 2251; environment, 2993, 2994; growth, university residence, 704; locus of control, 3222; pragmatism, 95, 1515; pragmatic attitudes, 86; pressure for, 647, 673; self-confidence, 2073

Intelligence, 1117, 2265, 2689: children, 2677; culturally disadvantaged, 72; culture fair, 468; developmental, 1055; evaluated, 247; social, 1096, 1099, 1100, 2555, 2564; verbal, 887

Intensity, 2285

Intent(ionality): accidental, 381; judgment of, 622

Interaction, 68, 237: aide-child, 577; analysis, 427, 1049; anxiousness, 2572; behavioral, 585; behavior description, 596; classroom, 1105, 1894, 1897; counselor-client, 1253; family, 597; group, 1722; interpersonal, 448; interracial, 1143, 1745; marital, 240, 3024, 2035; mother, 1300; mother-child, 1953; parent-adolescent, 640; parent-child, 646, 1301, 1955; pupil, 1027; supervisor, 1248; teachers, 333, 1029; verbal, 596, 1261

Interconcept distance, 1908

Interest(s), 194—203, 593, 707—711: effort, counselors, 1003; information seeking, 868; job, 709; judgment of, 626; occupations, 196, 199, 201, 3629, 3631; parental, 650; patterns, 472; political, 537; religious, 1580; residence counselor, 1019; school, 391; science, intermediate, children, 864; social, 249; value, 1535; work, 757

Intermarriage, racial, 90

Internal: cognition, 2187; scanning, 1914; sensation, 2187; work motivation, 2001

Internal-external control, 50, 56,

238, 267, 576, 810, 1368, 1393, 1396, 1399, 1401, 1405, 1046, 1413, 1434, 2049, 2181: university freshmen, 221

Internationalism, 1795

Interorganizational relations, 1893

Interpersonal, 621, 625: adequacy, peer counseling, 1973; adjustment, college student, 2409; administrative behavior, 1863; aggression, 1221; alienation, 1110; attitudes, 546; attraction, 426, 1711; behavior, 1720; cognitive-complexity, 433; communication, 1900, 2920; competenc(e)(y), 446, 1724; complexity, 47; conflict, 523, 1950, 2573; contact, 328; control, 2075; dependency, adults, 1715, 2574; distanc(e)(ing), 436, 451, 2596; effectiveness, 2576; envy, 439; etiology, 530; feedback, 1899; flexibility, 217; index, 447; interaction, 448; jealousy, 2575; judgment, 1717; orientation, 54, 67, 216; perception, 428, 433; perceptions, teacher-child, 2076; problem, 892; pursuing, 2596; reflexes, 448; regard, 681; relations, 51, 431, 464, 575, 1102, 1256, 1668, 2548, 2577, 2588; relations, counselors, 1003; relations, self-perceptions, 780; relations university residence, 704; relationships, 1716; relationships, locus of control, 2087; seniority, 428, 444; sensitivity, 1663, 1681, 1718, 2269, 2288; situations, 1721; skills, 431; style, 1489; support, 2578; trust, 954, 1504, 2914; value constructs, 2304

Interpretat(ing)(ion)(ive), 600, 689, 1448: data, 1607

Interracial: attitudes, 517, 1150, 1198; attitude, students, 535; interaction, 1745

Interrogative patterns, recognition, 380, 384

Intervention: acceptability, 3400; federal, 79

Interview(ing), 587, 589: assessment, 3162; behavior, counselor, 584; client reaction, 998; counseling, 699; home, 647; maternal, 927; rating, counseling, 699; re-

competence, basic, 380, 384; comprehension, 355; infant, 2935; informal, 378; negative, 2933; oral, 1275; performance, 1035; proficiency, 376; skills, 1597; street, 378

Late adolescent(s), 498: males, 646

Latency, 585

Laterality assessment, 1881, 2681, 2687, 2690, 3422

Law(s): abidingness, 287; and order, 1797; enforcement personnel, 3577, 3579, 3587; knowledge of, 1018

Leader(ship): behavior, 1241, 1333, 1866, 2084, 2843, 2845, 2872, 2884, 2896; creativity, 1925; firemen, 1549; influence, 1544; initiative, self-concept, 2056; -member exchange, 1986, 2915, 2916, 2926; motivational style, 2184; opinion, 2104; qualities, 338; satisfaction, 2345; students, 2349, 2684, 2844; style, 941; style, supervisors, 1023; teacher, 1057; technical competence, 1555

Learn(er)(ing), 494: attitude toward, 540, 2785; behavior, 2829; behavior, perception of, 838; behavior in classrooms, 838; children's, 521, 2677; climate, 1323; cognitive, 175; disabled, 2853; enthusiasm for, 540; environment, 473, 647, 673, 686, 1298, 1324, 1371, 2985, 3076, 3089, 3109, 3114; grades vs. true, 487; higher, 347; inflectional principals, 17; materials, 1325; memory, 8; preference, 3402; process, 488, 3431; readiness, 2193; self-concept, 1389, 3213, 3299; student perceptions, 175; style, 2216; tasks, 1868

Learning disabled, children, phonics, 2398

Lectures: controversial, 586; quality, 3085

Legibility, 1052, 2376

Leisure activities, 198, 268, 870, 2185, 3404, 3407

Lesson, evaluation, 1027

Length, 2224

Letter: discrimination, 1051; formation, 1052; identification, 12; sound translation, 1062

Level of arousal, 2291

Level of aspiration, self-concept, 2056

Level of regard, 227, 309, 431, 2353

Liberal-conservative, 95, 280, 1527

Liberal dimension, mother's, 2313

Liberalism, 555, 2258

Liberalism-conservatism, college students, 1835

Libertarian democracy, 1799

Library, attitude, 2758

Lie scale, 499

Life: change(s), 1290, 2522, 2532, 3009; changes, college students, 1942; events, 2581, 3111; experience, 1719, 3373; experiences, women's liberation, 861; history, 1288; imagined, 3193; inventory, 2836; irritants, 3075; meaningfulness in, 821, 3524; perspective, 2047; satisfaction, 33, 415, 2504, 2529; statuses, perception, 2047; stress, 2533, 2543; style, 268, 1800

Lifestyle orientation, 2186

Liking, 460, 2582

Line Meanings, 608

Linguistic competence, 1121

Listening, 1735, 2913: achievement, 1043; comprehension, 2688

Literacy: basic occupational, 1038; child understanding, 3257, 3337; functional, 1611

Literal reading comprehension, 1609

Locative prepositional, 377

Locus of conflict, 2085

Locus of control, 50, 221, 239, 310, 320, 1368, 1383, 1393, 1396, 1399, 1401, 1406, 1413, 1434, 1628, 2068, 2071, 2074, 2088—2091, 2093, 2094, 2102, 2150, 3166, 3171, 3178, 3222—3225, 3230, 3233—3240, 3244: administrators, 818; adolescents, 2072; adult(s), 2033, 2100, 3194, 3196, 3255, 3272, 3274; black children, 793; children, 754, 797, 799, 2041, 2092, 2101, 2146, 2148, 3182—3187, 3205, 3241, 3242, 3252; health, 2066, 3217—3219, 3251, 3339, 3340; intellectual, social physical, 2086; internal-external, 576, 2049, 2081, 3164; interpersonal relationships, 2087; mental health, 2096; peer counseling, 1973; preschool, primary,

2113; rehabilitation clients, 29; teacher, 3332—3334

Logic(al), 474, 884: ability, children, 3441; additions, 19; connectives, 123; operations, 2946

Loneliness, 1703—1705, 1729, 2552—2554, 2561, 2615: children, 2583

Long-term memory, 1601

Love: addiction, 2584; punishment, symbolic, 654; reward, symbolic, 654; romantic, 2599, 2600; sickness, 3012

Loving, styles, 1871

Lower class, 349: children, test anxiety, 1076

Loyalty: supervisor, 1005; teacher, 1883

Lunar effects, 3172

■ ■ ■

Machiavelliansim, 1492, 1517, 1721, 3486, 3487, 3514

Magic, 3539

Majors, college, 222, 662

Maladjustment, 2492

Malaise, African society, 65

Male(s): influence on female career choice, 710; need achievement, 728; self-esteem, 826; sex-role attitude, 2760; young adult, 636

Management, 388: strategy, classroom, 880; style, 1333

Manager(ial)(s): attitudes, 523, 1536; autocratic personality, 787; behavior, 3560; changes in practice, 1129; description, 1447; needs, 1348; positions, 3104; rating, 1560, 3580, 3585, 3586; sex-role stereotypes, 1482; traits, 2265

Manifest: alienation, 443, 1102; anxiety, 29, 1478, 1493, 1647, 2524, 3488; needs, 211, 2005; rejection, 496

Marginality, 249

Marijuana, 353, 1214, 1223: attitude toward, 1133

Marital: activities, 3013; alternatives, 3016; communication, 2972, 3017; conflict, 2973; dependency, 3029, 3046; instability, 3023; interaction, 3024, 3025; quality, 3026; relationships,

toward, 482
Risk orientations, 1786
Risk taking, 861, 1077, 1234, 2160, 2161, 2172, 2255, 2776
Rod and frame, 776, 815
Role(s), 3053: ambiguity, 1687, 2357, 2525, 3288, 3289, 3292; ambiguity, perceptions, 2121; choice, 869; concepts, counseling, 313, 3199; conflict, 1687, 2122, 2357, 2526, 2641, 3002, 3289, 3292; conflict, counselors, 314; conflict, perceptions, 2121, 2123; consistency, 1461; constructs, 219, 816; counselor's, 332; deviant, 3202; expectations, 3291; family, 302; female, attitude, 2742; force, negotiators, 324; graduate student, 2426; guidance director's, 318; identification, 331; mother, 652, 2970; orientation, 263; orientation, professional 539; peer, 2590; perception, teachers, 2038; primary, 713; projection, 2512; repertory, 1465; sick, 1239; strain, 1667; stress, 2525—2527; student, 2590; taking, 579, 1096, 1236, 1503, 3259; vocational, 3660; work, 2672
Romantic: attitudes, 2777; love, 295, 2599, 2600
Roommate preference, 262
Rule(s), 695: conformity, 967; -orientation behavior, 2158

■ ■ ■

Sad mood, 1670
Safety: practice, supervisor's, 1073; traffic, 1622
Sales person, rating, 3596, 3598
Salience, 1422: career, 3260, 3621, 3638; work, 2672; work role, 3665
Sampling procedures, 161
Satisfaction: attainment of students, 714; body image, 2044; body in adolescents, 756; client, 182, 999, 3059; college major, 872; college student, 663, 1961, 2407; communication, 2904; community, 3060; congregation, 3062; counseling, 3564; course, 175; employee, 164, 2362; environment, 1965; job, 709, 1575, 1577, 1578,

1581—1586, 1588, 1589, 1592, 1595, 1668, 2320, 2624, 2625, 2629—2637, 2657, 2659, 2668, 2670, 2675; leadership, 2345; life; 33, 415, 2504, 2529; marital, 648, 2967, 3007, 3020, 3027, 2038, 3035; Navy, 2661; need, 1356; occupational, 709; parental, 3008; pay, 2652; student, 159; task, 2663; training, 310, 320; university student, 705; work, 178, 2673; work schedule, 2660
Scales, recommended, 666
Scanning, 612: internal, 1914, 2932
Schedul(e)(ing), 694: modular, 1328
Schizophreni(a)(c)(s), 526, 1084, 1085, 1224, 1504, 2491: patients, improvement, 306; socialization, 1111
Scholastic: activities and attitude, 556; potential in women, 1739; women's potential, 1119
School(s), 491, 494, 497, 516, 532: acceptance, 1070; administrators, 528; administrator morale, 1680, 1978; attitude toward, 66, 155, 540, 541, 1136, 1149, 1181, 1825, 2778, 2779; attitude, peer counseling, 1973; beginners, black & white, 655; behavior, 1238; behavior adjustment, 1628; bureaucratic structure, 695; children, 629; climate, 3108; -community relations, 1827; competence, 460; counselor attitude, 1826; desegregated, 452; disadvantaged, 434; drop-out prediction, 476; elementary, 1723; elementary-inner city, 990; enthusiasm toward, 540; feelings toward, 1825; guidance evaluation, 687; history, 625; interest, 391; last year, 494; motivation, 737, 2004, 3151; nongraded, 574; nursing, 694; organization, 695; orientation, 547; orientation attitude, 534; perception of, 700, 3055; picture stories, 738; principal, 3107; psychologist stress, 2662; rating, 548; readiness, 469; related experiences and aspirations, 472; satisfaction, general, 2147; self-esteem, 2064; sentiment, 1179; situations, 700; situations, student survey of, 700; subjects, attitudes, 2745; sub-

jects, ratings intermediate grade, 871; success, prediction of, 71; work, 593
Science: aptitude, 1732; attitudes, 2793; interest, intermediate children, 864
Scientists, creative potential, 1933
Screening interviewee candidates, 1013
Seat belt: attitudes, 1828, 2780; beliefs, 1829
Second-language, elementary school English, 1598
Secondary: reading attitude, 1824; school, 1787; social studies, 600; student, 368, 369, 537, 549; students' attitudes, 93; students' political attitude, 537; teacher evaluation, 1030
Security, 502, 2317: child, 3037; job, 709, 1687
Seeking professional psychological help, 1764
Selection: counselor, 104; job, 3632; supervisors, 1017
Self-, 241, 250, 494, 499, 551: acceptance, 252, 759, 831, 1425, 1880, 2125; acceptance, social, 499; actualization, 214, 2367, 3285, 3286; adjustment, 409; aggression, 242; appraisal, 472; appraisal, curiosity, 2021; assessment depression, 1692; assessment of emotions, 2165; assurance, 1101, 1427, 2265; attitude, 1439; attitude of disabled, 752; centrality, 249; concept, 219, 230, 243, 252, 255, 300, 472, 755, 759, 787, 796, 798, 823, 824, 1279, 1376, 1389, 1394, 1395, 1402, 2108, 2109, 2123, 2127, 2129, 2130, 2171, 2239; concept, academic, 2030, 3153, 3301, 3303; concept, academic interest and satisfaction, 2056; concept, actual ideal, 748; concept, adolescent, 2103; concept, anxiety, 1381; concept, blood donor, 3174; concepts, children, 807, 3186, 3213, 3221, 3232, 3250, 3254, 3279, 3297; concept, college students, 2035, 3300, 3305; concept, counselor, 822; concept, crystallization, vocational, 2155; concept, global, 1398; concept, leadership and initiative, 2056;